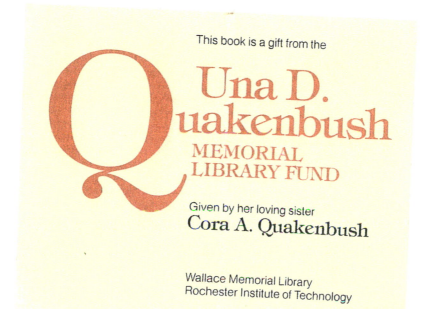

EMERGING

NEUROLOGICAL

INFECTIONS

EMERGING
NEUROLOGICAL
INFECTIONS

EDITED BY
CHRISTOPHER POWER
RICHARD T. JOHNSON

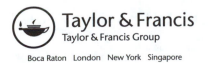

Taylor & Francis
Taylor & Francis Group

Boca Raton   London   New York   Singapore

Portions of Chapter 4 also appear in *Handbook of Dementing Illnesses, Second Edition*, edited by John C. Morris, James Galvin, and David Holtzman, © Taylor & Francis Group LLC.

Published in 2005 by
Taylor & Francis Group
6000 Broken Sound Parkway NW, Suite 300
Boca Raton, FL 33487-2742

International Standard Book Number-10: 0-8247-5423-9 (Hardcover)
International Standard Book Number-13: 978-0-8247-5423-5 (Hardcover)

Library of Congress Cataloging-in-Publication Data

Catalog record is available from the Library of Congress

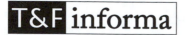

Taylor & Francis Group
is the Academic Division of T&F Informa plc.

Visit the Taylor & Francis Web site at
http://www.taylorandfrancis.com

As always, we are indebted
to our wives, Joan and Fran,
and our children
for their endurance and encouragement
for this and other projects that
we have pursued.

Contents

Foreword

When I attended medical school in the 1960s, we were required to write essay responses to questions on our examinations. I recall using the acronym CANDIE to help me focus on the major etiologic categories of disease: cancer, atherosclerosis, nutritional, degenerative, infectious, and endocrine. In the past 40 years, enormous advances have been achieved in understanding many of these domains. Cancer is a genetic disease, caused by mutations of DNA; atherosclerosis is an inflammatory process; nutritional deficiencies are definable, in large part, by socioeconomic circumstances; and degenerative diseases are associated with new definitions of cell death (apoptosis) and organ dysfunction. Endocrinopathies are now defined at the molecular and genetic level. The demographic features of these diseases have not changed measurably in any significant way since then.

Such is not the case with the infectious diseases. A number of new infectious diseases including HIV/AIDS have been described since 1980. Not only have new pathogens been identified for other diseases, but also new origins of infections, new locales in which they occur, and new diseases emerging from previously identified classes of agents have found their way into our everyday lives. *Emerging Neurological Infections* is a timely review of that subset of these disorders that affect the nervous system. Power and Johnson have sought the collaboration of world leaders in the areas outlined and have brought to attention the current state of understanding of disorders that have new forms of transmission and new neurologic findings. As a general class, infectious diseases are contagious, often activate latent defense mechanisms, which trigger new syndromes, and illustrate best the impact of our dependence on the environment for health and the ever-present danger of new, unprecedented, even fatal conditions.

Population health scientists assess the impact of disease on global health, and although cancer and cardiovascular disease are major culprits, it is the infectious diseases that remain the most important. In addition, they are the most unpredictable and, with globalization, potentially the most dangerous. A more proximate assessment of the importance of these infectious diseases is to survey how much has changed since Ken Tyler and I edited *Infectious Diseases of the Central Nervous System*, published in 1993.[a] Many of the topics in Power and

Johnson's book were unheard of then. And another ten years will almost certainly lead to the same conclusion but hopefully accompanied by more effective and less cumbersome means to diagnose, delineate, and manage these disorders. Indeed, they will represent a continued challenge to our very existence.

Joseph B. Martin, M.D., Ph.D.
Dean of the Faculty of Medicine
Harvard University

---

[a]Tyler KL and Martin JB. Infectious Diseases of the Central Nervous System. F.A. Davis Company, Philadelphia, PA 1993.

Preface

From winter, plague and pestilence, good lord, deliver us.
                                        Thomas Nashe
                                        (16ᵗʰ Century)

Infections of the nervous system are among the most vivid of all diseases because of their dramatic clinical presentations and ominous prognoses. Over the past 20 years, there has been remarkable progress in the recognition, understanding and treatment of neurological infections. As new infections have arisen, an appreciation has developed of factors influencing neurovirulence and the spread of different agents. The fields of microbiology and neuroscience have experienced revolutionary developments, ranging from seminal molecular and epidemiological advances to unforeseen neurological infections in humans and other species. Hence, it is timely to provide a book that merges these two disciplines, as we face new neurological infections due to microbial evolution (Enterovirus 71, drug resistant bacteria and viruses), a change in host (variant Creutzfeld-Jacob disease, Nipah Virus, HIV/AIDS), or expanding geographic locations of different infectious agents (Lyme disease, Japanese encephalitis Virus, West Nile virus). Infections of the nervous system have had a long and colorful history in terms of epidemics throughout the world including poliomyelitis, rabies, bacterial meningitides, arbovirus encephalitides together with those infections with prominent neurological complications such as measles, influenza, leprosy, tuberculosis, and most recently HIV/AIDS.

The underlying determinants of these past epidemics apply to today's emerging epidemics including changes in human demographics and behavior, technology and industry, economic development and land use, international travel and commerce, microbial adaptation with increased microbial virulence, and breakdown or absence of public health resources due to political priorities or poverty. However, the accelerated rate of appearance of new neurological infections in the last decade lies in several current global circumstances, not the least of which is the exponential rise in the global human population size, now 6.2 billion but expected to reach 10 billion by 2050. Indeed, as the population rises, there has been an increase in environmental pollution, trafficking of humans and animals and their products across international borders together with new food production practices. Major social upheavals also contribute to emerging infections including famine and war coupled with poverty or social inequality. Prime examples of burgeoning and emerging neurological infections include the HIV/AIDS epidemic, which has influenced most biomedical fields and exhibits a wide range of neurological manifestations, and the increased frequency of transmissible spongiform encephalopathies, such as vCJD. These two diseases reflect changing social and economic milieus respectively, which resulted in the emergence of diseases previously unknown in humans. Both diseases are zoonoses, likely contracted by humans through eating contaminated foods; simian immunodeficiency virus-infected bush meat was likely the source of HIV infection in humans while consumption of bovine spongiform encephalopathy-infected cattle tissues represents the most plausible explanation for vCJD in humans. However, other mechanisms of zoonotic infection have recently been shown to cause new or re-emerging neurological infections in humans including Nipah virus transmission from pigs to humans with fruit bats serving as the primary reservoir and West Nile virus from a mosquito or a bird transported from warmer climates.

Increased quantity and speed of travel by humans and the exportation of animals globally has provided ripe opportunities for neurotropic pathogens to spread across continents. Fifty years ago it would have taken months for live-stock to be shipped across oceans during which time sick human, or animals would have died or been culled while today's movements across continents occur in a matter of hours. Social developments over the past two decades have also contributed to the appearance of new diseases including increased global urbanization and changing trends in the workforce, with more women now working and subsequently greater dependence on day care. Similarly, select regions of the world, coping with increased population size, poverty, and war and already beset with other diseases, are now faced with the ever increasing HIV/AIDS epidemic and its accompanying opportunistic infections of the brain. These regions have few or diminishing resources to cope with the associated economic and social burdens.

Neurological infections are unique among infections because they are usually evolutionary cul-de-sacs for many pathogens, frequently resulting in the host being unable to support further pathogen replication and spread or, worse still, death. Unlike systemic infections, pathogens in the brain also pose a more ominous predicament for clinicians because of the brain's enhanced vulnerability due to its limited host defense mechanisms, which are largely dependent on innate immunity. In addition, delivery of drugs across the blood–brain barrier remains an obstacle, even when highly specific and effective drugs are available. Moreover, drug resistance has also become a pressing issue among neurological infections just as it is for systemic infections, including methacillin-resistant *Staphylococcus aureas* and drug-resistant tuberculosis and herpes virus infections. Other treatment strategies may also yield new infections including the proposed use of stem cells from human embryos or animal organs in xeno-transplantation. Nonetheless, we are in an era of hitherto unimagined tools for the diagnosis and treatment of diseases. The use of molecular tools for infectious disease epidemiology was barely in its infancy a decade ago, yet today it is the cornerstone of controlling disease outbreaks and monitoring ongoing epidemics. Indeed, a greater understanding of host susceptibility to infection has arisen through the identification of specific host genotypes associated with disease including single nucleotide polymorphisms. Neurological diagnostics and therapeutics have also evolved with the advent of improved neuroimaging, neurocognitive testing, and a wider availability to specific drugs for neurological infections. The approach taken herein is one of emphasizing the basis for emergence or resurgence of neurological infections together with recognition of the disease and its pathogenesis and finally, implementing the appropriate therapeutic and public health measures.

The present monograph contains chapters from authors who were selected for their internationally recognized expertise in areas related to emerging diseases and specific neurological infections. Thus, the spectrum of topics covered by the authors of each chapter ranges widely from determinants of emerging infections to new pathogens, new locations and disease manifestations of infectious neurological disease, drug resistance, and finally, potential interventions. The book begins with a chapter devoted to the origins of new infections that focuses on microbial evolution in relation to disease while in the second chapter, environmental factors that contribute to emerging infections are addressed. In Part II, new human pathogens are examined, concentrating on Nipah virus, prion diseases and neurotropic viruses causing hemorrhagic fevers. The spread of pathogen into new geographic domains is reviewed in Part III in respective chapters dealing with cerebral malaria, rabies, neurocysticercosis, borrelial infections, flaviviruses including West Nile and Japanese encephalitis viruses and African trypanosomias. New human diseases caused by previously recognized pathogens is the spotlight of Part IV in which enterovirus 71 encephalitis, campylobacter infection, and Guillain-Barré syndrome, and putative brain pathogens including human herpes virus-6, endogenous retroviruses, and other microbes linked to multiple sclerosis are considered. In view of the increased impact of drug resistant pathogens, Part V reviews the clinical aspects and mechanisms of drug resistance of herpes simplex virus, HIV-1, and nosocomial infections among neurological diseases. Finally, potential interventions including vaccine development and priority strategies are addressed in Part VI.

We anticipate that this book will provide a perspective of emerging neurological infections for those working or training in neurology, neurosurgery, infectious diseases, public health, pediatrics, and in related basic science disciplines. We hope, however, that this book will also contribute to the early identification and enhanced care of patients afflicted with neurological infections.

C. Power
R. T. Johnson

Acknowledgments

We thank all who contributed to the preparation of the monograph. In particular, we are beholden to the authors for their outstanding contributions. We also thank Jinnie Kim at Taylor & Francis and Belinda Ibrahim for their persistence and patient diligence in contacting the authors around the world with gentle reminders.

Contributors

Deborah S. Asnis
Flushing Hospital Medical Center, Flushing, New York, U.S.A.

B.J. Brew
St. Vincent's Hospital, Darlinghurst, Sydney, Australia

Ying-Chao Chang
Department of Pediatrics, Chang Gung Children's Hospital, Kaohsiung, Taiwan

Cheng-Yu Chen
Department of Radiology, Tri-Service General Hospital, and National Defense Medical Center, Taipei, Taiwan

Kaw-Bing Chua
Ministry of Health, Kuala Lumpur, Malaysia

Patricia K. Coyle
Department of Neurology, School of Medicine, Health Sciences Center, Stony Brook State University of New York, Stony Brook, New York, U.S.A.

Robert Crupi
Flushing Hospital Medical Center, Flushing, New York, U.S.A.

Larry E. Davis
Neurology Service, New Mexico VA Health Care System, and Department of Neurology, University of New Mexico School of Medicine, Albuquerque, New Mexico, U.S.A.

Nicholas Day
Director, Wellcome Trust, Oxford Tropical Medicine Research Programme, Faculty of Tropical Medicine, Mahidol University, Mahidol, Thailand; and Honorary Consultant Physician, Nuffield Department of Clinical Medicine, University of Oxford, John Radcliffe Hospital, Headington, Oxford, U.K.

xx   *Contributors*

Esteban Domingo
University of California–San Diego, San Diego, California, U.S.A.;
Centro de Biología Molecular "Severo Ochoa" (CSIC-UAM),
Universidad Autónoma de Madrid, Cantoblanco, Madrid, and Centro de
Investigación en Sanidad Animal (CISA-INIA), Valdeolmos, Madrid, Spain

Delia A. Enria
Instituto Nacional de Enfermedades Virales Humanas "Dr. Julio I. Maiztegui"
(INEVH)-Administración Nacional de Laboratorios e Institutos de Salud
(ANLIS), Monteagudo, Pergamino, Argentina

Paul W. Ewald
Department of Biology, University of Louisville, Louisville, Kentucky, U.S.A.

Mustafa A. Hammad
Department of Neurology, School of Medicine, Health Sciences Center, Stony
Brook State University of New York, Stony Brook, New York, U.S.A.

Chao-Ching Huang
Department of Pediatrics, National Cheng Kung University Hospital,
Tainan City, Taiwan

Alan C. Jackson
Departments of Medicine and Microbiology and Immunology,
Queen's University, Kingston, Ontario, Canada

J. B. Johnston
Robarts Research Institute, London, Ontario, Canada

Peter G. E. Kennedy
Division of Clinical Neurosciences, Department of Neurology,
Institute of Neurological Sciences, University of Glasgow,
Southern General Hospital, Glasgow, U.K.

C.T. Loy
St. Vincent's Hospital, Darlinghurst, Sydney, Australia

James A. Mastrianni
The University of Chicago, Chicago, Illinois, U.S.A.

Michael Mayne
Department of Pharmacology and Therapeutics, University of Manitoba,
Winnipeg, Canada

Catriona A. McLean
Department of Medicine, Monash University, Melbourne, Australia,
and Macfarlane Burnet Institute for Medical Research and Public Health,
Melbourne, Australia

Irving Nachamkin
Department of Pathology and Laboratory Medicine, School of Medicine,
University of Pennsylvania, Philadelphia, Pennsylvania, U.S.A.

Karen L. Roos
The John and Nancy Nelson Professor of Neurology, Department of Neurology,
Indiana University School of Medicine, Indianapolis, Indiana, U.S.A.

Firas G. Saleh
Department of Neurology, School of Medicine, Health Sciences Center, Stony
Brook State University of New York, Stony Brook, New York, U.S.A.

Kazim A. Sheikh
Department of Neurology, School of Medicine, Johns Hopkins University,
Baltimore, Maryland, U.S.A.

Chong-Tin Tan
Department of Medicine, University of Malaya, Kuala Lumpur, Malaysia

Richard B. Tenser
Departments of Neurology, and Microbiology and Immunology, Pennsylvania
State University College of Medicine, Hershey, Pennsylvania, U.S.A.

S. Tomlinson
St. Vincent's Hospital, Darlinghurst, Sydney, Australia

Steven L. Wesselingh
Department of Medicine, Monash University, Melbourne, Australia
and Macfarlane Burnet Institute for Medical Research
and Public Health, Melbourne, Australia

Mary Elizabeth Wilson
Associate Professor of Medicine, Harvard Medical School and Associate
Professor of Population and International Health, Harvard School of Public
Health, Mount Auburn Hospital, Cambridge, Massachusetts, U.S.A.

K. Thong Wong
Department of Pathology, University of Malaya, Kuala Lumpur, Malaysia

Edwina J. Wright
Department of Medicine, Monash University, Melbourne, Australia
and Macfarlane Burnet Institute for Medical Research
and Public Health, Melbourne, Australia

1

Microbial Evolution and Emerging Diseases

Esteban Domingo

University of California–San Diego, San Diego, California, U.S.A. and Centro de Biología Molecular "Severo Ochoa" (CSIC-UAM), Universidad Autónoma de Madrid, Cantoblanco, Madrid, and Centro de Investigación en Sanidad Animal (CISA-INIA), Valdeolmos, Madrid, Spain

The population evolves as the scattered group of novel individuals start coalescing into a synchronous chorus. The dominant version now becomes the one that won out in the competition, not the one written down on some preordained sheet of music.

William H. Calvin, 1989

1. INTRODUCTION: A HIGHLY DIVERSE AND DYNAMIC MICROBIAL WORLD

The advent of molecular techniques for the analysis of cellular and viral genomes has revealed an unsuspected degree of genetic diversity not only among representatives of the same species of pathogen from different origins but also within clonal populations (those recently derived from the same parental genome) of cells and subcellular replicons. There is a great diversity among organisms living today and probably there has been great diversity in the course of evolution of life on earth. The elucidation of the nucleotide sequence of entire genomes of differentiated organisms has suggested that interaction between cellular genomes and subcellular replicons (mobile elements, plasmids, viruses, etc.) must have been a common occurrence throughout the history of life on earth (1–3). As much as 44% of the human genome is made of heterogeneous arrays of genetic elements named transposons, mainly one class termed retrotransposons. These elements

1

share with retroviruses a reverse transcription step but lack an envelope gene and an extracellular step in their life cycle. Animal and plant species vary in their content of different types of transposons and other mobile elements, but current findings suggest that genetic elements that once probably had partly autonomous life cycles became integral parts of complex genomes (3). Truly genetically identical individuals are probably rare in nature. Most remarkable for the adaptive potential of pathogens is that the genetic variation observed is often associated with biological (phenotypic or behavioral) variation. That is, a good deal (and it is not wise to adventure a number) of the genetic variation is not selectively neutral but it has a certain probability of contributing to the survival capacity of the pathogen at some point during its life. The ways by which variation helps survival are extremely complex. Genetic changes may be neutral under the environmental conditions in which they occur but may be beneficial or detrimental in other environments. Despite immediate deleteriousness or even lethality, some types of replicons (mainly subcellular replicons) that depend on cells for replication, may survive by complementation with related genomes that supply required functions in *trans*. Genetic variation is blind with respect its biological purpose but it provides a repository of potentialities to be exploited when selective constraints so demand.

Viruses, bacteria, and eukaryotic unicellular pathogens generally have replication cycles which are more rapid than those of the majority of cells of the hosts they parasitize or infect. For this reason, microbial pathogens may have the possibility to adapt, through genetic variation and selection, to changing environments they encounter in their hosts. Environmental modifications that may affect short-term adaptation include physiological alterations such as inflammation, immune responses (humoral and cellular), immune debilitation, altered metabolic status, and also externally induced modifications (as a result of administration of drugs or vaccines, diet, etc.). The immune response of differentiated organisms represents a selective constraint that often drives antigenic variation of the infecting pathogen (Fig. 1). A condition for escape to the inactivating action of antibody molecules is either the preexistence or generation during replication of a variant antigenic form no longer recognized by the antibody molecules or recognized with a low affinity compatible with continuing pathogen replication. This new antigenic form which will dominate the population will generally be able to evoke also an antibody response either in the same host at a later time (depending on the duration of the infection), or in another individual, following transmission of the pathogen. Therefore, there is the potential of a continuous dynamics of immune responses and adaptive changes in the pathogen. This is just one (albeit one of the best known) of many facets of the interaction of pathogens with their hosts, in which the capacity of genetic variation and adaptation of the pathogen is manifested.

The molecular mechanisms by which pathogens express variant antigens range from point mutations at surface proteins in viruses to recombination events in some bacteria and protozoa (Secs. 2.1 and 2.2). The Darwinian principles of

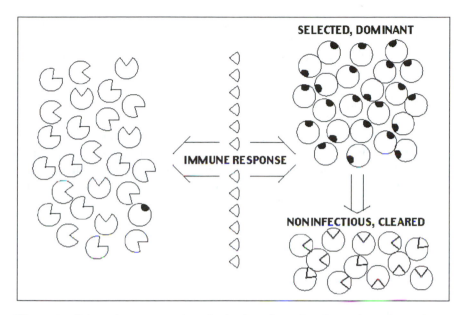

Figure 1 Schematic representation of selection of a variant form of a pathogen in the face of an immune response. A minority component (circle with black dot at the left) cannot be recognized by a molecular component of an immune response (i.e., antibody molecules, depicted as an alignment of quadrants in the middle). This variant form will become dominant while the previously dominant form will be unable to replicate and will be cleared or become a minority of the population. This scheme applies to many selective pressures discussed throughout this article.

genetic variation, competition, and selection, which have shaped all life forms as we know them on earth, underlie survival of pathogens, and the replacement of some forms of pathogens by others. Hypermutated measles virus finds a suitable niche in the human brain for replication to cause subacute sclerosing panencephalitis, and waves of influenza are often associated with antigenic variants of influenza virus [reassortants in antigenic "shift" and mutants in antigenic "drift" (Sec. 2.3)] [reviews of several examples for viruses in Ref. (4)]. Evolution of measles virus in some infants, antigenic variation of human influenza viruses, or the modification of cellular tropism of HIV-1 within infected individuals, are three out of several significant cases which illustrate the relevance of pathogen evolution to disease. Indeed, the progress of an infection in a differentiated organism can often be viewed as a microevolutionary process in which there is an accommodation of the pathogen to a changing environment as the infection progresses [evidence and reviews for different pathogens in Refs. (4–9)].

There are mechanisms other than genetic variation to counteract immune responses (9). Complex DNA viruses encode a number of proteins, some of which have a cellular homolog that may modulate host defense responses. These viral proteins can suppress major histocompatibility complex (MHC) class I and class II molecules required for T-cell recognition of infected cells; some are homologs of cytokines, chemokines or their receptors, and others may induce or inhibit apoptosis [reviews in Refs. (10,11)].

Variations of phenotypic traits among individuals of a group of living organisms were noted ever since the beginning of organized observations and experimental science, and eventually led to recognition of natural selection and Mendelian genetics. However, in the early times preceding modern science, variations were rarely the focus of attention since they were regarded as minor modifications of a "norm," the only one worthy of definition and description [review on evolution of thinking about biological variation in Ref. (12) and references therein]. This applies also to the early approaches taken for the study of viruses, bacteria and other pathogens. Pioneering work by Milkman (13) unveiled the extensive polymorphism of bacterial populations in nature, in an approach that followed the identification of polymorphic genomic loci in *Drosophila* (14) and humans (15). Contrary to a quite extended belief that the main source of genetic variation was the chromosomal reassortment associated with sexual reproduction, this early evidence and later developments throughout the twentieth century indicated that the same gene analyzed from individuals of one species may vary in its sequence and encoded proteins with higher frequency than suspected before procedures for nucleotide sequence sampling became available. There is great diversity of allelic forms at many genetic loci of organisms and this realization has exerted a remarkable influence in modern population genetics. Microbial pathogens are no exception. Molecular analyses of complete genomes and specific genomic regions have not ceased to document a great genetic diversity of cellular microbes (16,17). Pathogens are best described as "clouds" of variant forms gravitating around a "norm" which may also have a fleeting existence. Concepts such as species, strains, and genotypes are becoming increasingly harder to define (18–20). Plasticity blurs classification borders. Not only there is remarkable diversity within the microbial groups we know, but there is also the belief that a majority of microbial pathogens still remain unrecognized (21). This chapter addresses the molecular mechanisms of genetic variation of pathogens and some biological implications of pathogen variation related to disease emergence, with emphasis on highly variable RNA viruses, the source of many emergent and reemergent diseases covered in this book. It must be stressed, however, that the general principles that govern the adaptive dynamics of all types of pathogens are of a similar nature (8,22–24).

2. THE EVOLUTION OF MICROBIAL PATHOGENS

Evolutionary processes are amenable to experimental analysis with microbial pathogens because of their rapid replication and in many cases the frequent occurrence of genetic changes and adaptive responses to designed environments.

In contrast, minimal evolutionary processes in differentiated organisms very often take a long time under laboratory conditions. Microbes have become ideal objects for experimental studies on evolution.

2.1.   Mutation Rates of Cells, Viruses, and Intracellular Genetic Elements

The main mechanisms of genetic variation are mutation, several classes of genetic recombination, and chromosome or genome segment reassortment (Fig. 2). Drake (25) estimated mutation rates for some bacteria and bacteriophages (viruses which infect bacteria) that have DNA as their genetic material. From the frequency of reversion of conditionally lethal mutations, mutation rates of 2×10^{-10} substitutions per nucleotide copied were estimated for *Escherichia coli* and *Salmonella*

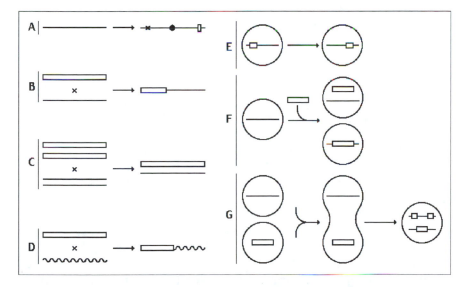

Figure 2   Schematic representation of some types of genetic modifications that underlie or affect adaptability of pathogens. (A) Mutation: Symbols on progeny genome indicate different types of mutations. (B) Homologous recombination. (C) Genome segment reassortment. (D) Nonhomologous recombination. (E) Intracellular transposition or rearrangement of genetic material. (F) Transfer into a cell of exogenous genetic material (i.e., infection, conjugation, etc.) that may remain as an episome or integrate into the cellular chromosome. (G) Gene transfers among distantly related cells (by cell-to-cell fusion, assimilation) may be a source of DNA variation. These and other forms of genetic variation and of transfer of genetic material among cells and subcellular replicons provide the molecular basis of the response of pathogens to selective forces, as discussed throughout this chapter.

typhimurium, and 7×10^{-12} for the fungus *Neurospora crassa* [reviewed in Ref. (26)]. The mutation rate for the DNA bacteriophages lambda and T4 of *E. coli* were estimated in 2×10^{-8} substitutions per nucleotide, two orders of magnitude higher than that of their host bacterium. Drake (27) also analyzed comparatively mutation rates of DNA-based microbes and documented that there is an approximately constant rate of 0.0033 spontaneous mutations per genome per replication round. These values are in contrast with mutation rates for RNA viruses and other RNA replicons which are in the range of 10^{-3}–10^{-5} substitutions per nucleotide copied (28–30) or an average of about one mutation per genome per replication round. This remarkable difference between DNA and RNA genomes led Holland et al. to emphasize a number of biological implications of the rapid evolution of RNA genomes in a relatively more static DNA biosphere (31).

The biochemical basis for the million-fold difference in mutation rates of RNA viruses as compared with their host organisms is the absence or low efficiency of proofreading repair activities associated with RNA-dependent RNA replicates and RNA-dependent DNA polymerases (reverse transcriptases). The three-dimensional structures of several such enzymes has not revealed the presence of any domain that could be assigned to a $3' \rightarrow 5'$ exonuclease, the activity needed for proofreading repair, which is present in most cellular DNA-dependent DNA polymerases (32,33). Biochemical tests have also failed to identify a $3' \rightarrow 5'$ proofreading exonuclease in viral RNA polymerases (34). A domain that may correspond to a nuclease activity has been identified in the emergent severe acute respiratory syndrome (SARS) virus, but its significance in fidelity of template-dependent polynucleotide synthesis is not known. Furthermore, a number of postreplicative repair pathways can correct misincorporated nucleotides on double-stranded DNA but not on RNA (35,36).

It has been estimated that the error rate during *E. coli* DNA replication would be 10^{-1}–10^{-2} if accuracy relied only on the stability of interactions associated with base pairing. The error rate would decrease to 10^{-5}–10^{-6} due to the effects of base selection together with the activity of a $3' \rightarrow 5'$ proofreading exonuclease, and to about 10^{-7} with the additional participation of proteins other than the polymerase itself in the polymerization complex. Finally, the error rate can reach levels of around 10^{-10} misincorporations per nucleotide with the contribution of postreplicative mismatch correction mechanisms [(35); review in Ref. (36)]. Studies of site-directed mutagenesis of reverse transcriptases have documented that some amino acid substitutions may increase the copying fidelity of this enzyme while other substitutions (the majority tested) decreased the copying fidelity [reviewed in Ref. (37)]. Therefore, and this is relevant to new antiviral strategies that exploit high mutation rates of viruses (discussed in Sec. 2.5), copying fidelity can be modified by structural modifications of the polymerases.

Error correction has an evolutionary basis. The tolerance of genomes to accept mutations while remaining functional decreases with genome complexity [(38,39); review in Ref. (26)]. In the sense used here, complexity can be equated with genome size provided no redundant information is encoded (23,26). Therefore, ensuring a copying fidelity during DNA synthesis, commensurate with the complexity of the genetic information to be maintained, required the evolutionary development of enzymatic activities for correction of nucleotide misincorporations. However, some cell types and some genetic elements that inhabit cells, display mutation rates orders of magnitude higher than those of the organisms that host them. High mutation rates occur during the process of somatic hypermutation of immunoglobulin genes, associated with affinity maturation of antibody molecules (40–42). Cancer development is a multi-step process, and in many types of tumors, high mutation rates contribute to phenotypic diversification of cells, with clonal selection of transformed cell subsets. Such cancer cell mutation, competition and selection events have been related to tumor cell adaptability and metastasis (43,44). Some DNA polymerases are specialized to bypass damaged DNA thereby preventing cell death that would follow inhibition of DNA replication. These polymerases show much reduced fidelity when copying undamaged DNA, and such reduced fidelity may be physiologically functional in processes such as immunoglobulin gene hypermutagenesis (45). Mutator bacteria, some times found in subpopulations associated with pathogenesis, have been characterized (46,47). High mutation rates in bacteria allowed faster adaptation to a given biological environment (46), an independent recognition of the adaptive value of the high mutation rates that characterize RNA replicons (compare with Sec. 2.5). There is evidence that some antibiotic treatments may select not only for antibiotic-resistant bacteria but also for mutator bacteria, thereby increasing the probability of selection of strains resistant to additional antibiotics used in subsequent treatments (48). The presence of subpopulations of mutator bacteria represents an added difficulty to the control of antibiotic-resistant bacteria (compare with Sec. 3.3).

Among intracellular elements, retroid agents [defined as those that encode a reverse transcriptase activity (49)] employ an error-prone retrotranscription step in their replication cycle (49). The mutation rate of retrotransposon Ty1 of *Saccharomyces* has been estimated in 2×10^{-5} substitutions per nucleotide copied (50). An appealing possibility is that because of their high mutation rates and mobility within cells, retroelements have contributed to cellular diversification and to the formation and adaptation of complex genomes, and perhaps to the accelerated evolution during some time periods of the evolution of life on earth (3,51). Some cell types have evolved defense mechanisms against excess copy numbers of mobile elements which are a potential source of perturbation of hereditary function due to excess foreign DNA. *Neurospora* and other fungal species include an expression system to induce mutations in some repeated nucleotide sequences in DNA, in a gene silencing process termed repeat-induced point (RIP) mutations [(52) and references therein; reviewed in Ref. (3)]. Genetic variation is a source of adaptability but may also be the cause of dysfunction, and cells and subcellular replicons must have evolved to find the adequate balance between variation and stability for long-term survival.

2.2. DNA and RNA Recombination and Rearrangements in Cells and Microbial Pathogens

The formation of new gene combinations is termed recombination. In its broadest terms it may involve covalent linkage of genetic material from two different parental genomes or between different sites of the same genome. It is a widespread process in most DNA organisms, as well as in subcellular, autonomous DNA and RNA genetic elements. In cells it underlies critical physiological and developmental processes, such as splicing, generation of diversity in immunoglobulin genes and T-cell receptors, modulation of gene expression through transposition in eukaryotes, "phase variation" (switch between stable states of gene expression) in bacteria, and repair pathways, among others [general reviews in Refs. (3,53,54)]. Recombination has been broadly divided into homologous and nonhomologous, each involving a number of mechanisms and proteins (Fig. 2). Homologous recombination occurs between genomic sites depicting high nucleotide sequence identity, such as in gene exchange during meiosis, in postreplicative repair of DNA, or between a chromosomal gene and its altered counterpart introduced in yeast by transformation. Homologous recombination may also take place during coinfection of the same cell by two variants of the same virus, thereby permitting selection of high fitness recombinants from two low fitness parental genomes. Recombination between similar 3' ends of a plant RNA virus and a subviral satellite RNA mediated repair of nonviral bases in satellite transcripts in plants (55). Mechanistically, homologous recombination may result from breakage and rejoining of nucleic acid fragments, or from the polymerase copying first one template molecule and then switching to continue copying another template molecule. This is termed the "copy choice" mechanism which appears to be frequently utilized by positive-strand RNA viruses and retroviruses, families of viruses which often display high frequencies of recombination per replication round [review and specific values in Refs. (56–59)].

Nonhomologous recombination encompasses a number of different mechanisms that share the absence of a requirement for extended regions of nucleotide sequence identity. Therefore, it may occur between nonidentical nucleotide sequences of the same genome or between unrelated genomes. It mediates DNA rearrangements in cells that may be involved in control of gene expression, in cell differentiation and in development. Nonhomologous recombination is exploited by bacteria and eukaryotic pathogens to evade immune recognition by the host. Phase variation in *S. typhimurium* involves the inversion of a DNA fragment which occurs at a frequency of 10^{-3}–10^{-5} per cell division [review in Ref. (3)]. DNA rearrangements are involved in the switching of variant surface glycoproteins of *Trypanosoma brucei*, the parasite that causes malaria in humans. In this case, the estimated frequency of expression switching is 10^{-6}–10^{-7} per cell division (60). Thus, a surface variant trypanosome present as a minority in the population can reinitiate a replicative process despite immune clearance of the dominant forms of the parasite (compare with Fig. 1). The continuous presence of low frequency variants allows the collectivity to survive and generate new mutant distributions, maintaining a reservoir of minority cellular genomes for survival.

Site-specific recombination is a type of protein-mediated nonhomologous recombination that requires a short stretch of nucleotide sequence identity. It is involved in integration into, and excision from, the bacterial chromosome of some temperate bacteriophages such as the prototype phage lambda. Transposition is still another class of recombination that mediates the movement of transposons along a genome without a requirement for nucleotide sequence identity. Transposons may move via DNA, as in the case of insertion elements in bacteria, or via an RNA intermediate, as in the case of retrotransposons (3,49,50).

Some lateral gene transfers necessitate cell-to-cell contacts to achieve conjugation, fusion or assimilation. In other cases, DNA needs to enter cells and this can be achieved by transformation or transfection, and more recently also by related artificial transfer means such as electroporation or ballistics. Viruses are also likely to have promoted lateral gene transfers through infection and transduction during cellular evolution, as suggested by present-day DNA and RNA tumor viruses, cytopathic variants of some flaviviruses, and several defective viruses that can acquire host sequences by nonhomologous recombination [examples of foreign gene capture in cells and viruses can be found in Refs. (3,4,23,61–63)].

The analysis of entire genomes of prokaryotes and eukaryotes suggest the widespread occurrence of recombination events in the process of construction of complex genomes. The yeast genome organization provides evidence of ancient duplicated chromosome blocks, frequent occurrence of chromosomal translocations, gene inversions, segmental duplications, and gene losses. The presence of interspersed blocks suggests multiple successive events to account for the yeast genome structure as we see it to date [(64,65) and references therein].

Recombination may have two disparate effects in evolution: it may rescue viable gene combinations from debilitated parents (a conservative activity) or it may produce new genomes from distant parents (an exploratory, risky but potentially innovative activity). Therefore, most types of cells have ample opportunity for genetic modification and exchanges between their genetic material and that of other cells or subcellular replicons.

2.3. Mutation, Recombination, and Reassortment as Sources of Microbial Variation

Mutation and recombination, the latter understood broadly to mean rearrangements and transfers of genetic material, occur universally during replication of pathogens albeit with different efficiency depending on each specific pathogen and its biological context. Statistical analyses of multilocus electrophoretic enzyme data of bacteria have indicated notable differences in the frequency of DNA transfer among bacteria (18). As an example, the rate of transfer of DNA sequences between strains is remarkably higher in *Neisseria gonorrhoea* than in *Salmonella* [as quantified by an "index of association" of 0.04 and 3.11, respectively, an index that would be zero for the random association of loci (18)]. Despite this difference, the two groups of bacteria display similar genetic variability. DNA transfers appear to be virtually absent in *Borrelia* (18). Large differences in recombination frequency are also found among viruses. In retroviruses and many positive-strand RNA viruses homologous recombination occurs at high frequencies. During picornavirus infections [a group of small RNA viruses which includes important human and animal pathogens such as poliovirus, hepatitis A virus and foot-and-mouth disease virus (FMDV)], recombination frequencies over the entire genome using selectable markers located in otherwise virtually identical parental viruses, have been estimated in 10–20% of the progeny. The recombination frequency decreases with the genetic distance between the parental viruses [reviews in Refs. (56,57)]. Recent estimates for a HIV-1-based vector system have confirmed minimum rates of 2.8 crossovers per genome per replication cycle (66). Recombination events may be favored in viral systems which naturally employ strand switching as a step in their replication cycles. Negative-strand RNA viruses do not seem to use (or use very infrequently) recombination during their natural infectious cycles, despite intragenome recombination events (internal deletions) that generate defective-interfering particles with high frequency (67,68). Recently, homologous recombination has been reported for the negative-strand RNA Tula hantavirus (69), an interesting observation that generalizes the occurrence of homologous recombination in viruses. The frequency of homologous recombination during natural evolution of hantaviruses and other negative-strand RNA viruses is unknown, and will certainly be the object of future studies.

Some animal and plant RNA viruses contain segmented genomes either of single-stranded RNA (typically the animal influenza viruses, arenaviruses, bunyaviruses, and several plant virus families) or double-stranded RNA (typically the reoviruses and rotaviruses). Reassortment together with within-segment rearrangements can contribute to diversity of segmented RNA viruses (4,70), and is a source of genetic variation additional to mutation and recombination (Fig. 2). Reassortment in viruses can be viewed as a parallel to chromosome reassortment during sexual reproduction, once thought to be the main (and even the only) source of variability in organisms that reproduce sexually. These sex-like processes must be distinguished from other types of gene transfers such as transformation, conjugation and transduction, that have been referred to as "parasexual" processes (18) and which may bring together genetic material of distant origins.

There have been occasional suggestions to attribute either to mutation or to recombination the most prominent role in general evolution or in the evolution of cellular and viral pathogens. Such assessments do not seem justified since the relative contribution of these two classes of genetic variation will depend on the extent of genetic diversification attained by the gene pool available as the substrate of evolution. Following gene (or genome) duplication in early stages of cellular life or in the evolution of animals (71) mutation must have followed duplication to shape-up functional diversification. Taking human immunodeficiency virus type 1 (HIV-1) as a present day, converse example, for homologous recombination to be of evolutionary value, the parental genomes must have diverged by mutation at some point, either within the human population or the simian populations that hosted the corresponding parental lentiviruses. A central role of recombination could be invoked only if mutation necessitated a recombination event, an unlikely possibility. The trend to detect an increasing number of natural HIV-1 recombinants in recent years (72) is likely to be not only the result of higher frequencies of reinfections as the AIDS epidemic advances, but also a consequence of an expanded mutant repertoire. An ample repertoire increases the chances of finding recombinants with sufficient relative fitness (a measure of relative replication capacity) for the virus to spread in the human population.

2.4. Main Steps in the Dynamics of Change of Microbial Populations

The following stages can be regarded as participating in the evolution of pathogens, as a result of intrinsic genetic variation and adaptive responses to environmental modifications inside and outside the infected host:

1. During replication, cells and subcellular replicons generate variants. As a result, in general, populations will be genetically heterogeneous: they will contain a repertoire of mutant and recombinant genomes in proportions that will be highly variable and dependent on features of the pathogen and its replicative circumstances [(intrinsic mutability, distance from a clonal origin, perception of environments as "coarse-grained" or "fine-grained"; description of early "grain" theory in Ref. (73), etc.]. The heterogeneity of bacterial populations extends to generate spectra of distinguishable clones, whose composition may vary in time, upon replication within infected individuals (74). For RNA viruses, quasispecies population structure and dynamics represent extreme forms of population heterogeneity (Sec. 2.5). The frequency of occurrence of mutation and recombination events is probably much larger than estimated from the variation that can be observed through genome isolation and analysis. Life forms we see to date, and variants of cells and subcellular replicons that we can isolate and study in the laboratory, are probably a successful minority out of many more unsuccessful trials.

2. Population subsets may often contain a different repertoire of variants. The latter will be ranked according to their fitness which is a relative and environmental-dependent parameter. In the limit case of a pathogen with a lethal mutation, its frequency will be zero unless its

replication strategy permits its maintenance by complementation. The larger the population that can be transmitted to the next round of infection (either in the same host or in another host individual) the larger the variant repertoire that can participate in selection when an environmental change occurs (Fig. 3). When the population size that is transmitted is small (in the extreme case, a single cell or replicon) the variant repertoire available will be dictated by the variation potential of the descendants of the founder replicon. In bottleneck transmissions from genetically heterogeneous parents, genetic drift (a change in the composition of the population which is relatively independent of fitness) has a great influence in the evolutionary outcome. However, the probability of participation in a bottleneck transmission will be higher for those pathogens that are more abundant in the parental pool. Therefore, there is a connection between fitness and the probability of being the founder genomes in a process of genetic drift (Fig. 3).

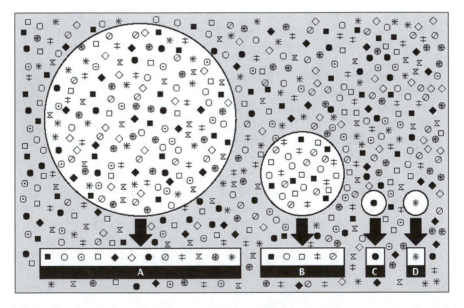

Figure 3 Populations of pathogens must be viewed as heterogeneous collections of genotypes and phenotypes. The population size that enters into an evolutionary process (circles of different size) may influence the outcome due to the different variant repertoire (A–D, bottom of the scheme) that participates in the process. (C, D) Severe genetic bottleneck since only one of the multiple mutants can generate progeny and participate in the following stages of evolution. Connections between population size, fitness variations, mutability, and genome complexity of pathogens are discussed in the text.

3. Upon subjecting the population of replicons to a selective pressure, minority components in the population, which are endowed with the capacity to replicate while overcoming the selective constraint, may become dominant. Dominance will generate a new variant distribution that may show a decreased replication capacity relative to the initial distribution. This is because the genetic changes required to overcome the selective constraint may incur a fitness cost. Then, a number of outcomes are possible: pathogen replication may be limited because of fitness loss or, if continued replication is allowed, additional genetic changes may improve fitness while retaining the phenotype needed to overcome the selective constraint. These fitness-enhancing modifications are often referred to as compensatory genetic changes, and they may act at the nucleic acid level (i.e., to restore higher order structures or protein-recognition signals) or at the protein level (i.e., to restore a catalytic activity or a protein–protein or protein–nucleic acid interaction). If the fitness cost of a mutation is high, then upon removal of the selective pressure reversion of the mutation may occur rapidly. Relative fitness, which embraces replication capacity, transmissibility, long-term potential to produce progeny, etc. [(75,76) and Sec. 2.5] and chance events will influence the possible spread of phenotypically altered pathogens (antibiotic-resistant bacteria, inhibitor-resistant protozoa or viruses) in the host populations (Sec. 3.3).

4. Events in (1)–(3) are the first stages of a process of genetic and phenotypic diversification that extends in time and must contemplate a complex array of interactions within and among the pathogen populations, diversity of host populations, interactions with the environment, including microenvironmental heterogeneity within individual hosts, and coevolutionary processes of the host organisms and the pathogens (3,77). Long-term evolution of pathogens is also affected by interactions among cells, and the lateral gene transfers that occasionally may have even bridged distant domains of life (3). Several facets of microbe–host interactions, that involve alternative pathways of penetration into cells, alteration of cell signaling and disruption of cellular functions, and microevolutionary processes of the parasites, among others, have been summarized in different chapters of (9,78–80).

This unavoidably sketchy account of events is based on a number of observations and models developed for different pathogens, mainly viruses and bacteria. The reader is referred to a number of articles and books that address these issues for various systems [(3,8,22,23,63) and references therein]. Because of the extensive studies carried out with RNA viruses (the research field best known to the author of this review), and also because underlying principles are similar for all pathogens, RNA virus population dynamics is briefly reviewed next.

2.5. RNA Viruses, the Paradigm of Extreme Heterogeneity and Potential for Rapid Evolution: Clouds, Fitness, Memory, and Error Catastrophe

A number of early observations in the decades of 1940s–1960s strongly suggested a considerable variation potential for viruses that use RNA as their genetic material [early work reviewed in Refs. (31,81)]. The studies by Weissmann and colleagues with bacteriophage Q documented a high mutation rate of about 10-4 substitutions per nucleotide (comparative values for DNA organisms discussed in Sec. 2.1), at a single extracistronic nucleotide position of the phage genome, despite the nucleotide belonging to a genomic region which is highly conserved among related bacteriophages (28,82). These early studies documented also a high complexity (meaning in this case digit complexity that refers to the presence of multiple genomic nucleotide sequences) in phage populations. Despite a clonal origin, the "wild type" (unmutated) genome represented at most 20% of the viral genomes that composed the populations examined (28,82,83). The phage genome had to be described as being "in a dynamic equilibrium" and consisting of a "weighted average of a large number of different individual sequences" (83). Complex and dynamic mutant distributions that characterize RNA viruses are termed viral quasispecies (26,84,85), in recognition of features of RNA viruses anticipated by the quasispecies theory formulated by Eigen and colleagues (86–89). Quasispecies theory was developed to describe self-organization and adaptation of simple RNA (or RNA-like) replicons that could exist as primitive life forms on earth. It constitutes a general theory of molecular evolution that has been extended to describe finite populations of replicons subjected to environmental changes (23,26,84,88,90). The emphasis of quasispecies theory on mutation, and its equivalence with other formulations of Darwinian evolution (91), justify its use as a framework to understand RNA virus evolution. Virologists use an extended definition of quasispecies to mean dynamic distributions of nonidentical but closely related mutant and recombinant viral genomes subjected to a continuous process of genetic variation, competition and selection, and which act as a unit of selection (92) (Fig. 4).

The biological significance of quasispecies for RNA viruses becomes apparent when considering genetic heterogeneity, population size and genome length of viruses as compared with cells (Table 1). The adaptive capacity of RNA viruses can be viewed in terms of occupation of sequence space. This refers to the total numbers of possible sequences theoretically available to a polymeric chain, be a nucleic acid or protein (93,94). Despite theoretical sequence spaces being unimaginably large numbers (for a virus of 10,000 nucleotides it is 410,000 or 106021), the capacity to occupy subsets of sequence space compatible with functionality is much greater for simple RNA replicons than for large DNA genomes. Adaptive movements are facilitated by the high connectivity among points of sequence space (26) which allows viruses to find pathways toward fitness peaks. The adaptive capacity of RNA viruses as compared with cells can also be viewed

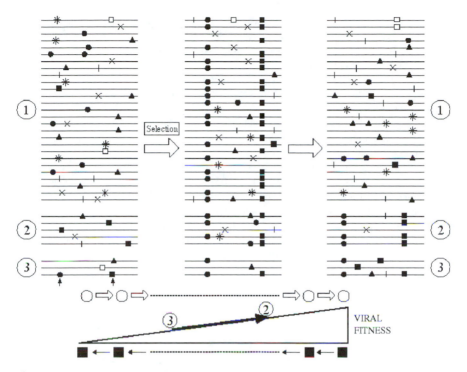

Figure 4 Scheme representing quasispecies distributions of genomes, quasispecies memory, and fitness variations. Individual genomes of a population are represented by horizontal lines and mutations are depicted as symbols on the lines. The abundance of different mutants has been divided arbitrary into three decreasing frequency levels ①, ②, and ③. Selection of a mutant class represented by the last genome of ③ (on the left) will result in a distribution dominated by the two mutations (indicated by arrows in the founder genome). Because selection involves replication and fitness gain, upon further replication in the absence of selective pressure, the selected genome may lose dominance, but will occupy level ②, defined as memory level (distribution on the right). This is depicted by movement ③ → ② in the triangle at the bottom, which serves also to illustrate that large population passages (empty circles and thick arrows) lead to fitness increase while repeated genetic bottlenecks (filled squares and thin arrows) lead to fitness losses. [Based on Refs. (111,112,115).]

considering the total possible number of mutants (disregarding fitness effects): a viral genome of 10,000 nucleotides has a total of 3×10^4 possible single mutants which is below the population size of many natural virus populations. In contrast, the total number of possible single mutants for a mammalian genome is about 10^{10}, well above the population size of mammalian species.

Work with animal and plant RNA viruses, notably extensive studies with HIV-1, have amply confirmed high mutation rates and quasispecies dynamics during RNA virus and retrovirus replication both in nature and in cell culture,

Table 1   Relevant Quantities for the Adaptive Capacity of RNA Viral Quasispecies as Compared with Complex Cellular Genomes

---

- Genetic heterogeneity in a virus
  The range is 1–100 mutations per individual genome, relative to the consensus nucleotide sequence defined with the same set of sequences (compare with Fig. 4)
- Virus population size
  Values are highly variable but can reach up to 1012 infectious units in a mammal at the peak of an infection
- Genome length
  For RNA viruses it is in the range of 3–32 kb. Critical for the impact of quasispecies dynamics is that this genome size is 102–103-fold smaller than that of a prokaryotic cell and 103–106-fold smaller than that of a eukaryotic cell
- Number of mutations required for a phenotypic change
  Many phenotypic changes that may be relevant to viral disease emergence and reemergence (host cell tropism variations, degree of virulence, sensitivity to antiviral inhibitors, etc.) are associated with one or a limited number of mutations
Quantities based in Refs. (4, 23,170) and references therein.

---

including double-stranded RNA viruses (95) [reviews in Refs. (4,7,12,22,26,29,61,81,84,85,87,92,96)].

Model studies with RNA viruses in cell culture and in vivo have unveiled a number of implications of quasispecies dynamics: fitness variations of viruses during disease processes, the effect of virus population size variation on viral fitness, memory in viral populations, deterministic and stochastic effects on viral evolution, the need of antiviral designs that take into consideration quasispecies dynamics, and new antiviral strategies based on virus entry into error catastrophe. The main conclusions of these studies are:

1. Fitness variations have been characterized and quantitated in vivo by infection-competition experiments in animals (97), and quantitated ex vivo with variant viruses isolated during infections of humans (24,29,98,99). The molecular and population basis of fitness variations have been approached with controlled experiments in cell culture. Large population passages of RNA viruses in a given environment tend to increase viral fitness when measured in that same environment (100,101). Repeated bottleneck events (that in cell culture are modeled as plaque-to-plaque transfers) tend to decrease viral fitness (102–105). Depending on the initial fitness, the virus population size that participates in the next rounds of viral replication may be a limiting factor for fitness gain (106,107). Low fitness virus subjected to bottleneck transfers shows a remarkable resistance to extinction despite accumulation of mutations in the viral genome (108–110). These complex effects of population size on viral fitness are summarized in Fig. 4.

2. Viruses may maintain a memory of their past evolutionary history in the form of minority genomes present in their mutant spectra. Work with the important animal pathogen FMDV has documented that genomes which were dominant at a given time may be outcompeted by fitter mutants but may remain at memory levels [(111–113); reviewed in Refs. (114,115)]. The memory level in the mutant spectrum will generally be higher than the level that the same genome would occupy if its presence depended only of mutational pressure. This is because memory is established as the next step to a process of selection in which the variants destined to become memory increase their relative fitness (112) (Fig. 4). Memory is a property of the quasispecies distribution as a whole since, as expected from its consisting of minority components of the mutant spectrum, memory is lost in the course of replication when genetic bottlenecks intervene (115). Quasispecies memory may have a number of biological implications for persistent infections such as those by HIV-1 and hepatitis C virus. It may allow a viral population to respond more effectively to a selective constraint that has been previously experienced by the same population, provided no genetic bottleneck intervened. The presence of memory genomes has opened the possibility of an extended diagnosis in that not only the dominant virus genomes but also minority genomes at memory levels can be detected and identified. Microarray-based techniques, currently under intense development, may provide an adequate technology for this purpose. The existence of memory in viral quasispecies could be predicted from quasispecies theory (111,112,115), and may be regarded as being a consequence of the dynamics of biological adaptive systems such as the immune system (116,117). In HIV-1 a "cellular" or "anatomical" memory derived from the retroviral integrative cycle, has been identified, in addition to the replicative memory previously defined with FMDV (118). Memory as defined with viruses, should also be found in populations of other microbial communities subjected to successive selective pressures that result in an alternative dominance of distinguishable genomes. Mutant spectra cannot be regarded merely as a random repertoire of mutants but rather as organized distributions affected by evolutionary history (115,116).

3. In the evolution of RNA viruses both deterministic and stochastic (probabilistic) effects are observed (119). The treatment of evolution as a deterministic process (in the sense that if a mutant with a selective advantage occurs, it will outgrow the previous mutant distribution) has at least two limitations. (a) Competition processes are vulnerable to statistical fluctuations derived from sampling effects that may modify the outcome anticipated by a deterministic theory (84). (b) The mutant spectrum may suppress high fitness individuals in ways which are difficult to predict (29,120). In addition, mutant generation is an elemen-

tary event subjected to quantum mechanical uncertainty underlying base-pairing properties of each base during nucleic acid replication (84,121). Despite these limitations, deterministic effects have been documented during RNA virus evolution. In competitions between two closely related quasispecies of vesicular stomatitis virus of the same relative fitness, a highly predictable behavior was found. Critical points at which the two populations may diverge in frequency were reached after nearly constant periods of time, and in all cases the winner population was the same (122). In addition, when the two competing populations were subjected to environmental perturbations (addition of defective-interfering particles, chemical mutagenesis or an increase in temperature) the same population always outgrew the other (123). The molecular interpretation of this deterministic evolutionary behavior was the decreased tolerance of the loser population to accept additional mutations for fitness gain. The authors coined the term "contingent neutrality" to describe mutations that while not affecting fitness, decrease the tolerance to additional mutations required for fitness gain (123). This concept has received support also from in silico experiments (124). Deterministic behavior can also be observed as a consequence of quasispecies memory, as evidenced by the systematic selection of specific antigenic variants of FMDV when they had occupied memory levels in evolving FMDV quasispecies (112). Therefore, theoretical treatments of virus evolution must consider both the deterministic and stochastic (or probabilistic) features observed experimentally (88,90,119).

4. Virus entry into error catastrophe by increasing the mutation rate during viral replication is now regarded as a promising antiviral strategy (125). It is based in the concept that for any given template-copying fidelity there is a maximum value for the complexity of genetic information that can be stably maintained. In this case complexity means the amount of genetic information that, for viruses with no redundant information, can be equated with genome length (compare with Sec. 2.1). There is considerable experimental evidence that mutation rates of RNA viruses are close to the maximum tolerable for the stability of the genetic information they carry. The maximum tolerable error rate is termed the "error threshold" (26,38,39,125). An increase in mutation rate by added chemical mutagens led to decreases in viral infectivity and in some cases to virus extinction (126–134). Interestingly, the nucleoside analog ribavirin, which was licensed to treat several human viral diseases, in some cases exerts its antiviral activity through enhanced mutagenesis and virus entry into error catastrophe (114,130,133). Most promising for the prospects of mutagenesis as an antiviral strategy has been the recent observation that pretreatment of mice with the mutagenic base analog 5-fluorouracil prevented the

establishment of a persistent infection with lymphocytic choriomeningitis virus in vivo (135). This constitutes a proof of principle that a designed antiviral strategy based on virus entry into error catastrophe may be feasible in vivo.

Two points are worth stressing to end this summary of quasispecies population dynamics. One is that an understanding of RNA viruses as quasispecies has represented a prolific stimulus for practical applications in virology. The presence of memory genomes as minority components in mutant spectra has encouraged development of new diagnostic procedures [(136) and point (2) above]. An understanding of the error threshold relationship developed as a consequence of quasispecies theory has led to the promising lethal mutagenesis approach in which the replicating virus but not the host cell may succumb to enhanced mutagenesis (62,115,125–134). Quasispecies dynamics has also provided a theoretical basis for the use of combination therapies and multi-component, multivalent vaccines as the preferred designs to treat and prevent infections associated with RNA viruses [(7,23,24,29) and references therein].

Quasispecies was formulated as a general theory and as such its domains of application are not restricted to RNA viruses. Certainly some DNA viruses show features of quasispecies dynamics. Recent examples are emergence of highly heterogeneous population of antibody-resistant mutants of the parvovirus minute virus of mice during its replication in vivo (137), and the presence of multiple variants of the complex DNA virus SIRV1 of the thermophilic archaeon *Sulfolobus* (138), with the implications of error-prone DNA synthesis for adaptation of DNA-based organisms to extreme environments. Earlier observations also led to suggestions that some DNA viruses at specific genetic loci could share with RNA viruses high mutation rates and quasispecies dynamics (23,139). Therefore, several lines of evidence suggest that distinct features of RNA genetics which stem from the combined impact of mutation rates, genome complexity and viral population size (Table 1), and which produce an extraordinary adaptive capacity, may be shared with some DNA viruses.

No matter how ample the opportunities for genetic novelty of cellular and subcellular pathogens are, they represent just one of several conditions necessary for infectious disease emergence.

3. THE EMERGENCE AND REEMERGENCE OF INFECTIOUS DISEASES

Cellular and subcellular replicons most often live and act as collectivities in permanent intragroup or intergroup interactions, with a constant interplay with their hosts (77,140). The behavior of an individual genome in a viral quasispecies (Sec. 2.5) can be profoundly modified by the surrounding mutant spectrum (22,23), much as the behavior of an individual bacterium in a biofilm is conditioned by the local environment created by the collectivity of bacteria [(141) and references therein]. Cell-to-cell communication among bacteria occurs through diffusible signal molecules that may even affect interacting eukaryotic cells (142).

The relationship of cellular and subcellular replicons with differentiated organisms need not be that of a pathogen. It may involve forms of symbiosis, such as commensalism or mutualism. Infectious disease may be regarded as a byproduct of an interaction with the host that leads to an abnormal outcome, from the point of view of the host. Understandably, microbiology research has been biased toward disease-causing agents. The pathogenic potential of all types of pathogens is highly conditioned by environmental alterations in the broadest sense possible. This interplay between environmental alterations and the adaptive capacity of microbes to favor the emergence of disease is discussed in the next sections.

3.1. The Complexities of Infectious Disease Emergence

About 50 human infectious diseases have been listed as emergent or reemergent over the last two decades, in addition to a number of diseases of animals and plants (143). In the following discussion, emergence refers to the first appearance of a disease previously unrecognized in the host population it affects; for example, human AIDS and SARS. Reemergence refers to the occurrence of a known disease, for the first time in a given geographical area, or that had been absent for long periods of time in that area; for example, foot-and-mouth disease outbreaks over the last years in Japan and the United Kingdom. Cellular and subcellular pathogens are not generated de novo, so that the emergence of a disease is due either to a contact of an existing microbe with a potential host that results in transmissible disease, or to some variant form of a pathogen that acquires new pathogenic potentials. Reemergence is some times used in a broader sense to signify a new wave of disease associated with a genetically altered pathogen, such as the seasonal increase of influenza associated with new mutant or reassortant influenza viruses (4).

Obviously, infectious disease emergence and reemergence represent a major concern for human health, and also for the sociological and economic impact of potentially devastating diseases of animals and plants. The recent 2001 outbreak of foot-and-mouth disease in the United Kingdom is an example (144). There is a consensus that infectious disease emergence is multifactorial in that a number of quite independent influences and chance occurrences, must converge to produce a disease emergence or reemergence. These events belong to the category of complex phenomena in which the final outcome (in this case disease emergence) cannot be anticipated merely by analyzing individually the participating elements (145). The difficulties of interpreting complex, emergent phenomena have been emphasized for disparate domains of science such as physics, evolution, or psychology (146–148). These difficulties apply to disease emergence in the sense that we are often limited to a historical account of events once they have occurred and that a scientific approach can only supply fragmentary information. For example, phylogenetic analyses can trace the close relatives of a pathogen, and these techniques have provided convincing evidence of a relationship between some human HIVs and simian counterparts. However, the phylogenetic relationship did not imply the emergence of AIDS. Similar uncertainties have been encountered to interpret the emergence of SARS (149), a new respiratory disease associated with a human coronavirus related to group 2 coronaviruses. A related virus was isolated from some colonies of civet cats. The human and civet cat viruses show remarkable genetic differences whose chance occurrence could contribute to the virus adaptation to the human host. However, contact of humans with civet cats (or other animals that may be reservoirs of related coronaviruses) could have also contributed to the emergence of SARS as a new human disease (149).

Despite these uncertainties derived from the complex nature of infectious disease emergence, a number of factors have been recognized as possible participants (Table 2). These factors can be divided broadly into three classes. (i) The adaptive potential of pathogens, mediated by molecular mechanisms discussed in Sec. 2. (ii) A number of ecological, sociological, and technological factors whose main influence consists in either rendering potential hosts more susceptible to infection (e.g., malnutrition in humans) or to increase the frequency of the interaction between pathogens and potential hosts (e.g., climatic alterations may cause flooding, and water surfaces may permit insect proliferation for the transmission of arboviruses; urban agglomerations favor person-to-person transmission of pathogens). (iii) Interactions among pathogens which generate new selective pressures. Some viral infections lead to immunosuppression, rendering the host more susceptible to other infectious agents. The increase in incidence of tuberculosis in the human population is believed to result partly of the circulation of antibiotic-resistant *Mycobacterium tuberculosis* (Sec. 3.3), facilitated by an increase in the number of immunocompromised individuals associated with the expansion of AIDS. Interference among related viruses both in cell culture and in vivo has been extensively documented, but new forms of inhibition [such as the delay of HIV-1 progression to AIDS by coinfection with hepatitis GBV-C virus (150)] have been recognized with new emergent pathogens.

3.2. The Variation Potential of Pathogens as a Factor in Disease Emergence

Changes in host cell tropism and host range of viruses have some times been associated with a single or a few amino acid replacements in the surface of viral capsids or envelopes. Since genomes differing minimally in genetic distance are frequently represented in the mutant distributions of viral quasispecies, they are likely to have played a role in emergence. Documented examples are amino acid replacements in structural and nonstructural (that are not found in the virus particle) proteins of Venezuelan equine encephalitis virus associated with the epizootic emergence of equine encephalitis from an enzootic reservoir of the virus (151). The canine parvovirus emerged as an important pathogen of dogs by mutation of a feline parvovirus as recently as in the 1970s (152). In a designed experiment, it has been demonstrated that the adaptation of an FMDV isolate from swine to the guinea-pig involved as critical mutation a single amino acid replacement in a nonstructural protein of the virus (153). For additional specific examples and reviews of the implications of pathogen genetic variation in disease emergence see Refs. (4,8,9,23,61,154–159).

3.3. Environmental Alterations and Medical Practices Favor the Manifestation of the Adaptive Potential of Pathogens: The Case of Antibiotic and Drug Resistance

Multiple factors, as those listed in Table 2, have as a net result the alteration of the traffic of pathogens and of the demography of vectors and hosts (157–160). As examples, the expansion of Rift valley virus followed dam constructions in several African countries, which originated water surfaces where larvae of insect vectors could proliferate. In addition, slave traffic from Africa to America resulted in the introduction of yellow fever virus and human T-cell leukemia virus type 1 (HTLV-1) in the American continent. The extensive use of blood transfusions without a diagnostic test available for the human hepatitis viruses, contributed during the mid-twentieth century to an expansion of hepatitis viruses, notably hepatitis C virus, in the human population. Pathogens may go unrecognized either because no diagnostic methods are available (161) or because mutations prevent recognition by current diagnostic tests (162).

Table 2   Some Factors Recognized as Potential Participants in Disease Emergence and Reemergence

- The adaptive potential of cellular and subcellular pathogens
- Sociological factors (malnutrition, urban agglomeration, poor hygiene, poverty, human migration, travel, high-risk practices such as drug abuse with the sharing of syringes, etc.)
- Ecological factors (environmental alterations resulting from global warming such as flooding or drought that results in altered patterns of distribution and migration of animals and insects, deforestation, dam construction with expansion of water surfaces, etc.)
- Medical practices (widespread use of antibiotics and antiviral agents, supply of contaminated blood or blood products, organ transplantation and xenotransplantation, etc.)
- The interactions among pathogens as they affect the host response (immunosuppression and ensuing opportunistic infections, etc.)

The extensive use of antibiotics to control bacterial infections and of antiviral agents to control viral infections has led to a dramatic increase in the proportions of antibiotic-resistant bacteria and of viruses with diminished sensitivity to inhibitors of virus replication. These are selective pressures that result from technological developments and medical practice. Resistance of bacteria to antibiotics, and of viruses to antiviral inhibitors, share some common features, and differ in some very fundamental aspects. Common features are that one or a limited number of mutations (or other genome alterations) are often sufficient to impart the resistance phenotype. The resistant pathogens often display decreased fitness relative to their sensitive counterparts, in the absence of the antibiotic or the antiviral agent. Therefore, sensitive pathogens often outcompete the resistant ones in the absence of antibiotic or antiviral agent. Fitness decrease may be compensated by additional mutations in target genes. The degree of resistance and fitness may increase if the pathogen still maintains some residual replication in the presence of the antibiotic or antiviral agent. Cross-resistance among different antibiotics or antiviral agents may be observed (63,156–160).

As distinctive features, resistance determinants in bacteria can map in chromosomal genes, plasmids, or mobile elements. Resistance to antiviral agents maps generally on the target gene of the viral genome. Antibiotic resistance determinants may undergo cross-species transmission, in particular from non-pathogenic bacteria to pathogenic bacteria. As a consequence, extensive use of antibiotics in agricultural practices (for food preservation) contributes a selective pressure for antibiotic resistance that may affect resistance frequency among pathogenic bacteria. In contrast, resistance to an inhibitor of a virus is often confined to the treated patients, and the transfer of resistance determinants to other viruses is unlikely.

Antibiotic resistance determinants are encoded in the bacterial chromosome, in conjugative plasmids, or mobile genetic elements. They have been associated with amino acid replacements in a variety of enzymes such as -lactamases, DNA gyrases, topoisomerases, catalase-peroxidases, etc. The extended-spectrum -lactamases (ESBL) phenotype is expanding worldwide, mainly among enterobacteria. Resistance may be associated also with alterations of cell wall biosynthesis and structure, which either prevent antibiotic entrance, or create false target sites for the binding of antibiotics. The active efflux of drugs from target cells may also decrease sensitivity to antibiotics, as extensively documented with bacteria and eukaryotic pathogens, including the recent study of fluoroquinolone resistance in *Listeria* (163). There are multiantibiotic resistance loci, some carried on pathogenicity islands, therefore with increased probability of spreading through flanking mobile elements [reviews in (63) and several chapters in Refs. (156–159)].

Eukaryotic cellular pathogens display also an ample repertoire of resistance mechanisms. Duplication and overexpression of a gene (without mutation in that gene) may be a determinant of resistance, such as in the multi-drug resistance gene of *Plasmodium chabandi* (164). A membrane transporter protein is associated with resistance of *Plasmodium falciparum* to chloroquine, with the possible participation of a membrane P glycoprotein (164).

Viruses resistant to inhibitors occur at high frequencies, mainly for RNA viruses (Sec. 2.5). Inhibitors targeting virus structural proteins (i.e., the WIN compounds against rhinoviruses) or viral enzymes (the HIV protease or reverse transcriptase) select for viruses with mutations that confer decreased sensitivity to one or several inhibitors [reviews in Refs. (24,165)]. The evasion potential of RNA viruses includes selection of mutants resistant to potent intracellular gene silencing mediated by double-stranded RNA (166). Resistance mutations often incur a fitness cost for the virus. However, continued residual replication often leads to additional, compensatory mutations in the viral genome, that result in fitness gain while maintaining the resistance phenotype. This is one of the reasons of an increasing circulation of viruses harboring mutations that confer resistance to inhibitors. Even in the case of reversion of the mutation causing the primary resistance, the constellations of mutations associated with fitness gain will render more likely the reacquisition of the resistance phenotype. This concept which applies to bacteria as well, has been supported by several observations [review in Refs. (136,167)].

This brief account of resistance mechanisms shows how the several molecular mechanisms of pathogen genetic variation (Sec. 2) provide an adequate machinery to respond to the presence of drugs aimed at impairing pathogen replication. Gene expression dosage, mutation and recombination can be exploited to produce pathogens with decreased sensitivity to one or multiple agents. If a chance for continuing replication is given (due to incorrect dosage or to insufficient inhibitory levels at sites where pathogens replicate) a pathogen will continue exploration of its allotted sequence space compatible with viability, to pursue its quest for survival. Such continuous dynamics of evolutionary exploration is in itself is an essential factor for disease emergence and reemergence.

4. CONCLUDING REMARKS

Infectious disease emergences and reemergences will continue, since they are an unavoidable consequence of the intrinsic capacity of pathogenic and nonpathogenic microbes to respond to and to overcome many natural and artificial (man-made) selective pressures (63,75,84,154–160). Continuous replication and fitness gains, reflected in increases of pathogen load and infectivity, must be regarded as potential determinants of pathogen persistence and, therefore, of genetic variation and diseases emergence and reemergence (98,99,168). A few things have been learned. Some human infections may have a zoonotic origin. Therefore surveillance of infectious diseases of animals may be important not only to control animal diseases, as important as this is, but also to anticipate possible transmissions to humans (169). Practices involving close contacts between human and animals (cohabitation, xenotransplantation, etc.) should be monitored. Understanding the molecular basis of adaptation of pathogens to new cell types and host organisms should be pursued experimentally. Preventive and therapeutic treatments should be designed taking into consideration the adaptive potential of pathogens. Vaccines should be multivalent (targeting independent B-cell and T-cell epitopes) and antibiotics and antiviral agents should be administered in combination. New anti-pathogen drugs are needed to increase the combinatorial potential of combination regimens. New diagnostic tools to refine the genotypic and phenotypic characterization of minority subpopulations of pathogens are needed to tailor therapeutic regimens to individual needs of patients. New antimicrobial approaches such as virus entry into error catastrophe should be pursued despite obvious difficulties that this and other approaches will face until a practical application becomes feasible. Research in the biochemistry of enzymes involved in pathogen replication has evidenced that the copying fidelity of polymerases can be decreased by structural alterations (37). Therefore, the design of error-enhancing drugs is becoming a possibility. Basic research together with increased surveillance of pathogen reservoirs provide some means to confront a really important challenge.

ACKNOWLEDGMENTS

I am indebted to many students and colleagues over many years for fruitful collaborations and discussions. Their names appear in the papers quoted in this review. The work in my laboratory has been supported by grants BMC2001-1823-C02-01, QLK2-2001-0082 from the EU, and Fundación R. Areces.

REFERENCES

1. Mount DW. Bioinformatics. Sequence and Genome Analysis. Cold Spring Harbor, NY: Cold Spring Harbor Laboratory Press, 2001.
2. Koonin EV, Makarova KS, Aravind L. Horizontal gene transfer in prokaryotes: quantification and classification. Annu Rev Microbiol 2001; 55:709–742.
3. Bushman F. Lateral DNA Transfer. Mechanisms and Consequences. Cold Spring Harbor, NY: Cold Spring Harbor Laboratory Press, 2002.
4. Domingo E, Webster RG, Holland JJ (eds). Origin and Evolution of Viruses. San Diego, CA: Academic Press, 1999.
5. Kimata JT, Kuller L, Anderson DB, Dailey P, Overbaugh J. Emerging cytopathic and antigenic simian immunodeficiency virus variants influence AIDS progression. Nat Med 1999; 5:535–541.
6. Nathanson N, Ahmed R, Gonzalez-Scarano F, Griffin DE, Holmes KV, Murphy FA, Robinson HL (eds). Viral Pathogenesis. Philadelphia: Lippincott-Raven, 1997.
7. Domingo E, Escarmís C, Menéndez-Arias L, Holland JJ. Viral quasispecies and fitness variations. In: Domingo E, Webster RG, Holland JJ, eds. Origin and Evolution of Viruses. San Diego, CA: Academic Press, 1999:141–161.

8. Stearns SC (ed.). Evolution in Health and Disease. Oxford: Oxford University Press, 1999.
9. Mims C, Nash A, Stephen J. Mims' Pathogenesis of Infectious Disease. San Diego, CA: Academic Press, 2001.
10. Alcami A, Koszinowski UH. Viral mechanisms of immune evasion. Trends Microbiol 2000; 8:410–418.
11. Xu XN, Screaton GR, McMichael AJ. Virus infections: escape, resistance, and counterattack. Immunity 2001; 15:867–870.
12. Domingo E. Vers une compréhension des virus comme systèmes complexes et dynamiques. Ann Méd Vét 1999; 143:225–235.
13. Milkman R. Electrophoretic variation in *Escherichia coli* from natural sources. Science 1973; 182:1024–1026.
14. Lewontin RC, Hubby JL. A molecular approach to the study of genic heterozygosity in natural populations. II. Amount of variation and degree of heterozygosity in natural populations of *Drosophila pseudoobscura*. Genetics 1966; 54:595–609.
15. Harris H. Enzyme polymorphisms in man. Proc R Soc Lond B Biol Sci 1966; 164:298–310.
16. Pace NR. A molecular view of microbial diversity and the biosphere. Science 1997; 276:734–740.
17. Morris CE, Bardin M, Berge O, Frey-Klett P, Fromin N, Girardin H, Guinebretiere MH, Lebaron P, Thiery JM, Troussellier M. Microbial biodiversity: approaches to experimental design and hypothesis testing in primary scientific literature from 1975 to 1999. Microbiol Mol Biol Rev 2002; 66:592–616.
18. Maynard Smith J, Smith N. The genetic population structure of pathogenic bacteria. In: Stearns SC, ed. Evolution in Health and Disease. Oxford: Oxford University Press, 1999:183–190.
19. van Regenmortel MHV, Fauquet CM, Bishop DHL, Carstens EB, Estes MK, Lemon SM, Maniloff J, Mayo MA, Mc Geoch DJ, Pringle CR, Wickner RB (eds). Virus Taxonomy. Seventh Report of the International Committee on Taxonomy of Viruses, San Diego, CA: Academic Press, 2000.
20. Cohan FM. What are bacterial species? Annu Rev Microbiol 2002; 56:457–487.
21. Relman DA. Sequence-based methods for pathogen discovery; the complex associations of microbes, microbial sequences, and host. In: Scheld WM, Craig WA, Hughes JM, eds. Emerging Infections. Vol. 4. Washington DC: ASM Press, 2000:69–81.
22. Nowak MA, May RM. Virus Dynamics. Mathematical Principles of Immunology and Virology. New York: Oxford University Press Inc., 2000.
23. Domingo E, Biebricher C, Eigen M, Holland JJ. Quasispecies and RNA Virus Evolution: Principles and Consequences. Austin: Landes Bioscience, 2001.
24. Domingo E, Mas A, Yuste E, Pariente N, Sierra S, Gutiérrez-Riva M, Menéndez-Arias L. Virus population dynamics, fitness variations and the control of viral disease: an update. Prog Drug Res 2001; 57:77–115.
25. Drake JW. Comparative rates of spontaneous mutation. Nature 1969; 221:1132.
26. Eigen M, Biebricher CK. Sequence space and quasispecies distribution. In: Domingo E, Ahlquist P, Holland JJ, eds. RNA Genetics. Vol. 3. Boca Raton, FL: CRC Press, 1988:211–245.
27. Drake JW. A constant rate of spontaneous mutation in DNA-based microbes. Proc Natl Acad Sci U S A 1991; 88:7160–7164.

28. Batschelet E, Domingo E, Weissmann C. The proportion of revertant and mutant phage in a growing population, as a function of mutation and growth rate. Gene 1976; 1:27–32.

29. Domingo E, Holland JJ. RNA virus mutations and fitness for survival. Annu Rev Microbiol 1997; 51:151–178.

30. Drake JW, Holland JJ. Mutation rates among RNA viruses. Proc Natl Acad Sci U S A 1999; 96:13910–13913.

31. Holland J, Spindler K, Horodyski F, Grabau E, Nichol S, VandePol S. Rapid evolution of RNA genomes. Science 1982; 215:1577–1585.

32. Bressanelli S, Tomei L, Roussel A, Incitti I, Vitale RL, Mathieu M, De Francesco R, Rey FA. Crystal structure of the RNA-dependent RNA polymerase of hepatitis C virus. Proc Natl Acad Sci U S A 1999; 96:13034–13039.

33. Steitz TA. DNA polymerases: structural diversity and common mechanisms. J Biol Chem 1999; 274:17395–17398.

34. Steinhauer DA, Domingo E, Holland JJ. Lack of evidence for proofreading mechanisms associated with an RNA virus polymerase. Gene 1992; 122:281–288.

35. Radman M, Dohet C, Bourguignon M-F, Doubleday OP, Lecomte P. High fidelity devices in the reproduction of DNA. In: Seeberg E, Kleppe K, eds. Chromosome Damage and Repair. New York: Plenum Publishing Corp., 1981:431–445.

36. Friedberg EC, Walker GC, Siede W. DNA Repair and Mutagenesis. Washington, DC: American Society for Microbiology, 1995.

37. Menéndez-Arias L. Molecular basis of fidelity of DNA synthesis and nucleotide specificity of retroviral reverse transcriptases. Prog Nucleic Acid Res Mol Biol 2002; 71:91–147.

38. Swetina J, Schuster P. Self-replication with errors. A model for polynucleotide replication. Biophys Chem 1982; 16:329–345.

39. Nowak M, Schuster P. Error thresholds of replication in finite populations mutation frequencies and the onset of Muller's ratchet. J Theor Biol 1989; 137:375–395.

40. Storb U, Shen HM, Michael N, Kim N. Somatic hypermutation of immunoglobulin and non-immunoglobulin genes. Philos Trans R Soc Lond B Biol Sci 2001; 356:13–19.

41. Storb U, Stavnezer J. Immunoglobulin genes: generating diversity with AID and UNG. Curr Biol 2002; 12:R725–R727.

42. Michael N, Martin TE, Nicolae D, Kim N, Padjen K, Zhan P, Nguyen H, Pinkert C, Storb U. Effects of sequence and structure on the hypermutability of immunoglobulin genes. Immunity 2002; 16:123–134.

43. Nicolson GL. Tumor cell instability, diversification, and progression to the metastatic phenotype: from oncogene to oncofetal expression. Cancer Res 1987; 47:1473–1487.

44. Strauss BS. The stability of the genome and the genetic instability of tumors. Perspect Biol Med 2000; 43:286–300.

45. Friedberg EC, Wagner R, Radman M. Specialized DNA polymerases, cellular survival, and the genesis of mutations. Science 2002; 296:1627–1630.

46. Giraud A, Matic I, Tenaillon O, Clara A, Radman M, Fons M, Taddei F. Costs and benefits of high mutation rates: adaptive evolution of bacteria in the mouse gut. Science 2001; 291:2606–2608.

47. de Visser JA. The fate of microbial mutators. Microbiology 2002; 148:1247–1252.

48. Giraud A, Matic I, Radman M, Fons M, Taddei F. Mutator bacteria as a risk factor in treatment of infectious diseases. Antimicrob Agents Chemother 2002; 46:863–865.

49. McClure MA. The retroid agents: disease, function and evolution. In: Domingo E, Webster RG, Holland JJ, eds. Origin and Evolution of Viruses. San Diego, CA: Academic Press, 1999:163–195.

50. Gabriel A, Willems M, Mules EH, Boeke JD. Replication infidelity during a single cycle of Ty1 retrotransposition. Proc Natl Acad Sci U S A 1996; 93:7767–7771.

51. Agur Z. Resilience and variability in pathogens and hosts. IMA J Math Appl Med Biol 1987; 4:295–307.

52. Graïa F, Lespinet O, Rimbault B, Dequard-Chablat M, Coppin E, Picard M. Genome quality control: RIP (repeat-induced point mutation) comes to Podospora. Mol Microbiol 2001; 40:586–595.

53. Cooper GM. The Cell. A Molecular Approach. Washington, DC: ASM Press, 2000.

54. Feil EJ, Spratt BG. Recombination and the population structures of bacterial pathogens. Annu Rev Microbiol 2001; 55:561–590.

55. Guan H, Simon AE. Polymerization of nontemplate bases before transcription initiation at the 3¢ ends of templates by an RNA-dependent RNA polymerase: an activity involved in 3¢ end repair of viral RNAs. Proc Natl Acad Sci U S A 2000; 97:12451–12456.

56. King AMQ. Genetic recombination in positive strand RNA viruses. In: Domingo E, Holland JJ, Ahlquist P, eds. RNA Genetics. Vol. II. Boca Raton, FL: CRC Press Inc., 1988.

57. Lai MMC. Genetic recombination in RNA viruses. Curr Top Microbiol Immunol 1992; 176:21–32.

58. Nagy PD, Simon AE. New insights into the mechanisms of RNA recombination. Virology 1997; 235:1–9.

59. An W, Telesnitsky A. HIV-1 genetic recombination: experimental approaches and observations. AIDS Rev 2002; 4:195–212.

60. Borst P, Fairlamb AH. Surface receptors and transporters of *Trypanosoma brucei*. Annu Rev Microbiol 1998; 52:745–778.

61. Baranowski E, Ruiz-Jarabo CM, Domingo E. Evolution of cell recognition by viruses. Science 2001; 292:1102–1105.

62. Baranowski E, Ruíz-Jarabo CM, Pariente N, Verdaguer N, Domingo E. Evolution of cell recognition by viruses: a source of biological novelty with medical implications. Adv Virus Res 2003: in press.

63. Chadwick DJ, Goode J (eds). Antibiotic Resistance: Origins, Evolution, Selection and Spread. Ciba Foundation Symposium 207. Chichester: John Wiley & Sons, 1997.

64. Lespinet O, Wolf YI, Koonin EV, Aravind L. The role of lineage-specific gene family expansion in the evolution of eukaryotes. Genome Res 2002; 12:1048–1059.

65. Richard GF, Cyncynatus C, Dujon B. Contractions and expansions of CAG/CTG trinucleotide repeats occur during ectopic gene conversion in yeast, by a MUS81-independent mechanism. J Mol Biol 2003; 326:769–782.

66. Zhuang J, Jetzt AE, Sun G, Yu H, Klarmann G, Ron Y, Preston BD, Dougherty JP. Human immunodeficiency virus type 1 recombination: rate, fidelity, and putative hot spots. J Virol 2002; 76:11273–11282.

67. Holland JJ. Defective viral genomes. In: Fields BM, Knipe DM, eds. Virology. New York: Raven Press, 1990:151–165.
68. Roux L, Simon AE, Holland JJ. Effects of defective interfering viruses on virus replication and pathogenesis in vitro and in vivo. Adv Virus Res 1991; 40:181–211.
69. Plyusnin A, Kukkonen SK, Plyusnina A, Vapalahti O, Vaheri A. Transfection-mediated generation of functionally competent Tula hantavirus with recombinant S RNA segment. EMBO J 2002; 21:1497–1503.
70. Desselberger U. Genome rearrangements of rotaviruses. Adv Virus Res 1996; 46:69–95.
71. Adoutte A, Balavoine G, Lartillot N, Lespinet O, Prud'homme B, de Rosa R. The new animal phylogeny: reliability and implications. Proc Natl Acad Sci U S A 2000; 97:4453–4456.
72. Thomson MM, Perez-Alvarez L, Najera R. Molecular epidemiology of HIV-1 genetic forms and its significance for vaccine development and therapy. Lancet Infect Dis 2002; 2:461–471.
73. Levins R. Evolution in Changing Environments. Princeton, NJ: Princeton University Press, 1968.
74. Schlager TA, Hendley JO, Bell AL, Whittam TS. Clonal diversity of *Escherichia coli* colonizing stools and urinary tracts of young girls. Infect Immun 2002; 70:1225–1229.
75. DeFilippis VR, Villarreal LP. An introduction to the evolutionary ecology of viruses. In: Hurst CJ, ed. Viral Ecology. San Diego, CA: Academic Press, 2000:125–208.
76. DeFilippis VR, Villarreal LP. Virus evolution. In: Knipes DM, Howley PM, Griffin DE, Lamb RA, Martin MA, Roizman B, Straus SE, eds. 4th ed. Fields Virology. Philadelphia: Lippincott-Raven, 2001:353–370.
77. Woolhouse ME, Webster JP, Domingo E, Charlesworth B, Levin BR. Biological and biomedical implications of the co-evolution of pathogens and their hosts. Nat Genet 2002; 32:569–577.
78. Klein B. Host–microbe interactions: fungi. Curr Opin Microbiol 2003; 6(3).
79. Sibley D. Host–microbe interactions: parasites. Curr Opin Microbiol 2003; 6(3).
80. Domingo E. Host–microbe interactions: viruses. Curr Opin Microbiol 2003; 6(3).
81. Domingo E, Holland JJ, Ahlquist P. RNA Genetics, I, II, III. Boca Raton: CRC Press, 1988.
82. Domingo E, Flavell RA, Weissmann C. In vitro site-directed mutagenesis: generation and properties of an infectious extracistronic mutant of bacteriophage Qb. Gene 1976; 1:3–25.
83. Domingo E, Sabo D, Taniguchi T, Weissmann C. Nucleotide sequence heterogeneity of an RNA phage population. Cell 1978; 13:735–744.
84. Domingo E, Holland JJ, Biebricher C, Eigen M. Quasispecies: the concept and the word. In: Gibbs A, Calisher C, García-Arenal F, eds. Molecular Evolution of the Viruses. Cambridge: Cambridge University Press, 1995:171–180.
85. Domingo E, Martínez-Salas E, Sobrino F, de la Torre JC, Portela A, Ortín J, López-Galindez C, Pérez-Breña P, Villanueva N, Nájera R, VandePol S, Steinhauer D, DePolo N, Holland JJ. The quasispecies (extremely heterogeneous) nature of viral RNA genome populations: biological relevance—a review. Gene 1985; 40:1–8.

86. Eigen M. Self-organization of matter and the evolution of biological macromolecules. Naturwissenschaften 1971; 58:465–523.

87. Eigen M. On the nature of virus quasispecies. Trends Microbiol 1996; 4:216–218.

88. Eigen M. Natural selection: a phase transition? Biophys Chem 2000; 85:101–123.

89. Eigen M, Schuster P. The Hypercycle. A Principle of Natural Self-Organization. Berlin: Springer, 1979.

90. Wilke CO, Ronnewinkel C, Martinetz T. Dynamic fitness landscapes in molecular evolution. Phys Rep 2001; 349:395–446.

91. Page KM, Nowak MA. Unifying evolutionary dynamics. J Theor Biol 2002; 219:93–98.

92. Domingo E. Quasispecies. In: Granoff A, Webster RG, eds. Encyclopedia of Virology. London: Academic Press, 1999:1431–1436.

93. Maynard Smith JM. Natural selection and the concept of a protein space. Nature 1970; 225:563–564.

94. Eigen M. Steps Towards Life. Oxford: Oxford University Press, 1992.

95. Jackwood DJ, Sommer SE. Identification of infectious bursal disease virus quasispecies in commercial vaccines and field isolates of this double-stranded RNA virus. Virology 2002; 304:105–113.

96. Nowak MA. What is a quasispecies? Trends Ecol Evol 1992; 4:118–121.

97. Carrillo C, Borca M, Moore DM, Morgan DO, Sobrino F. In vivo analysis of the stability and fitness of variants recovered from foot-and-mouth disease virus quasispecies. J Gen Virol 1998; 79:1699–1706.

98. Quiñones-Mateu ME, Arts EJ. HIV-1 fitness: implications for drug resistance, disease progression, and global epidemic evolution. In: Kuiken C, Foley B, Hahn BH, Marx P, McCutchan FE, Mellors J, Mullins JI, Sodroski J, Wolinsky S, Korber BT, eds. HIV-1 Sequence Compendium. Theoretical Biology and Biophysics Group. Los Alamos, NM: Los Alamos National Laboratory, 2002:134–170.

99. Ball SC, Abraha A, Collins KR, Marozsan AJ, Baird H, Quinones-Mateu ME, Penn-Nicholson A, Murray M, Richard N, Lobritz M, Zimmerman PA, Kawamura T, Blauvelt A, Arts EJ. Comparing the ex vivo fitness of CCR5-tropic human immunodeficiency virus type 1 isolates of subtypes B and C. J Virol 2003; 77:1021–1038.

100. Novella IS, Duarte EA, Elena SF, Moya A, Domingo E, Holland JJ. Exponential increases of RNA virus fitness during large population transmissions. Proc Natl Acad Sci U S A 1995; 92:5841–5844.

101. Escarmís C, Dávila M, Domingo E. Multiple molecular pathways for fitness recovery of an RNA virus debilitated by operation of Muller's ratchet. J Mol Biol 1999; 285:495–505.

102. Chao L. Fitness of RNA virus decreased by Muller's ratchet. Nature 1990; 348:454–455.

103. Duarte E, Clarke D, Moya A, Domingo E, Holland J. Rapid fitness losses in mammalian RNA virus clones due to Muller's ratchet. Proc Natl Acad Sci U S A 1992; 89:6015–6019.

104. Escarmís C, Dávila M, Charpentier N, Bracho A, Moya A, Domingo E. Genetic lesions associated with Muller's ratchet in an RNA virus. J Mol Biol 1996; 264:255–267.

105. Yuste E, Sánchez-Palomino S, Casado C, Domingo E, López-Galíndez C. Drastic fitness loss in human immunodeficiency virus type 1 upon serial bottleneck events. J Virol 1999; 73:2745–2751.

106. Novella IS, Elena SF, Moya A, Domingo E, Holland JJ. Size of genetic bottlenecks leading to virus fitness loss is determined by mean initial population fitness. J Virol 1995; 69:2869–2872.

107. Novella IS, Quer J, Domingo E, Holland JJ. Exponential fitness gains of RNA virus populations are limited by bottleneck effects. J Virol 1999; 73:1668–1671.

108. Escarmís C, Gómez-Mariano G, Dávila M, Lázaro E, Domingo E. Resistance to extinction of low fitness virus subjected to plaque-to-plaque transfers: diversification by mutation clustering. J Mol Biol 2002; 315:647–661.

109. Lázaro E, Escarmís C, Domingo E, Manrubia SC. Modeling viral genome fitness evolution associated with serial bottleneck events: evidence of stationary states of fitness. J Virol 2002; 76:8675–8681.

110. Lázaro E, Escarmís C, Pérez-Mercader J, Manrubia SC, Domingo E. Resistance of virus to extinction upon bottleneck passages: study of a decaying and fluctuating pattern of fitness loss. Proc Natl Acad Sci U S A 2003: in press.

111. Ruíz-Jarabo CM, Arias A, Baranowski E, Escarmís C, Domingo E. Memory in viral quasispecies. J Virol 2000; 74:3543–3547.

112. Ruíz-Jarabo CM, Arias A, Molina-París C, Briones C, Baranowski E, Escarmís C, Domingo E. Duration and fitness dependence of quasispecies memory. J Mol Biol 2002; 315:285–296.

113. Arias A, Lázaro E, Escarmís C, Domingo E. Molecular intermediates of fitness gain of an RNA virus: characterization of a mutant spectrum by biological and molecular cloning. J Gen Virol 2001; 82:1049–1060.

114. Airaksinen A, Pariente N, Menendez-Arias L, Domingo E. Curing of foot-and-mouth disease virus from persistently infected cells by ribavirin involves enhanced mutagenesis. Virology 2003; 311:339–349.

115. Domingo E. Viruses at the edge of adaptation. Virology 2000; 270:251–253.

116. Frank SA. The design of natural and artificial adaptive systems. In: Rose MR, Lauder GV, eds. Adaptation. San Diego, CA: Academic Press, 1996:451–505.

117. Ahmed R, Gray D. Immunological memory and protective immunity: understanding their relation. Science 1996; 272:54–59.

118. Briones C, Domingo E, Molina-Paris C. Memory in retroviral quasispecies: experimental evidence and theoretical model for human immunodeficiency virus. J Mol Biol 2003: in press.

119. Rouzine IM, Rodrigo A, Coffin JM. Transition between stochastic evolution and deterministic evolution in the presence of selection: general theory and application to virology. Microbiol Mol Biol Rev 2001; 65:151–185.

120. de la Torre JC, Holland JJ. RNA virus quasispecies populations can suppress vastly superior mutant progeny. J Virol 1990; 64:6278–6281.

121. Holland JJ, de La Torre JC, Steinhauer DA. RNA virus populations as quasispecies. Curr Top Microbiol Immunol 1992; 176:1–20.

122. Quer J, Huerta R, Novella IS, Tsimring L, Domingo E, Holland JJ. Reproducible nonlinear population dynamics and critical points during replicative competitions of RNA virus quasispecies. J Mol Biol 1996; 264:465–471.

123. Quer J, Hershey CL, Domingo E, Holland JJ, Novella IS. Contingent neutrality in competing viral populations. J Virol 2001; 75:7315–7320.

124. Wilke CO, Wang JL, Ofria C, Lenski RE, Adami C. Evolution of digital organisms at high mutation rates leads to survival of the flattest. Nature 2001; 412:331–333.

125. Eigen M. Error catastrophe and antiviral strategy. Proc Natl Acad Sci U S A 2002; 99:13374–13376.

126. Holland JJ, Domingo E, de la Torre JC, Steinhauer DA. Mutation frequencies at defined single codon sites in vesicular stomatitis virus and poliovirus can be increased only slightly by chemical mutagenesis. J Virol 1990; 64:3960–3962.

127. Lee CH, Gilbertson DL, Novella IS, Huerta R, Domingo E, Holland JJ. Negative effects of chemical mutagenesis on the adaptive behavior of vesicular stomatitis virus. J Virol 1997; 71:3636–3640.

128. Loeb LA, Essigmann JM, Kazazi F, Zhang J, Rose KD, Mullins JI. Lethal mutagenesis of HIV with mutagenic nucleoside analogs. Proc Natl Acad Sci U S A 1999; 96:1492–1497.

129. Loeb LA, Mullins JI. Lethal mutagenesis of HIV by mutagenic ribonucleoside analogs. AIDS Res Hum Retroviruses 2000; 13:1–3.

130. Crotty S, Maag D, Arnold JJ, Zhong W, Lau JYN, Hong Z, Andino R, Cameron CE. The broad-spectrum antiviral ribonucleotide, ribavirin, is an RNA virus mutagen. Nat Med 2000; 6:1375–1379.

131. Sierra S, Dávila M, Lowenstein PR, Domingo E. Response of foot-and-mouth disease virus to increased mutagenesis. Influence of viral load and fitness in loss of infectivity. J Virol 2000; 74:8316–8323.

132. Pariente N, Sierra S, Lowenstein PR, Domingo E. Efficient virus extinction by combinations of a mutagen and antiviral inhibitors. J Virol 2001; 75:9723–9730.

133. Crotty S, Cameron CE, Andino R. RNA virus error catastrophe: direct molecular test by using ribavirin. Proc Natl Acad Sci U S A 2001; 98:6895–6900.

134. Grande-Pérez A, Sierra S, Castro MG, Domingo E, Lowenstein PR. Molecular indetermination in the transition to error catastrophe: systematic elimination of lymphocytic choriomeningitis virus through mutagenesis does not correlate linearly with large increases in mutant spectrum complexity. Proc Natl Acad Sci U S A 2002; 99:12938–12943.

135. Ruiz-Jarabo CM, Ly C, Domingo E, Torre JC. Lethal mutagenesis of the prototypic arenavirus lymphocytic choriomeningitis virus (LCMV). Virology 2003; 308:37–47.

136. Domingo E, Ruíz-Jarabo CM, Arias A, Molina-Paris C, Briones C, Baranowski E, Escarmís C. Detection and biological implications of genetic memory in viral quasispecies. In: Matsumori A, Ruffy R, eds. Proceedings of the International Congress on Cardiomyopathies and Heart Failure. London, UK: Kluwer Academic Publishers, 2003: in press.

137. Lopez-Bueno A, Mateu MG, Almendral JM. High mutant frequency in populations of a DNA virus allows evasion from antibody therapy in an immunodeficient host. J Virol 2003; 77:2701–2708.

138. Prangishvili D, Stedman K, Zillig W. Viruses of the extremely thermophilic archaeon *Sulfolobus*. Trends Microbiol 2001; 9:39–43.

139. Smith DB, Inglis SC. The mutation rate and variability of eukaryotic viruses: an analytical review. J Gen Virol 1987; 68:2729–2740.

140. Futuyma DJ, Slatkin M (eds). Coevolution. Sunderland, MA: Sinauer Associates Inc., 1983.

141. Rice AR, Hamilton MA, Camper AK. Movement, replication, and emigration rates of individual bacteria in a biofilm. Microb Ecol 2002; 20:20.

142. Joint I, Tait K, Callow ME, Callow JA, Milton D, Williams P, Camara M. Cell-to-cell communication across the prokaryote-eukaryote boundary. Science 2002; 298:1207.

143. Brown C. Emerging diseases of animals. In: Scheld WM, Craig WA, Hughes JM, eds. Emerging Infections. Vol. 3. Washington, DC: ASM Press, 1999:153–163.

144. Samuel AR, Knowles NJ. Foot-and-mouth disease virus: cause of the recent crisis for the UK livestock industry. Trends Genet 2001; 17:421–424.

145. Martin B. The schema. In: Cowan GA, Pines D, Meltzen D, eds. Complexity. Metaphors, Models and Reality. Reading, MA: Addison-Wesley Publishing Co., 1994:263–285.

146. Bak P. How nature works. In: The Science of Self-Organized Criticality. New York: Springer-Verlag, 1996.

147. Holland JH. Emergence. From Chaos to Order. Reading, MA: Addison-Wesley Publishing Company, Inc., 1998.

148. Staddon JER. Adaptive Dynamics. Cambridge, MA: The MIT Press, 2001.

149. Holmes KV. SARS-associated coronavirus. N Engl J Med 2003; 348:1948–1951.

150. Stosor V, Wolinsky S. GB virus C and mortality from HIV infection. N Engl J Med 2001; 345:761–762.

151. Wang E, Barrera R, Boshell J, Ferro C, Freier JE, Navarro JC, Salas R, Vasquez C, Weaver SC. Genetic and phenotypic changes accompanying the emergence of epizootic subtype IC Venezuelan equine encephalitis viruses from an enzootic subtype ID progenitor. J Virol 1999; 73:4266–4271.

152. Parrish CR, Truyen U. Parvovirus variation and evolution. In: Domingo E, Webster RG, Holland JJ, eds. Origin and Evolution of Viruses. San Diego, CA: Academic Press, 1999:421–439.

153. Núñez JI, Baranowski E, Molina N, Ruiz-Jarabo CM, Sánchez C, Domingo E, Sobrino F. A single amino acid substitution in nonstructural protein 3A can mediate adaptation of foot-and-mouth disease virus to the guinea pig. J Virol 2001; 75:3977–3983.

154. Morse SS (ed.). Emerging Viruses. Oxford: Oxford University Press, 1993.

155. Morse SS (ed.). The Evolutionary Biology of Viruses. New York: Raven Press, 1994.

156. Lederberg J, Shope RE, Oaks SC. Emerging Infections. Microbial Threats to Health in the United States. Washington, DC: National Academy Press, 1992.

157. Scheld WM, Craig WA, Hughes JM (eds). Emerging Infections. Vol. 3. Washington, DC: ASM, 1999.

158. Scheld WM, Craig WA, Hughes JM (eds). Emerging Infections. Vol. 4. Washington, DC: ASM, 2000.

159. Scheld WM, Craig WA, Hughes JM (eds). Emerging Infections. Vol. 5. Washington, DC: ASM, 2001.

160. Hurst CJ (ed.). Viral Ecology. San Diego, CA: Academic Press, 2000.

161. Relman DA. New technologies, human–microbe interactions, and the search for previously unrecognized pathogens. J Infect Dis 2002; 186(suppl 2):S254–S258.

162. Weinberger KM, Bauer T, Bohm S, Jilg W. High genetic variability of the group-specific a-determinant of hepatitis B virus surface antigen (HBsAg) and the corresponding fragment of the viral polymerase in chronic virus carriers lacking detectable HBsAg in serum. J Gen Virol 2000; 81:1165–1174.

163. Godreuil S, Galimand M, Gerbaud G, Jacquet C, Courvalin P. Efflux pump Lde is associated with fluoroquinolone resistance in *Listeria* monocytogenes. Antimicrob Agents Chemother 2003; 47:704–708.

164. Cravo PV, Carlton JM, Hunt P, Bisoni L, Padua RA, Walliker D. Genetics of mefloquine resistance in the rodent malaria parasite *Plasmodium chabaudi*. Antimicrob Agents Chemother 2003; 47:709–718.

165. Richman DD (ed.). Antiviral Drug Resistance. New York: John Wiley and Sons Inc., 1996.

166. Gitlin L, Karelsky S, Andino R. Short interfering RNA confers intracellular antiviral immunity in human cells. Nature 2002; 418:430–434.

167. Lenski RE. The cost of antibiotic resistance from the perspective of a bacterium. In: Chadwick DJ, Goode J, eds. Antibiotic Resistance: Origins, Evolution, Selection and Spread. Ciba Foundation Symposium 207. New York: John Wiley and Sons, Inc., 1997:131–151.

168. Messenger SL, Smith JS, Orciari LA, Yager PA, Rupprecht CE. Emerging pattern of rabies deaths and increased viral infectivity. Emerg Infect Dis 2003; 9:151–154.

169. Haydon DT, Cleaveland S, Taylor LH, Laurenson MK. Identifying reservoirs of infection: a conceptual and practical challenge. Emerg Infect Dis 2002; 8:1468–1473.

170. Domingo E, Menéndez-Arias L, Quiñones-Mateu ME, Holguín A, Gutiérrez-Rivas M, Martínez MA, Quer J, Novella IS, Holland JJ. Viral quasispecies and the problem of vaccine-escape and drug-resistant mutants. Prog Drug Res 1997; 48:99–128.

2

Ecological Disturbances and Emerging Infections: Travel, Dams, Shipment of Goods, and Vectors

Mary Elizabeth Wilson

Associate Professor of Medicine, Harvard Medical School and Associate Professor of Population and International Health, Harvard School of Public Health, Mount Auburn Hospital, Cambridge, Massachusetts, U.S.A.

1. INTRODUCTION

Infectious diseases appear, disappear, wax, wane, and change in distribution and expression in response to multiple factors. Among these are the physicochemical environment, movement of microbial genetic material and species (humans and other animals, plants), and population characteristics (size, density, location, mobility, vulnerability). In the past two decades many previously unrecognized infectious diseases have been described in humans, as well as in plants and animals. There has been a tendency to react to these with surprise, followed by the assumption that something new has happened in the microbial world to lead to disease in humans. In fact, most infections that are considered new or emerging are caused by pathogens long present in animals, soil, or water. The milieu, in which the infections have appeared, increased in incidence, spread into new geographic areas, or become more virulent or resistant to antimicrobials is typically one that has been altered in subtle or profound ways by humans.

This chapter will look at the ecological context in which new infections appear and old ones change (1). The focus will be on travel, trade, and changes in the landscape. Several specific disease examples will illustrate how infections emerge. Notably, multiple factors (simultaneously or sequentially) are often involved and may act synergistically to contribute to emergence and spread.

2. TRAVEL AND TRADE

2.1. Travel

Human travel today is unprecedented in its volume, reach, and speed. According to the World Tourism Organization (WTO) 50.9 million international tourists arrived in the United States in 2000. In the 1990s more than 5000 airports had regularly scheduled international flights, linking urban areas throughout the world. In 1996, 2.5 billion persons passed through airports and more than 500 million persons crossed international borders on commercial airplane flights. Of course, airplanes are only one of the means of travel. For example, in 1999 an estimated 400 million international travelers entered the United States by land, ship, or air. In addition to travel for pleasure, movement of humans includes planned travel for business and education, military maneuvers, pilgrimages, seasonal migration for harvest and other employment, and population displacements because of war, economic need, social, political, ethnic and religious conflicts, environmental crises, extreme weather events, and other natural disasters (2).

2.1.1. Infections Carried and Spread by Travelers

Microbes that can be carried by humans and transmitted from person to person can be carried to any corner of the earth. A prime example is the human immunodeficiency virus (HIV), which emerged from a related virus in primates, but which subsequently has spread throughout the world—carried by humans and spread primarily through sexual contact (3). Transmission from mother to infant and via blood and tissues (transfusions, shared needles and other devices, transplantation) have been important contributors but have not matched the efficiency of the human carrier spreading the virus to others via sexual activities. Social, cultural, economic and political factors have influenced spread. Sexual tourism has facilitated movement of HIV transnationally, assisting its spread through wide, loosely connected regional and global networks. Travel is a key factor in the spread of HIV-1 genetic variants, potentially including drug-resistant strains (4).

The spread of HIV has also led to the emergence and recognition of other infections and different clinical expressions of well-known infections. For example, as HIV has moved into areas that are endemic for leishmaniasis and American trypanosomiasis, reactivation of latent infections and new manifestations of these infections have been recognized. Tuberculosis has increased in many populations globally, in part because of an increase in the number of humans co-infected with HIV and *Mycobacterium tuberculosis*.

Travel is a potent and efficient way to spread microbes carried by humans, especially when they do not cause symptoms (1). Besides HIV, other important examples of bloodborne viruses carried by humans include hepatitis B and hepatitis C. Persons infected with *M. tuberculosis* may have latent infection that can reactivate years or decades later. Even persons with active (and contagious) tuberculosis, may have symptoms that are sufficiently mild that they do not seek medical attention for many weeks or longer and can infect others in the interim.

Neisseria meningitidis: Travel and Spread of W135. Although *N. meningitidis* can colonize the nasopharynx of healthy persons without causing symptoms, it can also cause meningitis, fulminant sepsis, and death. Traditionally most human disease has been caused by serogroups A, B, and C, with serogroups W135, Y, and others playing a lesser role. Infected carriers can transmit the microbe to others, unaware that they are carrying and transmitting infection.

Traveling humans have played a key role in changes in the epidemiology of meningococcal infections in recent decades. In 1987, pilgrims to the Hajj in Saudi Arabia carried an epidemic strain (subgroup III-1) of serogroup A *N. meningitidis* to Mecca. Other pilgrims became colonized with the strain and introduced it into sub-Saharan Africa, where it caused waves of epidemic meningococcal disease there and elsewhere (5). A part of sub-Saharan Africa, the so-called "meningitis belt," has long experienced seasonal meningitis outbreaks, usually caused by serogroup A, during the dry season. In 1996, for example, an epidemic of serogroup A meningococcal infection caused more than 185,000 cases with a case fatality rate of about 10%. It is thought that irritation of the throat by dry, dusty air facilitates invasion by colonizing bacteria. Co-infection with other respiratory pathogens also appears to increase vulnerability to disease (6).

In recent years about 2 million pilgrims from approximately 140 different countries have gathered in Saudi Arabia for the annual Hajj (7). Pilgrims have close contact with each other and then return home. Because of outbreaks of meningococcal infections in pilgrims, Saudi Arabia began to require that all pilgrims receive the meningococcal vaccine prior to entry into the country for the Hajj. In the spring of 2000, an outbreak of *N. meningitidis* serogroup W135 appeared among pilgrims, and subsequently among their contacts in multiple countries (7). About 240 cases were reported in Saudi Arabia and another 90 cases were reported in 13 other countries. Researchers using serotyping, multilocus sequence typing, multilocus DNA fingerprinting, and other techniques showed that 15 isolates from the United Kingdom and 19 from France were indistinguishable but were distinct from the W135 isolates that cause sporadic infections in Europe (8,9). Reports from other countries are consistent with the international spread of infection caused by this clone of W135 (10,11). In the United Kingdom, the case fatality rate of confirmed meningococcal cases from the W135 outbreak strain was 20%, in contrast to 9% for other culture-confirmed cases of meningococcal disease reported in England and Wales from 1995 to 2000 (12).

Meningococcal Vaccines: Several different meningococcal vaccines are used globally. Many countries in Europe and Asia have used a bivalent vaccine (A and C); a quadrivalent vaccine (A, C, Y, W135) is used routinely in the United

States and in some other countries. The vaccines have been reported to have protective efficacy in the range of 80–90% against serogroups included, but they do not eliminate nasopharyngeal carriage of *N. meningitidis*. Because of the continuing outbreaks of W135 in 2001, Saudi Arabia now requires use of a quadrivalent vaccine (including W135) for pilgrims.

Researchers in Singapore cultured tonsillopharyngeal swab specimens from 373 returning Malay pilgrims in 2001 (13). All had received the quadrivalent meningococcal vaccine prior to the Hajj pilgrimage. Overall, 15% of pilgrims carried the single clone of W135 *N. meningitidis* on return from the Hajj. Of 40 with positive cultures who had a repeat culture done 5–6 months later, 55% continued to carry the W135 clone. Notably, 8% of household contacts also became infected with the W135 clone, with all infections having been acquired during the 1 month after the return of the pilgrims (14). A much lower rate of carriage, 0.8%, was found in a U.S. study of 727 pilgrims returning to New York JFK airport after travel to Saudi Arabia in 2001 (15,16). Reasons for the differences between the two populations in rates of acquisition of W135 are unknown but may include differences in living conditions, accommodations, and activities during the Hajj and in duration of stay.

Spread of W135 Beyond Population of Pilgrims and Their Contacts: Various *N. meningitidis* isolates differ in their invasiveness and capacity to cause epidemic disease, and specific clones have been identified in many outbreaks. *N. meningitidis* is transmitted from human to human by aerosol or direct contact with respiratory secretions of patients or healthy carriers. No animal or environmental reservoirs exist. The above studies demonstrate the key role played by travelers in the dissemination of clones to new populations. Initial cases of W135 infection were in pilgrims and their close contacts, but more recent studies would suggest that the clone has spread more widely to other populations (17). During 2002 an epidemic of W135 began in February in Burkina Faso; by May more than 12,500 cases and almost 1500 deaths had been reported to the World Health Organization. The events are being closely monitored and have important implications for meningococcal vaccination programs in sub-Saharan Africa, which traditionally have focused on preventing disease caused by serogroup A, and to a lesser extent, serogroup C (18).

Travelers Carry Microbial Genetic Material: Interactive Biological Units. In addition to carrying specific pathogens, travelers can carry microbial genetic material that can be introduced into a new area (19,20). Microbial genetic material in pathogens or in commensal flora may have resistance genes that can, through recombination or other microbial molecular maneuvers, influence pathogens in a new region (21). Increasingly, it is recognized that for many pathogens a limited number of clones that spread globally cause much of the serious disease (22). The availability of molecular markers has allowed researchers to identify the source and subsequent spread of specific pathogens, but also has made it possible sometimes to pinpoint a common origin of infections that occur in different countries or continents.

A human can be considered an interactive biological unit, an assemblage of microbial flora, genetic material, and immunologic responses (23). Travelers or migrating humans pick up microbes and microbial genetic material, provide a biological vessel for growth and immunological processing and can transport them and drop them off in another geographic area. Transmission to other humans may occur silently. Depending on the microbe and host characteristics, transmission to one or more new hosts may occur days to decades after the traveler acquired it. Means of transfer also depend on the biological characteristics of host and microbe, but may include airborne or respiratory spread (e.g., tuberculosis, measles, *N. meningitis*), sexual contact (e.g., HIV, HBV), bloodborne or mother-to-child transmission (e.g., HIV, HBV, HCV, malaria), or rarely, transplantation of tissues (e.g., HIV, *Trypanosoma cruzi*, CJD, rabies virus).

Travel is a process that involves more than the origin and the destination. The entire loop or itinerary can lead to relevant interactions (to the traveler and from the traveler). Not uncommonly a trip may include one or more forms of land transportation (e.g., car, bus, train), a period of time spent in a terminal, often standing in line in densely packed areas with recirculated air with people from multiple parts of the world, and one or multiple flights (perhaps with additional excursions through terminals en route). This leads to frequent en route transmission and is relevant in considering possible exposures when evaluating a sick patient. For example, MDR tuberculosis, SARS and influenza, among other infections, have been documented to be spread on airplanes, where air is recirculated (24,25).

2.1.2. Cruise Ships: Routes to Acquire and Disperse Infections

Large cruise ships are a special category. These vessels, or floating towns, which may hold a population of more than 3000 passengers and crew, pick up passengers from multiple origins (typically after air or other travel), may visit multiple ports where passengers interact with local populations, and may pick up and drop off passengers along their course. Although cruises are often thought of as outdoor experiences, much of the time is spent in indoor spaces—dining room, dance hall, exercise room, lecture halls, etc. Not surprisingly, these have proved to be a site of many outbreaks of infectious diseases (26), including food and waterborne infections, respiratory infections [(including several well-documented outbreaks of influenza (27–30), rubella, and legionnaire's disease (31), among others]. Of note is the fact that some of the cruises have a high percentage of persons who are elderly and have underlying medical problems, and so are at high risk for some infections, such as influenza. Multiple outbreaks of infections caused by Noroviruses (caliciviruses, formerly called Norwalk-like viruses) have hit cruise ships in the recent years (32).

2.1.3. Travelers and Immigrants: Need to Recognize Their Infections

The extent of travel and immigration today means that clinicians in every part of the world must be familiar with infections that occur in any part of the world—or have access to sources that help them to define what infections are possible, how and when they might manifest clinically, what risk they might pose to others (and through what routes of spread) and means for diagnosis and treatment. In the United States as of March 2000 the foreign-born population was estimated to be 28 million (U.S. Census 2000), up from about 10 million in 1970. Many undertake regular visits to family and relatives in their birth country. The foreign-born may have residua of past infections (such as latent tuberculosis) that can have clinical expression years later. In the United States to date about half of the cases of tuberculosis are in the foreign-born, reflecting primarily infections that were acquired before they moved to their country. Three cases of Chagas disease appeared in the United States in recipients of cadaveric organ transplantation (liver, pancreas, kidneys). The organ donor was an immigrant from Central America who harbored unrecognized infection with *T. cruzi* (33).

2.1.4. Travelers: A Sentinel Population

In 2000, an outbreak of 12 cases of eosinophilic meningitis caused by *Angiostrongylus cantonensis* occurred in medical students after visiting Jamaica. This infection, unfamiliar to most clinicians in the United States, has been reported primarily in Southeast Asia and the Pacific Basin in the past. Humans are incidental, dead end hosts and become infected by ingesting larvae of the worms in raw or undercooked snails or slugs, or in produce (such as lettuce) contaminated by them (34). The outbreak led to an investigation that identified *A. cantonensis* in both rats and snails in Jamaica (35), though the precise food source of the infection in the travelers was not confirmed. Publication of the description of the outbreak and clinical and laboratory findings has heightened awareness of this infection among clinicians.

  These cases also show the way that travelers can serve as a sentinel population, providing insights about pathogens or their profiles of resistance to antimicrobials in other geographic regions (23,36). Travelers may have manifestations that differ from a locally resident population (who may respond in different ways immunologically). Travelers may return home, where medical resources allow diagnostic and specialized testing that would be unavailable to a local population, thus permitting documentation about specific infections circulating in a distant or remote area. A network (GeoSentinel Network) currently systematically collects information about ill returned travelers and enters it into a database (37). This and other networks have helped to identify risky activities for particular infections (leptospirosis and ecochallenge) or increased risks in certain geographic regions (e.g., African trypanosomiasis in travelers; malaria and dengue outbreaks).

2.1.5. Dengue Fever

Continues to Spread: *Increase in Severe Infections*. Dengue is the most common vector-borne viral infection globally. The dynamic and worsening situation with dengue fever, caused by the mosquito-borne RNA virus, a flavivirus, illustrates how multiple factors can contribute to emergence of a disease. Dengue fever, which has caused major outbreaks for decades in Asia, is now expanding in distribution and causing more severe disease in the Americas (38). Dengue is found in tropical and subtropical regions worldwide, areas inhabited by more than 2.5 billion people, or approximately 40% of the world population (see Fig. 1). Four antigenically distinct viral serotypes, designated dengue 1, 2, 3, and 4, cause dengue fever, also known as breakbone fever because of the intense muscle aches and pains associated with infection. Infection with one serotype provides good long-lasting immunity to that serotype, but increases the likelihood of serious and complicated dengue (dengue hemorrhagic fever or dengue shock syndrome) if a person is subsequently infected with a different dengue serotype (39).

Mosquitoes Essential: *Ambient Temperature Affects Extrinsic Incubation*. Humans are the usual source of the dengue virus; although some primates can be infected but they do not play an important role in the epidemiology of dengue in most areas. Humans become infected when bitten by an infective mosquito. Not all species of mosquitoes are competent to transmit dengue. Even

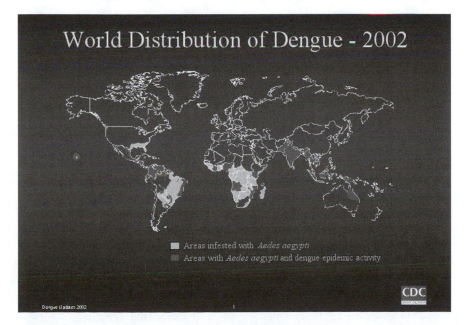

Figure 1   World distribution of dengue (CDC, 2002).

if a mosquito is competent to transmit the virus, the mosquito must feed on a person carrying the virus, survive long enough (usually 8–12 days) for the virus to replicate in the midgut, reach other tissues, and replicate in the salivary glands, and then must bite another human who is not already immune to the dengue serotype carried by the mosquito. The time it takes for the mosquito to become infective is highly dependent on the ambient temperature, for example 7 days at 90°F and 12 days at 86°F. A mosquito can also pass virus to offspring vertically, through infection of eggs. This means that mosquitoes can serve as reservoirs for the virus (40). Transovarial transmission may be important in maintaining the virus during periods between epidemics. The mosquito remains infectious for life and may infect more than one person. Viremia in humans, which may last as long as 7–8 days (typically 3–5 days), usually begins about 2 days before onset of symptoms. The levels of virus in the blood may be high. Plasma viral RNA levels in children in Thailand were as high as 10^9 RNA copies (41). Incubation period, or time between the bite of an infected mosquito and onset of symptoms, is typically 4–7 days. The virus can also be transmitted from mother to fetus (42) and probably via blood transfusion, but these means of transmission play a minor role in the overall epidemiology of infection.

Contemporary Urban Landscape Favors Transmission: Several factors are contributing to the worsening situation with dengue. Although each viral serotype probably evolved in geographic isolation, all four are now found in Asia, Africa, and in the Americas (43). The primary vector in most areas, *Aedes aegypti*, has expanded into larger regions and infests large portions of the tropics and subtropics. The vector is well adapted to human habits and habitats and lives in close association with humans, breeding in standing water in discarded plastic containers, flowerpots, used tires, water storage containers, and other vessels that litter the contemporary urban landscape. It inhabits urban areas, so has access to large and growing human populations, many living in urban or periurban slums where open water collection containers and other vessels provide ready breeding sites. Houses that lack screens or air conditioning provide the mosquitoes ready access to humans. More people are living in urban areas than ever before; urban growth is occurring preferentially in low latitude areas. In South America, 78% of the population lived in urban areas in 1995 and this is projected to increase to 88% by 2025. About 50% of the world population is now living in urban areas. More and more urban areas in tropical and subtropical areas are reaching the population size required for the ongoing circulation of dengue virus. This leads to a higher background rate of infection and increases the likelihood of severe and complicated infection if a second dengue serotype is introduced.

Human Population Size, Location, Density, Mobility, and Living Conditions: Size of the population as well as density may be important. Researchers have shown that during the past two centuries the number of dengue lineages has been increasing roughly in parallel with the size of the human population (44). A larger population in which the virus replicates allows increased opportunities for viral mutation, which enhances the likelihood of the appearance of more virulent strains. Large urban populations in hyperendemic regions also may provide more opportunities for intra-serotype recombination events when two viruses infect the same cell (45).

Large urban populations globally are now linked air travel, allowing frequent movement of viremic humans, who can introduce new serotypes and genotypes into regions where competent vectors reside. Dengue endemic countries in the Americas receive more than 50 million international arrivals each year (38). The wide distribution of *Ae. aegypti*, which also transmits yellow fever virus, in tropical and subtropical cities has also raised concern about outbreaks of urban yellow fever (46,47).

The presence of competent vectors, although necessary, is not sufficient to lead to major outbreaks of dengue fever. Recent studies in the border cities of Laredo (Texas) and Nuevo Laredo (Mexico) noted striking differences in the likelihood of serologic evidence of dengue infection, even though climatic conditions are similar in both cities (separated only by the Rio Grande River) and cross-border traffic is extensive (48). When researchers conducted surveys of randomly selected households on both sides they found residents of Nuevo Laredo were more likely to test positive for dengue IgM and IgG (16% and 48%, respectively) than residents of Loredo (1.3% and 23%) even though containers infested with *Ae. aegypti* were more common in Loredo than in Nuevo Laredo. Of note, air conditioning (AC) was more common in Laredo homes (82%) than in Nuevo Laredo (24%); absence of AC was significantly associated with dengue infection.

2.2. Trade

Human traffic—local, national, and international—contributes to the spread of infections in humans, plants, and animals, but trade likewise has a profound impact on infectious diseases in humans, plants, and animals. The planned cargo of ships and other vehicles is only a part of what is carried and what is biologically relevant in another ecosystem.

2.2.1. Food: Produce and Processed Foods

With the globalization of the food supply, the food chain has become very long. Prepared foods as well as produce from the fields in developing countries regularly and rapidly reach the tables in the United States and other industrialized countries (49). During some months of the year, up to 70% of some fresh produce consumed in the United States comes from developing countries (50). For example, between 1989 and 1992 during the winter months up to 33–70% of cantaloupes, 57–72% of green onions, and 20–64% of tomatoes sold in the United States were grown and harvested in Mexico. Common, familiar pathogens, such as *Salmonella*, *Shigella*, *Campylobacter*, and *Escherichia coli* are found in imported foods (as well as in domestically produced foods). The origin of an outbreak may be difficult to trace. Because of mass processing and distribution networks, outbreaks may affect consumers in multiple states or several countries (51). Imported foods have also been the source of unusual pathogens. In 1995, 1996, 1997, and 2000, outbreaks of diarrhea caused by a previously little known pathogen, *Cyclospora cayetanensis*, were linked to raspberries imported from Guatemala (52,53). Outbreaks also occurred in Canada. Outbreaks of *Shigella sonnei* infections in 1994 in the United Kingdom, Norway and Sweden were associated with lettuce grown in southern Europe (54).

Foods implicated in outbreaks go beyond fresh produce. An outbreak of cholera in 1991 in Maryland was linked to consumption of frozen fresh coconut milk imported from Thailand (55). Toxigenic *Vibrio cholerae* O1 was isolated from one of the unopened bags of the same brand of coconut milk used in preparing dishes eaten by the persons who developed cholera. *V. cholerae* O1 organisms can survive freezing.

Illnesses related to contaminated food include a spectrum of diseases, not just diarrheal illness. An outbreak of hepatitis A in the United States was traced to frozen strawberries from Mexico (56). Other systemic diseases that can follow ingestion of contaminated food include toxoplasmosis, typhoid fever, hemolytic-uremic syndrome (following infection with *E. coli* O157:H7), listeriosis, trichinosis, botulism, among others. Infections that are rare or unfamiliar may be misdiagnosed, and appropriate treatment and interventions to halt spread may be delayed.

Although food processed domestically can be the source of infection, foods prepared in developing countries may be more likely to be contaminated with pathogenic microbes, chemicals, or other substances because of conditions under which they are prepared and the lack of controls in some settings.

2.2.2. Live Animals

The main components of the international agricultural food trade are fruits and vegetables, meat and meat preparations, and dairy products and eggs. Live animals are also imported, many for pets. Nonhuman primates cannot be imported as pets, but about 9000 primates enter the country each year for scientific research and exhibition. In Miami alone, more than 30 million animals were imported in 1996 including 28.6 million fish, 1.1 million reptiles, 108,000 amphibians, 70,000 mammals, and 1400 birds (Stephanie Ostrowski, Division of Quarantine, CDC). A large but unknown number of rare and exotic animals also enter the United States illegally. The annual trade in illegal plants and animals is estimated to be $3 billion per year in the United States. In 1999, during the year when infections due to West Nile virus were first recognized in the United States with the epicenter in New York, 2770 birds were legally brought into the United States through JFK International Airport in New York and almost 18,000 passed through in transit.

The United States also participates in the global trade of live animals and exports prairie dogs, among other animals. The potential risks associated with this practice were highlighted in 2002 when an outbreak of tularemia was identified in prairie dogs at a distribution center in Texas that ships animals to other states and European and Asian countries (57). Prairie dogs can become infected with plague as well as tularemia, both infections that can cause life-threatening disease in humans. In addition to posing a risk to humans, microbes in imported animals can also threaten domestic and local wildlife populations in other regions (58).

Even more striking was the appearance in the summer of 2003 of a multi-state outbreak of human monkeypox, a zoonosis previously known to exist only in western and central Africa (58a; CDC 2003). Infection can resemble smallpox, though has a lower mortality. The outbreak was traced to prairie dogs (from the United States) that had been housed with animals from Ghana. The implicated shipment from Ghana arrived on April 9 in Texas. Included were 792 small animals of nine species, including six genera of African rodents that might have been the source of monkeypox. These included rope squirrels (*Funiscuirus* sp.), tree squirrels (*Heliosciurus* sp.), Gambian giant rats, brushtail porcupines (*Atherurus* sp.), dormice (*Graphiurus* sp.), and striped mice (*Hybomys* sp.). CDC laboratory testing confirmed presence of monkeypox in some of animals from this shipment (Gambian rat, dormice, rope squirrels). Of these animals, 77% were traced to distributors in six states; 23% could not be traced beyond point of entry in Texas because of inadequate records. Most human cases resulted from exposure to prairie dogs sold as pets in the Midwest. As of July 30, 2003, 72 cases in six states were under investigation and 37 cases had been confirmed by laboratory testing.

The relocation of raccoons and other animals in the 1970s from Florida to the southeastern United States (Virginia and West Virginia) to stock hunting clubs, introduced a rabies variant into animals in the mid-Atlantic states. Rabies subsequently spread through a large part of the north-eastern United States (about 1 million square km), an area with about 90 million human residents and many suburban communities with large raccoon populations. The spillover effects have been disruptive and extremely costly because of exposures of cats, dogs and other animal populations to rabies and human–raccoon interactions, leading to expanded use of post-exposure rabies preventive therapy with rabies vaccine and rabies immune globulin. In New York State alone, where the raccoon rabies variant reached the state from Pennsylvania in 1990, the estimated cost to prevent rabies between 1993 and 1998 was $13.9 million (59). More than $10 million of the total was spent on post-exposure prophylaxis treatment, which cost an average of $1136 per person treated in 1998.

2.2.3. Vectors

Mosquito Dispersal: Mosquitoes and other arthropods that serve as vectors for important human pathogens, such as malaria, yellow fever, dengue, and others have been transported from one continent to another for centuries (60). *Ae. aegypti*, the main vector for dengue and yellow fever viruses in the Americas, is believed to have been introduced into the Americas on slave ships from West Africa from the 15th through the 17th centuries. Introductions of this vector to the New World may also have occurred via European ships from Spain and Portugal. Water storage containers on ships provided a habitat in which the mosquitoes could flourish. After *Ae. aegypti* was introduced into the New World, it became established in temperate and tropical areas. Because of the threat posed by yellow fever epidemics, an intensive campaign was organized by the Pan American Health Organization starting in 1947 to eradicate *Ae. aegypti* in the Americas. By the late 1960s, the vector had been eliminated from most areas except Venezuela and United States (see Fig. 2). A side benefit was a halt in dengue outbreaks in areas where the vector had been eliminated. The support for the vector control programs, however, faltered, and *Ae. aegypti* reinfested areas where it had been controlled and spread to new areas. Today the mosquito is found in most tropical and subtropical areas of the Americas.

An anopheline mosquito, *Anopheles gambiae*, an efficient transmitter of malaria found in Africa, was discovered in a grassy field between a railway and a river in Natal, Brazil in 1930 (61). It probably reached Brazil via boats that made mail runs between Dakar, Senegal and Natal, Brazil, covering the 3300 km in less than 100 hr. No efforts were untaken to control the vector initially, and over the

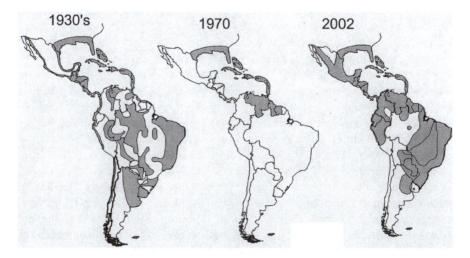

Figure 2   *Aedes aegypti* distribution in the Americas (CDD, 2002).

ensuing years it spread along the coastal region and inland. Natal, an ocean port and terminus of two railway lines and a hub for truck, car and river transport, was well situated for the dissemination of the anopheline mosquito into the region. Malaria already existed in the region, but the local vectors were not particularly efficient vectors. *A. gambiae*, in contrast, bred in close proximity to humans and sought human blood meals. In 1938 and 1939, major outbreaks of malaria occurred in this region, killing more than 20,000 persons. An intensive campaign to eliminate the vector was undertaken and, though expensive, was successful (61). This example illustrates that not just the presence of a competent vector but the species of vector can change the epidemiology of a vector-borne infection.

Aedes albopictus, a competent vector for dengue and other viruses, has been introduced into a number of countries by shipping and trade. The first recognized introduction into North America was in 1985, when it was found in Texas (62,63). It probably reached Texas via used tires shipped from north Asia. Within 12 years it had spread to 678 counties in 25 states in the United States. Its dispersal followed interstate highways; it presumably was carried with human traffic and trade (64). As of 2002, *A. albopictus* had been introduced into Brazil, the Dominican Republic, Guatemala, Honduras, Panama, Mexico, Cuba, Bolivia, El Salvador, Nicaragua, and Colombia in the Western Hemisphere and was continuing to spread in New World and Old. *A. albopictus* was the vector implicated in the 2001 dengue outbreak in Hawaii.

Although mosquitoes and other insects can be carried by planes, trucks, and other forms of transport, most successful mosquito invasions in the past resulted from ship transport. Modern ships with container vessels are effective in dispersing immature stages of mosquitoes.

Mosquitoes can survive airplane flights and can survive long enough after to take at least one blood meal, as has been demonstrated by the occasional cases of so-called "airport malaria" occurring close to international airports receiving flights from tropical areas. In an experiment carried out many years ago, beetles, house flies, and mosquitoes were placed in special cages and inserted into the wheel bays of 747 aircraft and carried along on flights lasting up to 7 hr. Despite temperatures as low as -62°F (-52°C) outside and 44–77°F (8–25°C) in the wheel bays, survival rates were >99% for the beetles, 93% for the flies, and 84% for the mosquitoes (65).

Vehicles can transport vectors over land. *Glossinia palpalis*, a vector for African trypanosomiasis (African sleeping sickness), can fly up to 21 km but can be transported much longer distances on animals and in vehicles (60).

Pesticide Resistance: Insects resistant to pesticides can also be dispersed and can transfer resistance genes to mosquitoes and pests in other areas (66–68). The potential impact of resistance of mosquitoes and other pests on human health is obvious, but insects also play a key role in the spread of many infections among plants (including food crops) and animals (69).

2.2.4. Bats

Bats, some species of which can carry rabies, West Nile, Nipah and other viruses as well as the fungus *Histoplasma capsulatum*, can undergo geographic translocation, using human conveyances for long-distance movement (70). Bats can alight on ships or can roost on ships in port and be carried long distances. Many examples have been documented when bats from one country or continent end up in another, having been transported in a container, e.g., with fruit, lettuce, and timber. Bats occasionally enter aircraft and are carried long distances. A bat of African origin flew out of a suitcase of a traveler on his return to Los Angeles. He had closed his suitcase in the dark in a hut within Kruger National Park in South Africa 3 days earlier.

2.2.5. Shipping

Ships participate in the global dissemination of a number of species (71). In addition to bats and mosquitoes, rodents and other animals that may be carriers or intermediate hosts for human pathogens have reached new ports aboard ships, inside containers, along with shipped goods, or elsewhere on or below deck. Ships carry ballast to help maintain stability. Although historically, ships used rocks and other material as ballast (term comes from Middle English word meaning "useless load"), ships today use water as ballast. Water is pumped in and discharged in multiple different locations in ports or in open sea. The amount of water can be huge. A large tanker, for example, may be able to carry 200,000 cm3 of water. In Australia, an estimated 60 million tons of ballast is discharged into 40 ports each year. The United States receives an estimated 79 million tons of ballast water from overseas each year (71). Ballast contains water, sediment, and plants and animals less than 1 cm that are adjacent to the ship at the time the ballast water is taken on. Ships may transport more than 3000 species of plants and animals around in the world in ballast water. In a study of ships traveling between Coos Bay, Oregon and Japan, investigators identified 367 different taxa in ballast water (72). Although most released organisms may be unable to survive in a new environment, some do. These invasive species may be harmful and destructive in a new ecosystem, where natural predators may be absent.

In the early 1990s when a cholera epidemic was spreading in Latin America, researchers isolated toxigenic *V. cholerae* O1 from ballast, bilge and sewage from three of 14 cargo ships docking at Gulf of Mexico ports. The ships had recently been in ports in Brazil, Colombia, and Chile (73).

3.   CHANGES IN LAND USE

3.1.   Geography of Infectious Diseases

Pathogens that are transmitted from person to person may be influenced by temperature and humidity, and the epidemiology of disease may have a striking seasonal pattern in some parts of the world (e.g., influenza in temperate regions, meningococcal meningitis in sub-Saharan Africa). Pathogens that require an arthropod vector to carry the pathogen from one host to another or that require an intermediate host for completion of parts of the development cycle are typically closely linked to geoclimatic and physicochemical conditions in the environment and have geographically focal distributions (74). Pathogens that live in the soil, such as *Coccidioides immitis*, have certain constraints for survival. It should also be recognized that soil, water, vegetation, animals, and arthropods may harbor a plethora of microbes, as yet undefined, that are potentially pathogenic for humans. These are most likely to be present in areas where no or limited human exploration has occurred so far. Removal of or replacement of vegetation, disruption of soil (75), changes in land use, alterations in water management (e.g., dams, irrigation, creation of artificial lakes) may change local ecology, affect dispersal, and enhance survival and abundance of some species and lead to loss of others (76,77). In a number of instances, one consequence of such a change was infection of humans with pathogens, often previously unknown. One example was the appearance of cases of lethal Venezuelan hemorrhagic fever, caused by a previously unknown virus, Guanarito virus, after development of lands in Venezuela (78).

Arthropods, such as mosquitoes, require certain temperatures, moisture, and breeding conditions to survive and to flourish. They are intimately tied to the landscape. Likewise, ticks are embedded in the landscape (79). Types of vegetation and presence of animals will affect distribution and abundance.

3.2. Roads

The building of roads, integral to the development of regions, has multiple consequences, some perverse (80,81). These include the fragmentation of habitats leading to loss of species diversity, easier movement of some species from one region to another (especially for those that can hitch a ride with/on/under vehicles), breaching of barriers that may have limited species spread, changes in human and viral traffic (82), and introductions of invasive species (including plants and animals) and new arthropod vectors (83). A growing network of roads in Africa may have facilitated bushmeat trade and human contact with primates (84).

3.3. Building of Dams

3.3.1. Schistosomiasis

The schistosome parasite requires a specific snail as an intermediate host, in order to complete its development cycle. Not all snails are competent to permit the development of the parasite. A schistosome-infected snail releases thousands of free-swimming forms of the parasite into the water. These cercariae, if they come into contact with a human, can penetrate intact skin over a period of 30 sec to 10 min. The parasites undergo development in the human (or other) host, mate, and produce eggs. A byproduct of the presence of the parasites and eggs in the human may be the development of the disease schistosomiasis, which is commonly chronic and debilitating, and occasionally fatal. The eggs, excreted by infected humans in urine or feces, hatch into larval forms and infect snails, to continue the cycle, under the right circumstances. Eggs must reach water with competent snails. Water and snails are essential for the completion of the cycle—as is human contact with untreated water, typically streams, ponds, and lakes.

The building of dams in several instances has led to increases in schistosomiasis in human populations (85). In Egypt the completion of the dam at Aswan in 1933 and the High Dam in 1970 along with the institution of perennial irrigation, was associated with an increase in schistosomiasis. In four areas, surveyed in 1934 and again in 1937, for example, the prevalence of *Schistosoma haematobium* had increased from 2–11% to 44–75%. In the 1980s, extensive agricultural development was carried out in the Senegal River basin with the development of two major dams. The first human case of schistosomiasis was identified in 1988. Two years later, the prevalence of schistosomiasis had reached 45–70%. A survey in 1990 found that 91% of people were infected (86).

In Cote d'Ivoire, baseline schistosomiasis prevalence was available in areas surrounding two large dams (Kossou and Taabo), which became operational in the 1970s. Prevalence of *S. haematobium*, as determined from studies in schoolchildren in 1992, increased from 14% to 53% around Lake Kossou and from 0% to 73% around Lake Taabo. At the same time, prevalence of *Schistosoma mansoni* around Lake Taabo showed little change between 1979 and 1992 (3% and 2%) (87).

In China the Three Gorges Dam across the Yangtze River, scheduled to be completed in 2009, is a massive undertaking that will create a lake 640 km long (88). It is expected to displace at least 1.3 million persons and have direct impact on another 20 million who live in the region (89). In all, up to 60–80 million persons who live in the area may be affected. *Schistosoma japonicum* is endemic in China. One million people and 70,000 cattle are estimated to be infected. Many scientists have voiced concerns about the potential for schistosomiasis to spread and have recommended enhanced surveillance. The dam will elevate the water table, create new waterways and also potentially allow movement of snails around the gorges via canals (90).

In Nigeria, more than 246 dams were constructed between 1970 and 1995. Of the 323 dams in Nigeria as of 1995, 106 were characterized as large, 27 medium-sized, and 192 as small (91). In a review published in 2002, the author found that only 47 (15%) of the dams in Nigeria had been surveyed for presence of snail intermediate hosts.

3.2.2. Malaria

Water is essential for the breeding of mosquitoes, vectors for many human infections. In Ethiopia, a goal of a rural development program was to improve food production by constructing micro dams and introducing irrigation systems in the Tigray region, an area plagued by drought and erratic rainfall. Researchers undertook a 1 year longitudinal survey of malaria incidence in eight communities living near dams and eight control communities at similar altitudes but beyond the flight range of mosquitoes that might breed in standing water created by dams. They found that malaria was significantly more common in villages close to dams than in control villages (14.0 episodes/1000 child months vs. 1.9 in control villages) (92). Malaria was hypoendemic in all of the sites studied, but the risk of malaria in dam-adjacent and control populations was significantly higher at lower altitudes. Examples of increases in malaria related to development projects have been noted in other malaria endemic regions, e.g., Sri Lanka, Burundi. A recent review acknowledges the many examples of settings in which water irrigation schemes have been associated with increases in malaria, especially in areas of unstable transmission, but also notes that in areas where malaria transmission is stable, introduction of irrigation may have little impact on malaria and may lead to substantial benefits through more wealth, improved health care, and greater use of insecticide-treated bednets (93).

3.2.3. Other Consequences of Dams and Changes in Land Use

Although the impact of dams on human schistosomiasis and malaria has been repeatedly described, dams have multiple environmental and social impacts and may influence burden and types of infectious diseases in a region through several mechanisms (85,94). Populations displaced by the building of the dam (or attracted to the area because of opportunities for agricultural development) may end up in an area with different infectious disease risks. They may lack immunity to these infections; they may encounter unfamiliar risks and lack knowledge about preventive strategies. Displaced persons may live in crowded, substandard housing and may lack basic sanitation and access to clean water and a balanced, adequate diet. Migration may disrupt health care and vaccination schedules.

Other factors related to land use and agricultural practices can also influence vector populations and hence potential risk of human infection. Japanese encephalitis virus, which causes sporadic and epidemic encephalitis in Asia, is transmitted by *Culex* mosquitoes. One recent study linked increase in mosquito larvae abundance of *Culex vishnui* in dose-related way to use of inorganic fertilizers in rice fields. Use of manure and other organic fertilizers on rice fields was associated with lower levels of mosquito breeding (95).

4. SUMMARY AND PERSPECTIVES FOR THE FUTURE

As illustrated by the many examples above, infectious diseases are dynamic. The global environment to date favors the changes in old infections and the appearance and recognition of new ones. Multiple factors contribute to the emergence of infections; typically human activities, directly or indirectly, are the most potent factors driving disease emergence. The last two decades, during which HIV has spread throughout the world, and many zoononses, including Nipah encephalitis, variant Jakob Creutzfeldt disease, hemorrhagic colitis related to *E. coli* O157:H7, SARS, avian influenza H5 N1, and West Nile virus infections, have been recognized for the first time or have moved into new populations, should not be viewed as a transient period of unusual disease instability. The factors that have contributed to the appearance or increase in many infections, including microbial adaptation and change, changing environment and ecosystems, economic development and land use, human demographics and behavior, technology and industry, travel and trade, poverty and social inequality, war and famine, and breakdown of public health measures and lack of political will, as discussed in the recent report on microbial threats by the Institute of Medicine, are not likely to be reversed or changed in a substantial way in the near future (96). What has become clear is that the interconnectedness of the world today requires a global response. One source of optimism is that tools of communication and science today offer opportunities unavailable in past decades. Still, they must be harnessed and used for good. Any meaningful response must draw on knowledge from multiple disciplines. In addition, it is essential to keep a broad view and long time frame when considering potential impacts from technological interventions.

REFERENCES

1. Wilson ME. Infectious diseases: an ecological perspective. Br Med J 1995; 311:1681–1684.
2. Wilson ME. Travel and emergence of infectious diseases. Emerg Infect Dis 1995; 1:39–45.
3. Hahn BH, Shaw GM, De Cock KM, Sharp PM. AIDS as zoonoses: scientific and public health implications. Science 2000; 287:607–614.
4. Perrin L, Kaiser L, Yerly S. Travel and the spread of HIV-1 genetic variants. Lancet Infect Dis 2003; 3:22–27.
5. Moore PS, Reeves RW, Schwartz B, Gellin BG, Broome CV. Intercontinental spread of an epidemic group A *Neisseria meningitidis* strain. Lancet 1989; 2:260–263.
6. Moore PS, Hierholzer J, DeWitt W, Gouan K, Djore D, Lippeveld T, Plikaytis B, Broome DV. Respiratory viruses and mycoplasma as cofactors for epidemic group A meningococcal meningitis. J Am Med Assoc 1990; 264(10):1271–1275.
7. Centers for Disease Control and Prevention. Serogroup W-135 meningococcal disease among travelers returning from Saudi Arabia—United States, 2000. MMWR Morb Mortal Wkly Rep 2000; 49:345–346.
8. Taha MK, Achtman M, Alonso JM, Greenwood B, Ramsay M, Fox A, Gray S, Kaczmarski E. Serogroup W135 meningococcal disease in Hajj pilgrims. Lancet 2000; 356:2159.
9. Popovic T, Sacchi CT, Reeves MW, Whitney AM, Mayer LW, Noble CA, Ajello GW, Mostashari F, Bendana N, Lingappa J, Hajjeh R, Rosenstein NE. *Neisseria meningi-*

tidis serogroup W135 isolates associated with the ET-37 complex. Emerg Infect Dis 2000; 6:428–429.

10. Aguilera J-F, Perrocheau A, Meffre C, Hahne S, W135 Working Group. Outbreak of serogroup W135 meningococcal disease after the Hajj pilgrimage, Europe, 2000. Emerg Infect Dis 2002; 8(8):761–767.

11. Mayer LW, Reeves MW, Al-Hamdan N, Sacchi CT, Taha MK, Ajello GW, Roble CA, Tondella MLC, Whitney AM, Al-Mazrou Y, Al-Jefri M, Mishkhis A, Sabban S, Caugant DA, Lingappa J, Rosenstein NE, Popovic T. Outbreak of W135 meningococcal disease in 2000: not emergence of a new W135 strain but clonal expansion within the electrophoretic type-37 complex. J Infect Dis 2002; 185:1596–1605.

12. Hahne SJM, Gray SJ, Aguilera J-F, Crowcroft N, Nichols T, Kaczmarski EB, Ramsay ME. W135 meningococcal disease in England and Wales associated with Hajj 2000 and 2001. Lancet 2002; 359:582–583.

13. Wilder-Smith A, Barkham TMS, Earnest A, Paton NI. Acquisition of W135 meningococcal carriage in Hajji pilgrims and transmission to house contacts: prospective study. Br Med J 2002; 325:365–366.

14. Wilder-Smith A, Barkham TMS, Ravindran S, Earnest A, Paton NI. Persistence of W135 *Neisseria meningitidis* carriage in returning Hajj pilgrims: risk for early and late transmission to household contacts. Emerg Infect Dis 2003; 9(1):123–126.

15. Centers for Disease Control and Prevention. Risk for meningococcal disease associated with the Hajj 2001. MMWR Morb Mortal Wkly Rep 2001; 50:97–98.

16. Centers for Diseases Control and Prevention. Update: assessment of risk for meningococcal disease associated with the Hajj 2001. MMWR Morb Mortal Wkly Rep 2001:50:221–222.

17. Wilder-Smith A, Barkham TMS, Paton NI. Sustained outbreak of W135 meningococcal disease in east London, UK [Letter]. Lancet 2002; 360:644–645.

18. World Health Organization. Meningococcal vaccines: polysaccharide and polysaccharide conjugate vaccines. Wkly Epidemiol Rep 2002; 77:331–338.

19. O'Brien TF, Pla MDP, Mayer KH, Kishi H, Gilleece E, Syvanen M, Hopkins JD. Intercontinental spread of a new antibiotic resistance gene on an epidemic plasmid. Science 1985; 230:87–88.

20. Okeke IN, Edelman R. Dissemination of antibiotic-resistant bacteria across geographic borders. Clin Infect Dis 2001; 33:364–369.

21. O'Brien TF. Emergence, spread, and environmental effect of antimicrobial resistance: how use of an antimicrobial anywhere can increase resistance to any antimicrobial anywhere else. Clin Infect Dis 2002; 34(suppl 3):S78–S84.

22. Sa-Leao R, Tomasz A, Santos Sanches I, Brito-Avo A, Vilhelmsson SE, Kristinsson KG, de Lencastre H. Carriage of internationally-spread epidemic clones of *Streptococcus pneumoniae* with unusual drug resistance patterns in children attending day care centers in Lisbon, Portugal. J Infect Dis 2000; 182:1153–1160.

23. Wilson ME. The traveller and emerging infections: sentinel, courier, transmitter. J Appl Microbiol 2003; 94:1S-11S.

24. Kenyon TA, Volway SE, Khle WW, Onorato IM, Castro KG. Transmission of multidrug resistant *Mycobacterium tuberculosis* during a long airplane flight. N Engl J Med 1996; 334:933–938.

25. Moser MR, Bender TR, Margolis HS, Noble GR, Kendal AP, Ritter DG. An outbreak of influenza aboard a commercial airliner. Am J Epidemiol 1979; 110:1–6.

26. Minooee A, Richman L. Infectious diseases on cruise ships. Clin Infect Dis 1999; 29:737–744.

27. Centers for Disease Control and Prevention. Update: influenza activity—United States, 1997–1998 season. MMWR Morb Mortal Wkly Rep 1997; 46:1094–1098.

28. Centers for Disease Control and Prevention. Update: outbreak of influenza A infection: Alaska and the Yukon Territory, July–August 1998. MMWR Morb Mortal Wkly Rep 1998; 47:685–688.

29. Centers for Disease Control and Prevention. Influenza B virus outbreak on a cruise ship—northern Europe, 2000. MMWR Morb Mortal Wkly Rep 2001; 50:137–140.

30. Miller JM, Tam TW, Maloney S, Fukuda K, Cox N, Hockin J, Kertesz D, Klimov A, Cetron M. Cruise ships: high-risk passengers and the global spread of new influenza viruses. Clin Infect Dis 2000; 31:433–438.

31. Castellani Pastoris M, Monaco RL, Goldoni P, Mentore B, Balestra G, Ciceroni L, Visca P. Legionnaires' disease on a cruise ship linked to the water supply system: clinical and public health implications. Clin Infect Dis 1999; 28:33–38.

32. Centers for Disease Control and Prevention. Outbreaks of gastroenteritis associated with noroviruses on cruise ships—United States, 2002. MMWR Morb Mortal Wkly Rep 2002; 51(13):1112–1115.

33. Centers for Disease Control and Prevention. Chagas disease after organ transplantation—United States, 2001. MMWR Morb Mortal Wkly Rep 2002; 51(10);210–212.

34. Slom TJ, Cortese MM, Gerber SI, Jones RC, Holtz TH, Lopez AS, Zambrano CH, Sufit RL, Sakolvaree Y, Chaicumpa W, Herwaldt BL, Johnson S. An outbreak of eosinophilic meningitis caused by *Angiostrongylus cantonensis* in travelers returning from the Caribbean. N Engl J Med 2002; 346:668–675.

35. Lindo JF, Waugh C, Hall J, Cunningham-Myrie C, Askley D, Eberhard ML, Sullivan JJ, Bishop HS, Robinson DG, Holtz T, Robinson RD. Enzootic *Angiostrongylus cantonensis* in rats and snails after an outbreak of human eosinophilic meningitis, Jamaica. Emerg Infect Dis 2002; 8:324–326.

36. Hakanen A, Jousimies-Somer H, Siitonen A, Huovinen P, Kotilainen P. Fluoroquinolone resistance in *Campylobacter jejuni* isolates in travelers returning to Finland: association of ciprofloxacin resistance to travel destination. Emerg Infect Dis 2003; 9(2):267–270.

37. Freedman DO, Kozarsky PE, Weld LH, Cetron M. GeoSentinel: the global emerging infections sentinel network of the International Society of Travel Medicine. J Travel Med 1999; 6:94–98.

38. Wilson ME, Chen LH. Dengue in the Americas. Dengue Bull 2002; 26:44–61.

39. Halstead SB, O'Rourke EJ. Dengue viruses and mononuclear phagocytes. I. Infection enhancement by non-neutralizing antibody. J Exp Med 1977; 146:201–217.

40. Joshi V, Mourya DT, Sharma RC. Persistence of dengue-3 virus through transovarial transmission passage in successive generations of *Aedes aegypti* mosquitoes. Am J Trop Med Hyg 2002; 67(2):158–161.

41. Sudiro TM, Zivny J, Ishiko H, Green S, Vaughn D, Kalayanarooj S, Nisalah N, Normal JE, Ennis FA, Rothman AL. Analysis of plasma viral RNA levels during acute dengue virus infection using quantitative competitor reverse transcription-polymerase chain reaction. J Med Virol 2001; 63(1):29–34.

42. Chye JK, Lim CT, Ng KB, Lim JMH, George R, Lam SK. Vertical transmission of dengue. Clin Infect Dis 1997; 25:1374–1375.

43. Gubler DJ. Resurgent vector-borne diseases as a global health problem. Emerg Infect Dis 1998; 4(3):442–450.

44. de Zanotto PM, Gould EA, Gao GF, Harvey PH, Holmes EC. Population dynamics of flaviviruses revealed by molecular phylogenies. Proc Natl Acad Sci U S A 1996; 93:548–553.

45. Worobey M, Rambaut A, Holmes EC. Widespread intra-serotype recombination in natural populations of dengue virus. Proc Natl Acad Sci U S A 1999; 96:7352–7357.

46. Van der Stuyft P, Gianella A, Pirard M, Cespedes J, Lora J, Peredo C, Peligrino JL, Vorndam V, Bollaert M. Urbanisation of yellow fever in Santa Cruz, Bolivia. Lancet 1999; 353:1558–1562.

47. Monath TP. Facing up to re-emergence of urban yellow fever. Lancet 1999; 353:1541.

48. Reiter P, Lathrop S, Bunning M, Biggerstaff B, Singer D, Tiwari T, Baber L, Amador M, Thirion J, Hayes J, Seca C, Mendez J, Ramirez B, Robinson J, Rawlings J, Vorndam V, Waterman S, Gubler D, Clark G, Hayes E. Texas lifestyle limits transmission of dengue virus. Emerg Infect Dis 2003; 9:86–89.

49. Hedberg CW, MacDonald KL, Osterholm MT. Changing epidemiology of foodborne disease: a Minnesota perspective. Clin Infect Dis 1994; 18:671–682.

50. Osterholm MT. Cyclosporiasis and raspberries—lessons for the future. N Engl J Med 1997; 336(22):1597–1599.

51. Mahon BE, Ponka A, Hall WN, Komatsu K, Dietrich SE, Siitonen A, Cage G, Hayes PS, LambertFair MA, Bean NH, Griffin PM, Slutsker L. An international outbreak of *Salmonella* infections caused by alfalfa sprouts grown from contaminated seeds. J Infect Dis 1997; 175(4):876–882.

52. Herwaldt BL. *Cyclospora cayetanensis*: a review, focusing on the outbreaks of cyclosporiasis in the 1990s. Clin Infect Dis 2000; 31(4):1040–1057.

53. Herwaldt BL, Beach JM. The return of *Cyclospora* in 1997: another outbreak of cyclosporiasis in North American associated with imported raspberries. *Cyclospora* Working Group. Ann Intern Med 1999; 130(3):210–220.

54. Frost JA, McEvoy MB, Bentley CA, Andersson Y, Rowe B. An outbreak of *Shigella sonnei* infection associated with consumption of iceberg lettuce. Emerg Infect Dis 1995; 1:6–9.

55. Taylor JL, Tuttle J, Pramukul T, O'Brien K, Barrett TJ, Jolbitado B, Lim YL, Vugia D, Morris JG Jr, Rauxe RV, Dwyer DM. An outbreak of cholera in Maryland associated with imported commercial frozen fresh coconut milk. J Infect Dis 1993; 167:1330–1335.

56. Centers for Disease Control and Prevention. Hepatitis A associated with consumption of frozen strawberries—Michigan, March 1997. MMWR Morb Mortal Wkly Rep 1997; 46(13):288–295.

57. Center for Disease Control and Prevention. Public health dispatch: outbreak of tularemia among commercially distributed prairie dogs. MMWR Morb Mortal Wkly Rep 2002(31):688.

58. Daszak PA, Cunningham AA, Hyatt AD. Emerging infectious diseases of wildlife—threats to biodiversity and human health. Science 2000; 287:443–449.

58a. Centers for Disease Control and Prevention. Update: multistate outbreak of monkeypox—Illinois, Indiana, Kansas, Missouri, Ohio, and Wisconsin, 2003. MMWR Morb Mortal Wkly Rep 2003; 52(27):642–646.

59. Chang H-GH, Eidson M, Noonan-Toly C, Trimarchi CV, Rudd R, Wallace BJ, Smith PF, Morese DL. Public health impact of reemergence of rabies, New York. Emerg Infect Dis 2002; 8(9):909–913.

60. Lounibos LP. Invasions by insect vectors of human disease. Ann Rev Entomol 2002; 47:233–266.

61. Soper FL, Wilson DB. *Anopheles gambiae* in Brazil, 1930–1940. New York City: The Rockefeller Foundation, 1943.

62. Sprenger D, Wuithiranyagool T. The discovery and distribution of *Aedes albopictus* in Harris County, Texas. J Am Mosq Control Assoc 1986; 2:217–219.

63. Moore CG, Francy DB, Eliason DA, Monath TP. *Aedes albopictus* in the United States: rapid spread of a potential disease vector. J Am Mosq Control Assoc 1988; 4:356–361.

64. Moore CG, Mitchell DJ. Aedes albopictus in the United States: ten-year presence and public health implications. Emerg Infect Dis 1997; 3(3):329–334.

65. Russell RC. Survival of insects in the wheel bays of a Boeing 747B aircraft on flights between tropical and temperate airports. Bull World Health Org 1987; 65:659–662.

66. Hemingway J, Ranson H. Insecticide resistance in insect vectors of human disease. Ann Rev Entomol 2000; 45:371–391.

67. Daborn PJ, Yen JL, Bogwitz MR, Goff GL, Feil E, Jeffers S, Tiget N, Perry T, Hecket D, Batterham P, Feyereisen R, Wilson TG, ffrench-Constant RH. A single P450 allele associated with insecticide resistance in *Drosophila*. Science 2002; 297:2253–2256.

68. Denholm I, Devine GJ, Williamson MS. Insecticide resistance on the move. Science 2002; 297:2222–2223.

69. Bram RA, George JE, Reichard RE, Tabachnick WJ. Threat of foreign arthropod-borne pathogens to livestock in the United States. J Med Entomol 2002; 39:405–416.

70. Constantine DG. Geographic translocation of bats: known and potential problems. Emerg Infect Dis 2003; 9(1):17–21.

71. Ruiz GM, Rawlings TK, Dobbs FC, Drake LA, Mullady T, Huq A, Colwell RR. Invasion biology: global spread of microorganisms by ships. Nature 2000; 408:49–50.

72. Carlton JT, Geller JB. Ecological roulette: the global transport of non-indigenous marine organisms. Science 1993; 261:78–82.

73. McCarthy SA, McPhearson RM, Guarino AM. Toxigenic *Vibrio cholerae* O1 and cargo ships entering Gulf of Mexico. Lancet 1992; 339:624–625.

74. Wilson ME. Geography of infectious diseases. In: Cohen J, Powderly W, eds Infectious Diseases 2nd ed. London: Mosby International, 2004, pp. 1419–1427.

75. Schneider E, Hajjeh RA, Spiegel RA, Jibson RW, Harp EL, Marshall GA, Gunn RA, McNeil MM, Pinner RW, Baron RC, Hutwagner LC, Crump C, Kaufman L, Reef SE, Feld,man GM, Pappigianis D, Werner SB. A coccidioidomycosis outbreak following the Northridge, California, earthquake. J Am Med Assoc 1997; 277:904–908.

76. Wilson ME. Environmental change and infectious diseases. Ecosystem Health 2000; 6:7–12.

77. Wilson ME, Levins R, Spielman A (eds). Disease in evolution: global changes and emergence of infectious diseases. Ann N Y Acad Sci 1994:740:1–503.

78. Tesh RB, Jahrling PB, Salas R, Shope RE. Description of Guanarito virus (Arenaviridae: *Arenavirus*), the etiologic agent of Venezuelan hemorrhagic fever. Am J Trop Med Hyg 1994; 50:452–459.

79. Wilson ME. Prevention of tick-borne diseases. Med Clin N Am 2002; 86(2):219–238.

80. Former RTT, Alexander LE. Roads and their major ecological effects. Ann Rev Ecol Syst 1998; 29:207–231.

81. Hourdequin M. Ecological effects of roads. Conserv Biol 2000; 14:18–19.
82. Nisbett RA, Monath TP. Viral traffic, transnational companies and logging in Liberia, West Africa. Global Change Human Health 2001; 2(1):18–19.
83. Dutta P, Khan SA, Sharma CK, Doloi P, Hazarika NC, Mahanta J. Distribution of potential dengue vectors in major townships along the national highways and trunk roads of northeast India. SE Asian J Trop Med Public Health 1998; 29:173–176.
84. Peeters M, Courgnaud V, Abela B, Auzel P, Pourrut X, Bibollet-Ruche F, Loul S, Liegeois F, Butel C, Koulagna D, Mpoudi-Ngole E, Shaw GM, Shan GH. Delaporte E. Risk to human health from a plethora of simian immunodeficiency viruses in primate bushmeat. Emerg Infect Dis 2002; 8:451–457.
85. Lerer LB, Scudder T. Health impacts of large dams. Environ Impact Assess Rev 1999; 19:113–123.
86. Picquet M, Ernould JC, Vercruysse J, Southgate VR, Mbaye A, Sambou B, Niang M, Rollinson D. The epidemiology of human schistosomiasis in the Senegal river basin. Trans R Soc Trop Med Hyg 1996; 90:340–346.
87. N'Goran EK, Diabate S, Utzinger J, Sellin B. Changes in human schistosomiasis levels after the construction of two large hydroelectric dams in Central Cote d'Ivoire. Bull WHO 1997; 75:541–545.
88. Sleigh A, Jackson S. Public health and public choice: dammed off at China's Three Gorges? Lancet 1998; 351:1449–1450.
89. Xing-jian W, Sian-xiang Y, Yu-hai D, Gui-yang Y, Liu-yan C, Zheng-ming S. Impact of environmental change and schistosomiasis transmission in the middle reaches of the Yangtze River following the Three Gorges construction project. SE Asian J Trop Med Public Health 2000; 30(3):549–555.
90. Hotez PJ, Zheng F, Long-qi X, Ming-gang C, Shuhua X, Shu-xian L, Blair D, McManus DP, Davis GM. Emerging and reemerging helminthiases and the public health of China. Emerg Infect Dis 1997; 3:303–310.
91. Ofoezie IE. Human health and sustainable water resources development in Nigeria: schistosomiasis in artificial lakes. Nat Resour Forum 2002; 26:150–160.
92. Ghebreyesus, TA, Haile M, Witten KH, Getachew A, Yahannes AM, Yohannes M, Teklehaimanot HD, Lindsay SW, Byass P. Incidence of malaria among children living near dams in northern Ethiopia: community based incidence survey. Br Med J 1999; 319:663–666.
93. Ijumba JN, Lindsay SW. Impact of irrigation on malaria in Africa: paddies paradox. Med Vet Entomol 2001; 15:1–11.
94. Hunter JM. Inherited burden of disease: agricultural dams and the persistence of bloody urine (*Schistosomiasis hematobium*) in the Upper East Region of Ghana, 1959–1997. Soc Sci Med 2003; 56:219–234.
95. Sunish IP, Reuben R. Factors influencing the abundance of Japanese encephalitis vectors in ricefields in India—I. Abiotic. Med Vet Entomol 2001; 15:381–392.
96. Smolinski MS, Hamburg MA, Lederberg J (eds). Microbial Threats to Health: Emergence, Detection, and Response. Washington, DC: Institute of Medicine of the National Academies, The National Academies Press, 2003. Website: http://www.nap.edu.

3

Nipah Encephalitis

Chong-Tin Tan

Department of Medicine, University of Malaya, Kuala Lumpur, Malaysia

K. Thong Wong

Department of Pathology, University of Malaya, Kuala Lumpur, Malaysia

Kaw-Bing Chua

Ministry of Health, Kuala Lumpur, Malaysia

1. INTRODUCTION

The Nipah virus (NiV) is a novel virus that emerged to cause serious morbidity and mortality in hundreds of humans, and even more animals in Malaysia and Singapore. The vast majority of animals involved were pigs. The outbreak of human NiV infection started around September of 1998 in several pig farms just outside Ipoh, a city in the northern part of peninsular Malaysia. In this epicenter, there were about 27 patients with 15 fatalities (1).

The outbreak spread when infected pigs were unwittingly sent to other pig farms across the country, including several farms in an area about 300 km south (2). This area comprising *Sikamat, Kampung Sungai Nipah, Kampung Sawah* and *Bukit Pelanduk*, was to become the second—and most severely affected—epicenter of the outbreak. The virus was named "Nipah" after *Kampung Sungai Nipah* (Nipah river village) because patients' specimens from this village yielded the first viral isolates. It was estimated that more than 180 people were involved here (3). Later from pig farms around *Sepang* and *Sungei Buloh*, and abattoirs in neighboring Singapore, there were a handful more cases reported (3,4).

Published sources quote a prevalence in Malaysia of 265 cases of acute NiV encephalitis, the most serious form of the infection, with 105 fatalities, giving a mortality of nearly 40% (5). It was thought that these figures do not adequately describe the extent of the outbreak because it did not take into account the asymptomatic and mildly symptomatic, non-encephalitic seroconvertors that number about 89 cases (6). Although this group could arguably include endemic infections prior to the outbreak or even false-positive serology results (7), the estimated total number of infected people was thought to be closer to 354 (8).

2. EPIDEMIOLOGY

Preliminary observations by investigators into this outbreak revealed there was a link between sick pigs and their handler. This was confirmed by epidemiologic studies that demonstrated that direct contact with pigs or fresh pig products was responsible for most viral transmissions to humans (9). Among 110 NiV-infected patients studied, a significantly higher number of 59% vs. 24% of controls reported increased numbers of sick or dying pigs on farms where they worked (5). Moreover, patients were significantly more likely than controls (86% vs. 50%) to be involved with activities requiring direct contact with pigs. There were also reports of infection, albeit at a lower rate, among abattoir workers, pork sellers, and army personnel involved with culling of infected pigs (10–13).

Subsequently, a nationwide surveillance of pig farms, and culling of sick pigs stopped the outbreak in Malaysia (1). In Singapore, the banning of pig imports from Malaysia, and abattoir closure also ended the outbreak there (1,11). Possible transmission to humans from infected cats and dogs was suggested in a small number of patients (5,14).

The fact that virus could be isolated from patients' urine and tracheal secretions suggests that human-to-human transmission is possible (15). However, viral transmission to health care workers was thought to be generally low (16,17). Among 288 Malaysian health workers who were directly involved with the outbreak, only three were found to have IgG antibodies to NiV. However, IgM antibodies and serum neutralization tests were negative, so these cases were thought to represent false positives (16). Intriguingly, one of these cases is a nurse who had cared for an infected patient but remained asymptomatic. She apparently had no other activities, which could have exposed her to infection. Her brain MR scan showed many discrete lesions very similar to those seen in acute NiV encephalitis (18,19). Thus, this case provided compelling evidence that human-to-human transmission is possible albeit rare. The higher prevalence in males, especially from the Chinese ethnic group, is due to the fact that this group more than others are traditionally involved in pig farming (20).

In the early stages, endemic Japanese encephalitis (JE) was seriously considered as a likely cause of the outbreak rather than a new virus. Most patients admitted to the hospital had signs and symptoms suggestive of viral encephalitis. Other evidence that appeared to support JE as a causative agent included the apparent detection of JE antibodies in some patients, and the fact that the victims were associated with pig farming and/or live around these farms.

Nonetheless, several observations at the beginning of the outbreak in Ipoh suggested otherwise. Infection predominantly involved adults rather than children. There was a clustering of cases in members of the same household, which suggested an infection with a high attack rate in contrast to JE virus, which causes symptomatic encephalitis only in one out of 300 infected [It was shown later that more than half of patients had family members affected as well, confirming a high attack rate (20).] Moreover, many patients had previous immunization against JE (9). A high proportion of patients were in direct contact with pigs as opposed to uninfected individuals living in the same neighborhood, thus arguing against a mosquito-borne disease. Despite a massive operation to clear the affected areas of mosquitoes, infection continued unabated. Finally, there was a history of illness in the pigs belonging to affected farmers (3).

3. VIROLOGY

Analysis of the entire NiV genomic sequence established that it belongs to the family *Paramyxoviridae*, subfamily *Paramyxovirinae*, which also includes measles, mumps, and Hendra (HeV) (21–23). The total length of the NiV viral genome is 18,246 nucleotides, the largest paramyxoviral genome described so far. There is a high degree of nucleotide homology in the various genes of HeV and NiV that exceeds 70%, and a high amino acid identity of more than 80% in most genes (23). The nucleoprotein genes of HeV and NiV, for example, have a homology of 78%. On the contrary, these viruses have no more than 49% similarity to other members of the *Paramyxovirinae* subfamily (24). Thus, it was suggested that a new genus *Henipavirus* (*He*ndra + *Nipa*h) be created to accommodate these new paramyxoviruses (25,26).

Ultrastructurally, like all paramyxoviruses, NiV has a viral envelope derived from the host's cell membrane (Fig. 1). Therefore, the virus shape is pleomorphic with a variable diameter of >40 nm, and a single-fringe envelope formed by surface projections on the envelope. The helical-shaped nucleocapsid within the envelope that incorporates the viral RNA, exhibits the typical paramyxoviral "herringbone" appearance with negative staining (27).

4. ACUTE CLINICAL MANIFESTATIONS

The incubation period was thought to range from a few days to 2 weeks (20,28). A significant number of people exposed to the virus became symptomatic. The ratio of symptomatic to asymptomatic seroconvertors was estimated to be about 3:1 (14). A wide spectrum of clinical manifestations ranging from fever, headache

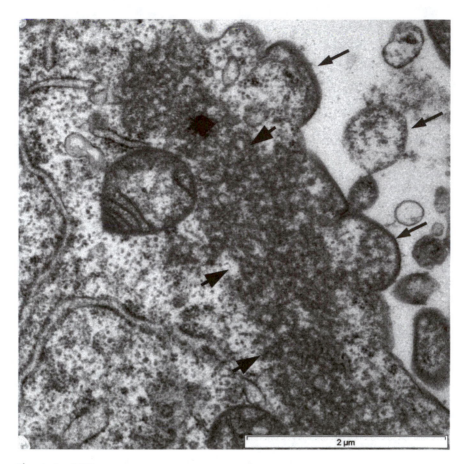

Figure 1 NiV paramyrovaus.

and drowsiness, to a severe, fatal acute encephalitic syndrome had been reported (4,9,20,28,29). The main presenting features were fever, headache, dizziness, vomiting, and reduced level of consciousness. The frequency of clinical signs based on 103 patients, the largest number of admissions to a single hospital, is shown in Table 1 (28). In this cohort, the age range was 4–75 years, with a mean of 38 years, 88% were males, and 78% were pig farmers or hired farm workers.

Distinctive clinical features were areflexia, hypotonia, and prominent autonomic changes such as tachycardia and hypertension. Segmental myoclonus was characterized by focal, rhythmic jerking of muscles, frequently involving the diaphragm and limbs (Table 1), and was more commonly associated with severe disease (20,28).

There appeared to be involvement of the respiratory tract in some patients with a range of 14–24% reported to have cough and/or abnormal chest x-rays

Table 1 Frequency of Clinical Signs in Nipah Encephalitis

Signs	%
Drowsiness	85
Confusion	69
Hyporeflexia	59
Myoclonus	54
Diaphragmatic muscle	20
Limb muscles	17
Facial muscles	3
Diaphragmatic and limbs muscles	7
Limb and facial muscles	3
Diaphragmatic and facial muscles	2
Diaphragmatic, limb and facial muscles	2
Tachycardia (heart rate >120 bpm)	53
Hypertension	52
Ptosis	30
Sweating (profuse or segmental)	27
Nystagmus	25
Hypotonia	25
Dysconjugate eye movement	16
Babinski's sign	16
Paralysis	15
Neck stiffness	12
Cranial nerve(s) palsy	9
Cerebellar signs	3

(Reprinted with permission from ASEAN Neurological Association.)

(20,28). In the Singapore series of 11 patients, three were clinically thought to have atypical pneumonia with abnormal chest x-rays (4).

5. LABORATORY INVESTIGATION FINDINGS

In more than 75% of patients, cerebrospinal fluid (CSF) was abnormal showing elevated protein levels and/or raised white cell counts on repeat examinations (20). Both protein levels and white cell counts were elevated in 39% of patients at first examination. Glucose levels were within normal limits. All these features are non-specific and could be found in many primary viral encephalitides.

IgM and IgG antibody detection in serum and CSF were critical to the diagnosis of NiV infection in many cases (1,7). These enzyme-linked immunosorbent assays (ELISA) have a high specificity, and were therefore useful for screening patients with suspected NiV infection (7). Serum neutralization tests where available was useful as a confirmatory test. For IgM, by day 4 of infection seroconversion was about 65%, by day 12 it was 100%, and it persisted for at least 3 months in most patients. For IgG, there was 100% seroconversion by day 25 of illness (30).

About 9% of patients' CSF were found to be positive for IgM to JE virus. This could reflect the endemicity of JE infection or recent immunization, rather than a dual infection. In fact, none of the autopsy brains revealed any immunohistochemical (IHC) evidence for JE (8). The breakdown in blood–brain barrier associated with disseminated vasculitis seen in NiV encephalitis may have further contributed to the significant rate of positive JE antibodies in the CSF (31).

The most common electroencephalography abnormality was continuous diffuse, symmetrical slowing with or without focal discharges. The degree of slowing correlated with severity of disease. Independent bitemporal periodic complexes were common among those deeply comatosed, and were associated with 100% mortality (32).

Blood examination in patients revealed thrombocytopenia (30–66%), leukopenia (11–60%), raised alanine (33–61%) and aspartate (42–60%) amino-transferases, but blood urea, creatinine, and electrolyte levels generally remained normal (20,28). These changes were attributed to non-specific systemic changes in very ill patients.

Virus isolation would be confirmatory of NiV infection, and many different cell cultures, including Vero cells, are susceptible to the virus. Cytopathic effects are characterized by syncytial formation as would be expected with paramyx-oviruses. Ultrastructural features such as the types and distribution of viral nucle-ocapsid aggregates, and viral envelope characteristics may help to distinguish NiV from HeV and other paramyxoviruses (27). Direct visualization by electron microscopy in negatively stained preparations of CSF specimens to detect virus was found to be useful for diagnosis but may not be able to positively confirm NiV infection (33).

6. RADIOLOGIC FINDINGS

Brain MR imaging proved to be a useful diagnostic aid in acute NiV encephali-tis (34,35). Typically, in acute NiV encephalitis the brain showed multiple, dis-seminated, small discrete hyperintense lesions, best seen in the FLAIR sequence, mainly in the subcortical and deep white matter, and occasionally in the cortex (Fig. 2). These lesions, which measured 2–7 mm were likely to be the necrotic plaques noted in postmortem tissues. Similar changes were also seen in 16% of asymptomatic patients suggesting that subclinical cerebral involvement was not uncommon in this group (18). Many months later in uncomplicated acute NiV encephalitis, these lesions were still present but may remain the same or become smaller in size (34,36). Cortical lesions may become more prominent (36).

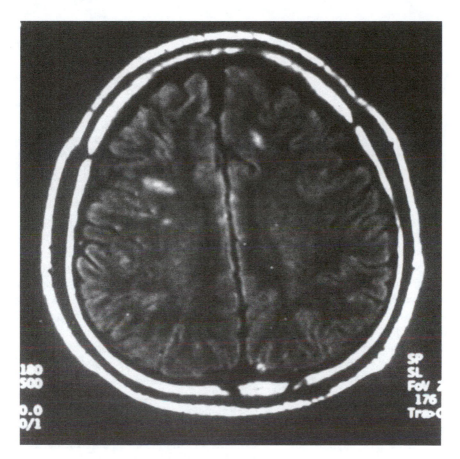

Figure 2 Brain encephalitis FLAIR sequence.

7. PATHOLOGY AND PATHOGENESIS

7.1. Pathology

The macroscopic features were generally non-specific, although occasional small lesions suggestive of necrosis may be observed in the brain. A few cases may have evidence of raised intracranial pressure but the majority did not (37). This finding correlated well with brain MR scans in which neither mass effect nor brain edema was detected in 31 patients studied (34).

7.1.1. Blood Vessels

Medium-sized to small blood vessels (both arteries and veins) in major organs, including the brain, lung and kidney, were susceptible to infection. The earliest lesion seemed to be the formation of multinucleated syncytium in the endothelium often without accompanying inflammation (Fig. 3A). These lesions were encountered in only 27% of autopsies probably because most fatal cases represented terminal stages of the disease (37). More commonly seen was true vasculitis (as opposed to perivascular cuffing) characterized by endothelial ulceration, fibrinoid necrosis, and intramural infiltration by neutrophils, macrophages and other inflammatory cells (Fig. 3B) (9,37). Vasculitis was frequently associated with thrombosis and vascular occlusion.

Staining by IHC often demonstrated the presence of viral antigens within endothelium, syncytium and smooth muscle in the tunica media (37). Furthermore, viral nucleocapsids could be identified in the endothelium by electron microscopy (24,27,37).

7.1.2. Central Nervous System

The most severely affected organ is the brain, which showed widespread vascular lesions, including in the meninges (37). Large arteries such as the middle cerebral artery, however, did not appear to be involved. Near many vasculitic vessels, with or without thrombosis, there were small areas of necrosis and ischemia called necrotic plaques (Fig. 3C). These plaques, which could be found in both the gray and white matter, were probably caused by a combination of microinfarction and direct viral infection. Neuronal infection was evidenced by cytoplasmic, and less frequently, nuclear inclusions, which were shown to comprise viral antigens (Fig. 3D) and paramyxoviral nucleocapsids (27,37). Cytoplasmic inclusions were eosinophilic, discrete, and may be multiple. Nuclear inclusions were waxy and surrounded by a thin rim of chromatin at the edge of the nuclear membrane, thus resembling other paramyxoviral inclusions. More rarely, ependyma and other glial cells may show IHC evidence of viral infection. Perivascular cuffing and neuronophagia could also be seen particularly in cases that died after more than a week of illness.

7.1.3. Other Organs

Outside the CNS, except perhaps in the liver, vasculitis and parenchymal lesions could be found in all the major organs including lung, kidney, and heart (37). Vasculitis-induced thrombosis and occlusion may result in infarction. Furthermore, parenchymal lesions in the lung, lymph node, and spleen may be associated with multinucleated giant cells possibly derived from macrophages and other cells. IHC confirmed the presence of viral antigens in most affected tissues.

7.2. Pathogenesis

After exposure to NiV possibly via the aerodigestive tract, primary viral replication was presumed to have occurred, perhaps in the lung and spleen (37). Following this, viremia must have occurred, spreading the virus systemically resulting in disseminated vasculitis, which was found in numerous organs simultaneously. Endothelium may have been a secondary viral replication site after viremia has set in. In the brain, damage to the blood–brain barrier due to vasculitis probably facilitated viral escape into the parenchyma to infect neurons. This was evident from the fact that viral antigens were usually located near vasculitis. Overall, this pattern appeared to be the same in most other organs examined. Whether or not virus can penetrate an intact vessel to cause parenchymal infection is presently unknown.

Severe and predominant CNS involvement may explain why symptomatic patients usually presented with neurologic manifestations. This combination of vasculitis-induced ischemia/microinfarction and direct neuronal infection is a unique feature of acute NiV encephalitis, and perhaps also HeV encephalitis, which is not found in other primary viral encephalitides (37).

8. TREATMENT

Ribavirin, a very broad-spectrum virustatic agent, which showed some efficacy against viruses such as respiratory syncytial virus, influenza and measles was tried empirically on NiV-infected patients (38,39). In an open-label trial of 140 patients with 54 patients as controls (patients who refused treatment or otherwise not given the drug) there were 45 deaths (32%) in the ribavirin group vs. 29 deaths (54%) in the control arm, representing a reduction in mortality of 36% (39). Although this trial was disadvantaged by the use of historical controls, it does suggest that ribavirin may be useful in the treatment of acute NiV encephalitis. There were no apparent serious side effects in this trial.

9. PROGNOSIS, SEQUELAE, AND COMPLICATIONS

Severe brain stem involvement indicated by tachycardia and abnormal doll's-eye reflex, hypertension and high fever appeared to be associated with poor prognosis (20,28). The presence of viable virus in the CSF, which could suggest high viral replication, was also associated with high mortality (40). Concomitant diabetes mellitus was also related to high mortality, probably due to immunosuppression (41).

Most surviving patients (>50%) recovered more-or-less completely with no serious sequelae (20). In one rare case, the patient recovered from a coma to be able to walk and communicate, but developed a fatal intracerebral hemorrhage shortly after.

9.1. Relapsed and Late-Onset Encephalitis

A small number of patients suffered a second or even a third neurologic episode following what appeared to be complete recovery. These relapsed NiV encephalitis patients constitute about 7.5% of the total number of survivors (6).

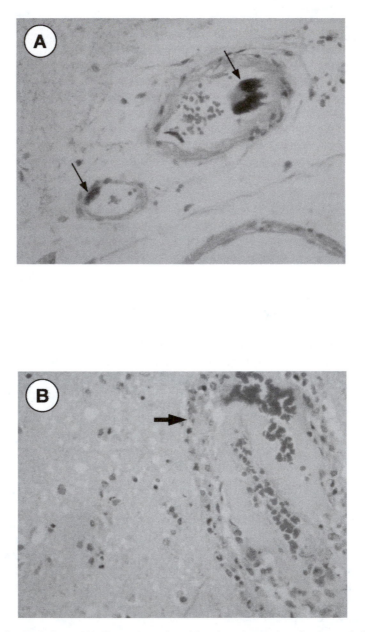

Figure 3 Pathology. (A) Formation of multinucleated synctium in the endothelium. (B) Vasculitis characterized by ulceerationn, necioses, and infiltration by neutrophils, etc. (C) Necrotic plagues. (D) Cytoplasmic and nuclear inclusions in neuronal infection.

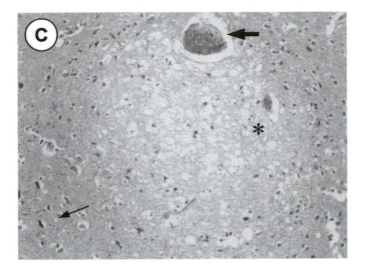

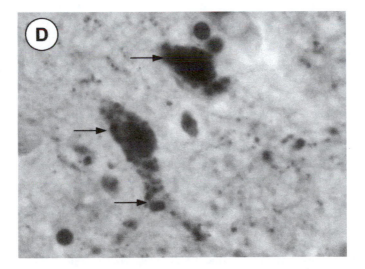

Furthermore, about 3.4% who were either asymptomatic or only had mild non-encephalitic illness initially also developed similar neurologic episodes (late-onset NiV encephalitis) for the first time after recovery from acute infection. Clinical, radiologic, and pathologic findings suggested that essentially relapsed and late-onset NiV encephalitis was the same disease process that was distinct from acute NiV encephalitis (6,34). The symptoms appeared after an average of 8.4 months following viral exposure. The common clinical features in relapsed and late-onset encephalitis were fever, headache, seizures, and focal neurological signs. There was an 18% mortality. Brain MR imaging typically showed patchy areas of confluent cortical lesions that were distinct from acute NiV encephalitis (6).

The demonstration of neuronal viral antigen in brains of fatal cases suggested that relapsed and late-onset NiV encephalitis were due to recurrent infections rather than post-infectious demyelination (6). Relapsed NiV encephalitis is probably analogous to the single human case of HeV encephalitis in which 13 months following meningitis associated with drowsiness, he developed fatal encephalitis (42). HeV antigen was demonstrated in the brain. Nonetheless, in both relapsed/late-onset NiV encephalitis and HeV encephalitis, the respective viruses have not been isolated (6,42).

Late-onset NiV encephalitis appears to resemble subacute sclerosing panencephalitis (SSPE), an infection due to measles virus, in that in both diseases the initial infection is non-encephalitic and neurologic complications appear late. However, in contrast to SSPE which is relentless, some patients with late-onset NiV encephalitis may recover, although the long-term prognosis remains to be seen (6).

The factors that determine the occurrence of relapsed and late-onset NiV encephalitis are still unknown. Possibilities include viral genomic mutations in, and alteration in host's immune response to, residual foci of viruses. In the case of SSPE, pathogenesis is associated with viral genomic mutations (43). It is well known that measles infection is associated with immunosuppression (44). Like measles, NiV could possibly also cause immune suppression but its contribution to disease severity and pathogenesis of acute and relapse/late-onset NiV encephalitis is unknown. More recent studies suggest that some NiV proteins could evade or interfere with interferon activity (45,46).

10.   INFECTION IN ANIMALS

NiV-infected pigs develop a distinctive clinical syndrome now given the name "Porcine Respiratory and Encephalitis Syndrome" or "Barking Pig Syndrome" (2). As the name suggests, pigs developed a characteristic loud barking cough, neurological signs, and fever. However, many pigs whether symptomatic or not generally recovered (2). In both natural and experimental infection, the main pathology in the pig was found in the respiratory system and meninges (47).

There was evidence of tracheitis, peri-bronchial inflammation, and pneumonia. Viral antigens could be demonstrated by IHC. These findings could explain the severe pulmonary symptoms in pigs as well as provide support for the suggestion that aerosol spread of NiV from pig to human represents an important mode of transmission.

Meningitis was characterized by edema and vasculitis. Encephalitis was rare, consisting of mild perivascular lymphocytic cuffing and glial foci. No necrotic foci similar to that in human cases were apparent. Apart from pigs, other animals including the cat, dog, and horse were reported to show evidence of infection, including systemic vasculitis (1,7,47,48).

The general absence of encephalitis and the predominant respiratory involvement in the infected pig and cat seem to indicate that these animals are probably not good animal models for the human infection. The guinea-pig should be investigated as an animal model for NiV since HeV infection of this animal by a high-dose subcutaneous route produced encephalitis (49). The golden hamster was recently investigated as a suitable model for acute NiV infection with promising results. In addition to systemic vasculitis, encephalitis was demonstrated in infected tissues (unpublished observations).

11. THE BAT AS RESERVOIR HOST: IMPLICATIONS FOR FUTURE OUTBREAKS

There is now evidence that the reservoir of NiV is most likely the fruit bat. In Tioman island off the coast of peninsular Malaysia, NiV has been isolated from urine (*Pteropus hypomelanus*) (50). Moreover, serum neutralizing antibodies were found in 4–31% of bat species, particularly *P. hypomelanus* and *P. vampyrus* (48). These may represent antibodies raised against NiV or other unidentified but related virus. There were recent reports of similar antibodies detected in *P. lylei* in Cambodia, and *Pteropus* species in Indonesia (51).

A serologic survey of Tioman island's residents living in close proximity to bat populations yielded no positive results indicating that the risk of human exposure to NiV directly from bats is low (52). Nonetheless, there should be continuing vigilance for new outbreaks of NiV infection particular in the tropics where fruits bats abound. There is a suggestion that major environmental changes may have disrupted the bat's natural habitat and feeding patterns resulting in their encroachment into fruit orchards and pig farms (53). Accidental transmission to pigs could be via half-eaten fruits dropped off by bats near farms, which were subsequently ingested by pigs. Indeed, viruses have been isolated from such fruits (50).

Forty viruses have been isolated from bat species in as many years recently. Four including NiV and HeV, were new members of the *Paramyxoviridae* family isolated from fruit bats over the last 6 years (54). One of these new paramyxoviruses, Tioman virus, found in the same bats' urine as NiV (55), causes vasculitis in mice but has so far not been known to cause human disease (unpublished observations). But the implications of novel viruses that could jump species from bats or other animals to humans to cause severe disease are immense. Questions have been raised with regard to the safety of human populations living near bat colonies, how viral transmission occurred and what factors determine it, and why these outbreaks have happened now (54).

ACKNOWLEDGMENTS

We acknowledge with gratitude the contribution and assistance from staff of the University of Malaya, Hospitals in the Ministry of Health, Centers for Disease Control and Prevention (Atlanta, Georgia, USA) in our research efforts. Some of the research findings quoted in this paper were supported in part by the Malaysian R&D grant no. 06-02-03-0743 and 06-02-03-0744.

REFERENCES

1. CDC. Update: outbreak of Nipah virus—Malaysia and Singapore, 1999. MMWR Morb Mortal Wkly Rep 1999; 48:335–337.
2. Mohd Nor MN, Gan CH, Ong BL. Nipah virus infection of pigs in peninsular Malaysia. Rev Sci Tech 2000; 19:160–165.
3. CDC. Outbreak of Hendra-like virus—Malaysia and Singapore, 1998–1999. MMWR Morb Mortal Wkly Rep 1999; 48:265–269.
4. Paton NI, Leo YS, Zaki SR, Auchus AP, Lee KE, Ling AE, Chew SK, Ang B, Rollin PE, Umapathi T, Sng I, Lee CC, Lim E, Ksiazek TG. Outbreak of Nipah-virus infection among abattoir workers in Singapore. Lancet 1999; 354:1253–1256.
5. Parashar UD, Sunn LM, Ong F, Mounts AW, Arif MT, Ksiazek TG, Kamaluddin MA, Mustafa AN, Kaur H, Ding LM, Othman G, Radzi HM, Kitsutani PT, Stockton PC, Arokiasamy J, Gary Jr HE, Anderson LJ. Case–control study of risk factors for human infection with the new zoonotic paramyxovirus, Nipah virus, during a 1998–1999 outbreak of severe encephalitis in Malaysia. J Infect Dis 2000; 181:1755–1759.
6. Tan CT, Goh KJ, Wong KT, Sarji SA, Chua KB, Chew NK, Murugasu P, Loh YL, Chong HT, Tan KS, Thayaparan T, Kumar S, Jusoh MR. Relapse and late-onset Nipah encephalitis. Ann Neurol 2002; 51:703–708.
7. Daniels P, Ksiazek TG, Eaton BT. Laboratory diagnosis of Nipah and Hendra infections. Microbes Infect 2001; 3:289–295.
8. Wong KT, Shieh WJ, Zaki SR, Tan CT. Nipah virus infection, an emerging paramyxoviral zoonosis. Springer Semin Immunopathol 2002; 24:215–228.
9. Chua KB, Goh KJ, Wong KT, Adeeba K, Tan PSK, Ksiazek TG, Zaki SR, Paul G, Lam SK, Tan CT. Fatal encephalitis due to Nipah virus among pig-farmers in Malaysia. Lancet 1999; 354:1257–1259.
10. Ali R, Mounts AW, Parashar UD, Sahani M, Lye MS, Isa MM, Balathevan K, Arif MT, Ksiazek TG. Nipah virus among military personnel involved in pig culling dur-

ing an outbreak of encephalitis in Malaysia, 1998–1999. Emerg Infect Dis 2001; 7:759–761.

11. Chew MH, Arguin PM, Shay DK, Goh KT, Rollin PE, Shieh WJ, Zaki SR, Rota PA, Ling AE, Ksiazek TG, Chew SK, Anderson LJ. Risk factors for Nipah virus infection among abattoir workers in Singapore. J Infect Dis 2000; 181:1760–1763.

12. Sahani M, Parashar U, Ali R, Das P, Lye MS, Isa MM, Arif MT, Ksiazek TG, Sivamoorthy M. Nipah virus infection among Abbatoir workers in Malaysia, 1998–1999. Int J Epidemiol 2001; 30:1017–1020.

13. Premalatha GD, Lye MS, Arokiasamy J, Parashar U, Rahmat R, Lee BY, Ksiazek TG. Assessment of Nipah virus transmission among pork sellers in Seremban, Malaysia. Southeast Asian J Trop Med Public Health 2000; 31:307–309.

14. Tan KS, Tan CT, Goh KJ. Epidemiological aspects of Nipah virus infection. Neurol J Southeast Asia 1999; 4:77–81.

15. Chua KB, Lam SK, Goh KJ, Hooi PS, Ksiazek T, Kamarulzaman A, Olson J, Tan CT. The presence of Nipah virus in respiratory secretions and urine of patients during an outbreak of Nipah virus encephalitis in Malaysia. J Infect 2001; 42:40–43.

16. Mounts AW, Kaur H, Parashar UD, Ksiazek TG, Cannon D, Arokiasamy JT, Anderson LJ, Lye MS. A cohort study of health care workers to assess nosocomial transmissibility of Nipah virus, Malaysia, 1999. J Infect Dis 2001; 183:810–813.

17. Chan KP, Rollin PE, Ksiazek TG, Leo YS, Goh KT, Paton NI, Sng EH, Ling AE. A survey of Nipah virus infection among various risk groups in Singapore. Epidemiol Infect 2002; 128:93–98.

18. Tan KS, Sarji SA, Tan CT, Abdullah BJ, Chong HT, Thayaparan T, Koh CN. Patients with asymptomatic Nipah virus infection may have abnormal cerebral MR imaging. Neurol J Southeast Asia 2000; 5:69–73.

19. Tan CT, Tan KS. Nosocomial transmissibility of Nipah virus. J Infect Dis 2001; 184:1367.

20. Goh KT, Tan CT, Chew NK, Tan PSK, Kamarulzaman A, Sarji SA, Wong KT, Abdullah BJ, Chua KB, Lam SK. Clinical features of Nipah virus encephalitis among pig farmers in Malaysia. N Engl J Med 2000; 342:1229–1235.

21. Yu M, Hansson E, Shiell B, Michalski W, Eaton BT, Wang LF. Sequence analysis of the Hendra virus nucleoprotein gene: comparison with other members of the subfamily *Paramyxovirinae*. J Gen Virol 1998; 79:1775–1780.

22. Harcourt BH, Tamin A, Halpin K, Ksiazek TG, Rollin PE, Bellini WJ, Rota PA. Molecular characterization of the polymerase gene and genomic termini of Nipah virus. Virology 2001; 287:192–201.

23. Harcourt BH, Tamin A, Ksiazek TG, Rollin PE, Anderson LJ, Bellini WJ, Rota PA. Molecular characterization of Nipah virus, a newly emergent paramyxovirus. Virology 2000; 271:334–349.

24. Chua KB, Bellini WJ, Rota PA, Harcourt BH, Tamin A, Lam SK, Ksiazek TG, Rollin PE, Zaki SR, Shieh W-J, Goldsmith CS, Gubler DJ, Roehrig JT, Eaton BT, Gould AR, Olson J, Field H, Daniels P, Ling AE, Peters CJ, Anderson LJ, Mahy BWJ, Nipah virus: a recently emergent deadly paramyxovirus. Science 2000; 288:1432–1435.

25. Wang LF, Yu M, Hansson E, Pritchard L, Shiell B, Michalski W, Eaton BT. The exceptionally large genome of Hendra virus: support for creation of a new genus within the family *Paramyxoviridae*. J Virol 2000; 74:9972–9979.

26. Wang LF, Harcourt BH, Yu M, Tamin A, Rota PA, Bellini WJ, Eaton BT. Molecular biology of Hendra and Nipah viruses. Microbes Infect 2001; 3:279–287.

27. Hyatt A, Zaki SR, Goldsmith CS, Wise TG, Hengstberger SG. Ultrastructure of Hendra virus and Nipah virus within cultured cells and host animals. Microbes Infect 2001; 3:297–306.

28. Chong HT, Kunjapan SR, Thayaparan T, Tong JMG, Petharunam V, Jusoh MR, Tan CT. Nipah encephalitis outbreak in Malaysia, clinical features in patients from Seremban. Neurol J Southeast Asia 2000; 5:61–67.

29. Lee KE, Umapathi T, Tan CB, Tjia HTL, Chua TS, Oh HML, Fock KM, Kurup A, Tan AKY, Lee WL. The neurological manifestations of Nipah virus encephalitis, a novel paramyxovirus. Ann Neurol 1999; 46:428–432.

30. Ramasundram V, Tan CT, Chua KB, Chong HT, Goh KJ, Chew NK, Tan KS, Thayaparan T, Kunjapan S, Petharunam V, Loh YL, Ksiazek TG. Kinetics of IgM and IgG seroconversion in Nipah virus infection. Neurol J Southeast Asia 2000; 5:23–28.

31. Chong HT, Tan CT, Karim N, Wong KT, Kumar S, Abdullah W, Chua KB, Lam SK, Goh KJ, Chew NK, Petharunam V, Kunjapan SR, Thayaparan T. Outbreak of Nipah encephalitis among pig-farm workers in Malaysia 1998/1999: was there any role for Japanese encephalitis? Neurol J Southeast Asia 2001; 6:129–134.

32. Chew NK, Goh KJ, Tan CT, Sarji SA, Wong KT. Electroencephalography in acute Nipah encephalitis. Neurol J Southeast Asia 1999; 4:45–51.

33. Chow VT, Tambyah PA, Yeo MW, Phoon MC, Howe J. Diagnosis of nipah virus encephalitis by electron microscopy of cerebrospinal fluid. J Clin Virol 2000; 19:143–147.

34. Sarji SA, Abdullah BJ, Goh KJ, Tan CT, Wong KT. Magnetic resonance imaging features of Nipah encephalitis. AJR Am J Roentgenol 2000; 175:437–442.

35. Lim CC, Sitoh YY, Hui F, Lee KE, Ang BS, Lim E, Lim WE, Oh HM, Tambyah PA, Wong JS, Tan CB, Chee TS. Nipah viral encephalitis or Japanese encephalitis? MR findings in a new zoonotic disease. AJNR Am J Neuroradiol 2000; 21:455–461.

36. Lim CC, Lee KE, Lee WL, Tambyah PA, Lee CC, Sitoh YY, Auchus AP, Michael Lin BK, Hui F. Nipah virus encephalitis: serial MR study of an emerging disease. Radiology 2002; 222:219–226.

37. Wong KT, Shieh WJ, Kumar S, Norain K, Abdullah W, Guarner J, Goldsmith CS, Chua KB, Lam SK, Tan CT, Goh KJ, Chong HT, Jusoh R, Rollin PE, Ksiazek TG, Zaki SR. Nipah virus infection: pathology and pathogenesis of an emerging paramyxoviral zoonosis. Am J Pathol 2002; 161:2153–2167.

38. Snell J. Ribavirin-current status of a broad spectrum antiviral agent. Expert Opin Pharmacother 2001; 2:1317–1324.

39. Chong HT, Kamarulzaman A, Tan CT, Goh KJ, Thayaparan T, Kunjapan SR, Chew NK, Chua KB, Lam SK. Treatment of acute Nipah encephalitis with ribavirin. Ann Neurol 2001; 49:810–813.

40. Chua KB, Lam SK, Tan CT, Hooi PS, Goh KJ, Chew NK, Tan KS, Kamarulzaman A, Wong KT. High mortality in Nipah encephalitis is associated with presence of virus in cerebrospinal fluid. Ann Neurol 2000; 48:802–805.

41. Chong HT, Tan CT, Goh KJ, Tan KS, Chew NK, Ramasundram V, Loh YL, Thayaparan T. Occupational exposure, age, diabetes mellitus and outcome of acute Nipah encephalitis. Neurol J Southeast Asia 2001; 6:7–11.

42. O'Sullivan JD, Allworth AM, Paterson DL, Snow TM, Boots R, Gleeson LJ, Gould AR, Hyatt AD, Bradfield J. Fatal encephalitis due to novel paramyxovirus transmitted from horses. Lancet 1997; 349:93–95.

43. Cattaneo R, Schmid A, Spielhofer P, Kaelin K, Baczko K, ter Meulen V, Pardowitz J, Flanagan S, Rima BK, Udem SA, Billeter MA. Mutated and hypermutated genes of persistent mesles viruses which caused lethal human brain diseases. Virology 1989; 173:415–425.

44. Griffin DE, Bellini WJ. Measles virus. In: Field's Virology. Fields B, et al., eds. Philadelphia: Lippincott-Raven, 1996:1267–1312.

45. Rodriguez JJ, Parisien JP, Horvath CM. Nipah virus V protein evades alpha and gamma interferons by preventing STAT1 and STAT2 activation and nuclear accumulation. J Virol 2002; 76:1476–1483.

46. Park MS, Shaw ML, Munoz-Jordan J, Cros JF, Nakaya T, Bouvier N, Palese P, Garcia-Sastre A, Basler CF. Newcastle disease virus (NDV)-based assay demonstrates interferon-antagonist activity for the NDV V protein and the Nipah virus V, W and C proteins. J Virol 2003; 77:1501–1511.

47. Hooper P, Zaki S, Daniels P, Middleton D. Comparative pathology of the diseases caused by Hendra and Nipah viruses. Microbes Infect 2001; 3:315–322.

48. Johara MY, Field H, Rashdi AM, Morissy C, van der Heide B, Rota P, Adzhar AB, White J, Daniels P, Jamaluddin A, Ksiazek TG. Nipah virus infection in bats (Order Chiroptera) in Peninsular Malaysia. Emerg Infect Dis 2001; 7:439–441.

49. Williamson MM, Hooper PT, Selleck PW, Westbury HA, Slocombe RFS. A guinea-pig model of Hendra virus encephalitis. J Comp Pathol 2001; 124:273–279.

50. Chua KB, Koh CL, Hooi PS, Wee KF, Khong JH, Chua BH, Chan YP, Lim ME, Lam SK. Isolation of Nipah virus from Malaysian island flying-foxes. Microbes Infect 2002; 4:145–151.

51. Olson JG, Rupprecht C, Rollin PE, An US, Niezgoda M, Clemins T, Walston J, Ksiazek TG. Antibodies to Nipah-like virus in bats (*Pteropus lylei*), Cambodia. Emerg Infect Dis 2002; 8:987–988.

52. Chong HT, Tan CT, Goh KJ, Lam SK, Chua KB. The risk of human Nipah virus infection directly from bats (*Pteropus hypomelanus*) is low. Neurol J Southeast Asia 2003; in press.

53. Chua KB, Chua BH, Wang CW. Anthropogenic deforestation, El Nino and the emergence of Nipah virus in Malaysia. Malaysian J Pathol 2002; 24:15–21.

54. Eaton BT. Introduction to current focus on Hendra and Nipah viruses. Microbes Infect 2001; 3:277–278.

55. Chua KB, Wang LF, Lam SK, Crameri G, Yu M, Wise T, Boyle D, Hyatt AD, Eaton BT. Tioman virus: a novel paramyxovirus isolated from fruit bats in Malaysia. Virology 2001; 283:215–219.

4

Prion Diseases and Dementia

James A. Mastrianni
The University of Chicago, Chicago, Illinois, U.S.A.

1. INTRODUCTION

The prion diseases (PrD) are a group of unusual neurodegenerative disorders that affect both humans and animals, are associated with a variety of phenotypes, and are transmissible. The earliest description of PrD was that of Creutzfeldt and then Jakob in the early 1900s (1,2) as a progressive dementia associated with gait abnormalities and extensive vacuolation and astrocytic gliosis on pathologic review of the brain. In the mid-1950s, while studying primitive cultures in the Highlands of New Guinea, Carleton Gajdusek recognized and described a disease the Fore people, living in this region, called "kuru." Sufferers of kuru developed a progressive gait ataxia, unusual behavior, and a relatively rapid progression to death. Gajdusek's studies suggested that this disease was the result of a transmissible agent carried within the brain of the affected individual that was horizontally transmitted rituals that involved cannibalism. Women and children were most affected by the disease, due likely to their greater contact with infectious tissue during both the preparation of the feast and the ritualistic ceremony. Pathologic examination of the kuru brain revealed the same pattern of vacuolation (also called spongiform change) that was observed in the disease described by Creutzfeldt and Jakob. Most importantly, however, this same pathology was astutely recognized by the veterinarian William Hadlow as the same pathology present in scrapie, a known transmissible disease of sheep associated with similar features of gait dysfunction, behavioral changes, and a rapid progression to death. It was natural to speculate that CJD (Creutzfeldt–Jakob disease) and kuru were similarly transmissible, which was confirmed in the mid-1960s (3,4). These results led to the recognition of several other transmissible spongiform encephalopathies (TSEs). Until relatively recently, the infectious agent of the TSEs was considered to be a slow virus (5), yet despite considerable effort, evidence for a virus has not materialized. Instead, a wealth of data has accumulated to implicate an abnormal isoform of the prion protein (PrP) as the etiologic agent in these diseases (6). Several years after Gajdusek received the first Nobel Prize for linking the transmissible nature of these diseases, Stanley Prusiner captured the second TSE-related Nobel Prize for his discovery of the prion, the infectious protein of PrD.

2. PRION PROTEIN

The prion protein is a cell surface glycoprotein encoded by the PrP gene (*PRNP*), located on the short arm of chromosome 20. It is abundantly expressed in neurons, but is also present in several peripheral tissues including heart, lung, and white blood cells, among others (7). In its normal state, PrP is expressed in a nonpathogenic conformation (PrP^c) and translocated to the cell surface where it is anchored to the outer membrane by a glycosylphosphatidylinositol (GPI) tail (Fig. 1). It contains two asparagine-linked glycosylation sites and a single disulfide bond. The primary function of PrP is unknown, although evidence supports several possible roles, including synapse formation (8,9), signal transduction (10), and copper delivery to cells (11–14). The underlying feature of PrD is the conversion of the primarily (α-helical, nonpathogenic PrP^c isoform to the predominantly (β-sheet, pathogenic scrapie isoform (PrP^{Sc}). Compared with PrP^c, PrP^{Sc} is insoluble in detergent solutions and is relatively resistant to protease digestion, a feature allows the detection of the abnormal protein in the brain of affected patients (Fig. 2).

How is PrP^{Sc} initially generated? While "infection" with PrP^{Sc} is often considered to be the primary method for initiation of disease, it is, in fact, the least common. Only iatrogenic CJD and variant CJD are known to occur by exogenous introduction of PrP^{Sc}, whereas the majority of human PrD cases appear to be sporadic without genetic linkage and cannot be traced to an infectious source (Fig. 3). A spontaneous conversion of PrP^c to PrP^{Sc} within the brain of a healthy individual is the most likely scenario, although the reasons for this spontaneous event have not been elucidated. It is likely that predisposing genes or environment (or even aging itself) may predispose to the conversion process. The genetic forms of PrD are well known and are most easily explained as the result of a destabilizing mutation in PrP that predisposes PrP^c to convert to PrP^{Sc}. Along the same lines, a somatic mutation has been postulated as a potential cause of sporadic PrD. Regardless of the mode, once PrP^{Sc} is generated, it acts as a conformational template that complexes with PrP^c and converts it to additional PrP^{Sc} (Fig. 4). Accumulation of PrP^{Sc} in the brain generally correlates with disease progression,

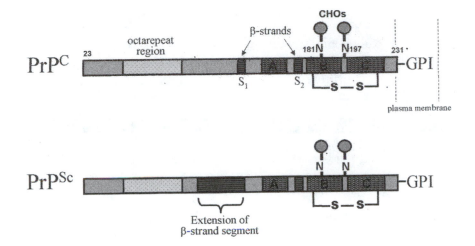

Figure 1 General organization of PrP^c and PrP^{Sc}. PrP^c is a 253 amino acid protein encoded by the *PRNP* gene on chromosome 20. The mature form of PrP^c has the first and last 22 amino acids removed in the ER during processing. Additional processing in the ER includes the attachment of a glycosylphosphatidylinositol moiety for anchoring to the membrane, glycosylation at two asparagine (N)-linked glycosylation sites, and a disulfide bridge. Three alpha-helical regions are designated A, B, and C whereas two short beta-strand segments are labeled S_1 and S_2. An octarepeat region is composed of five repeating motifs of the sequence [Pro-(His/Gln)-Gly-Gly-Gly-(-/Gly)-Trp-Gly-Gln]. Conversion of PrP^c to PrP^{Sc} results from the extension of β-strand into the region of the protein that is without obvious structure in PrP^c. This results in β-sheet formation, protein aggregation, and, presumably, the infectious property of PrP^{Sc}.

although the actual mechanism of cell death in PrD is not yet understood. As with other neurodegenerative diseases, the usual suspects of apoptosis, cellular inflammation (cytokines in particular), and oxidation, have been implicated.

3. DOPPEL, THE PRION-LIKE PROTEIN

Recent studies have identified a second gene that may be linked to PrD. Downstream from the *PRNP* gene is the prion-like protein (*PRND*) gene, so named because its gene product has over 30% homology with the C-terminal region of PrP (15). As in PrP, doppel has three (α-helices, two short β-strands, and two glycosylation sites, but rather than one, there are two disulfide bonds. Overall, the three dimensional structure of doppel (Dpl) is similar to that of PrP^c, suggesting a potential overlap of function (16). No mutations have yet been found in *PRND* that are consistently associated with human PrD, although several poly-morphisms have been identified (17,18). While no studies in humans have yet

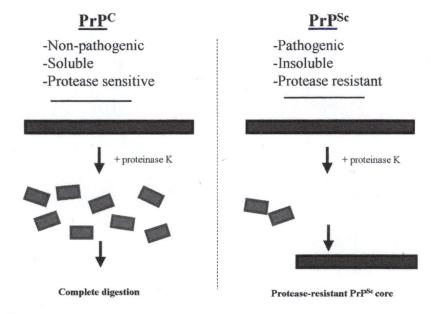

Figure 2   Comparison of the physicochemical properties of PrP^C and PrP^{Sc}. The altered conformation of PrP^{Sc} induces the protein to aggregate and develop a relative resistance to protease digestion. A protease-resistant core can be demonstrated by Western blot of brain extracts obtained from the brain of patients with PrD.

shown an upregulation of doppel in PrD, there is evidence that over-expression of doppel in transgenic mice promotes cerebellar cell death and the development of ataxia (19,20). The role of doppel as a modifier of PrD is currently under study.

4.   CLINICAL AND PATHOLOGIC SUBTYPES OF PrD

In contrast to most other neurodegenerative diseases, with the exception, perhaps, of the frontotemporal dementias (FTDs), PrD is associated with several clinico-pathologic profiles. This became obviously apparent once the *PRNP* gene was discovered and a specific antibody to PrP was generated. With the advent of these tools, several individuals originally diagnosed with Alzheimer's or other nonspecific diseases were subsequently recognized to be PrD. Additionally, the demonstration of GSS-type amyloid plaques in diseases not previously considered to be GSS, broadened the scope of that disease, in particular. These findings further emphasized that common pathologic features could be observed in diseases with quite disparate clinical presentations.

While it is clear that PrP^{Sc} is associated with a major conformational shift from α-helical to β-sheet structure, recent studies suggest that there may be sev-

Generation of PrP^Sc

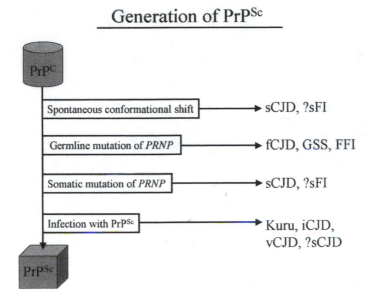

Figure 3 Several possible mechanisms may lead to the generation of PrP^Sc. The presence of a mutation of the *PRNP* gene results in mutated PrP^C that may be predisposed to the abnormal conformation by the presence of a destabilizing mutation of PRNP carried in the germline or by a somatic mutation occurring within a single neuron later in life. PrP^C may spontaneously adopt the PrP^Sc isoform by an unknown risk, which

eral conformational variants of PrP^Sc, each of which may produce a particular "strain" or phenotype of PrD (21,22). Five distinct clinicopathologic phenotypes of PrD, based in part on the clinical presentation of disease, but primarily on the brain pathology, have thus far emerged; these include (1) kuru, (2) Creutzfeldt–Jakob disease (CJD), (3) Gerstmann–Sträussler–Scheinker syndrome (GSS), (4) fatal insomnia (FI), and (5) new variant CJD (vCJD). Although kuru is no longer observed because cannibalism has ostensibly ceased, it is mentioned for its historical significance. The pathologic picture of kuru is characterized by the presence of dense-core amyloid plaques, also known as "kuru plaques," deposited primarily within the cerebellum, although they may be diffusely spread throughout the brain. GSS is also a plaque-forming disease, although the plaques in this case are typically of the multicentric type, in which an amyloid core is surrounded by smaller satellites of amyloid. Depending on the specific GSS subtype, these plaques may also be isolated to the cerebellum, cerebrum, or diffusely spread throughout both. Spongiform change is significantly less prominent in GSS than it is in CJD and kuru. CJD is typically devoid of plaques, yet replete with diffuse spongiform change. Occasionally, in perhaps less than 10% of cases, small round

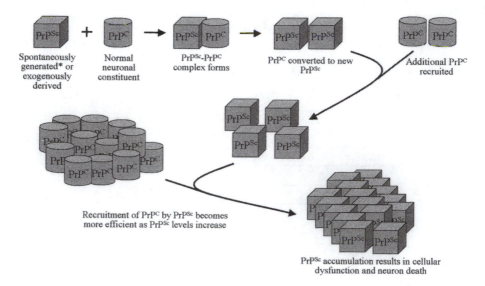

Figure 4   Once generated, PrP^{Sc} complexes with PrP^{C}, by protein–protein association, and converts it to additional PrP^{Sc}. Propagation of PrP^{Sc} may proceed geometrically because of the doubling with each conversion cycle. The actual ratio of molecular conversion is not known, although this concept helps to explain the rapid rate of neuronal death and disease progression.

kuru-type plaques may be evident on detailed inspection. Fatal insomnia was initially defined on the basis of its unique clinical phenotype and subsequently determined to be a PrD, based on genetic studies of the familial form of FI (FFI). This occurred because the pathology is uncharacteristic of PrD, consisting primarily of gliosis and neuron loss within the thalamus and brainstem, while spongiform change is minimal to absent. In recent years, a new subtype of PrD that carries a fifth pathologic variant, defined by the presence of dense-core amyloid plaque deposits surrounded by a halo of spongiform change, labeled "florid plaques" has emerged. This subtype, labeled vCJD, is unique among the PrDs, as it represents a human PrP thought to result from the ingestion of beef contaminated with bovine spongiform encephalopathy (BSE). The clinical features of the current human subtypes are detailed in the following sections.

5. CREUTZFELDT–JAKOB DISEASE

5.1. Sporadic CJD (sCJD)

The first case of CJD was described by Hans Creutzfeldt in 1921 as "spastic pseudosclerosis" (1). A year later, Alfons Jakob (2) described the "sponge-like" pathologic features in the brain of a patient that had similar clinical features as the one described by Creutzfeldt, which was fortuitous since the overall clinical features of Creutzfeldt's patient was inconsistent with CJD. Today, CJD is defined by the presence of extensive spongiform change throughout the gray matter of the cerebrum, cerebellum, and deep nuclei. CJD is by far the most common subtype of PrD. Still, the worldwide incidence of disease is only ~1 per million per year. While this reported incidence has been steady for over 25 years, its accuracy is lowered by the less than rigorous efforts to track disease occurrence prior to the emergence of vCJD in 1995. Surveillance efforts have since increased and new numbers will likely be generated.

CJD most often presents in the 6th or 7th decade, although a handful of teenagers and nonagenarians have been reported. There is no obvious gender bias, as observed in Alzheimer's disease. The "classic tetrad" of CJD includes a rapidly progressive dementia, ataxia, myoclonus, and an abnormal electroencephalogram (EEG). It should be noted, however, that a host of neurologic signs and symptoms may be present. These include, but are not limited to, diffuse and focal weakness, aphasia, painful neuropathy, choreiform movements, hallucinations, supranuclear ophthalmoplegia, cortical blindness, amyotrophy, and alien hand syndrome (23–27). Thus, while the classic tetrad represents the core features that help to establish the diagnosis of CJD, they are not the sole features observed in sCJD and, more importantly, they may not be the presenting features, making it often difficult to diagnose CJD early in the disease course. Criteria for the diagnosis of "definite," "probable," and "possible" CJD have been recently proposed by the World Health Organization (Table 1). Estimates of the sensitivity and specificity of these criteria for defining "probable CJD" have been recently reported to be approximately 65% and 95%, respectively, while inclusion of the "possible CJD" category changes these figures to 91% and 28%, respectively, suggesting that the criteria for possible CJD increases the sensitivity but reduces specificity (28). Overall, it was estimated that 12% of CJD was missed by these criteria, supporting the need for better diagnostic methods.

The most common presenting feature is cognitive decline, which occurs in about 70% of patients, either alone or in combination with ataxia, while ~25% will present only with ataxia, and a smaller percentage will develop cortical blindness, referred to as the Heidenhain variant (29). Pyramidal and extrapyramidal features may be present at onset in about 1–2% of cases, yet eventually develop in approximately 50% of patients during the course of disease. In general, most cases of CJD develop subacutely over the course of several weeks, although about 10% of cases will have a more abrupt onset that suggests encephalitis, stroke, or acute inflammatory disease of the brain. A prodromal period, characterized by vague complaints of fatigue, vertigo, headache, sleep disturbance, and anxiety, may be apparent in 25% of patients prior to the onset of clinically obvious disease. The most common feature at time of onset is memory loss or confusion. This may be evident only when the patient has to perform unfamiliar tasks or is placed in unfamiliar situations. The patient may complain of problems in concentrating, difficulty in performing calculations in the head, or

Table 1 WHO Criteria for the Diagnosis of sCJD

Definite CJD:
1. Diagnosed by standard neuropathological techniques and/or;
2. Immunocytochemically and/or Western blot confirmed protease-resistant PrP and/or
3. Presence of scrapie-associated fibrils
Probable CJD:
1. Progressive dementia, *and*;
2. At least 2 of the following four clinical features:
   a. myoclonus
   b. visual or cerebellar disturbance
   c. pyramidal/extrapyramidal signs
   d. akinetic mutism
and
3. Periodic discharges on the EEG, *and/or* a positive 14-3-3 CSF assay, and a clinical duration to death < 2 years;
4. Routine investigations should not suggest an alternative diagnosis;
Possible CJD:
1. Progressive dementia *and*;
2. At least 2 of the following four clinical features:
   a. myoclonus
   b. visual or cerebellar disturbance
   c. pyramidal/extrapyramidal signs
   d. akinetic mutism
and
3. No EEG available or atypical EEG, and;
4. Duration < 2 years

maintaining train of thought. Such vague complaints may quickly escalate to specific impairments of immediate and/or delayed recall, aphasia, constructional apraxias, and any other cortical based function, thereby mimicking the early stages of AD. These features alone may bring the patient to medical attention, although the onset of physical or behavioral symptoms often provide the greatest motive for seeking medical assistance. Ataxia commonly presents within weeks of the onset of dementia, although a delay until midway into the course of disease is not uncommon. As mentioned, about one-quarter of CJD patients present exclusively with ataxia. Gait or truncal ataxia is the most prominent feature, although appendicular ataxia may appear simultaneously or shortly follow. Other signs and symptoms of ataxia include vertigo, nystagmus, ocular dysmetria, intention tremor, and dysarthria.

Once symptoms become prominent enough to bring the patient to medical attention, the disease generally takes an accelerated course. Dementia becomes more obvious, as cortical involvement of disease expands. Examination at this time may show impairment of short- and long-term memory, difficulty with expressive and/or receptive language (dysphasia), problems with calculations (dyscalculia), difficulty in carrying out a complex motor movement (dyspraxia), or loss of the ability to write (dysgraphia). Often, the presenting feature is most obviously and severely affected by the time other features of disease appear. Because of the relatively rapid rate of progression, it is not uncommon to hear reports from family members that the patient had mild confusion and memory problems one week and by the next week was unable to recognize family members. If ataxia is present, its progression will be evident primarily by an increased frequency of falls, which eventually confines the patient to a wheel chair. Incoordination of swallowing, manifested initially as coughing during eating or drinking, may also become evident at this point, as does the risk for aspiration pneumonia, a common cause of death in these patients. Other features of disease, including pyramidal and extrapyramidal signs and symptoms, sensory changes, pseudobulbar signs, oculomotor disturbances, and a multitude of other possible neurologic features, may appear at this time, as may the loss of bowel and bladder control.

More than 75% of CJD patients will develop myoclonus, which typically appears at the mid or late stage of disease. This appears as a spontaneous or stimulus-induced irregular multifocal jerking of large muscle groups. Startle myoclonus may be induced by a loud noise, such as from clapping the hands or dropping a book on the table, or following a tactile stimulus. In some cases, this response may be so prominent that simply walking into the room, initiating speech during a quiet period, or turning on the light in a dark room may provoke the response. As with the Moro response in an infant, the CJD patient may exhibit repetitive jerking of all four limbs for several seconds after the stimulus.

In the final stage of disease, the typical picture is one of a bedridden, akinetic, and mute patient. Sleep–wake cycles may be evident and myoclonus may be prominent. Death typically results from aspiration pneumonia or urosepsis secondary to the debilitated state. Total disease duration is generally under 6 months, although less typical cases may extend beyond a year.

5.2. Laboratory Investigations for CJD

Currently, there is no single diagnostic test for CJD, although considerable effort is underway to develop a simple assay for detecting PrP^{Sc} from blood or CSF. Certain studies, however, are useful in providing support for the diagnosis of CJD. Early in the course of disease, the EEG may show nonspecific slow wave activity, but with disease progression, a characteristic pattern of periodic paroxysms of triphasic or sharp waves with a frequency of 0.5–2 Hz, against a slow background will appear (30–32) (Fig. 5). Roughly, only 70% of pathologically proven sCJD patients will demonstrate periodic sharp wave complexes (PSWCs) on the EEG, due in part to the lack of typical EEG changes in the ataxic forms of

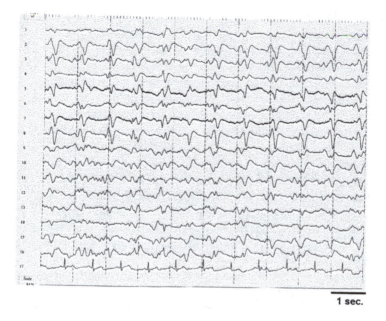

1 sec.

Figure 5   The typical pattern of periodic sharp or slow wave complexes (PSWCs) of CJD consist of triphasic type waves occurring at a regular period of every 0.5–2 sec. Initially, these may appear unilaterally or focally, then spread bilaterally. In this case, the periodic activity is primarily left sided (top half of EEG in typical "double banana" orientation), but smaller amplitude complexes are beginning to appear in the right hemisphere. This patient presented with language dysfunction early in the disease.

sCJD, but also because PSWCs may not be present in the early stage of disease and often disappear once the disease reaches the end stages, leaving a somewhat narrow window of opportunity (30,33,34). It is important, therefore, to repeat the EEG at regular intervals, perhaps weekly, to increase the capture rate, if suspicion of CJD is high.

Brain imaging with MRI is done primarily to rule out structural or vascular abnormalities as a cause for the observed clinical features. In the early stage of disease mild to moderate generalized atrophy may be present on T_1-weighted images. Early estimates suggested that in 10–15% of cases, T_2-weighted images may demonstrate hyperintensity of the basal ganglia (35–37). Recent estimates suggest that up to 80% of cases may carry this sign, although a rigorous study to determine the true sensitivity and specificity of this sign has not yet been provided. In our experience, this sign is somewhat MR-operator dependent and therefore used with caution. In contrast, diffusion-weighted MRI (DWI) promises greater sensitivity and specificity in this regard (38–42). In some reports, increased signal in DWI appeared within the cortical ribbon even prior to deep structures (43). Anatomical studies suggest that the hyperintense signal on DWI correlates with the spongiform and/or gliotic pathology of the brain (42,44). This finding has also been noted in a few cases of familial CJD (45,46) and in a single report of possible iatrogenic CJD (47). Hyperintensity of the basal ganglia and head of the caudate is most commonly observed in sCJD, while pulvinar hyperintensity may be seen in variant CJD (discussed later). PET or SPECT scanning appears to be of limited usefulness in CJD patients, as the findings show nonspecific and diffuse cortical hypoactivity that may, in some cases, show a frontal predominance (48,49). In some reports, a reduction in perfusion to specific brain regions correlated with the clinical symptoms observed in the patient (i.e., left frontal and occipital cortex hypoactivity in a patient with language and visual deficits) (50,51). Thus, in contrast to the noted utility of PET and SPECT to discriminate frontotemporal dementia from AD, there is no typical diagnostic pattern for CJD. One exception, however, is in the diagnosis of FI, which is associated with a specific reduction in activity within the thalamus (discussed later).

Because of the progressive nature of the disease and the need to rule out an active and potentially treatable CNS infection or inflammatory process, CSF examination is routinely performed as part of the evaluation. An immunologic response is not present in the CSF, although a minor elevation in protein is common. In recent years, several proteins from the CSF have been studied as markers for PrD, including S-100 (52,53), neuron specific enolase (NSE) (54,55) and the 14-3-3 protein (52,56,57), none of which are specific for CJD. The 14-3-3 protein, however, appears to have the greatest overall sensitivity and specificity as a marker for PrD, but it carries with it limitations. The 14-3-3 proteins are abundant in the nervous system and function in signal transduction, cell cycle regulation, apoptosis, and the cellular stress response (58,59). As neurons die, 14-3-3 is released from the dying neurons into the CSF where it can be detected. It is important to note that 14-3-3 is not a specific marker for PrD, but rather a marker for cell death. Because the rate of cell death associated with PrD is rapid, the 14-3-3 protein accumulates in CSF to a significant level. Sporadic CJD, which has the most rapid rate of progression, is more likely to be associated with elevated 14-3-3 protein than the slowly progressive familial forms. It should also be noted that false positive and negative results occur with the 14-3-3 test. Also, as with EEG testing, an initially negative 14-3-3 may convert to a positive result upon repeated testing. Some reports suggest the test to be 95% specific and sensitive in a well-selected population of patients with a high suspicion of PrD (52,56,57), whereas others report much lower sensitivity and specificity (60–62). Conditions that result in a high false positive rate include herpes encephalitis and hypoxic brain damage due to stroke (56,63), although elevated levels of 14-3-3 have also been reported with Hashimoto's encephalopathy (64), Alzheimer's disease (62), and multiple sclerosis (65). It has been suggested that certain isoforms of 14-3-3, in particular the γ-isoform, may be more specific for PrD (66).

A more appropriate test would be the detection of PrP^{Sc} from CSF, however, attempts to isolate measurable quantities of protease-resistant PrP^{Sc} from the CSF of patients have been unsuccessful, although PrP^c can be detected by Western blot (67). Intracerebral inoculation of CSF from patients with PrD to nonhuman primates has, however, successfully transmitted disease (68), indicating that prions are present but perhaps at levels too low to be detected by Western analysis. Methods to detect PrP^{Sc} by an ELISA-based system predicted to have higher sensitivity than Western, analysis, are currently under development.

5.3. Familial CJD

About one in every 8–10 CJD patients show an autosomal dominant pattern of inheritance due to a mutation of the *PRNP* gene. There are now over 25 mutations of the *PRNP* gene associated with PrD (Table 3 and Fig. 6). Most mutations are single base pair mismatches that induce a change in coding of a single amino acid in PrP but do not change the overall length of the protein, while a series of variable length insertions of the gene act to substantially increase the size of PrP, and two point mutations result in a foreshortened PrP, by the generation of a premature stop translation signal. Most familial forms of PrD are associated with a relatively younger age at onset compared with sCJD, with approximately 90% occurring under the age of 60 and the majority occurring under 50 years; a feature that helps to distinguish familial from sCJD, the latter presenting typically in the 60s and 70s. A further distinction is the protracted course of fCJD, which extends from about 1 to 3 years, compared with the 4–6-month duration of sCJD. This prolonged course contributes to the reduced recognition and frequent misdiagnosis of fCJD, as it may closely resemble AD or other slowly evolving dementia. It is, therefore, of critical importance to obtain a detailed family history as part of the evaluation of patients with suspected PrD. Since the onset of familial PrD occurs relatively early in life, there is likely to be evidence of other family members with a similar disease; however, because of inaccuracies in making the diagnosis, the family history may include a variety of neurological conditions, including Huntington's disease, amyotrophic lateral sclerosis, multiple sclerosis, Alzheimer's disease, and Parkinson's disease, among others. It is also important to determine if a parent died at a young age from an unrelated condition or accident, thereby masking the presence of a genetic disease in the family. There are several mutations of *PRNP* that are associated with the CJD phenotype (Table 2). Details of the specific clinical phenotypes of several of these mutations can be found elsewhere (see Ref. 69), although the E200K mutation will be discussed as an example of a point mutation, and the insertion/deletion mutations will be discussed as a group.

5.3.1. fCJD (E200K)

One of the first mutations of *PRNP* to be described, which is also the most commonly represented mutation of *PRNP* worldwide, is a coding change of glutamate (E) to lysine (K) at codon 200 (E200K) (70). Carriers of this mutation most com-

Table 2 Diagnostic Studies for Evaluation of PrD Subtypes

Disease	EEG	Neuroimaging	CSF Studies	Biopsy*
sCJD	~70% of cases have PSWCs	Non-specific atrophy; T_2 hyperintensity of basal ganglia in some; Increased signal in basal ganglia or cortex with DWI	14-3-3 positive in most cases of highly probable CJD, although not diagnostic on its own. May need to repeat to increase sensitivity. Mild, non-specific protein elevation common in all PrD	Frontal cortex shows spongiform change; Negative in tonsils and lymphoid organs
fCJD	Mutation-dependent: V2101, and E200K carriers, generally positive, most others, negative	Similar to sCJD, but may be mutation dependent	Less consistent results with fCJD, some 14-3-3 positive, most not	Mutation-dependent, but most will have positive spongiform change by frontal cortex biopsy; Studies of lymphoid tissues lacking
iCJD	Slow waves	Insufficient data	Insufficient data	—
GSS	Typically, no PSWC's	Non-specific, ?cerebellar atrophy; Insufficient data on DWI	14-3-3 typically negative	May show regional pathology, cerebellar or frontal plaque path
FI	Slow waves	PET useful—thalamic hypometabolism	Insufficient data	Minimal biopsy pathology at cortex, may therefore be unhelpful
vCJD	Slow waves	T_2 hyperintensity of pulvinar and proton-weighted; Increased signal on DWI	< 50% 14-3-3 positive	Tonsils, lymph nodes may contain protease-resistant PrP; Cerebral cortex shows florid plaque pathology

*Biopsy often reserved for younger patients and those w/o other findings consistent with PrD

monly develop a CJD-like presentation of dementia, ataxia, myoclonus, and a periodic EEG. The pathology of the brain is also characteristic of typical CJD, with diffuse vacuolation (spongiosis) of the cerebral and cerebellar cortex and deep nuclei. This mutation is most prevalent in a population of Libyan Jews now living in Israel (71). Other clusters of the E200K mutation have also been recognized in Slovakia, Morocco, and Chile (72,73). While most mutations of *PRNP* result in disease onset before age 55, carriers of the E200K mutation show an age-dependent risk to disease, with 65% of carriers affected by age 55, and nearly 100% by age 90 (74,75). Because of the late onset of disease in some carriers, death may occur from diseases of older age prior to developing CJD, accounting for the "skipped generation" observed in some families.

5.3.2. Insertions and Deletions of *PRNP*

Within the amino terminal end of PrP, from amino acid 51 to 91, there are five repeating stretches of eight amino acids each, known also as the octarepeat region. These repeats are rich in glycine, in contrast to the glutamate repeats of the trinucleotide diseases (Fig. 6). Insertions of from 1 to 9 repeats are known, most of which are associated with a fCJD phenotype, with the exception of the longest inserts of 7, 8, and 9 repeats, which are associated primarily with GSS-like pathology (76–79), although exceptions have been noted (80). Unlike the trinucleotide repeat diseases, anticipation is not observed with these repeats and the insert length is unaffected during meosis (81). Longer insertions appear to be associated with an earlier onset (30s rather than 50s) and have a more protracted course of disease than short insertions (120 vs. 5 months) (82,83). The clinical phenotype of patients carrying an insertion of *PRNP* is quite variable, but commonly presents with atypical features such as dysphasia, apraxia, and a personality disorder, and eventual development of dementia. Cerebellar ataxia, pyramidal, and extrapyramidal features are also prevalent, while myoclonus is observed in roughly half of cases, and PSWCs on the EEG are present in less than 30%. In general, focal or diffuse spongiform change is present at autopsy, but the neuropathologic features are quite variable in that some families or members within a family have little or no spongiform pathology (76,77,84). One could speculate that the long insertions allow greater flexibility of PrP that may allow for the generation of multiple conformers of PrP^{Sc}, which ultimately lead to the development of different disease phenotypes.

5.4. Laboratory Investigations for fCJD

Diagnostic testing in fCJD is less helpful than in sCJD. The EEG is less likely to show periodic discharges, although this depends partly on the associated mutation. For instance, Lanska et al. (31) reported that nearly 100% of 29 carriers of the E200K mutation studied had an EEG with PSWCs, whereas those carrying

Table 3 Mutations and Polymorphisms of PRNP

Codon Affected	Amino Acid Change	Phenotype
Disease Associated Point Mutations		
102	Pro (P) → Leu (L)	GSS
105	Pro (P) → Leu (L)	GSS
117	Ala (A) → Val (V)	GSS
131	Gly (G) → Val (V)	GSS
145	Tyr (Y) → Stop	GSS
160	Gln (Q) → Stop	GSS
178	Asp (D) → Asn (N)	CJD or FI [a]
180	Val (V) → Ile (I)	CJD
183	Thr (T) → Ala (A)	CJD/atypical
187	His (H) → Arg (R)	CJD
198	Phe (F) → Ser (S)	GSS
200	Glu (E) → Lys (K)	CJD
208	Arg (R) → His (H)	CJD
210	Val (V) → Ile (I)	CJD
211	Glu (E) → Gln (Q)	CJD
217	Gln (Q) → Arg (R)	GSS
232	Met (M) → Arg (R)	CJD/GSS
Non-disease Associated Polymorphisms		
23	Pro (P) → Ser (S)	--
129	Met (M) → Val (V)	Modifier
171	Asn (N) → Ser (S)	Schizophrenia?[b]
188	Thr (T) → Arg (R)	--
219	Glu (E) → Lys (K)	Protective?
Insertional Mutations		
* Octarepeat	- 1	normal
"	+ 1	CJD
"	+ 2	CJD
"	+ 4	CJD
"	+ 5	CJD
"	+ 6	CJD
"	+ 7	CJD
"	+ 8	GSS/HD-like
"	+ 9	GSS

*[Pro-(His/Gln)-Gly-Gly-Gly-(-/Gly)-Trp-Gly-Gln] X 5
[a]FI is seen when codon 129 is Met, and fCJD occurs when 129 is Val.
[b]Polymorphism reported in normal controls and some patients with schizophrenia.

the mutation at codon 178 have a much lower frequency. Imaging studies may also be similar to those observed with sCJD, yet positive findings may be less common. Scattered reports of CSF levels of 14-3-3 protein vary depending on the series and associated mutation (45,85–88) although, in general, it is less likely to

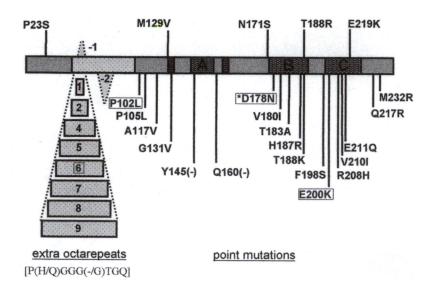

Figure 6 Mutations and polymorphisms of *PRNP*. Three major types of mutations are known: insertions that increase the length of the protein, deletions or stop mutations that shorten or truncate the protein, and point mutations that change the sequence of amino acids but do not alter the length of the mature protein. A single deletion of one octarepeat (24 base pairs, 8 amino acids) is considered a nonpathogenic polymorphism, whereas the remaining polymorphisms (denoted at the top of the gene schematic) may influence the risk to disease or the ultimate phenotype; the Ml29V polymorphism is best characterized. Debate exists about the N171S polymorphism, which has been reported in normals and some members of a family with schizophrenia. The T188R is recently reported without clear distinction as to its role in disease, and the E219K has been proposed to be protective. Numbers indicate the amino acid mutated and letters indicate the change in coding (left side of number is original coding). Boxed mutations indicate those with true linkage to disease, defined by LOD scores greater than 3.0. In most others, the number of families is too low to attain linkage, but association with disease within families is 100%. Octarepeat insertions include 1–9, except three, inserts. Letter codes are the following: A = alanine, D = aspartate, E = glutamate, F = phenylalanine, G = glycine, H = histidine, I = isoleucine, K = lysine, L = leucine, P = proline, Q = glutamine, R = arginine, S = serine, T = threonine, V = valine, Y = tyrosine, (-) = stop signal.

be positive than in sCJD. It appears that mutations associated with a phenotype that more closely resembles the rapidly progressive sCJD, such as what is seen with the E200K and V210I mutations, are more likely to feature positive results from EEG, MRI, and the 14-3-3 tests. Genetic testing for these mutations could be used as supportive evidence for fCJD, although this service is not commercially available. Only a few centers in the country perform gene sequencing on a research basis. It is important, however, not to substitute genetic testing for a complete diagnostic evaluation, to avoid missing a potentially treatable disease.

6. GERSTMANN–STRÄUSSLER–SCHEINKER SYNDROME

This subtype of PrD was initially described by Josef Gerstmann in 1928 (89) and later detailed in collaboration with Ernst Straussler and Isaak Scheinker in 1936 (90). GSS is an exclusively genetic form of PrD. Although one report suggested a sporadic form of GSS, this was later shown to be associated with a mutation of the *PRNP* gene (91,92). In fact, the analysis of families with GSS assisted in the initial linkage of *PRNP* to PrD (93,94).

GSS typically begins in the 4–6th decade, heralded by the insidious onset of cerebellar ataxia, manifest typically as unsteady gait and mild dysarthria. Psychiatric or behavioral symptoms are atypical. Neurological examination may reveal signs of pyramidal and/or extrapyramidal involvement. Cognitive dysfunction is generally not apparent early on, which attests to the cerebellar focus of this disease, although with progression, bradyphrenia, or slowness of thought processing, may be evident. Over the next 3–5 years, the disease progresses at a relatively leisurely, but relentless pace. Cerebellar dysfunction produces severe dysarthria, gait and appendicular ataxia, ocular dysmetria, and eventual dyscoordination of swallowing. Extrapyramidal involvement is common also and include bradykinesia, increased muscle tone with or without cogwheeling, and masked facies, although a rest tremor is uncommon. With continued progression of disease, cognitive decline, particularly with respect to concentration and focus, may become evident. Compared with CJD, patients with GSS will be wheel chair bound sooner and show cognitive impairment later in the course of their disease. In the terminal stage of disease, the patient becomes bedridden from the disabling ataxia, is unable to swallow because of dyscoordination, and is unable to communicate because of the profound dysarthria, yet insight into his/her condition may persist.

Ancillary studies are generally uninformative in GSS. The EEG may exhibit slow waves, but it does not demonstrate PSWCs. The number of studies regarding 14-3-3 protein in GSS are too few to report, but because of the slower rate of disease progression, it is likely that this test would not be helpful. In addition, brain imaging by MRI and especially DWI, has not been studied in detail.

A definite diagnosis of GSS is made following pathologic review of the brain. The presence of plaque deposits to which anti-PrP antibodies are immunoreactive is the defining pathologic hallmark of GSS. In general, gliosis is associated with plaques, and spongiform change is minimal compared with CJD. The plaques are PAS positive and show birefringence under polarized light following Congo red staining. Multiple plaque types have been observed, although

Pathology   **Associated Diseases**

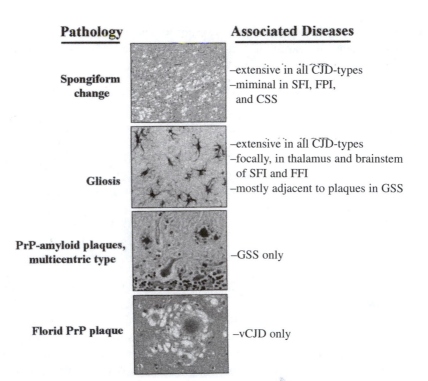

Spongiform
change

–extensive in all CJD-types
–miminal in SFI, FPI,
    and CSS

Gliosis

–extensive in all CJD-types
–focally, in thalamus and brainstem
    of SFI and FFI
–mostly adjacent to plaques in GSS

PrP-amyloid plaques,
multicentric type

–GSS only

Florid PrP plaque

–vCJD only

Figure 7   Pathologic features observed in PrD. Spongiform change and gliosis are common to several forms of PrD, whereas amyloid plaques composed of PrP are deposited in specific patterns depending on the subtype of disease. The spongiform pathology and vCJD section are hematoxylin and eosin stains. Gliosis was detected by anti-GFAP stain, and GSS plaque was demonstrated with anti-PrP antibody. (Photomicrograph of vCJD kindly provided by Dr. J.W. Ironside, University of Edinburgh.)

the most common is the multicentric plaque, which consists of a dense central amyloid core surrounded by smaller amyloid satellites (Fig. 7). In some varieties of GSS, plaques are confined primarily to the cerebellum, while in others both cerebrum and cerebellum are involved. The plaques are composed of amino and carboxy terminal truncated polypeptides spanning the region anywhere from amino acid 50 to ~150 of the PrP holoprotein (95).

The above description of GSS is most characteristic of the P102L mutation, which also happens to be the first *PRNP* mutation described (93), the most common GSS-related mutation worldwide, and the mutation carried by the family initially described by Gerstmann (96). With the development of a specific antibody to human PrP, identification of GSS plaques became easier, and in some cases, revealed that patients previously diagnosed at autopsy with AD, actually had GSS (97). The combination of antibody availability and identification of the *PRNP* gene led to the recognition of GSS-associated mutations with presentations less typical of the classic GSS description. Mutations that cosegregate with GSS (Table 1) include point mutations at codons 102, 105,117, 145,160, 198, and 217, and insertions of 7–9 repeats within the octarepeat segment of PrP.

The largest known GSS kindred carries a phenylalanine (F) to serine (S) mutation at amino acid 198 (98). The presentation in these patients is similar to that of the P102L mutation, and includes progressive ataxia, dysarthria, and mild short-term memory problems, often associated with extrapyramidal signs of bradykinesia and rigidity, and less often pyramidal tract signs. Ocular findings include supranuclear gaze palsy, jerky pursuits, and gaze-evoked nystagmus in all directions. Myoclonus is variably present. Pathologically, GSS plaques are diffusely spread throughout the cerebellum and cerebrum. In addition, -positive neurofibrillary tangles are found primarily in frontal, parahippocampal, and insular cortex, in addition to the cingulate gyrus (99). Interestingly, an asymptomatic carrier of this kindred died at 42 years of age from other causes, but was found on autopsy to have numerous PrP plaque deposits in cerebellar but not cerebral cortex, illustrating that this disease begins in the cerebellum, and pathology begins in advance of symptom onset.

An interesting point mutation associated with GSS occurs at amino acid 145 of PrP. This mutation converts a tryrosine to a stop codon, thereby resulting in the expression of PrP truncated at amino acid 145 (100). The patient reported with this mutation had a 20-year course of memory problems, leading eventually to severe dementia and death at age 59. This patient was clinically diagnosed with Alzheimer's disease prior to analysis of the *PRNP* gene. The pathology was consistent with GSS, although PrP deposits had an unusual distribution, in that they were concentrated in and around small and medium sized blood vessels, giving this disease the label of "vascular variant" (101). In addition, NFTs were evident throughout the cerebral cortex. Recently, a similar truncation mutation, with an early stop signal at 160 has been identified, the clinical features of which appeared consistent with Alzheimer's disease (personal communication, Thomas Bird, University of Washington, Seattle).

Other GSS mutations have been associated with the onset of spastic paraparesis (P105L) (102), dementia rather than ataxia as the primary feature (Al 17V) (103), and neurofibrillary tangles in addition to plaques, as in the F1985 and Q217R mutations (104).

7. FATAL INSOMNIA

Fatal insomnia was not initially considered to be a PrD. In fact, in the early descriptions of this disease, it was argued that the lack of spongiform pathology made it unlikely to be a PrD (105). Genetic analysis of families with FI, and those previously diagnosed with a disorder known as thalamic dementia were later found to carry a mutation of the *PRNP* gene that results in a change in coding from aspartate (D) to asparagine (N) at codon 178 (106–111). Interestingly, this mutation was not specifically associated with FFI, but rather fCJD with a somewhat variable phenotype. A specific genotype–phenotype correlation emerged when it was astutely observed that the polymorphic codon 129 on the same allele as the D178N mutation predicted whether the CJD or FI phenotype was present; VI29 was associated with the fCJD phenotype, while M129 was always present in FFI (112). Further, analysis of the pathogenic prion protein (PrP^{Sc}) by limited proteolysis and Western analysis of each disease indicated that the protein conformations also differ between these two diseases. There are now well over 20 kindreds identified throughout the world with FFI. Fatal insomnia is not, however, an exclusively familial disease; evidence for a sporadic form of FI was provided in 1999 with the recognition of a patient with the classic presentation of FI, characteristic pathology on autopsy, and transmission characteristics to susceptible transgenic mice, but no mutation of the *PRNP* gene (113). Additional examples of sporadic FI (sFI) followed (114), providing strong evidence for a nongenetic form of FI. Interestingly, although these patients were homozygous for Met at codon 129, the electrophoretic pattern of the protease-resistant PrP from each was comparable to that seen in FFI, suggesting that the conformation, rather than the sequence of PrP is the ultimate determinant of strain or phenotype of prion disease.

The classic phenotype of FI is fairly stereotypical. Occurring in mid life is the insidious or subacute onset of insomnia, initially manifest as a mild, then more severe, reduction in overall sleep time. When sleep is achieved, vivid dreams are common. A disturbance in autonomic function then emerges, which may manifest as elevated blood pressure, episodic hyperventilation, excessive lacrimation, sexual and urinary tract dysfunction, and/or a change in basal body temperature. Signs of brainstem involvement, such as decreased upgaze, skew deviations, abnormal saccadic movements, or dysarthric speech, may also appear in some patients. With continued progression over the next few to several months, patients will develop truncal and/or appendicular ataxia. Mental status may show reduced speed of processing, as is commonly observed in subcortical dementing states, and variable degrees of memory impairment, but compared with other more prominent features of disease, cognitive capacity is relatively spared until late in the course. Advancing disease results in progressively greater loss of total sleep time, worsening ataxia, and more profound confusion, leading ultimately to an awake but stuporous state as death approaches. As with most forms of PrD, debilitation leading to feeding difficulties and loss of airway protection is the most common immediate cause of death. The typical duration of disease is 12–16 months.

The presentation described above is striking and should be easily recognizable, however; since insomnia is common and FI is rare, it is not generally considered until obvious signs of brainstem involvement and/or ataxia develop. Further, the insomnia is not always obvious early in the disease, and may require overnight polysomnographic sleep studies to document a reduction in total sleep time. The insomnia that does develop is poorly responsive to hypnotics, although a temporary benefit may be realized initially, however, it soon becomes refractory to therapy. As with GSS, the EEG does not show PSWCs but may show diffuse slowing, and detection of the 14-3-3 protein in the CSF has not been thoroughly studied in this form of PrD. Anatomical imaging studies are generally unhelpful in the diagnosis of this PrD subtype, although PET typically shows a focal reduction in metabolic activity in the thalamus (Fig. 8). This finding may be detected early in the course and it correlates well with the underlying pathology, which is characterized by the presence of mild or absent spongiform change, but prominent neuronal dropout and astrocytic gliosis centered primarily within the thalamus and inferior olivary nucleus of the brainstem (105,115). The specificity of the pathology is remarkable in that gliosis and neuronal dropout is confined to the anteromedial and dorsolateral nuclei of the thalamus, in addition to the inferior olivary nucleus.

8. THE POLYMORPHIC CODON 129

In addition to autosomal dominant forms of familial PrD, polymorphisms of the *PRNP* gene also appear to play a role in directing the phenotype of several forms of PrD, and modifying the risk to development of disease. The polymorphic

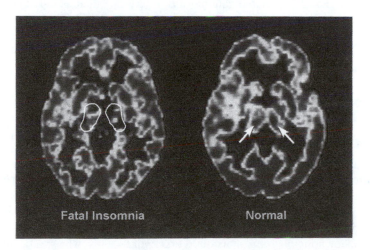

Figure 8 PET scan of FI compared with age-matched control. An early and consistent finding in FI is the reduced rate of fluorodeoxyglucose uptake within the thalami. The thalamus is the primary site of pathology in both familial and sporadic forms of FI.

codon at position 129 may be either ATG, which encodes methionine (Met) or GTG, which encodes valine (Val). In the general Caucasian population, the allelic frequency of Val is 0.34, while that of Met is 0.66, and the resulting genotype distribution is 37% Met/Met, 12% Val/Val, and 51% Met/Val. In contrast to the relatively equal proportion of heterozygous and homozygous genotypes in the normal population, several genetic surveys from the United Kingdom, France, Italy, and the United States, agree that from 80% to 90% of patients with sCJD carry the homozygous Met/Met or Val/Val state, suggesting that homozygosity is a risk factor for development of PrD (116,117). Homozygosity at codon 129 is also over-represented in patients who develop iCJD and vCJD. In fact, all vCJD cases thus far reported are homozygous for Met.

In addition to disease risk, the genotype at 129 appears also to direct the phenotype of both sporadic and familial PrD. The best demonstration of the phenotypic influence of the polymorphic 129 amino acid is in the case of the dominant D178N mutation described in the section on FFI. In other cases of familial PrD, homozygosity may reduce the age at onset of disease and shorten the course of disease (98).

In sCJD, the Met/Met genotype is more typically associated with a rapidly progressive dementia and cerebral spongiform pathology, while the Val/Val genotype is associated with hindbrain pathology and an ataxic onset. Interestingly, it was noted that gel electrophoresis of the protease-resistant PrP^{Sc} from Met/Met patients differed from Val/Val patients in that the former migrates slower through the gel than the latter. The slower migrating form is designated type 1 PrP^{Sc} and the faster, type 2. The majority of Met/Met cases carry type 1 PrP^{Sc} and the Val homozygotes carry type 2 PrP^{Sc}, while heterozygotes have a roughly equal split of type 1 and type 2. The classification of PrP^{Sc} types and their association to phenotype continue to evolve, and in the case of vCJD, issues and debates over differences in the glycosylation pattern of the protease-resistant fraction of PrP^{Sc} from these brains, adds new levels of complexity, and hopefully, improved understanding to this field.

9. ACQUIRED PrD

Acquired PrD results from the horizontal transmission of prions to humans. Kuru, which was propagated during cannibalistic rituals, is the quintessential example of acquired PrD. With the banning of cannibalistic practices, this disease has been largely eliminated, leaving two major forms of acquired PrD in humans; iatrogenic (i) CJD and new variant (v) CJD. Iatrogenic CJD, caused by the transmission of prions via contaminated biologicals, has been known for many years, and constituted the principle form of acquired PrD until recently, when vCJD, thought to originate from cattle affected by BSE took the spotlight as a major threat for spreading CJD among humans. More recently, deer and elk have been detected with a naturally occurring PrD known as chronic wasting disease (CWD) that is raising concerns about a new threat to humans.

9.1. Iatrogenic CJD

The potential for transmission of CJD via contaminated biologicals or medical instruments was initially recognized in 1974 when a recipient of a corneal transplant developed CJD, the same disease diagnosed years earlier in the donor (118). Three years later, two patients who underwent stereotaxic localization of a seizure focus with a depth electrode that was used in a CJD patient 2 months earlier, developed CJD (119). Although the electrode was subjected to standard sterilization procedures, the conditions required for inactivation of prions are much more rigorous than those required for common bacterial and viral agents. Proof that the electrode was the source of infection came from the subsequent transmission of CJD to a chimpanzee following implantation of the electrode into its cerebral cortex (120). Since these initial cases of iCJD, several others have been reported, the most onerous of which was the contamination of human growth hormone (hGH) derived from cadaveric pituitaries used to treat children with hypopituitarism and related short stature. To date, more than 130 individuals from the United States, United Kingdom, France, South America, Australia, and New Zealand have developed CJD as a result of such injections (121–125). The children that received the greatest number of injections were at greatest risk for developing CJD (126). In contrast to sCJD, patients with iCJD due to contaminated hGH typically develop cerebellar ataxia, rather than memory problems as an early feature, and the EEG shows a diffuse slow wave pattern rather than PSWCs (127). With the introduction of recombinant hGH in 1985, the rate of hGH-related iCJD has declined precipitously. However, since an incubation period of up to 30 years is possible, an occasional patient may still be present.

The second most common form of iCJD is that resulting from the use of contaminated dura mater grafts. More than 110 patients throughout the world developed iCJD after receiving dural tissue grafts originating from a single supplier in Germany whose preparative process was inadequate to eliminate prions from infected tissues (128–130). Iatrogenic CJD has also been attributed to contamination of neurosurgical instruments in five cases (131,132) and gonadotrophic hormone injections in four patients (133–135).

9.2. vCJD

In 1996, Will et al. (136) reported 10 cases of PrD with unique clinical and pathologic features that they labeled vCJD. The appearance of this new strain of PrD followed closely on the heels of an epidemic of BSE, commonly referred to as mad cow disease (137). Early speculation that vCJD was the result of BSE transmission to humans was met with resistance but eventually substantiated (138–140). Several lines of evidence now suggest that humans with vCJD were infected with BSE. The cause of the BSE epidemic appeared to result from a change in the rendering practice as a cost-cutting measure, which likely reduced the clearance of prions from offal produced from cows afflicted with the disease. When this was used in meat and bone meal (MBM) preparations that were fed to cattle, in effect as a form of cow cannibalism, the disease was spread at an alarming rate. In a move to eliminate BSE from the United Kingdom, the Ministry of Agriculture Fisheries and Food (MAFF) ordered the slaughter of 2 million cattle and banned the feeding to cattle of cattle-derived MBM.

Several features distinguish vCJD from other forms of PrD. First and foremost is the population at risk. For unclear reasons, but probably related in part to the time of exposure and host susceptibility to disease, vCJD predominantly affects teens and young adults, with an average age at onset of 29 years (range of 18–53 years) (141). It should be noted, however, that a 74-year-old man was diagnosed with vCJD, raising questions about the true extent of this disease. Second, the onset of symptoms in vCJD is commonly psychiatric or behavioral (especially depression and apathy) and, in many cases, a persistent painful sensory syndrome, rather than confusion and memory impairment. These early features may persist for several weeks or months until ataxia and then dementia emerge as prominent features. Third, the pathology of vCJD is distinct and characterized by the presence of diffusely distributed florid plaques; defined as large PrP-amyloid deposits, circumscribed by extensive vacuolation. With respect to the diagnostic work-up, the EEG is generally not periodic and the 14-3-3 test is positive in less than 50% of cases (143,144), making these studies even less useful than in sCJD. The MRI, on the other hand, appears to have some utility in the diagnosis of this form of PrD; T_2 images typically show hyperintensity of the pulvinar and proton-weighted division of the thalamus (145). This contrasts with the caudate and basal ganglia signal hypersensitivity observed in sCJD.

At the time of writing, well over 140 individuals from the United Kingdom, two from France, and one from Ireland have been diagnosed with vCJD. No cases have yet been diagnosed in the United States, with the exception of a woman in Florida who was born and raised in the United Kingdom.

While the connection of vCJD to BSE is clear, the mechanism of exposure is less clear. The time of exposure is not known, although the period of greatest risk to exposure was between 1989 and 1994, at the height of the BSE epidemic. Although the period of exposure may be estimated, history tells us that CJD can be delayed by up to 30 years following exposure, as was demonstrated with hGH-related iCJD. Because of this, it appears that we are not yet able to determine if the incidence of vCJD has peaked or it is still the beginning of a potential epidemic. Are those who have been affected by vCJD the most susceptible of the population, or the ones who received the greatest exposure? These questions are currently unanswered. In response to the BSE threat, surveillance centers in the United Kingdom have been established to better monitor the disease, and in the United States, the CDC has begun to establish voluntary reporting of PrD. BSE had not been detected in the United States, until December 2003, when a single cow in the state of Washington was detected with the disease. The cow was traced back to Canada, where BSE had been previously reported. This sentinel cow triggered a change in the standards by which cows are screened for BSE and allowed to enter the food supply. An additional threat to humans and natural wildlife is a PrD of deer and elk known as CWD.

This disease is naturally occurring in the western United States and is spreading north and south at a relatively rapid pace. The USDA has begun a screening program of animals in the wild in which those herds that are positive for CWD are culled and killed. It is not known that CWD is transmissible to humans, but prior to the emergence of vCJD, it was wrongly predicted that the risk of BSE transmission to humans was unlikely, because of a potential species barrier. While a species barrier may exist, it is not absolute.

10. DIFFERENTIAL DIAGNOSIS

It should be clear that PrD may take on several forms and presentations, some of which may still be undiscovered. Because of this, and the fact that dementia, psychiatric symptoms, and a movement disorder may occur alone or in combination, several neurodegenerative and infectious diseases should be considered at the time of presentation. These include, but are not limited to Alzheimer's disease, dementia with Lewy bodies (DLB), frontotemporal dementia (FTD), Huntington's disease (HD), and spinocerebellar ataxia (SCA). Herpes and other viral encephalitides, in addition to bacterial causes, should also be considered, although rarely does PrD present with the abrupt onset seen in these conditions. In some patients, a stroke-like onset has been repeated, but appropriate imaging studies should help to rule out a vascular etiology. A variety of other potentially treatable diseases need to be considered, including autoimmune diseases such as Hashimoto's thyroiditis and related encephalopathy, limbic encephalitis, and CNS or systemic vasculitides. A cerebellar paraneoplastic syndrome due to antibody secretion of anti-Purkinje cell antibodies (anti-Yo antibodies) from an occult lung tumor should be ruled out. The ataxia of GSS may be mistaken for multiple sclerosis or SCA, especially since this disease may affect younger patients. Toxin-related causes should be considered in the differential diagnosis, especially bismuth and lithium toxicity, both of which can induce mental status changes and cerebellar ataxia, in addition to producing an EEG that mimics the PSWCs observed in CJD. Overall, the diagnostic work-up for PrD is one of exclusion of other potentially treatable diseases. A systematic approach will generally include MRI, lumbar puncture, EEG, metabolic studies, a careful search for more common bacterial or viral pathogens, inflammatory and autoimmune panels, possibly an angiogram, and heavy metal studies.

11. THERAPY FOR PrD

Currently, there exists no treatment for prion-related diseases; management is largely symptomatic. Seizures can be treated with general anticonvulsants (diphenylhydantoin, carbamazepine), whereas myoclonus may be treated with more selective agents (clonazepam). Psychiatric symptoms are best controlled with atypical antipsychotics (risperidal, olanzepine, quietipine, etc.), although these and other behavior-modifying agents may be minimally effective.

At the time of this writing, there is an active and aggressive search underway for effective therapeutic agents. A variety of substances, including amphotericin B (146–148), dapsone (149,150), pentosan polysulfate (151–153), cyclic tetrapyrroles (154), Congo red (155–157), sulfated polyamines (115), anti-PrP antibodies (158), quinacrine, and chlorpromazine (159,160) have shown some effect. The mechanisms by which these agents inhibit prions are quite varied and not well defined, although theories include blocking the misfolding of PrP^C to PrP^{Sc}, inhibiting or disassembling PrP amyloid, sequestering PrP^C away from PrP^{Sc}, or perhaps by affecting the degradation of one or both isoforms. While many of these substances have shown promise in the inhibition of prion generation in cell culture assay systems or cell free systems, their efficacy in treating or inhibiting the onset of PrD in experimental animal models has been modest and is best demonstrated when the agent is administered just prior to inoculating the animal with prions. This feature speaks to the predicted difficulty of treatment of these diseases once symptoms have started. As such, those at risk, especially carriers of a *PRNP* mutation, would benefit most from a therapy that could be administered prophylactically far in advance of symptom onset. This finding also emphasizes the need to develop a sensitive assay with which to test patients who are potentially "incubating" prions prior to manifestation of symptoms.

REFERENCES

1. Creutzfeldt HG. Uber eine eigenartige herdformige Erkrankung des Zentralnervensystems. Z Gesamte Neurol Psychiatrie 1920; 57:1–18.
2. Jakob A. Über eine der multiplen Sklerose klinisch nahestehende Erkrankung des Zentralnervensystems (spastische Pseudosklerose) mit bemerkenswertem anatomischem Befunde. Mitteilung eines vierten Falles. Med Klin 1921; 17:372–376.

3. Gajdusek DC, Gibbs CJ Jr, Alpers M. Experimental transmission of a kuru-like syndrome to chimpanzees. Nature 1966; 209:794–796.

4. Gibbs CJ Jr, Gajdusek DC, Asher DM, Alpers MP, Beck E, Daniel PM, Matthews WB. Creutzfeldt–Jakob disease (spongiform encephalopathy): transmission to the chimpanzee. Science 1968; 161:388–389.

5. Sigurdsson B. Rida, a chronic encephalitis of sheep with general remarks on infections which develop slowly and some of their special characteristics. Br Vet J 1954; 110:341–354.

6. Prusiner SB. Prions (Les Prix nobel lecture). In: Frangsmyr T, eds. Les Prix Nobel. Stockholm, Sweden: Almqvist and Wiksell International, 1998:268–323.

7. Bendheim PE, Brown HR, Rudelli RD, Scala LJ, Goller NX, Wen GY, Kascsak RJ, Cashman NR, Bolton DC. Nearly ubiquitous tissue distribution of the scrapie agent precursor protein. Neurology 1992; 42:149–156.

8. Collinge J, Whittington MA, Sidle KC, Smith CJ, Palmer MS, Clarke AR, Jefferys JGR. Prion protein is necessary for normal synaptic function. Nature 1994; 370:295–297.

9. Whittington MA, Sidle KCL, Gowland I, Meads J, Hill AF, Pahner MS, Jefferys JGR, Collinge J. Rescue of neurophysiological phenotype seen in PrP null mice by transgene encoding human prion protein. Nat Genet 1995; 9:197–201.

10. Mouillet-Richard S, Ermonval M, Chebassier C, Laplanche JL, Lehmann S, Launay JM, Kellermann O. Signal transduction through prion protein. Science 2000; 289:1925–1928.

11. Brown DR, Qin K, Herms JW, Madlung A, Manson J, Strome R, Fraser PE, Kruck T, von Bohlen A, Schulz-Schaeffer W, Giese A, Westaway D, Kretzschmar H. The cellular prion protein binds copper in vivo. Nature 1997; 390:684–687.

12. Hornshaw MP, McDermott JR, Candy JM. Lakey JH, Copper binding to the N-terminal tandem repeat region of mammalian and avian prion protein: structural studies using synthetic peptides. Biochem Biophys Res Commun 1995; 214:993–999.

13. Pauly PC, Harris DA. Copper stimulates endocytosis of the prion protein. J Biol Chem 1998; 273:33107–33110.

14. Stockel J, Safar J, Wallace AC, Cohen FE, Prusiner SB. Prion protein selectively binds copper (U) ions. Biochemistry 1998; 37:7185–7193.

15. Moore RC, Lee IY, Silverman GL, Harrison PM, Strome R, Heinrich C, Karunaratne A, Pasternak SH, Chishti MA, Liang Y, Mastrangelo P, Wang K, Smit AF, Katamine S, Carlson GA, Cohen FE, Prusiner SB, Melton DW, Tremblay P, Hood LE, Westaway D. Ataxia in prion protein (PrP)-deficient mice is associated with upregulation of the novel PrP-like protein doppel. J Mol Biol 1999; 292:797–817.

16. Mo H, Moore RC, Cohen FE, Westaway D, Prusiner SB, Wright PE, Dyson HJ. Two different neurodegenerative diseases caused by proteins with similar structures. Proc Natl Acad Sci USA 2001; 98:2352–2357.

17. Peoc'h K, Guerin C, Brandel JP, Launay JM, Laplanche JL. First report of polymorphisms in the prion-like protein gene (PRND): implications for human prion diseases. Neurosci Lett 2000; 286:144–148.

18. Schroder B, Franz B, Hempfling P, Selbert M, Jurgens T, Kretzschmar HA, Bodemer M, Poser S, Zerr I. Polymorphisms within the prion-like protein gene

(PRND) and their implications in human prion diseases, Alzheimer's disease and other neurological disorders. Hum Genet 2001; 109:319–325.

19. Moore RC, Mastrangelo P, Bouzamondo E, Heinrich C, Legname G, Prusiner SB, Hood L, Westaway D, DeArmond SJ, Tremblay P. Doppel-induced cerebellar degeneration in transgenic mice. Proc Natl Acad Sci USA 2001; 98:15288–15293.

20. Rossi D, Cozzio A, Flechsig E, Klein MA, Rulicke T, Aguzzi A, Weissmann C. Onset of ataxia and Purkinje cell loss in PrP null mice inversely correlated with Dpl level in brain. EMBO J 2001; 20:694–702.

21. Peretz D, Scott MR, Groth D, Williamson RA, Burton DR, Cohen FE, Prusiner SB. Strain-specified relative conformational stability of the scrapie prion protein. Protein Sci 2001; 10:854–863.

22. Safar J, Wille H, Itri V, Groth D, Serban H, Torchia M, Cohen FE, Prusiner SB. Eight prion strains have PrP^{Sc} molecules with different conformations. Nat Med 1998; 4:1157–1165.

23. Brown P, Cathala F, Castaigne P, Gajdusek DC. Creutzfeldt–Jakob disease: clinical analysis of a consecutive series of 230 neuropathologically verified cases. Ann Neurol 1986; 20:597–602.

24. Kitagawa Y, Gotoh F, Koto A, Ebihara S, Okayasu H, Ishii T, Matsuyama H. Creutzfeldt–Jakob disease: a case with extensive white matter degeneration and optic atrophy. J Neurol 1983; 229:97–101.

25. MacGowan DJ, Delanty N, Petito F, Edgar M, Mastrianni J, DeArmond SJ. Isolated myoclonic alien hand as the sole presentation of pathologically established Creutzfeldt–Jakob disease: a report of two patients. J Neurol Neurosurg Psychiatry 1997; 63:404–407.

26. Salazar AM, Masters CL, Gajdusek DC, Gibbs CJ Jr. Syndromes of amyotrophic lateral sclerosis and dementia: relation to transmissible Creutzfeldt–Jakob disease. Ann Neurol 1983; 14:17–26.

27. Worrall BB, Rowland LP, Chin SSM, Mastrianni JA. Amyotrophy in prion diseases. Arch Neurol 2000; 57:33–38.

28. Brandel JP, Delasnerie-Laupretre N, Laplanche JL, Hauw JJ, Alperovitch A. Diagnosis of Creutzfeldt–Jakob disease: effect of clinical criteria on incidence estimates. Neurology 2000; 54:1095–1099.

29. Heidenhain A. Klinische und anatomische utersuchungen uber eine eigenartige erkrankung des zentralnervensystems im praesenium. Z Ges Neurol Psychiatry 1929; 118:49.

30. Chiafalo N, Fuentes AN, Galvez S. Serial EEG findings in 27 cases of Creutzfeldt–Jakob disease. Arch Neurol 1980; 37:143–145.

31. Lanska DJ. Diagnosis of Creutzfeldt–Jakob disease: effect of clinical criteria on incidence estimates. Analysis of EEG and CSF 14-3-3 proteins as aids to the diagnosis of Creutzfeldt–Jakob disease. Neurology 2001; 56:1422–1423.

32. Steinhoff BJ, Racker S, Herrendorf G, Poser S, Grosche S, Zerr I, Kretzschmar H, Weber T. Accuracy and reliability of periodic sharp wave complexes in Creutzfeldt–Jakob disease. Arch Neurol 1996; 53:162–166.

33. Kuritzky A, Davidovitch S, Sandbank U, Bechar M. Normal EEG in Creutzfeldt–Jakob disease. Neurology 1980; 30:1134–1135.

34. Lee RG, Blair RDG. Evolution of EEG and visual evoked response changes in Jakob–Creutzfeldt disease. Electroencephalogr Clin Neurophysiol 1973; 35:133–142.

35. Milton WJ, Atlas SW, Lavi E, Mollman JE. Magnetic resonance imaging of Creutzfeldt–Jakob disease. Ann Neurol 1991; 29:438–440.

36. Poser S, Mollenhauer B, Kraubeta A, Zerr I, Steinhoff BJ, Schroeter A, Finkenstaedt M, Schulz-Schaeffer WJ, Kretzschmar HA, Felgenhauer K. How to improve the clinical diagnosis of Creutzfeldt–Jakob disease. Brain 1999; 122:2345–2351.

37. Yoon SS, Chan S, Chin S, Lee K, Goodman RR. MRI of Creutzfeldt–Jakob disease: asymmetric high signal intensity of the basal ganglia. Neurology 1995; 45:1932–1933.

38. Bahn MM, Parchi P. Abnormal diffusion-weighted magnetic resonance images in Creutzfeldt–Jakob disease. Arch Neurol 1999; 56:577–583.

39. Demaerel P, Heiner L, Robberecht W, Sciot R, Wilms G. Diffusion-weighted MRI in sporadic Creutzfeldt–Jakob disease. Neurology 1999; 52:205–208.

40. Kropp S, Finkenstaedt M, Zerr I, Schroter A, Poser S. Diffusion-weighted MRI in patients with Creutzfeldt–Jakob disease. Nervenarzt 2000; 71:91–95.

41. Matoba M, Tonami H, Miyaji H, Yokota H, Yamamoto L. Creutzfeldt–Jakob disease: serial changes on diffusion-weighted MRI. J Comput Assist Tomogr 2001; 25:274–277.

42. Na DL, Suh CK, Choi SH, Moon HS, Seo DW, Kim SE, Na DG, Adair JC. Diffusion-weighted magnetic resonance imaging in probable Creutzfeldt–Jakob disease: a clinical-anatomic correlation. Arch Neurol 1999; 56:951–957.

43. Tribl GG, Strasser G, Zeitlhofer J, Asenbaum S, Jarius C, Wessely P, Prayer D. Sequential MRI in a case of Creutzfeldt–Jakob disease. Neuroradiology 2002; 44:223–226.

44. Mittal S, Farmer P, Kalina P, Kingsley PB, Halperin J. Correlation of diffusion-weighted magnetic resonance imaging with neuropathology in Creutzfeldt–Jakob disease. Arch Neurol 2002; 59:128–134.

45. Huang N, Marie SK, Kok F, Nitrini R. Familial Creutzfeldt–Jakob disease associated with a point mutation at codon 210 of the prion protein gene. Arq Neuropsiquiatr 2001; 59:932–935.

46. Nitrini R, Mendonca RA, Huang N, LeBlanc A, Livramento JA, Marie SK. Diffusion-weighted MRI in two cases of familial Creutzfeldt–Jakob disease. J Neurol Sci 2001; 184:163–167.

47. Rabinstein AA, Whiteman ML, Shebert RT. Abnormal diffusion-weighted magnetic resonance imaging in Creutzfeldt–Jakob disease following corneal transplantations. Arch Neurol 2002; 59:637–639.

48. Matsuda M, Tabata K, Hattori T, Miki J, Ikeda S. Brain SPECT with 123I-IMP for the early diagnosis of Creutzfeldt–Jakob disease. J Neurol Sci 2001; 183:5–12.

49. Watanabe N, Seto H, Shimizu M, Tanii Y, Kim YD, Shibata R, Kawaguchi M, Tsuji S, Morijiri M, Kageyama M, Wu YW, Kakishita M, Kurachi M. Brain SPECT of Creutzfeldt–Jakob disease. Clin Nucl Med 1996; 21:236–241.

50. Kirk A, Ang LC. Unilateral Creutzfeldt–Jakob disease presenting as rapidly progressive aphasia. Can J Neurol Sci 1994; 21:350–352.

51. Mathews D, Unwin DH. Quantitative cerebral blood flow imaging in a patient with the Heidenhain variant of Creutzfeldt–Jakob disease. Clin Nucl Med 2001; 26:770–773.

52. Beaudry P, Cohen P, Brandel JP, Delasnerie-Laupretre N, Richard S, Launay JM, Laplanche JL. 14-3-3 Protein, neuron-specific enolase, and S-100 protein in cere-

brospinal fluid of patients with Creutzfeldt–Jakob disease. Dement Geriatr Cogn Disord 1999; 10:40–46.

53. Otto M, Wiltfang J, Schutz E, Zerr L, Otto A, Pfahlberg A, Gefeller O, Uhr M, Giese A, Weber T, Kretzschmar HA, Poser S. Diagnosis of Creutzfeldt–Jakob disease by measurement of S100 protein in serum: prospective case–control study. BMJ 1998; 316:577–582.

54. Jimi T, Wakayama Y, Shibuya S, Nakata H, Tomaru T, Takahashi Y, Kosaka K, Asano T, Kato K. High levels of nervous system-specific proteins in cerebrospinal fluid in patients with early stage Creutzfeldt–Jakob disease. Clin Chim Acta 1992; 211:37–46.

55. Kropp S, Zerr I, Schulz-Schaeffer WJ, Riedemann C, Bodemer M, Laske C, Kretzschmar HA, Poser S. Increase of neuron-specific enolase in patients with Creutzfeldt–Jakob disease. Neurosc Lett 1999; 261:124–126.

56. Hsich G, Kenney K, Gibbs CJ, Lee KH, Harrington MG. The 14-3-3 brain protein in cerebrospinal fluid as a marker for transmissible spongiform encephalopathies. N Engl J Med 1996; 335:924–930.

57. Zerr I, Bodemer M, Gefeller O, Otto M, Poser S, Wiltfang J, Windl O, Kretzschmar HA, Weber T. Detection of 14-3-3 protein in the cerebrospinal fluid supports the diagnosis of Creutzfeldt–Jakob disease. Ann Neurol 1998; 43:32–40.

58. Aitken A, Collinge DB, van Heusden BP, Isobe T, Roseboom PH, Rosenfeld G, Soll J. 14-3-3 Proteins: a highly conserved, widespread family of eukaryotic proteins. Trends Biochem Sci 1992; 17:498–501.

59. Aitken A, Jones D, Soneji Y, Howell S. 14-3-3 Proteins: biological function and domain structure. Biochem Soc Trans 1995; 23:605–611.

60. Chapman T, McKeel DW, Morris JC. Misleading results with the 14-3-3 assay for the diagnosis of Creutzfeldt–Jakob disease. Neurology 2000; 55:1396–1397.

61. Satoh J, Kurohara K, Yukitake M, Kuroda Y. The 14-3-3 protein detectable in the cerebrospinal fluid of patients with prion-unrelated neurological diseases is expressed constitutively in neurons and glial cells in culture. Eur Neurol 1999; 41:216–225.

62. Tschampa HJ, Neumann M, Zerr I, Henkel K, Schroter A, Schulz-Schaeffer WJ, Steinhoff BJ, Kretzschmar HA, Poser S. Patients with Alzheimer's disease and dementia with Lewy bodies mistaken for Creutzfeldt–Jakob disease. J Neurol Neurosurg Psychiatry 2001; 71:33–39.

63. Lee KH, Harrington MG. Premortem diagnosis of Creutzfeldt–Jakob disease by cerebrospinal fluid analysis. Lancet 1996; 348:887.

64. Hernandez-Echebarria H, Saiz A, Grauss F, Tejada J, Garcia JM, Clavera B, Fernandez F. Detection of 14-3-3 protein in the CSF of a patient with Hashimoto's encephalopathy. Neurology 2000; 54:1539–1540.

65. Martinez-Yelamos A, Saiz A, Sanchez-Valle R, Casado V, Ramon JM, Graus F, Arbizu T. 14-3-3 Protein in the CSF as prognostic marker in early multiple sclerosis. Neurology 2001; 57:722–724.

66. Takahashi H, Iwata T, Kitagawa Y, Takahashi RH, Sato Y, Wakabayashi H, Takashima M, Kido H, Nagashima K, Kenney K, Gibbs CJ Jr, Kurata T. Increased levels of epsilon and gamma isoforms of 14-3-3 proteins in cerebrospinal fluid in patients with Creutzfeldt–Jakob disease. Clin Diagn Lab Immunol 1999; 6:983–985.

67. Wong BS, Green AJ, Li R, Xie Z, Pan T, Liu T, Chen SG, Gambetti P, Sy MS. Absence of protease-resistant prion protein in the cerebrospinal fluid of Creutzfeldt–Jakob disease. J Pathol 2001; 194:9–14.

68. Brown P, Gibbs CJ Jr, Rodgers-Johnson P, Asher DM, Sulima MP, Bacote A, Goldfarb LG, Gajdusek DC. Human spongiform encephalopathy: the National Institutes of Health series of 300 cases of experimentally transmitted disease. Ann Neurol 1994; 35:513–529.

69. Mastrianni JA. The prion diseases: Creutzfeldt–Jakob, Gerstmann–Sträussler–Scheinker, and related disorders. J Geriatr Psychiatry Neurol 1998; 11:78–97.

70. Goldfarb L, Korczyn A, Brown P, Chapman J, Gajdusek DC. Mutation in codon 200 of scrapie amyloid precursor gene linked to Creutzfeldt–Jakob disease in Sephardic Jews of Libyan and non-Libyan origin. Lancet 1990; 336:637–638.

71. Meiner Z, Gabizon R, Prusiner SB. Familial Creutzfeldt–Jakob disease—codon 200 prion disease in Libyan Jews. Medicine 1997; 76:227–237.

72. Brown P, Gálvez S, Goldfarb LG, Nieto A, Cartier L, Gibbs CJ Jr, Gajdusek DC. Familial Creutzfeldt–Jakob disease in Chile is associated with the codon 200 mutation of the PRNP amyloid precursor gene on chromosome 20. J Neurol Sci 1992; 112:65–67.

73. Goldfarb LG, Mitrova E, Brown P, Toh BH, Gajdusek DC. Mutation in codon 200 of scrapie amyloid protein gene in two clusters of Creutzfeldt–Jakob disease in Slovakia. Lancet 1990; 336:514–515.

74. Chapman J, Ben-Israel J, Goldhammer Y, Korczyn AD. The risk of developing Creutzfeldt–Jakob disease in subjects with the *PRNP* gene codon 200 point mutation. Neurology 1994; 44:1683–1686.

75. Spudich S, Mastrianni JA, Wrensch M, Gabizon R, Meiner Z, Kahana I, Rosenmann H, Kahana E, Prusiner SB. Complete penetrance of Creutzfeldt–Jakob disease in Libyan Jews carrying the E200K mutation in the prion protein gene. Mol Med 1995; 1:607–613.

76. Duchen LW, Poulter M, Harding AE. Dementia associated with a 216 base pair insertion in the prion protein gene. Clinical and neuropathological features. Brain 1993; 116:555–567.

77. Goldfarb LG, Brown P, McCombie WR, Goldgaber D, Swergold GD, Wills PR, Cervenakova L, Baron H, Gibbs CJJ, Gajdusek DC. Transmissible familial Creutzfeldt–Jakob disease associated with five, seven, and eight extra octapeptide coding repeats in the *PRNP* gene. Proc Natl Acad Sci USA 1991; 88:10926–10930.

78. Goldfarb LG, Brown P, Vrbovská A, Baron H, McCombie WR, Cathala F, Gibbs CJ Jr, Gajdusek DC. An insert mutation in the chromosome 20 amyloid precursor gene in a Gerstmann–Sträussler–Scheinker family. J Neurol Sci 1992; 111:189–194.

79. Owen F, Poulter M, Lofthouse R, Collinge J, Crow TJ, Risby D, Baker HF, Ridley RM, Hsiao K, Prusiner SB. Insertion in prion protein gene in familial Creutzfeldt–Jakob disease. Lancet 1989; 1:51–52.

80. Moore RC, Xiang F, Monaghan J, Han D, Zhang Z, Edstrom L, Anvret M, Prusiner SB. Huntington disease phenocopy is a familial prion disease. Am J Hum Genet 2001; 69:1385–1388.

81. Group THsDCR. A novel gene containing a trinucleotide repeat that is expanded and unstable on Huntingdon's disease chromosomes. Cell 1993; 72:971–983.

82. Capellari S, Vital C, Parchi P, Petersen R, Ferrer X, Jarnier D, Pegoraro E, Gambetti
     P, Julien J. Familial prion disease with a novel 144-bp insertion in the prion protein
     gene in a Basque family. Neurology 1997; 49:133–141.
83. Goldfarb LG, Cervenakova L, Brown P, Gajdusek DC. Genotype-phenotype corre-
     lations in familial spongiform encephalopathies associated with insert mutations.
     In: Court L, Dodet B, eds. Transmissible Subacute Spongiform Encephalopathies:
     Prion Diseases. Paris: Elsevier, 1996:425–431.
84. van Gool W, Hensels G, Hoogerwaard E, Wiezer J, Wesseling P, Bolhuis P.
     Hypokinesia and presenile dementia in a Dutch family with a novel insertion in the
     prion protein gene. Brain 1995; 118(Pt. 6):1565–1571.
85. Butefisch CM, Gambetti P, Cervenakova L, Park KY, Hallett M, Goldfarb LG.
     Inherited prion encephalopathy associated with the novel PRNP H187R mutation:
     a clinical study. Neurology 2000; 55:517–522.
86. Harder A, Jendroska K, Kreuz F, Wirth T, Schafranka C, Karnatz N, Theallier-Janko
     A, Dreier J, Lohan K, Emmerich D, Cervos-Navarro J, Windl O, Kretzschmar HA,
     Nurnberg P, Witkowski R. Novel twelve-generation kindred of fatal familial insom-
     nia from Germany representing the entire spectrum of disease expression. Am J
     Med Genet 1999; 87:311–316.
87. Mastrianni JA, Capellari S, Telling GC, Han D, Bosque P, Prusiner SB, DeArmond
     SJ. Inherited prion disease caused by the V210I mutation: transmission to trans-
     genic mice. Neurology 2001; 57:2198–2205.
88. Rosenmann H, Meiner Z, Kahana E, Halimi M, Lenetsky E, Abramsky O, Gabizon
     R. Detection of 14-3-3 protein in the CSF of genetic Creutzfeldt–Jakob disease.
     Neurology 1997; 49:593–595.
89. Gerstmann J. Über ein noch nicht beschriebenes Reflex—phanomen bei einer
     Erkrankung des zerebellaren Systems. Wien Med Wochenschr 1928; 78:906–908.
90. Gerstmann J, Straussler E, Scheinker L. Über eine eigenartige hereditär-familiäre
     Erkrankung des Zentralnervensystems zugleich ein Beitrag zur frage des vorzeiti-
     gen lokalen Alterns. Z Neural 1936; 154:736–762.
91. Liberski PP, Barcikowska M, Cervenakova L, Bratosiewicz J, Marczewska M,
     Brown P, Gajdusek DC. A case of sporadic Creutzfeldt–Jakob disease with a
     Gerstmann–Sträussler–Scheinker phenotype but no alterations in the PRNP gene.
     Acta Neuropathol (Berl) 1998; 96:425–430.
92. Liberski PP, Bratosiewicz J, Barcikowska M, Cervenakova L, Marczewska M,
     Brown P, Gajdusek DC. A case of sporadic Creutzfeldt–Jakob disease with a
     Gerstmann–Sträussler–Scheinker phenotype but no alterations in the PRNP gene.
     Acta Neuropathol (Berl) 2000; 100:233–234.
93. Hsiao K, Baker, HF, Crow, TJ, Poulter M, Owen F, Terwilliger, JD, Westaway D,
     Ott J, Prusiner SB. Linkage of a prion protein missense variant to
     Gerstmann–Sträussler syndrome. Nature 1989; 338:342–345.
94. Hsiao KK, Westaway DA, Prusiner SB. An amino acid substitution in the prion pro-
     tein of ataxic Gerstmann–Sträussler syndrome. Am J Hum Genet 1988; 43:A87.
95. Ghetti B, Piccardo P, Frangione B, Bugiani O, Giaccone G, Young K, Prelli F,
     Farlow MR, Dlouhy SR, Tagliavini F. Prion protein amyloidosis. Brain Pathol
     1996; 6:127–145.
96. Kretzschmar, HA, Honold G, Seitelberger F, Feucht M, Wessely P, Mehraein P,
     Budka H. Prion protein mutation in family first reported by Gerstmann, Sträussler,
     and Scheinker. Lancet 1991; 337:1160.

97. Heston LL, Lowther DLW, Leventhal CM. Alzheimer's disease: a family study. Arch Neurol 1966; 15:225–233.

98. Dlouhy SR, Hsiao K, Farlow MR, Foroud T, Conneally PM, Johnson P, Prusiner SB, Hodes ME, Ghetti B. Linkage of the Indiana kindred of Gerstmann–Sträussler–Scheinker disease to the prion protein gene. Nat Genet 1992; 1:64–67.

99. Ghetti B, Tagliavini F, Hsiao K, Dlouhy SR, Yee RD, Giaccone G, Conneally PM, Hodes ME, Bugiani O, Prusiner SB, Frangione B, Farlow MR. Indiana variant of Gerstmann–Sträussler–Scheinker disease. In: Prusiner SB, Collinge J, Powell J, Anderton B, eds. Prion Diseases of Humans and Animals. London: Ellis Horwood, 1992:154–167.

100. Kitamoto T, Iizuka R, Tateishi J. An amber mutation of prion protein in Gerstmann–Sträussler syndrome with mutant PrP plaques. Biochem Biophys Res Coramun 1993; 192:525–531.

101. Ghetti B, Piccardo P, Spillantini MG, Ichimiya Y, Porro M, Perini F, Kitamoto T, Tateishi J, Seiler C, Frangione B, Bugiani O, Giaccone G, Prelli F, Goedert M, Dlouhy SR, Tagliavini F. Vascular variant of prion protein cerebral amyloidosis with -positive neurofibrillary tangles: the phenotype of the stop codon 145 mutation in *PRNP*. Proc Natl Acad Sci USA 1996; 93:744–748.

102. Kitamoto T, Amano N, Terao Y, Nakazato Y, Isshiki T, Mizutani T, Tateishi J. A new inherited prion disease (PrP-P105L mutation) showing spastic paraparesis. Ann Neurol 1993; 34:808–813.

103. Hsiao KK, Cass C, Schellenberg GD, Bird T, Devine-Gage E, Wisniewski H, Prusiner SB. A prion protein variant in a family with the telencephalic form of Gerstmann–Sträussler–Scheinker syndrome. Neurology 1991; 41:681–684.

104. Hsiao K, Dlouhy S, Farlow, MR, Cass C, Da Costa M, Conneally M, Hodes ME, Ghetti B, Prusiner SB. Mutant prion proteins in Gerstmann–Sträussler–Scheinker disease with neurofibrillary tangles. Nat Genet 1992; 1:68–71.

105. Lugaresi E, Medori R, Montagna P, Baruzzi A, Cortelli P, Lugaresi A, Tinuper P, Zucconi M, Gambetti P. Fatal familial insomnia and dysautonomia with selective degeneration of thalamic nuclei. N Engl J Med 1986; 315:997–1003.

106. Brown P, Goldfarb LG, Kovanen J, Haltia M, Cathala F, Sulima M, Gibbs CJ Jr, Gajdusek DC Phenotypic characteristics of familial Creutzfeldt–Jakob disease associated with the codon 178[Asn] *PRNP* mutation. Ann Neurol 1992; 31:282–285.

107. Goldfarb LG, Brown P, Haltia M, Cathala F, McCombie WR, Kovanen J, Cervenakova L, Goldin L, Nieto A, Godec, MS, Asher DM, Gajdusek DC. Creutzfeldt–Jakob disease cosegregates with the codon 178[Asn] *PRNP* mutation in families of European origin. Ann Neurol 1992; 31:274–281.

108. Goldfarb LG, Haltia M, Brown P, Nieto A, Kovanen J, McCombie WR, Trapp S, Gajdusek DC. New mutation in scrapie amyloid precursor gene (at codon 178) in Finnish Creutzfeldt–Jakob kindred. Lancet 1991; 337:425.

109. Medori R, Montagna P, Tritschler HJ, LeBIanc A, Cortelli P, Tinuper P, Lugaresi E, Gambetti P. Fatal familial insomnia: a second kindred with mutation of prion protein gene at codon 178. Neurology 1992; 42:669–670.

110. Medori R, Tritschler H-J, LeBIanc A, Villare F, Manetto V, Chen HY, Xue R, Leal S, Montagna P, Cortelli P, Tinuper P, Avoni P, Mochi M, Baruzzi A, Hauw JJ, Ott J, Lugaresi E, Autilio-Gambetti L, Gambetti P. Fatal familial insomnia, a prion dis-

ease with a mutation at codon 178 of the prion protein gene. N Engl J Med 1992; 326:444–449.

111.   Petersen RB, Tabaton M, Berg L, Schrank B, Torack RM, Leal S, Julien J, Vital C, Deleplanque B, Pendlebury WW, Drachman D, Smith TW, Martin JJ, Oda M, Montagna P, Ott J, Autilio-Gambetti L, Lugaresi E, Gambetti P. Analysis of the prion protein gene in thalamic dementia. Neurology 1992; 42:1859–1863.

112.   Goldfarb LG, Petersen RB, Tabaton M, Brown P, LeBlanc AC, Montagna P, Cortelli P, Julien J, Vital C, Pendelbury WW, Haltia M, Wills PR, Hauw JJ, McKeever PE, Monari L, Schrank B, Swergold GD, Autilio-Gambetti L, Gajdusek DC, Lugaresi E, Gambetti P. Fatal familial insomnia and familial Creutzfeldt–Jakob disease: disease phenotype determined by a DNA polymorphism. Science 1992; 258:806–808.

113.   Mastrianni JA, Nixon R, Layzer R, Telling GC, Han D, DeArmond SJ, Prusiner SB. Prion protein conformation in a patient with sporadic fatal insomnia. N Engl J Med 1999; 340(21):1630–1638.

114.   Parchi P, Capellari S, Chin S, Schwarz HB, Schecter NP, Butts JD, Hudkins P, Burns DK, Powers JM, Gambetti P. A subtype of sporadic prion disease mimicking fatal familial insomnia. Neurology 1999; 52:1757–1763.

115.   Gambetti P, Medori R, Manetto V, Petersen R, LeBlanc A, Tritschler HJ, Monari L, Tabaton M, Autilio-Gambetti L. Fatal familial insomnia: a prion disease with distinctive histopathological and genotype features. In: Guilleminault C, Lugaresi E, Montagna P, Gambetti P, eds. Fatal Familial Insomnia: Inherited Prion Diseases, Sleep, and the Thalamus. New York: Raven Press, 1994:27–32.

116.   Owen F, Poulter M, Shah T, Collinge J, Lofthouse R, Baker H, Ridley R, McVey J, Crow T. An in-frame insertion in the prion protein gene in familial Creutzfeldt–Jakob disease. Mol Brain Res 1990; 7:273–276.

117.   Palmer MS, Dryden AJ, Hughes JT, Collinge J. Homozygous prion protein genotype predisposes to sporadic Creutzfeldt–Jakob disease. Nature 1991; 352:340–342.

118.   Duffy P, Wolf J, Collins G, Devoe A, Streeten B, Cowen D. Possible person to person transmission of Creutzfeldt–Jakob disease. N Engl J Med 1974; 290:692–693.

119.   Bernouilli C, Siegfried J, Baumgartner G, Regli F, Rabinowicz T, Gajdusek DC, Gibbs CJ Jr. Danger of accidental person to person transmission of Creutzfeldt–Jakob disease by surgery. Lancet 1977; 1:478–479.

120.   Gibbs CJ Jr, Asher DM, Kobrine A, Amyx HL, Sulima MP, Gajdusek DC. Transmission of Creutzfeldt–Jakob disease to a chimpanzee by electrodes contaminated during neurosurgery. J Neurol Neurosurg Psychiatry 1994; 57:757–758.

121.   Billette de Villemeur T, Beauvais P, Gourmelon M, Richardet JM. Creutzfeldt–Jakob disease in children treated with growth hormone. Lancet 1991; 337:864–865.

122.   Billette de Villemeur T, Deslys J-P, Pradel A, Soubrié C, Alpérovitch A, Tardieu M, Chaussain J-L, Hauw J-J, Dormont D, Ruberg M, Agid Y. Creutzfeldt–Jakob disease from contaminated growth hormone extracts in France. Neurology 1996; 47:690–695.

123.   Billette de Villemeur T, Gelot A, Deslys, JP, Dormont D, Duyckaerts C, Jardin L, Denni J, Robain O. Iatrogenic Creutzfeldt–Jakob disease in three growth hormone recipients: a neuropathological study. Neuropathol Appl Neurobiol 1994; 20:111–117.

124. Brown P, Gajdusek DC, Gibbs CJ Jr, Asher DM. Potential epidemic of Creutzfeldt–Jakob disease from human growth hormone therapy. N Engl J Med 1985; 313:728–731.

125. Croxson M, Brown P, Synek B, Harrington MG, Frith R, Clover G, Wilson J, Gajdusek DC. A new case of Creutzfeldt–Jakob disease associated with human growth hormone therapy in New Zealand. Neurology 1988; 38:1128–1130.

126. Fradkin JE, Schonberger LB, Mills JL, Gunn WJ, Piper JM, Wysowski DK, Thomson R, Durako S, Brown P. Creutzfeldt–Jakob disease in pituitary growth hormone recipients in the United States. JAMA 1991; 265:880–884.

127. Brown P, Preece MA, Will RG. "Friendly fire" in medicine: hormones, homografts, and Creutzfeldt–Jakob disease. Lancet 1992; 340:24–27.

128. Anonymous, From the Centers for Disease Control and Prevention. Creutzfeldt–Jakob disease associated with cadaveric dura mater grafts—Japan, January 1979–May 1996. JAMA 1998; 279:11–12.

129. Thadani V, Penar PL, Partington J, Kalb R, Janssen R, Schonberger LB, Rabkin CS, Prichard JW. Creutzfeldt–Jakob disease probably acquired from a cadaveric dura mater graft. Case report. J Neurosurg 1988; 69:766–769.

130. Willison HJ, Gale AN, McLaughlin JE. Creutzfeldt–Jakob disease following cadaveric dura mater graft. J Neurol Neurosurg Psychiatry 1991; 54:940.

131. Masters CL, Harris JO, Gajdusek DC, Gibbs CJ Jr, Bernouilli C, Asher DM. Creutzfeldt–Jakob disease: patterns of worldwide occurrence and the significance of familial and sporadic clustering. Ann Neurol 1978; 5:177–188.

132. Will RG, Matthews WB. Evidence for case-to-case transmission of Creutzfeldt–Jakob disease. J Neurol Neurosurg Psychiatry 1982; 45:235–238.

133. Cochius JI, Hyman N, Esiri MM. Creutzfeldt–Jakob disease in a recipient of human pituitary-derived gonadotrophin: a second case. J Neurol Neurosurg Psychiatry 1992; 55:1094–1095.

134. Cochius JI, Mack K, Burns RJ, Alderman CP, Blumbergs PC. Creutzfeldt–Jakob disease in a recipient of human pituitary-derived gonadotrophin. Aust N Z J Med 1990; 20:592–593.

135. Healy DL. and Evans J, Creutzfeldt–Jakob disease after pituitary gonadotrophins. Br J Med 1993; 307:517–518.

136. Will RG, Ironside JW, Zeidler M, Cousens SN, Estibeiro K, Alperovitch A, Poser S, Pocchiari M, Hofman A, Smith PG. A new variant of Creutzfeldt–Jakob disease in the UK. Lancet 1996; 347:921–925.

137. Prusiner SB. Prion diseases and the BSE crisis. Science 1997; 278:245–251.

138. Baker HF, Ridley RM, Wells GAH. Experimental transmission of BSE and scrapie to the common marmoset. Vet Rec 1993; 132:403–406.

139. Bruce ME, Will RG, Ironside JW, McConnell L, Drummond D, Suttie A, McCardle L, Chree A, Hope J, Birkett C, Cousens S, Fraser H, Bostock CJ. Transmissions to mice indicate that 'new variant' CJD is caused by the BSE agent. Nature 1997; 389:498–501.

140. Hill AF, Desbruslais M, Joiner S, Sidle KCL, Gowland L, Collinge J, Doey LJ, Lantos P. The same prion strain causes vCJD and BSE. Nature 1997; 389:448–450.

141. Andrews NJ, Farrington CP, Cousens SN, Smith PG, Ward H, Knight RS, Ironside JW, Will RG. Incidence of variant Creutzfeldt–Jakob disease in the UK. Lancet 2000; 356:481–482.

142. Supattapone S, Wille H, Uyechi L, Safar J, Tremblay P, Szoka FC, Cohen FE, Prusiner SB, Scott MR. Branched polyamines cure prion-infected neuroblastoma cells. J Virol 2001; 75:3453–3461.

143. Will RG, Zeidler M, Brown P, Harrington M, Lee KH, Kenney KL. Cerebrospinal-fluid test for new-variant Creutzfeldt–Jakob disease. Lancet 1996; 348:955.

144. Zeidler M, Stewart GE, Barraclough CR, Bateman DE, Bates D, Burn DJ, Colchester AC, Durward W, Fletcher NA, Hawkins SA, Mackenzie JM, Will RG. New variant Creutzfeldt–Jakob disease: neurological features and diagnostic tests. Lancet 1997; 350:903–907.

145. Zeidler M, Sellar RJ, Collie DA, Knight R, Stewart G, Macleod MA, Ironside JW, Cousens S, Colchester AC, Hadley DM, Will RG, Colchester AF. The pulvinar sign on magnetic resonance imaging in variant Creutzfeldt–Jakob disease. Lancet 2000; 355:1412–1418.

146. Mange A, Nishida N, Milhavet O, McMahon HE, Casanova D, Lehmann S. Amphotericin B inhibits the generation of the scrapie isoform of the prion protein in infected cultures. J Virol 2000; 74:3135–3140.

147. McKenzie D, Kaczkowski J, Marsh R, Aiken J. Amphotericin B delays both scrapie agent replication and PrP-res accumulation early in infection. J Virol 1994; 68:7534–7536.

148. Xi YG, Ingrosso L, Ladogana A, Masullo C, Pocchiari M. Amphotericin B treatment dissociates in vivo replication of the scrapie agent from PrP accumulation. Nature 1992; 356:598–601.

149. Guenther K, Deacon RM, Perry VH, Rawlins JN. Early behavioural changes in scrapie-affected mice and the influence of dapsone. Eur J Neurosci 2001; 14:401–409.

150. Manuelidis L, Fritch W, Zaitsev I. Dapsone to delay symptoms in Creutzfeldt–Jakob disease. Lancet 1998; 352:456.

151. Caughey B, Raymond GJ. Sulfated polyanion inhibition of scrapie-associated PrP accumulation in cultured cells. J Virol 1993; 67:643–650.

152. Diringer H, Ehlers B. Chemoprophylaxis of scrapie in mice. J Gen Virol 1991; 72:457–460.

153. Ladogana A, Casaccia P, Ingrosso L, Cibati M, Salvatore M, Xi YG, Masullo C, Pocchiari M. Sulphate polyanions prolong the incubation period of scrapie-infected hamsters. J Gen Virol 1992; 73:661–665.

154. Priola SA, Raines A, Caughey WS. Porphyrin, phthalocyanine antiscrapie compounds [see comments]. Science 2000; 287:1503–1506.

155. Caughey B, Race RE. Potent inhibition of scrapie-associated PrP accumulation by Congo red. J Neurochem 1992; 59:768–771.

156. Ingrosso L, Ladogana A, Pocchiari M. Congo red prolongs the incubation period in scrapie-infected hamsters. J Virol 1995; 69:506–508.

157. Milhavet O, Mange A, Casanova D, Lehmann S. Effect of Congo red on wild-type and mutated prion proteins in cultured cells. J Neurochem 2000; 74:222–230.

158. Peretz D, Williamson RA, Kaneko K, Vergara J, Leclerc E, Schmitt-Ulms G, Mehlhorn IR, Legname G, Wormald MR, Rudd PM, Dwek RA, Burton DR, Prusiner SB. Antibodies inhibit prion propagation and clear cell cultures of prion infectivity. Nature 2001; 412:739–743.

159. Doh-Ura K, Iwaki T, Caughey B. Lysosomotropic agents and cysteine protease inhibitors inhibit scrapie-associated prion protein accumulation. J Virol 2000; 74:4894–4897.

160. Korth C, May BC, Cohen FE, Prusiner SB. Acridine and phenothiazine derivatives as pharmacotherapeutics for prion disease. Proc Natl Acad Sci USA 2001; 98:9836–9841.

5

Arenaviral Hemorrhagic Fevers: Argentine Hemorrhagic Fever and Lassa Fever

Delia A. Enria

Instituto Nacional de Enfermedades Virales Humanas "Dr. Julio I. Maiztegui" (INEVH)-Administración Nacional de Laboratorios e Institutos de Salud (ANLIS), Monteagudo Pergamino, Argentina

1. INTRODUCTION

The family Arenaviridae comprises several RNA spherical to pleomorphic viruses, including various important causative agents of hemorrhagic fever in Africa and America. The prototype virus of this family, lymphocytic choriomeningitis (LCM) has a worldwide distribution corresponding to the widespread presence of its reservoir, *Mus musculus*, and produces diseases in humans characterized by a febrile syndrome with occasional central nervous system (CNS) involvement. There are currently at least 19 arenaviruses recognized, but only six have been associated with human illness: in South America, Junin virus (Argentine hemorrhagic fever, AHF), Machupo virus (Bolivian hemorrhagic fever, BHF), Guanarito (Venezuelan hemorrhagic fever, VHF) and Sabia (hemorrhagic fever in Brazil); in Africa, Lassa virus (Lassa fever), and the above-mentioned LCM (Fig. 1, Table 1) (1).

2. THE VIRUSES

Based on the serologic properties, genetic data, and geographic distribution, arenaviruses have been divided in two main groups: Old World, and New World, or Tacaribe complex (2–4).

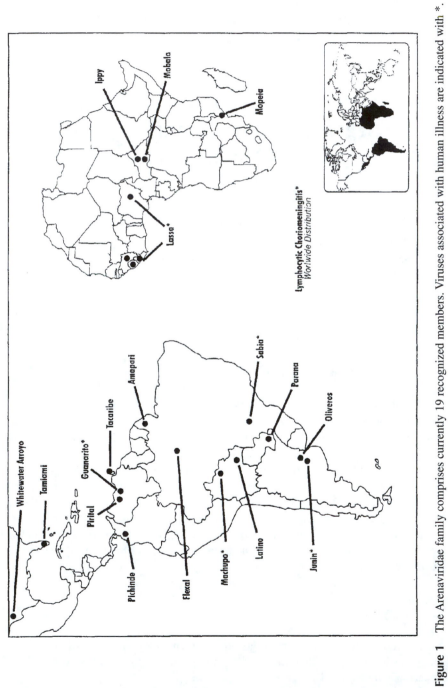

Figure 1 The Arenaviridae family comprises currently 19 recognized members. Viruses associated with human illness are indicated with *.

Table 1 Principal Characteristics of the Members of the Arenaviridae Family (For Each Virus, the Principal Reservoir Is Indicated)

Virus	Principal reservoir	Geographic distribution	Human illness
Old World arenavirus			
Ippy virus	*Arvicanthis sp.*	Central African Republic	No
Lassa virus	*Mastomys sp.*	West Africa	Hemorrhagic fever
Lymphocytic choriomeningitis virus	*Mus musculus*	Probably worldwide	Febrile syndrome, aseptic meningitis
Mobala virus	*Praomys sp.*	Central Africa Republic	No
Mopeia virus	*Mastomys natalensis*	Mozambique, Zimbabwe	No
New World arenavirus			
Amapari virus	*Neacomys guianae*	Brazil	No
Flexal virus	*Oryzomys spp.*	Brazil	Laboratory infection
Guanarito virus	*Zygodontomys brevicauda*	Venezuela	Hemorrhagic fever
Junin virus	*Calomys musculinus*	Argentina	Hemorrhagic fever
Latino virus	*Calomys callosus*	Bolivia	No
Machupo virus	*Calomys callosus*	Bolivia	Hemorrhagic fever
Paraná virus	*Oryzomys buccinatus*	Paraguay	No
Pichinde virus	*Oryzomys albigularis*	Colombia	Laboratory infection
Pirital virus	*Sigmodon alstoni*	Venezuela	No
Oliveros virus	*Bolomys obscurus*	Argentina	No
Sabiá virus	*Unknown*	Brazil	Hemorrhagic fever
Tacaribe virus	*Artibeus spp.*	Trinidad	Laboratory infection
Tamiami virus	*Sigmodon hispidus*	United States	No
White water Arroyo virus	*Neotoma albigula*	United States	Probably severe disease

The viruses belonging to New World group are closely related, according to complement fixation (CF) and immunofluorescence tests, but the cross-reactions with Old World viruses are limited. The molecular phylogenetic analyses have also shown that Old World and New World arenaviruses occupy two different clades. The New World arenaviruses comprise three lineages of evolution, named A, B, and C. The lineage A includes Flexal, Paraná, Pichinde, Pirital, and Tamiami viruses. The lineage B includes the four agents of South American hemorrhagic fevers (Junin, Mapucho, Guanarito, and Sabia), as well as Tacaribe and Tamiami viruses. Lineage C includes Latino and Oliveros virus (5). In a recent report, white water Arroyo virus is recognized as a product of genetic recombination between lineage A and lineage B virus (6). Among the Old World arenaviruses, LCM is the most closely related to New World viruses.

2.1. Morphology

Virions are spherical or pleomorphic particles between 50 and 300 nm in diameter, with a lipoprotein envelope, from which club-shaped projections of 8–10 nm are projected (7). The virions are relatively unstable and can be rapidly inactivated by ultraviolet or gamma irradiation, heating at 56°C or through exposition to pH outside the 5.0–8.5 range. On the contrary, the presence of a lipid envelope makes them susceptible to the inactivation by solvents or detergents (8,9). The presence of electro-dense granules that have been identified as ribosomes from cell origin, gives to these viruses the characteristic "sandy appearance," from which the "arenaviruses" name is derived (10). The genome consists of two single-stranded RNA molecules, named L (large) and S (small). Although the viruses show some differences in the segment lengths, the genome general organization is similar for all of them (11).

The S segment encodes for the principal structural components: the nucleoprotein (N or NP) and a precursor glycoprotein (GPC), which by post-transcriptional cleavage encodes the two glycoproteins of the viral envelope (G1 or GP1, and G2 or GP2). The L segment codes for an RNA-dependent polymerase, and for a small protein (Z) with potential capacity for combining with metals (12–16).

Arenaviruses have an original strategy of genomic codification, named "ambisense." The ambisense codification provides a mechanism of genetic expression with temporal regulation: the mRNAs corresponding to the NP and L can be transcripts from the incoming S and L segments, and the mRNAs corresponding to GPC and Z are only transcripts from an anti-genomic RNA, that is also an intermediate product of the synthesis of genomic RNA (17,18).

2.2. Laboratory Hosts

2.2.1. Infection in Cell Cultures

The arenaviruses grow in a variety of cell lines derived from mammals. In vitro propagation is usually done in fibroblasts; BHK-21 and Vero cells are the most commonly used. In general, the infection with arenaviruses is non-cytolitic (19–21). Junin virus multiplies effectively in BHK-21 cells and in mouse fibroblast without cytopathic effects However, Junin virus multiplication in Vero cells produces a marked cytopathic action, characterized by cellular rounding, cytoplasmatic vacuolization, nuclear pyknosis, and final cellular detachment. Vero cells are an appropriate cell culture system for obtaining plaques under agarose or methylcellulose for Junin virus and the other arenaviruses.

2.2.2. Infection in Animals

In their natural reservoir, the arenaviruses establish a persistent infection when they have acquired the virus in utero or a few days after birth (22,23). The viral

persistence allows the maintenance of the virus in nature. In *C. musculinus* experimentally infected with Junin virus, antigenic variants and mutants with different
phenotypes have been isolated in conjunction with chronic infection. However, it
is not yet clear if these variants are the cause or the consequence of the persistence (24). The presence of defective viral genomes is another potential variable
involved in the persistence (25).

Many studies have been done in experimental animals with the objective of
explaining the physiopathologic findings in humans. It has been established that
the infection of adult mice with LCM produces an acute disease that ends with
death or the recovery of the animal, depending on the dose, inoculation route, and
the genetic background of the rodent. On the contrary, the infection of newborn
or adult immunosuppressed mice results in a persistent infection. The inoculation
of adult hamsters results in an acute disease, including immunosuppressed animals. In both guinea-pigs and primates, the lethal dose is highly dependent on the
viral strain (26).

Suckling mice are highly susceptible to different strains of Junin virus. In
all cases, the animals develop a meningoencephalitis, with viral antigen
detectable in cortical neurons, meninges, and choroid plexus. The damage in the
CNS is due to the cellular immune response. Infection of athymic mice produces
an asymptomatic persistent infection, with high viral titers in cerebrum, in the
absence of CNS lesions. Adult guinea-pigs infected with pathogenic strains of
Junin virus develop a hemorrhagic illness, similar to the human disease. The
guinea-pig model has been the object of many studies and is one of the assays
used to evaluate the virulence of Junin virus strains (22,27,28). Junin virus infection of primates such as *Callithrix jacchus* or *Macaccus rhesus* also results in a
disease similar to that observed in humans with fever, anorexia, weight lost, pete-
quiae in the skin and organs, and disseminated hemorrhages. Immune serum is
effective in controlling the hemorrhagic illness, but it is associated with the development of a late neurological syndrome (LNS) (29–31).

Lassa virus infection of rhesus monkeys and guinea-pigs shows common
pathologic findings, that include hepatic necrosis and regeneration, lymphoid
necrosis in spleen and lymph nodes, myocarditis, focal arteritis, renal tubular
necrosis, and late mononuclear choriomeningoencephalitis (32,33).

3. EPIDEMIOLOGY AND ECOLOGY

All arenaviruses, with the exception of Tacaribe virus that is linked to bats, are
maintained in nature by the chronic infection of different species of rodents
(34,35). With the exception of LCM, the arenaviruses have a restricted geographic distribution (Fig. 1). The specificity of the relationship virus–host is a distinctive characteristic. In each region, the virus can infect different species of
rodents, but there is always one that behaves as the principal reservoir due to the
density, the prevalence, and the characteristic of the infection. The relationship

between the virus and the reservoir is a highly evolved form of parasitism that has occurred as the result of a long-term co-evolution (36). The Old World arenaviruses are related to rodents of the *Muridae*, subfamily *Murinae* (Old World rat and mice), and the New World arenaviruses to rodents of the family *Muridae*, subfamily Sigmodontinae (New World rat and mice) (Table 1).

3.1. Transmission

It is considered that Junin virus is maintained among the reservoir populations mainly by horizontal transmission (22,37,38). The vertical transmission of Junin virus seems to produce a deleterious effect, according to some experimental studies (39). A similar pattern is considered for Machupo virus (34). However, the maintenance of Guanarito virus seems to have a different pattern, and the experimental studies suggest that the horizontal transmission may have a deleterious effect in the reproduction of *Zygodontomys brevicauda* (40). For both Lassa and LCM, the vertical transmission is considered the most relevant way of perpetuation (34,41).

Although the exact mechanism of transmission from the rodents to the humans is unknown, there is strong experimental evidence suggesting that this transmission occurs mainly by inhalation of aerosols from the excreta of infected rodents (42–44).

Argentine hemorrhagic fever is not usually contagious from person to person, although in some circumstances this form of transmission can occur. There is viremia during the acute febrile period and Junin virus has also been isolated from urine and maternal milk (45). On the contrary, the possibility of inter-human transmission has been suggested in a group of women who are assumed to have acquired the illness from their convalescent spouses as a consequence of intimate contacts (46). For BHF, the inter-human transmission has been more frequently reported in familial and community clusters (47–50). For VHF, there are no reports of person-to-person transmission (51). For Lassa fever, in one outbreak there were evidence of inter-human transmission, but in general this has been difficult to evaluate due to the constant presence of infected *Mastomys* (52).

3.2. Geographic Distribution

Argentine hemorrhagic fever is endemic in the humid pampas of Argentina, and the endemo-epidemic area has been progressively expanding since the emergence of the disease in the 1950s (Fig. 2) (53). The BHF endemic area is restricted to El Beni department, in the north-eastern part of Bolivia (50). Venezuelan hemorrhagic fever was originally restricted to Guanarito county, in the south of Portuguesa State of Venezuela, but the endemic area is also expanding (51,54)

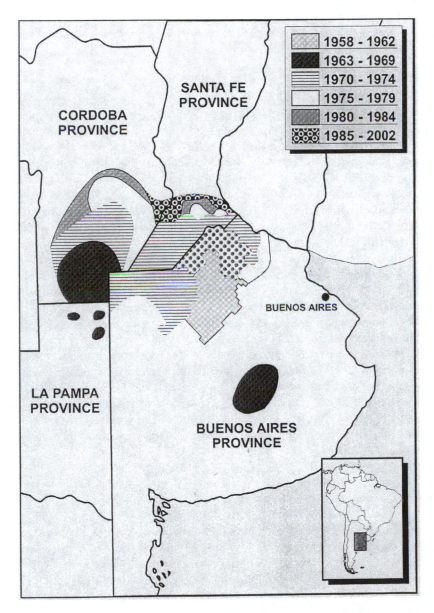

Figure 2 Endemic region and geographic extension of Argentine hemorrhagic fever (AHF). The area has been expanding since the discovery of Junin virus in 1958.

There is only one natural infection with Sabia virus in a case occurring in Sao Paulo State in Brazil (55).

Lassa fever is a disease that is characteristic of occidental Africa, and the most affected countries include Sierra Leona, Guinea, Liberia, and Nigeria (56).

3.3. Incidence

Argentine hemorrhagic fever has produced annual outbreaks without interruption since the discovery of Junin virus in 1958. It has a focal distribution that can also be correlated with the focal distribution of the infected rodents. The incidence rates in some areas can be as low as 1/100,000, but in regions of major activity could reach 140/100,000, and 355/100,000 adult males. The rates are higher during the initial period of 5–10 years in new areas and then decline. However, in areas considered historical, isolated cases can occur. This classical epidemiologic pattern has been modified since 1991 through the selective vaccination of adults at higher risk with a live attenuated Junin virus vaccine (57).

Bolivian hemorrhagic fever was an important public health problem during the 1960s. The initial explosive outbreaks resulted in effective and intensive rodents control programs with subsequent interruption of community outbreaks. There were no reported BHF since mid-1970s, although it is believed that sporadic cases still occur. In 1993, and after 20 years of quiescence, the reemergence of the disease was reported. This reemergence included an intrafamiliar outbreak in 1994 in which six of the seven affected members died (50). For VHF, the alternation of periods of low and high incidence has been described (51). Only one case of natural infection, and two laboratorial infections with Sabia virus has been reported (55,58,59). Lassa fever is considered a very frequent disease in the endemic region of Occidental Africa. In the most affected area of Sierra Leona, Lassa fever could be responsible for a quarter of the hospital admissions and deaths (60).

3.4. Seasonal Distribution and Risk Factors

Although AHF cases can occur during the whole year, annual outbreaks are registered during autumn and winter, with a peak in the month of May. The classical epidemiologic pattern of AHF is of a disease four times more frequent in men than in women, and is also more frequent (90%) among rural than in urban inhabitants. The children of less than 14 years comprise around 10% of the annual cases (57).

Bolivian hemorrhagic fever has also a seasonal distribution, with the majority of cases presenting during the dry season, coincident with the peak in agricultural activities. Most sporadic BHF cases have been male rural workers, while the familial and community outbreaks have comprised both genera and all age groups, and have been related to the rodents invasion of towns (47). Cases of VHF are reported during the whole year, but the outbreaks occurred during the major agricultural activities, with a peak between November and January (51).

Lassa fever is a common illness of both adults and children. The pattern of similar distribution of diseases in men, women, and children has been regarded as evidence that the peri-domestic exposition to the virus is probably very important. Similarly, the lack of biosafety measures in the care of the patients has played an important in the inter-human transmission (61).

4. FACTORS IN THE EMERGENCE OF ARENAVIRAL HEMORRHAGIC FEVERS

Many of the factors linked to the emergence of these "new" illnesses caused by "old" viruses are unknown. Several hypotheses have been suggested, but the great majority have not been proved in the field, given the difficulties and the financial costs of the long-term studies required.

The model Junin virus, AHF, has been the best studied. It has been suggested that the emergence of AHF in the 1950s was the result of the alterations produced in the ecosystem as a result of the agricultural practices. These changes have benefited the growth of *C. musculinus* populations. The humid pampas of Argentina is a patchwork of intensively cultivated areas; bordered by roads, railways, wire fence, etc. Six species of small rodents coexist in the region, and five of them belong to the Sigmodontinae subfamily: *C. musculinus, C. laucha, Akodon azarae, N. benefactus* and *Oligoryzomys flavescens.* The Murinae subfamily is represented by the introduced species *M. musculus.* It is considered that the rodent communities of the pre-agricultural pampas were dominated by *Akodon, Bolomys* and *Oligoryzomys* (37,45,62–64). Both *Bolomys* and *Akodon* live almost exclusively in rural habitats and are dominant over *Calomys* species. *Calomys musculinus* can easily invade modified habitats. They are more frequently captured in rural habitats, but they are also found in cultivated fields, before and after harvesting. They are rarely captured in urban habits (65–67).

A long series of environmental variables has been related to the fluctuating rodent populations, although the issue is still controversial. Climate is one of the factors that more probably influences the rodent population densities and, therefore, is very likely to contribute to cycles in the incidence of South American hemorrhagic fevers. In the Argentine humid pampas, it has been suggested that the cold and humid winters as well as the hot and dry summers would result in a decrease, while the warm and dry winters and the chilly and rainy summers would contribute to the increase in the rodent's densities. Other factors that has been considered important are the increment or decreases in the harvest, and the type of crop; the burning or the burning and cut of the linear habitats, that give refuge to the rodents, and the intensity in the use of herbicides and insecticides (45,62,63).

On the contrary, the description of the geographic limits of Junin virus activity is based mainly on the distribution of the disease, and not of the virus. The principal reservoir of Junin virus is found in most central and north-western Argentina, and its distribution exceeds widely the known AHF endemic area. A gradient of infection with Junin virus has been described in *C. musculinus* within the endemic region. The prevalence of Junin virus infection in *C. musculinus* is higher in the newly involved areas, and has been reported as low or absent outside the endemic area (67). However, Junin virus has been isolated from rodents trapped in areas without human cases in the last 10 years and in areas where the disease has not been recognized yet, suggesting the possibility of new extensions of the endemic region and of the reemergence in areas currently considered historic (68). Junin virus infection of *C. musculinus* has a focal distribution. The reasons for this particular pattern are not cleared. The complete elucidation of the factors responsible for AHF emergence and progressive extension deserves further investigation.

The reservoir of Machupo virus, *C. callosus*, is found preferably in the areas where prairies are connected with the forest. *Calomys callosus* can also live in urban areas, and has the capacity of invading houses, especially in the flood areas, and looking for lands at higher altitudes. It is considered that the outbreaks affecting towns and cities would arise during epizootics, especially when the densities of rodents reach unusual levels and invade urban areas (47,48,69).

For VHF, the deforestation of some areas for agriculture use has been the factor linked to the emergence. Both *Z. brevicauda* (reservoir of Guanarito virus), and *Sigmodon alstoni* (reservoir of Pirital virus) have been captured in the cultivated field, in their borders and in those of the roads. Only exceptionally, are these viruses found in urban habitats. Venezuelan hemorrhagic fever outbreaks have been associated with the increase in the densities of *Z. brevicauda* that occur when densities of *S. alstoni* decreased. This suggests that interspecies competence plays a role in the emergence of the illness (40). The role of peri-domestic exposition to Lassa is considered important, with the densities of rodents being much higher inside the houses than in the agricultural and forest areas. Human infections would be increased by the common practice of hunting and eating rodents, and by the preservation of food in open places (61).

5. CLINICAL DESCRIPTION

The hemorrhagic fevers caused by the viruses Junin, Guanarito, and Mapucho (and probably also Sabia) produce similar clinical pictures, while Lassa human infection has a distinct clinical presentation. Argentine hemorrhagic fever will be used as a model of this description.

5.1. Argentine Hemorrhagic Fever

Argentine hemorrhagic fever is characterized by hematological, cardiovascular, renal, neurological, and immunologic manifestations (70). The incubation period is between 6 and 14 days, with a range of 4–21 days. The disease begins with a prodromal phase, characterized by the insidious onset of unspecific symptoms such as malaise, headaches, and moderate fever (38–39∞C). During the following days, myalgias, low backache, arthralgias, retro-orbital pain, epigastic pain, dizziness, nauseas, and vomiting may appear. Constipation or diarrhea may be also present. During this phase, hemorrhages are limited to bleeding of the gums, epistaxis or metrorrhagia in women. The almost constant absence of productive cough, sore throat, or nasal congestion is very useful for distinguishing the initial symptoms of AHF from those of respiratory infections.

During the first week, on the physical examination there is an erythematous exanthema in the face, neck and upper part of the trunk. In the skin of the axillary regions or in the superior aspects of the arms, there are frequently isolated petechiae. Conjunctival congestion and periorbital edema may also be present. The oropharyngeal membranes are congested, and there is congestion of the vessels bordering the gums, which may bleed spontaneously or under a slight pressure. Over the soft palate, there is an enanthem characterized by the presence of petechiae and small vesicles. In the laterocervical regions, there may be enlarged lymph nodes that are not painful. Signs of pulmonary abnormalities are generally absent, although some patients report cough. Relative bradycardia and orthostatic hypotension are frequently found. Generally, there is no hepatomegaly or splenomegaly, and jaundice is rare. At the end of the first week of illness, different degrees of dehydration may occur.

During the second week of illness, 70–80% of the cases begin to improve. The remaining 20–30% enters in a hemorrhagic/neurological phase, characterized by severe hemorrhages or neurological manifestations, shock and superimposed bacterial infections that appear between 8 and 12 days after the onset of symptoms. Profuse bleeding may occur in the form of hematemesis, melena, hemoptysis, epistaxis, hematomas, metrorrhagia, or hematuria. Acute renal failure is uncommon, but may arise in terminal cases or after prolonged periods of shock, and is secondary to acute tubular necrosis. Superimposed bacterial infections such as pneumonia and septicemia can also complicate the clinical course, usually appearing after 8 days from onset of symptoms. Patients destined to survive begin to improve by the third week of illness, and the convalescence may last up to 3 months. Temporary hair loss is common. Many patients have asthenia, irritability and memory changes (57).

5.1.1. Neurological Alterations in AHF

In AHF, the nervous system is compromised in almost all cases during the acute phase, and the patients may have alterations from both the CNS, and the peripheral. The symptoms most frequently found include headaches, myalgias, insomnia, somnolence, and anxiety. A decrease in muscular tonicity, particularity of the lower limbs, is frequently seen. The muscular masses are soft, with an increased sensitivity to the compression in half of the cases. This decrease in the muscular tonicity may persist, although diminishing, up to the third week of illness.

A decrease or complete absence of deep tendon reflexes follows the decrease in tone early in the course of infection and is almost invariable found in 80% of the patients. The patellar reflexes are the more frequently reduced. In the upper extremities, the decrease in deep tendon reflexes is not frequent, and a decrease in all four limbs is very rare. A noticeable variability in the reflexes is seen during the first week. In more than 30% of the patients, irregular, arrhythmic tremor of the hands and tongue are observed. Most patients have dysgraphia, even the cases in which the tremor is not important. The disappearance of the dysgraphia and the tremor is coincident with the clinical recovery. The Romberg sign is seen in almost 30% of the cases, although the clinical importance is minimal given that in the standing position the patients are insecure, even with opened eyes. On the contrary, most patients have orthostatic hypotension. The gait alterations include an increase in the base with tremors; a mild separation of the upper extremities; and short, irregular steps. More than 25% of the patients have ataxia, both from the upper and the lower extremities. The severe neurological manifestations seen in one-third of the cases during the second week of illness consist of mental confusion, increased irritability and excitation; these are followed by delirium, generalized convulsions and coma. During convalescence, many patients have asthenia, irritability and memory changes; these are transitory and disappear gradually over a period of 1–3 months. Around 10% of AHF patients treated with immune plasma develop an LNS (71,72).

5.1.2. The Late Neurological Syndrome of AHF

From the very first description of AHF, it was recognized that some patients might present a neurological disease that appeared after the acute phase. This disease was known among inhabitants and physicians of the AHF endemic area as a "relapse." This entity was then named LNS of the AHF. This LNS occurs after an interval free of symptoms of around 4–6 weeks (range 3–90 days) from the acute period, and is characterized by a febrile syndrome, mainly with cerebellar trunk manifestations. A controlled clinical trial showed an association between AHF treatment with immune plasma and the LNS (73). Subsequent studies reinforce that the LNS is seen only in the surviving AHF cases who have received treatment with immune plasma. No cases have been registered among AHF patients who have recovered without specific treatment (71,72). A single case has been observed in a patient who was treated late in the course of illness with intravenous ribavirin (74). The onset of the symptoms is insidious. The majority of the patients (90%) begin with mild to moderate headaches, nausea, vomiting, and dizziness. During the following days, 70% of the cases refer tinnitus, blurred vision, and gait impairment. Almost half of the cases have diplopia, nervousness, and changes in behavior.

At physical examination, all cases have fever and more than half have paralysis of the VI nerve, nistagmus, and cerebellar ataxia. Deep tendon reflexes can be normal or decreased, but in a small percentage, a frank increase in tone is found. In a minority of patients, dysarthria with pyramidal and extrapiramidal signs are also seen. Paresis and paralysis have been recorded in around 5% of patients. In one fatal case, the disease presented as an ascendant paralysis that caused respiratory insufficiency (71,72).

5.2. Differential Findings with the Other South American Arenaviral Hemorrhagic Fevers

In a nosocomial outbreak of BHF of high lethality occurring in a high altitude area, jaundice was found in some cases (47–49). Cases with VHF refer sore throat frequently among initial symptoms (51). In the unique natural infection with Sabia virus seen so far, extensive hepatic necrosis was found (55).

5.3. Lassa Fever

Lassa fever is prevalent in both males and females within all age groups. The disease begins after 3–21 days of incubation (mean 10 days) with the insidious onset of fever, generalized weakness, severe headaches, generally frontal, and malaise (61,75–78). Other common symptoms include aching in the large joints, low backache, non-productive cough, sore throat, retrosternal chest pain, abdominal pain, and a variety of other generalized symptoms. Vomiting and diarrhea are also referred. On physical examination, conjunctivitis with or without conjunctival hemorrhages, facial and neck swelling in florid cases, pharyngitis or diffuse inflamed and swollen posterior pharynx and tonsils, sometimes with exudates but exceptionally with petechiae have been described. In half of the patients, tenderness of the abdomen is found (79).

The bleeding is often mild, and is seen as nose, mouth, and genitourinary or gastrointestinal tract. Severe bleeding has been described in only 15–20% of the patients, with vaginal bleeding in pregnant women been potentially hemodynamically significant. No characteristical rashes have been described in Lassa fever, although in white-skinned patients maculo-papular or petechial rashes have been observed.

During the second week of illness, up to a third of Lassa fever cases progress to a severe illness, with the frequent presence of persisting vomiting and diarrhea. Hypotension and tachycardia are observed. Elevated respiratory rates are also frequent, with pleural effusion being common. Pericardial effusions are only occasionally seen in the terminal stages. These pleural and pericardial effusions have been linked to the severe retrosternal or epigastric pain referred by many patients.

5.3.1.   Neurological Abnormalities in Lassa Fever

Neurological signs in the early stages are limited to a fine tremor, most marked in the lips and tongue. With the progression of the illness, neurological signs are more infrequent than in AHF, but carry a poor prognosis. Patients with severe illness may deteriorate rapidly, progressing from confusion to a severe encephalopathy with or without seizures, but without focal signs. It is not clear to what extent these represent direct effect of Lassa virus on the CNS, secondary immune-mediated effects or non-specific metabolic ones common to any critically ill patient. Other underlying health problems may affect the clinical course as well (80,81).

Sensorineural deafness in one or both ears is the major chronic sequelae of Lassa fever and may occur in almost 30% of cases. The onset is invariably during the convalescent phase of the illness. There is no correlation with the severity of the acute disease, the level of viremia or aspartate aminotransferase (AST). About half of the patients recover by 3–4 months after onset, but the alteration is permanent in the other. It is unclear whether the damage is due to viral neurotropism, thrombosis, vasculitis, focal hemorrhage, or some other viral or immune response-related phenomenon. Depression and cerebellar signs, such as tremors and ataxia have also been reported during convalescence, but they are uncommon and resolve with time (82).

6.   CLINICAL LABORATORY STUDIES

Clinical laboratory studies are very useful to establish an early diagnosis in South American hemorrhagic fevers (Fig. 3). During the acute phase, there are low white cell and platelet counts (ranging from 50,000 to 100,000 mm^3). The sedimentation rate is normal or decreased. Almost constantly, there is protein in the urine, with alteration in the sediment, with the presence of hyaline-granular casts, red blood cells, and round cells with cytoplasmatic inclusions. Serum creatinine and urea are normal or increased in proportion to dehydration and shock in the severely ill patient. In AHF, AST, creatine phosphokinase (CPK), and lactate dehydrogenase (LDH) are commonly slightly increased, but hyperbilirubinemia or hyperamylasemia is rare (57). In patients with LNS, the hematological alterations that are characteristic of the acute phase are not seen, and in some cases presenting early in the convalescence, a moderate increase in the white cell counts can be seen, similarly to the other cases that do not develop the LNS. During the acute phase, the CSF is normal, even in the severe neurological forms of the disease. This differs from the findings in LNS cases, in which a moderate increase in the number of cells (mean: 100, range 20–400), mainly lymphocytes, is seen. Glucose is normal, and the total protein is normal or slightly increased (0.40–0.80 g/dL) (72). Junin virus isolation attempts or reverse transcription-polymerase chain reaction (RT-PCR)

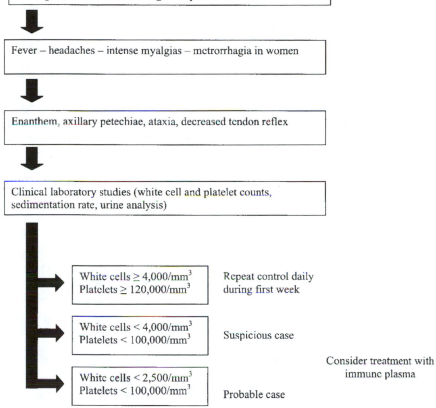

Figure 3 Algorithm for the detection of Argentine hemorrhagic fever (AHF). The AHF algorithm could also be effective for the early detection of the other South American hemorrhagic fevers.

from blood or CSF in LNS cases have been consistently negative. Junin virus-specific antibodies in CSF are always present in titers similar or even higher than those in serum.

In Lassa fever, thrombocytopenia is mild to moderate (usually not less than 100,000 mm^3). The while cell counts are generally normal, although a mild diminution with lymphopenia may occur (83). Severely ill patients are more likely to be thrombocytopenic, are usually lymphopenic, and may have an elevated WBC count with neutrophilia. In these patients, a moderate hemoconcentration and proteinuria could also be seen. The AST is often elevated and higher values are predictive of a poor prognosis. A similar association is found with the level of viremia. DIC is not a common finding (84).

7. OTHER COMPLEMENTARY EXAMINATIONS

More than 50% of the patients with Lassa fever have abnormal non-specific electrocardiograms (61). The alterations that have been found in neurophysiologic diagnostic tests during the acute phase of AHF comprise: (a) diminished sensory conduction velocities; (b) prolonged distal motor latency; (c) slight diminished speed of motor conduction; (d) diminished amplitude of the evoked motor potential; and (e) diminished amplitude of the evoked sensory potential. These findings suggest that during the acute period of AHF, there is predominantly axonal injury within the peripheral nerve (85).

In AHF, there are no characteristic alterations in the EEG. There is a tendency for the basic cortical rhythm to exhibit dysynchronization with minimal response to the opening of the eyelid. In some cases, the discordance between the somnolence seen, and the absence of typical modifications in the drawing of sleeping are striking (73). The study of auditory evoked potentials in LNS cases has shown abnormalities consisting of morphologic alterations of the components and a prolonged central conduction time, indicative of a structural alteration of the brainstem (86).

In a small series of AHF cases studied by MRI during the acute phase, the only alteration seen was a slight edema of the cerebellar cortex. In LNS cases, edema was limited to the cerebellar cortex without alteration in the white matter (87). Atrophy of the cerebellum was found in a severe LNS case more than 2 years after the illness.

8. DIFFERENTIAL DIAGNOSIS

During the prodromal phase, the clinical manifestations of South American hemorrhagic fevers are non-specific and the differential diagnosis includes dengue, DHF typhoid fever, hepatitis, infectious mononucleosis, leptospirosis, hantavirus infections, and rickettsioses. Malaria and yellow fever should also be considered in endemic areas. Diseases presenting with hematological or neurological alterations, such as intoxications, rheumatic diseases, and blood dyscrasias may also be taken into consideration. Within endemic areas or among patients with a history of travel to the specific geographic regions, a febrile syndrome with leucopenia and thrombocytopenia is suspicious of a South American hemorrhagic fever (Fig. 3).

At the initial stages, the non-specific presentation of Lassa fever needs to be differentiated of most febrile illnesses found in West Africa, including malaria, typhoid, and bacillary dysentery.

9. ETIOLOGIC DIAGNOSIS

Viremia is present throughout the acute febrile period in all the arenaviral hemorrhagic fevers and the viruses can be isolated from blood and tissues (particularly lymphoid tissues) of fatal cases. Isolation is usually performed in Vero cells, but other cellular lines or hosts, such as suckling mice or guinea-pigs (for AHF) or suckling hamsters (for BHF) can be used (88,89). In AHF, co-cultivation of peripheral blood mononuclear cells improves the sensitivity of virus recovery (90). The presence of virus can also be determined by RT-PCR. In AHF, RT-PCR has been successfully applied and plays an important role in establishing the etiologic diagnosis before the appearance of the specific antibodies, particularly in fatal cases. For Lassa fever, a sensitive assay exists, but strain variation and the problems linked to cross-contamination pose practical problems. Fatal cases can also be diagnosed by immunohistochemistry on fixed tissues (91).

The serologic diagnosis can be done by CF, immunofluorescence, and ELISA and neutralization tests. Complement fixation has been widely employed in the past, but has a low sensitivity. ELISA tests for the detection of IgG antibodies in paired serum samples (one from acute period and the other from convalescence) is the method of choice for the diagnosis of AHF. Neutralization tests are very important to confirm the specificity of the reactions. For BHF, antigen detection ELISA and IgM ELISA have been successfully applied (92). Acute Lassa fever is best diagnosed in early phases by combining ELISA for IgM antibody and antigen. IgG ELISA antibodies takes longer to develop (approximately 3 weeks), but appear earlier than the neutralizing antibodies, that are often detected several weeks after disease resolves; the final response is low in titer (61).

10. PATHOLOGY AND PATHOPHYSIOLOGY

Pathologic descriptions of arenavirus infections in humans are limited to a few necropsy series. Gross and microscopic pathologic findings in these human cases are generally similar among different arenavirus infections. Common gross findings at postmortem examinations include ecchymoses and petechial hemorrhages involving skin, conjunctivae, mucous membranes, and internal organs. The degree of hemorrhage varies, and sometimes can be minimal or absent. Conjunctival swelling, pleural and pericardial effusions, and ascites are frequently present (33,93–95).

Microscopically, congestion and variable degrees of necrosis are usually observed in all organ systems. Necrosis is most prominent in the liver and spleen, but is also frequently found in adrenal gland, kidney, and gastrointestinal mucosa. The most consistent histophatologic feature is seen in the liver and consists of multifocal hepatocellular necrosis with cytoplasmic eosinophilia, councilman body formation, nuclear pyknosis, cytolysis, and fatty metamorphosis. Inflammatory cell infiltrates in necrotic areas are usually mild and, when present, consist of a mixture of mononuclear cells and neutrophils. The spleen usually shows depletion of follicles and focal necrosis. Other pathologic features that may be present in arenavirus infections include mild interstitial pneumonitis, diffuse alveolar damage, myocarditis, and acute renal tubular necrosis.

Because none of these pathologic features are specific, a confirmatory test such as immunohistochemistry is essential to a definitive tissue diagnosis, and such studies have also demonstrated a wide spectrum of tissue tropism. In Lassa fever, the localization of viral antigens can be summarized as the following: (1) hepatocytes, especially those in the areas of necrosis; (2) cells of the mononuclear phagocytic system such as Kupffer cells in hepatic sinusoids, alveolar macrophages, and endothelial cells; (3) mesothelial cells lining pericardium, pleura, peritoneum, and serosal surfaces of other organs; and (4) specialized cells involved in hormone secretion, including those in adrenal gland, ovary, uterus, placenta, and breast (91,96).

In AHF, ultrastructural and immunohistochemical studies revealed characteristic intracellular inclusions that were more prominent in lymphatic tissues, coincident with the presence of Junin virus antigens. In the kidney, a large number of virus-like intracytoplasmic particles are found in distal and collecting tubules coincident with severe tissue necrosis and large quantities of Junin virus antigen as demonstrated by immunofluorescence. Morphologic studies of the bone marrow indicate that an acute and transient arrest of hemopoiesis occurs, with bone marrow hypocellulary, but without permanent hematological sequelae in survivors (97–100).

During the progression to severe illness, there are clinical evidences of capillary leakage, that seems to be more prominent in Lassa fever cases, in which there are effusions in the peritoneum, pleura and pericardia, progressing to facial (but not lower extremity) edema, pulmonary edema with adult respiratory distress syndrome (ARDS), and hypovolemic shock. ARDS is a frequent cause of death in Lassa infection, and have been reported late in the course of fatal AHF cases. Encephalopathy, but not encephalitis, is prominent in severe neurological AHF patients and in some with Lassa fever. There is little or no virus found in CNS, and no evidence of parenchymal damage in the brain. Leaky capillaries and edema may well explain this process (61).

A common characteristic of arenavirus infections, and particularly of the hemorrhagic fevers, is the lack of histological lesions to explain the altered organ function and death. This is the origin of the concept that arenaviruses induce an alteration of the cellular functions without morphologic changes.

In the South American hemorrhagic fevers, particularly in AHF, the pathophysiology seems to be the result of direct viral action, in contrast to the mouse models of LCM virus infection in which immunopathologic cell action causes encephalitis and B-cell products result in chronic immune complex disease. In AHF, several studies have demonstrated that immune complexes, complement activation or DIC are not relevant pathogenic mechanisms (101). Mediators released or activated as a result of the virus–cell interactions, such as lymphokines, vasoactive mediators, and proteolytic enzymes may explain some of the observed alterations. Hemorrhagic manifestations are considered to be the result of the thrombocytopenia, abnormal platelet function induced by a plasma component, and alterations of the blood coagulation with fibrinolysis activation.

The hemostatic alterations found include prolongation of activated partial thromboplastin time (APTT), low levels of factors VIII, IX and XI, increased values of factor V, von Willebrand factor, and fibrinogen; and mild decreases in antithrombin III, and plasminogen. Endothelial cell involvement is also suspected, based on the fact that Junin virus replicates in cultured endothelial cells and that in human disease there are increased levels of von Willebrand factor (102–104).

Argentine hemorrhagic fever is also characterized by an acute transitory immunodeficiency. There is a lag in the humoral immune response, with antibodies appearing during the second week of illness, coincident with the recovery of patients. During the acute phase, cell-mediated immunity is also depressed, as it has been shown by tests of delayed-type hypersensitivity to non-viral recall antigens and lymphocyte proliferation stimulated by mitogens. During this acute period, there are also changes in the T-cell subpopulations that return to normal values in convalescence (105,106).

In addition, during the initial phase of AHF, very high titers of endogenous interferon (IFNα) have been demonstrated circulating in the serum of the patients. The titers of IFNα are significantly higher in cases developing severe forms of the illness, and are considered a marker link to fatal evolution. Tumor necrosis factorα (TNF-α) levels are also elevated, particularly in fatal cases. Another study suggested the association between histocompatibility antigens and the severity of the disease (107–109).

Several physiopathogenic mechanisms have been suggested to explain the LNS seen in AHF patients treated with immune plasma. The humoral immune response is different in patients with LNS, and they present a delayed primary response, but achieving higher titers of neutralizing antibodies than the other surviving cases, even those that have not received immune plasma. The ratio between antibodies titers in serum and CSF paired samples may suggest local synthesis of antibodies (72,105). The search of Junin virus by isolation attempts (even by the most sensitive test, such as co-cultivation) and RT-PCR from blood, lymphoid tissues and CSF has been consistently negative. The higher titers of NT antibodies and the CSF–serum ratio in LNS cases may suggest the possibility of a more prolonged antigenic stimulation, probably through a longer persistence of the virus or antigens at the CNS. Although the interval free of symptoms had led to the consideration of the LNS as a post-infectious encephalomyelitis, the absence of lesion in the white matter, as shown by MRI, has ruled out this possibility (87).

Lassa fever has a similar pathogenesis as South American hemorrhagic fevers. Although platelet counts do not fall to the low levels found in the other arenaviral hemorrhagic fevers, an extensive inhibition of platelet aggregation mediated by soluble serum factors is found (83,91). There is a rapid B-cell response to Lassa virus, with a classic IgG and IgM antibody responses that often coexist with high viremia in both humans and primates. Neutralizing antibodies appear late in the course of illness, and their levels are low. Thus, the clearance of Lassa virus and the recovery of infection are not mediated by antibody, and presumably depend on CMI response. In experimental models, a lack of protection with passive transfer of antibodies has been shown; and splenic cell transfer was linked to clearance of viremia and survival. On the contrary, the sensorineural deafness during convalescence has been suggested to be the result of an immune-mediated injury (61).

11. TREATMENT

11.1. Specific Treatment

For AHF, a specific treatment is available and consists of the transfusion of immune plasma upon a standardized amount of neutralizing antibodies to Junin virus. Immune plasma reduces the case-fatality rate from 15–30% to less than 1% provided that it is transfused during the first 8 days from onset of symptoms, but is of no benefit to patients when they are treated after the first week of illness (71,110). For the other South American hemorrhagic fevers, the specific treatment suggested is intravenous ribavirin. This may also prove useful in the treatment of AHF patients (110,111). For Lassa fever; also the specific treatment is the nucleoside analog ribavirin. Patients with poor prognostic indicators (high AST or viremia levels) should be treated intravenously, and the suggested dose is 30 mg/kg initially, 15 mg/kg every 6 hr for 4 days, and 7.5 mg/kg every 8 hr for six more days. Oral ribavirin in less severe form has also shown efficacy. There are evidences indicating that is more effective when given early in the course of illness (112–114).

11.2. General Supportive Measures

Supportive treatment consists of adequate hydration, symptomatic measures, and proper management of the neurological alterations, blood losses, shock, and superimposed infections. There is no specific indication for the use of steroids. Medication should be given by the oral or intravenous route. Intramuscular and subcutaneous injections are contraindicated because of the risk of hematomas.

In the AHF endemic area, several observations have been made: pneumonia is the most common secondary bacterial infection and is often accompanied by radiographic changes and an increase in fever, but not by leukocytosis; it usually responds to ampicillin. Other common secondary infection is oral candidosis that is treated with nystatin. Platelet transfusions have been used, but the complex nature of the coagulopathy and clinical experience suggest they are not useful. Transfusions are needed occasionally, but most of the severe forms are neurological. It is useful to sedate agitated patients with diphenhydramine or diazepam; diazepam also provides some protection against seizures. Seizures are generally treated with phenytoin. Cerebral edema may require both steroids and mannitol.

12. BIOSAFETY MEASURES

The patients with arenaviral hemorrhagic fevers are viremic during the acute period and the virus can be transmitted by parental inoculation. The South American hemorrhagic fevers are not considered highly contagious in the endemic areas where they occur. Nosocomial transmission has not been described for AHF, but was observed at least in one outbreak for BHF. Nevertheless, unusual patients capable of disseminating both Junin and Machupo viruses to hospital staff and families have been described. Nosocomial transmission of Lassa fever has been also reported. The absence of parental precautions has caused serious epidemics in African hospitals. Moreover, transmission to hospital staff or other patients was related to close contact with infected secretions, blood or tissues from hospitalized patients with Lassa fever. There is no credible epidemiologic evidence of airborne transmission (115–119).

Outside the endemic area where they occur, it is suggested to use small-particle aerosol precautions to treat these patients, but emphasizing that the most important measures would be those preventing parenteral and droplet exposure to blood and body fluids.

During convalescence, patients are not generally contagious. Hemorrhagic fever patients have transmitted virus to spouses sometimes during convalescence. Thus, intimate contact should be limited and condoms should be used during sex for at least 1 month. Lassa virus has been isolated from urine for several weeks and the use of disinfectant in the toilet before voiding is advised. For the manipulation of potentially infected samples in the laboratory, biosafety-2 measures are adequate. However, in all procedures capable of aerosol production, the use of biosafety cabinet is indicated. Virus cultures should be handled under biosafety level 3 and outside the respective endemic areas, under biosafety level 4. All persons working in relation to Junin virus should be immune. Candid #1 live attenuated Junin virus vaccine is available for seronegative personnel. The same consideration would be considered for personnel working with Machupo virus.

13. PREVENTION AND CONTROL

Rodent control has been successful in the control of BHF outbreaks occurring in towns, but sporadic cases still occur after rural exposure or contact with a case (120). The control of the rodent reservoir of Junin virus is impractical given the large geographic zones involved and the difficulties of intervening in local agricultural economies. Control of human contact with rodents is also not feasible. For this reason, almost since the discovery of the disease, all efforts for prevention have been directed toward the development of a vaccine (121).

The remarkable progress achieved with the discovery of the XJ Clone 3 vaccine candidate in the 1960s, prompted the development of a live attenuated Junin virus vaccine through the effort of an international collaborative project initiated in the late 1970s. Candid #1 vaccine was the final result of this project. Candid #1, the first vaccine against an arenavirus, was shown to be safe, highly immunogenic and effective for the prevention of AHF. Moreover, Candid #1 showed promise in preventing two natural arenaviral hemorrhagic fevers and thus potentially diminishing the medical significance of Junin and Machupo viruses as bioterrorism agents (122,123). Vaccination of high-risk population corroborated the results obtained in phases I, II, and III trials, and indicated that the vaccine will also be immunogenic under field conditions. Studies of antibody persistence showed stability of antibody positivity for at least 10 years after immunization. The long-term protection afforded by only one dose of Candid #1 argues in favor of its excellence for the control of AHF.

The observed changes in the current profile of AHF cases attributable to the impact of selected vaccination of high risk people, is indicative that a broader strategy of vaccination to protect the whole population at risk should be evaluated. This objective could be accomplished with a full operation of vaccine production facilities at the INEVH, in Pergamino, Argentina. With sufficient supplies of Candid #1 vaccine, the definitive control of AHF may be envisioned. However, the disease cannot be eradicated because Junin virus reservoirs are rodents, and even with good vaccine coverage, small outbreaks and isolated AHF cases may be expected (123).

The widespread control of the *Mastomys* species reservoir of Lassa virus in West Africa is also unfeasible as a broad approach for controlling the illness. The improvement of housing, and the educational campaigns to avoid rodents as food source, and for proper food storage might reduce the domestic rodent population. Rodent trapping in villages with a high transmission rate may have some impact on disease outbreaks. Barrier nursing in affected hospitals should be emphasized as well as adequate burial procedures of fatal cases. The control of Lassa fever in Africa will only be achieved with the availability of an effective vaccine. The studies of potential vaccines to Lassa fever began in the 1980s, through the development of a recombinant vaccine candidate using vaccinia vector. This approach gave promising results in experimental models, but the use of inactivated candidates has not been successful. Available evidence suggests that a successful vaccine against Lassa fever should induce protective cellular immune responses (124–126).

ACKNOWLEDGMENTS

The author wishes to thank Adriana Salas, Mara Eraso, and Marcelo Biglieri for their secretarial assistance.

REFERENCES

1. Clegg JCS, Bowen MP, Buchmeier MJ, Gonzalez JP, Lukashevich IS, Peters CJ, Rico-Hesse R, Romanowsky V. Family Arenaviridae. In: van Regenmortel MHV, Fuquet CM, Bishop DHL, Carstens EB, Estes MK, Lemon SM, Maniloff J, Mayo MA, McGeoch DJ, Pringle CR, Wickner RB, eds. Virus Taxonomy. Seventh Report of the International Committee on Taxonomy of Viruses. Orlando: Academic Press, 2000.

2. Rowe WP, Pugh WE, Webb PA, Peters CJ. Serological relationship of the Tacaribe complex of viruses to lymphocytic choriomeningitis virus. J Virol 1970; 5:289–292.

3. Casals J, Buckley SM, Cedeno R. Antigenic properties of the arenaviruses. Bull World Health Organ 1975; 52:421–427.

4. Wulff H, Lange JV, Webb PA. Interrelationships among arenaviruses measured by indirect immunofluorescence. Intervirology 1978; 9:344–350.

5. Bowen MD, Peters CJ, Nichol ST. The phylogeny of New World (Tacaribe complex) arenaviruses. Virology 1996; 219:285–290.

6. Charrel RN, Feldman H, Fullhorst CF, Khelifa R, de Chesse R, de Lamballerie X. Phylogeny of New World arenaviruses based on the complete coding sequences of the small genomic segment identified an evolutionary lineage produced by intrasegmental recombination. Biochem Biophys Res Commun 2002; 296:1118–1124.

7. Pedersen IR. Structural components and replication of arenaviruses. Adv Virus Res 1979; 24:277–330.

8. Buchmeier MJ, Clegg JCS, Franze-Fernanadez MT. Family Arenaviridae. In: Fauquet FA, Fauquet CM, Bishop DHL, eds. Virus Taxonomy: Sixth Report of the International Committee on Taxonomy of Viruses. New York: Springer Verlag, 1995:319–323.

9. Peters CJ. Arenaviruses. In: Horzinek MC, Osterhaus ADME, eds. Viral Infections of Vertebrates, Virus Infections of Rodents and Lagomorphs. Vol. 5. Amsterdam: Elsevier, 1994:321–341.

10. Rowe WP, Murphy FA, Bergold GH, Casals J, Hotchin J, Johnson KM, Lehman-Grube F, Mims CA, Traub E, Webb PA. Arenaviruses: proposed name for a newly defined virus group. J Virol 1970; 5:651–652.

11. Southern PJ. Arenaviridae: the viruses and their replication. In: Fields BN, Knipe DM, Howley PM, eds. Fields Virology. 3rd ed. Philadelphia: Lippincott Raven, 1996:1505–1519.

12. Auperin DD, Galinski M, Bishop DH. The sequences of the N protein and intergenic region of the S-RNA of Pichinde arenavirus. Virology 1984; 134:208–219.

13. Salvato MS, Shimomaye EM. The completed sequence of lymphocytic choriomeningitis virus reveals a unique RNA structure and a gene for a zinc finger protein. Virology 1989; 173:1–10.

14. Iapalucci S, Lopez N, Franze-Fernandez MT. The 3', end termini of the Tacaribe arenavirus subgenomic RNAs. Virology 1991; 182:269–278.

15. Wilson SM, Clegg JC. Sequence analysis of the S RNA of the African arenavirus Mopeia: an unusual secondary structure feature in the intergenic region. Virology 1991; 180:543–552.

16. Meyer BJ, Southern PJ. Concurrent sequence analysis of 5' and 3' RNA termini by intramolecular circulanzation reveals 5' nontemplated bases and 3' terminal hetero-

geneity for lymphocytic choriomeningitis virus mRNAs. J Virol 1993; 67:2621–2627.

17. Bishop DHL. Arenaviridae and their replication. In: Fields BN, Knipe DM, Howley PM, eds. Virology. 2nd ed. New York: Raven Press, 1990:1231–1243.

18. Meyer BJ, de la Torre JC, Southern PJ. Arenavirus: genomic RNAs, transcription and replication. In: Oldstone MBA, ed. Arenavirus I: The Epidemiology, Molecular and Cell Biology of Arenaviruses. New York: Springer Verlag, 2002:139–158.

19. Johnson KM, Wiebenga NH, MacKenzie RB. Virus isolations from human cases of hemorrhagic fever in Bolivia. Proc Soc Exp Biol Med 1965; 118:113–118.

20. Van der Groen G, Webb PA, Johnson KM, Lange SV, Lindsay H, Elliott L. Growth of Lassa and Ebola viruses in different cell lines. In: Pattyn SR, ed. Ebola Virus Hemorrhagic Fever. Amsterdam: Elsevier/North Holland, 1978.

21. Howard CR. Arenaviruses. Amsterdam: Elsevier, 1986:23–46.

22. Sabattini MS, Gonzalez de Rios LE, Diaz G, Vega VR. Infección natural y experimental de roedores con virus Junin. Medicina (B Aires) 1977; 37:149–161.

23. Webb PA, Justines G, Johnson KM. Infection of wild and laboratory animals with Machupo and Latino viruses. Bull World Health Organ 1975; 52:493–499.

24. Weissenbacher MC, Laguens RP, Coto CE. Argentine hemorrhagic fever. Curr Top Microbiol Immunol 1987; 134:79–116.

25. Buchmeier MJ, Welsh RM, Dutko FJ. The virology and immunobiology of lymphocytic choriomeningitis virus infection. Adv Immunol 1980; 30:275–331.

26. Oldstone MBA. Biology and pathogenesis of lymphocytic choriomeningitis virus infections. In: Oldstone MBA, ed. Arenaviruses II: The Molecular Pathogenesis of Arenavirus Infections. New York: Springer-Verlag, 2002:83–117.

27. Contigiani MS, Sabattini MS. Virulencia diferencial de cepas de virus Junin por marcadores biológicos en ratones y cobayos. Medicina (B Aires) 1977; 37:244–251.

28. Kenyon RH, Green DE, Maiztegui JI, Peters CJ. Viral strain dependent differences in experimental Argentine hemorrhagic fever (Junin virus) infection of guinea pigs. Intervirology 1988; 29:133–143.

29. McKee KT Jr, Mahlandt BG, Maiztegui JI, Eddy GA, Peters CJ. Experimental Argentine hemorrhagic fever in rhesus macaques: virus strain dependent clinical response. J Infect Dis 1985; 152:218–221.

30. Green DE, Mahlandt BG, McKee KT Jr. Experimental Argentine hemorrhagic fever in rhesus macaques: virus specific variations in pathology. J Med Virol 1987; 22:113–133.

31. Weissenbacher MC, Calello MA, Colillas OJ, Rondinone SN, Frigerio MJ. Argentine hemorrhagic fever: a primate model. Intervirology 1979; 1:363–365.

32. Walker DH, Johnson KM, Lange JV, Gardner JJ, Kiley MP, McCormick JB. Experimental infection of rhesus monkeys with Lassa virus and a closely related arenavirus, Mozambique virus. J Infect Dis 1982; 146:360–368.

33. Walker DH, Murphy FA. Pathology and pathogenesis of arenavirus infections. Curr Top Microbiol Immunol 1987; 133:89–113.

34. Childs JC, Peters CJ. Ecology and epidemiology of arenaviruses and their hosts. In: Salvato MS, ed. The Arenaviridae. New York: Plenum Press, 1993:331–373.

35. Salazar-Bravo J, Ruedas LA, Yates TL. Mammalian reservoirs of arenaviruses. In: Oldstone MBA, ed. Arenavirus I: The Epidemiology, Molecular and Cell Biology of Arenaviruses. New York: Springer-Verlag, 2002:25–64.

36. Bowen MD, Peters CJ, Nichol ST. Phylogenetic analysis of the Arenaviridae: patterns of virus evolution and evidence for cospeciation between arenaviruses and their rodent hosts. Mol Phylogenet Evol 1997; 8:301–316.

37. Sabattini MS, Contigiani MS. Ecological and biological factors influencing the maintenance of arenaviruses in nature, with special reference to the agent of Argentinean haemorrhagic fever. In: International Symposium on Tropical Arboviruses and Haemorrhagic Fevers, Belem, Brazil, April 14–18, 1980. Rio de Janeiro: Academia Brasileira de Ciencias, 1982:251–262.

38. Mills JN, Ellis BA, Childs JE, McKee KT, Maiztegui JI, Peters CJ, Ksiazek TG, Jahrling PB. Prevalence of infection with Junin virus in rodent populations in the epidemic area of Argentine hemorrhagic fever. Am J Trop Med Hyg 1994; 51:554–562.

39. Vitullo AD, Hodara V V, Merani MS. Vertical transmission of Junin virus in experimentally infected adult Calomys musculinus. Intervirology 1990; 31:339–344.

40. Fulhorst CF, Bowen MD, Salas RA, Duno G, Utrera A, Ksiazek TG, de Manzione NMC, de Miller E, Vázquez C, Peters CJ, Tesh RB. Natural rodent host associations of Guanarito and Pirital viruses (family Arenaviridae) in central Venezuela. Am J Trop Med Hyg 1999; 61:325–330.

41. Traub E. Epidemiology of lymphocytic choriomeningitis in a mouse stock observed for four years. J Exp Med 1939; 69:801–817.

42. Danes L, Benda R, Fuchsova M. Experimental inhalation infection with the lymphocytic choriomeningitis virus (WE strain) of the monkeys of the Macacus cynomolgus and Macaccus rhesus species. Bratisl Lek Listy 1963; 43:21–34.

43. Stephenson EH, Larson EW, Dominik JW. Effect of environmental factors on aerosol-induced Lassa virus infection. J Med Virol 1984; 14:295–303.

44. Kenyon RH, McKee KT Jr, Zack PM. Aerosol infection of rhesus macaques with Junin virus. Intervirology 1992; 33:23–31.

45. Sabattini MS, Maiztegui JI. Adelantos en Medicina: Fiebre Hemorrágica Argentina. Medicina (B Aires) 1970; 30(suppl 1): 111–128.

46. Briggiler AM, Enria D, Feuillade MR, Maiztegui JI. Contagio interhumano e infección inaparente por virus Junin en matrimonios del área endémica de fiebre hemorrágica Argentina. Medicina (B Aires) 1987; 47:565.

47. Johnson KM, Halstead SB, Cohen SN. Hemorrhagic fevers of South-east Asia and South America: a comparative appraisal. Prog Med Virol 1967; 9:105–158.

48. Kuns ML. Epidemiology of Machupo virus infection. II. Ecological and control studies of hemorrhagic fever. Am J Trop Med Hyg 1965; 14:813–816.

49. Peters CJ, Kuehne RW, Mercado R, Le Bow RH, Spertzel RO, Webb PA. Hemorrhagic fever in Cochabamba, Bolivia, 1971. Am J Epidemiol 1974; 99:425–433.

50. Kilgore PE, Peters CJ, Mills JN. Prospects for the control of Bolivian hemorrhagic fever. Emerg Infect Dis 1995; 1:97–100.

51. de Manzione N, Salas RA, Paredes H. Venezuelan hemorrhagic fever: clinical and epidemiologic studies of 165 cases. Clin Infect Dis 1998; 26:308–313.

52. Keenlyside RA, McCormick JB, Webb PA, Smith E, Elliott L, Johnson KM. Case–control study of Mastomys natalensis and humans in Lassa virus infected households in Sierra Leone. Am J Trop Med Hyg 1983; 32:829–837.

53. Maiztegui JI, Feuillade MR, Briggiler AM. Progressive extension of the endemic area and changing incidence of Argentine hemorrhagic fever. Med Microbiol Immunol 1986; 175:149–152.

54. Salas R, de Manzione N, Tesh RB. Venezuelan hemorrhagic fever. Lancet 1991; 338:1033–1036.

55. Coimbra TLM, Nassar ES, Burattini MN. New arenavirus isolated in Brazil. Lancet 1994; 343:391–392.

56. McCormick JB, Webb PA, Krebs JW. A prospective study of the epidemiology and ecology of Lassa fever. J Infect Dis 1987; 155:437–444.

57. Enria DA, Briggiler AM, Feuillade MR. An overview of the epidemiological, ecological and preventive hallmarks of Argentine haemorrhagic fever (Junin virus). Bull Inst Pasteur 1998; 96:103–114.

58. Vasconcelos PFC, Travassos da Rosa APA, Rodrigues SG. Infeccao humana pelo virus SP 114202 (Arenavirus: familia Arenaviridae): Aspectos clinicos e laboratorais de uma nova doenca. Rev Inst Med Trop Sao Paulo 1994; 35:521–525.

59. Barry M, Russi M, Armstrong L. Treatment of a laboratory-acquired Sabia virus infection. N Engl J Med 1995; 333:294–296.

60. McCormick JB, King IJ, Webb PA. A case–control study of the clinical diagnosis and course of Lassa fever. J Infect Dis 1987; 155:445–455.

61. McCormick JB, Fisher-Hoch SP. Lassa fever. In: Oldstone MBA, ed. Arenavirus I: The Epidemiology, Molecular and Cell Biology of Arenaviruses. New York: Springer-Verlag, 2002:75–110.

62. Maiztegui JI, Sabattini MS. Extensión progresiva del área endémica de Fiebre hemorrágica Argentina. Medicina (B Aires) 1977; 37(suppl 3):162–166.

63. de Villafañe G, Kravetz FO, Donadio O, Persich R, Knecher L, Torrs MP, Fernández N. Dinámica de las comunidades de roedores en agroecosistemas pampásicos. Medicina (B Aires) 1977; 37:128–140.

64. Crespo JA. Relaciones entre estados climáticos y la ecología de algunos roedores de campo (cricetidae). Rev Argent Zoogeográfica (B Aires) 1944; 41, 137–144.

65. Mills JN, Ellis BA, McKee KT, Maiztegui JI, Childs JE. Habitat associations and relative densities of rodent populations in cultivated areas of central Argentina. J Mammol 1991; 72:470–479.

66. Ellis BA, Mills JN, Childs JE, Muzzini MC, McKee KT, Enria DA, Glass GE. Structure and floristics of habitats associated with five rodent species in an agroecosystem in central Argentina. J Zool Lond 1997; 243:437–460.

67. Mills JN, Ellis BA, McKee KT, Calderon GE, Maiztegui JI, Nelson GO, Ksiazek TG, Peters CJ, Childs JE. A longitudinal study of Junin virus activity in the rodent reservoir of Argentine hemorrhagic fever. Am J Trop Med Hyg 1992; 47:749–763.

68. García JB, Morzunov SP, Levis S, Rowe J, Calderón G, Enria DA, Sabattini MS, Buchmeier MJ, Bowen MD, St. Jeor S. Genetic diversity of Junin virus in Argentina: geographic and temporal patterns. Virology 2000; 272(suppl 1):127–136.

69. Musser GG, Carleton MD. Family Muridae. In: Wilson DE, Reeder DM, eds. Mammal Species of the World, a Taxonomic and Geographic Reference. Washington, DC: Smithsonian Institution, 1993:501–755.

70. Maiztegui JI. Clinical and epidemiological patterns of Argentine hemorrhagic fever. Bull World Health Organ 1975; 52:567–575.

71. Maiztegui JI, Fernández NJ, Damilano AJ. Efficacy of immune plasma in treatment of Argentine haemorrhagic fever and association between treatment and a late neurological syndrome. Lancet 1979; 2:1216–1217.

72. Enria DA, de Damilano AJ, Briggiler AM, Ambrosio AM, Fernández NJ, Feuillade MR, Maiztegui JI. Sindrome neurologico tardio en enfermos de fiebre hemorrágica Argentina tratados con plasma immune. Medicina (B Aires) 1985; 45:615–620.

73. Biquard C, Figini HA, Monteverde DA, Somoza MJ, Alvarez F. Neurological manifestations in Argentine hemorrhagic fever. Medicina (B Aires) 1977; 37(suppl 3):193–199.

74. Enria DA, Briggiler AM, Levis S, Vallejos D, Maiztegui JI, Canonico PG. Tolerance and antiviral effect of ribavirin in patients with Argentine hemorrhagic fever. Antiviral Res 1987; 7:353–359.

75. Frame JD. Clinical features of Lassa fever in Liberia. Rev Infect Dis 1989; 2:S783–S789.

76. Frame JD, Baldwin JM, Gocke DJ, Troup JM. Lassa fever, a new virus disease of man from West Africa. I. Clinical description and pathological findings. Am J Trop Med Hyg 1970; 19:670–676.

77. Mertens PE, Patton R, Baum JJ, Monath TP. Clinical presentation of Lassa fever cases during the hospital epidemic at Zorzor, Liberia, March–April 1972. Am J Trop Med Hyg 1973; 22:780–784.

78. Monath TP, Maher M, Casals J, Kissling RE, Cacciapuoti A. Lassa fever in the Eastern Province of Sierra Leone, 1970–1972. II. Clinical observations and virological studies on selected hospital cases. Am J Trop Med Hyg 1974; 23:1140–1149.

79. Peters CJ, Zaki SR, Rollin PE. Viral hemorrhagic fevers. In: Fekety R, Mandell GL, eds. Atlas of Infectious Diseases. Vol. 8. External Manifestations of Systemic Infections. Philadelphia: Current Medicine, 1997:10.1–10.26.

80. Solbrig MV, McCormick JB. Lassa fever: central nervous system manifestations. J Trop Geogr Neurol 1991; 1:23–30.

81. Solbrig MV. Lassa virus and central nervous system diseases. In: Salvato MS, ed. The Arenaviridae. New York: Plenum Press, 1993:325–330.

82. Cummins D, McCormick JB, Bennett D. Acute sensorineural deafness in Lassa fever. JAMA 1990; 264:2093–2096.

83. Fisher-Hoch S, McCormick JB, Sasso D. Hematologic dysfunction in Lassa fever. J Med Virol 1988; 26:127–135.

84. Cummins D, Bennett D, Fisher-Hoch SJ. Electrocardiographic abnormalities in patients with Lassa fever. J Trop Med Hyg 1989; 92:350–355.

85. D'Avino P, Enria D, Briggiler A, Vallejos D, Maiztegui J, Sica REP. Velocidad de conducción nerviosa periférica en pacientes con Fiebre Hemorrágica Argentina (FHA). Medicina (B Aires) 1987; 47(suppl 6):565–566.

86. Cristiano E, Huerta M, D'Avino P, Enria D, Briggiler A, Maiztegui J. Potenciales evocados auditivos de tronco cerebral en períodos alejados de la Fiebre Hemorrágica Argentina (FHA). Medicina (B Aires) 1985; 45(suppl 4):409.

87. Nagel J, Enria, Briggiler A, Maiztegui J. Resonancia magné tica nuclear del nervioso central en la Fiebre Hemorrágica Argentina (FHA). XXXI Congreso Argentino de Neurología, Rosario, Octubre 14–17, 1992. Libro de Resúmenes, 1992:89.

88. Peters CJ, Webb PA, Johnson KM. Measurement of antibodies to Machupo virus by the indirect fluorescent technique. Proc Soc Exp Biol Med 1972; 142:526–531.

89. Peters CJ, Jahrling PB, Liu CT. Experimental studies of arenaviral hemorrhagic fevers. Curr Top Microbiol Immunol 1987; 134:5–68.

90. Ambrosio AM, Enria DA, Maiztegui JI. Junin virus isolation from lymphomononuclear cells of patients with Argentine hemorrhagic fever. Intervirology 1986; 25:97–102.

91. Zaki SR, Peters CJ. Viral hemorrhagic fevers. In: Connor DH, Chandler FW, Schwartz DA, eds. The Pathology of Infectious Diseases. Norwalk, CT: Appleton & Lange, 1997:347–364.

92. Peters CJ. Human infection with arenaviruses in the Americas. In: Oldstone MBA, ed. Arenaviruses I: The Epidemiology, Molecular and Cell Biology of Arenaviruses. New York: Springer-Verlag, 2002:65–74.

93. Elsner B, Schwarz ER, Mando OG. Pathology of 12 fatal cases of Argentine hemorrhagic fever. Am J Trop Med Hyg 1973; 22:229–236.

94. Child PL, MacKenzie RB, Johnson KM. Bolivian hemorrhagic fever. A pathologic description. Arch Pathol 1967; 83:434–445.

95. Walker DH, McCormick JB, Johnson KM. Pathologic and virologic study of fatal Lassa fever in man. Am J Pathol 1982; 107:349–356.

96. Shieh W-J, Greer PW, Ruo SL. Lassa fever: an immunopathologic study with pathogenetic and diagnostic implications (abstract). Lab Invest 1997; 76:141A.

97. Maiztegui JI, Laguens RP, Cossio PM, Casanova MB, de la Vega MT, Ritacco V, Segal A, Fernández NJ, Arana RM. Ultrastructural and immunohistochemical studies in five cases of Argentine hemorrhagic fever. J Infect Dis 1975; 132:35–43.

98. Gonzalez PH, Cossio PM, Arana RM, Maiztegui JI, Laguens RP. Lymphatic tissue in Argentine hemorrhagic fever. Arch Pathol Lab Med 1980; 104:250–254.

99. Cossio P, Laguens R, Arana R, Segal A, Maiztegui J. Ultrastructural and immunohistochemical study of the human kidney in Argentine haemorrhagic fever. Virchows Arch 1975; 368:1–9.

100. Ponzinibio C, Gonzalez PH, Maiztegui JI, Laguens RP. Estudio morfológico de la médula ósea humana en Fiebre Hemorrágica Argentina. Medicina (B Aires) 1979; 39:441–446.

101. De Bracco MME, Rimoldi MT, Cossio PM, Rabinovich A, Maiztegui J, Caraballal G, Arana R. Argentine hemorrhagic fever. Alterations of the complement system and anti-Junin-virus humoral response. N Engl J Med 1978; 299:216–221.

102. Molinas FC, de Bracco MME, Maiztegui JI. Coagulation studies in Argentine hemorrhagic fever. J Infect Dis 1981; 143:1–6.

103. Molinas FC, Maiztegui JI. Factor VIII: C and Factor VIII R: Ag in Argentine hemorrhagic fever. Thromb Haemost 1981; 46(2):525–527.

104. Heller MV, Marta RF, Sturk A, Maiztegui JI, Hack CE, ten Cate JW, Molinas FC. Early markers of blood coagulation and fibrinolysis activation in Argentine hemorrhagic fever. Thromb Haemost 1995; 73:368–373.

105. Enria D, Garcia Franco S, Ambrosio A, Vallejos D, Levis S, Maiztegui JI. Current status of the treatment of Argentine hemorrhagic fever with immune plasma. Med Microbiol Immunol 1986; 175:169–172.

106. Vallejos DA, Ambrosio AM, Feuillade MR, Maiztegui JI. Lymphocyte subsets alteration in patients with Argentine hemorrhagic fever. J Med Virol 1989; 27:160–163.

107. Levis SC, Saavedra MC, Ceccoli C, Feuillade MR, Enria DA, Maiztegui JI, Falcoff R. Correlation between endogenous interferon and the clinical evolution of patients with Argentine hemorrhagic fever. J Interferon Res 1985; 5:383–389.

108. Heller MV, Saavedra MC, Falcoff R, Maiztegui JI, Molinas FC. Increased tumor necrosis factor-alpha levels in Argentine hemorrhagic fever (letter). J Infect Dis 1992; 166:1203–1204.

109. Saavedra M, Feuillade M, Levis S, Maiztegui JI, Haas E. Antigenos de histocompatibilidad en la Fiebre Hemorrágica Argentina. Medicina (B Aires) 1985; 45:342.

110. Enria D, Maiztegui JI. Antiviral treatment of Argentine hemorrhagic fever. Antiviral Res 1994; 23:23–31.

111. Kilgore PE, Ksiazek TG, Rollin PE. Treatment of Bolivian hemorrhagic fever with intravenous ribavirin. J Infect Dis 1997; 24:718–722.

112. Jahrling PB, Hesse RA, Eddy GA, Johnson KM, Callis RT, Stephen EL. Lassa fever infection in rhesus monkeys. Pathogenesis and treatment with ribavirin. J Infect Dis 1980; 141:580–589.

113. McCormick JB, King IJ, Webb PA, Scribner CS, Craven RB, Johnson KM, Elliott LH. Lassa fever. Effective therapy with ribavirin. N Engl J Med 1986; 314:20–26.

114. Fisher-Hoch SP, Gborie S, Parker L. Unexpected adverse reactions during a clinical trial in rural West Africa. Antiviral Res 1992; 19:139–147.

115. Helmick CG, Webb PA, Scribner CL, Krebs JW, McCormick JB. No evidence for increased risk of Lassa fever infection in hospital staff. Lancet 1986; 8517:1202–1205.

116. Peters CJ, Jahrling PB, Khan AS. Management of patients infected with high-hazard viruses: scientific basis for infection control. Arch Virol 1996; 11(suppl):1–28.

117. Management of patients with suspected viral hemorrhagic fever. MMWR Morb Mortal Wkly Rep 1988; 37:1–15.

118. Update: management of patients with suspected viral hemorrhagic fever—United States. MMWR Morb Mortal Wkly Rep 1995; 44:475–479.

119. Douglas RG, Wiebenga NH, Couch RB. Bolivian hemorrhagic fever probably transmitted by personal contact. Am J Epidemiol 1965; 82:85–91.

120. Mercado RR. Rodent control programmes in areas affected by Bolivian haemorrhagic fever. Bull World Health Organ 1975; 52:691–696.

121. de Guerrero LB. Vacunas experimentales contra la Fiebre Hemorrágica Argentina. Medicina (B Aires) 1977; 37(suppl 3):252–259.

122. Barrera-Oro JG, Eddy GE. Characteristics of candidate live attenuated Junin virus vaccine. In: Kurstak E, Marusyk RG, Maramorosch K, eds. Presented at Fourth International Conference on Comparative Virology, Banff, Canada, October 17–22, 1982:S4–S10.

123. Enria DA, Barrera Oro JG. Junin virus vaccines. In: Oldstone MBA, ed. Arenaviruses II. The Molecular Pathogenesis of Arenavirus Infections. New York: Springer-Verlag. Curr Top Microbiol Immunol 2002; 263:239–264.

124. Auperin DD. Construction and evaluation of recombinant virus vaccines for Lassa fever. In: Salvato MS, ed. The Arenaviridae. New York: Plenum Press, 1993:259–280.

125. Clegg, JCS, Sanchez A. Vaccines against arenaviruses and filoviruses. In: Levine MM, Woodrow GC, Kaper JB, eds. New Generation Vaccines. 2nd ed. New York: Marcel Dekker, 1997:749–765.

126. Whitton JL. Designing arenaviral vaccines. In: Oldstone MBA, ed. Arenaviruses II: The Molecular Pathogenesis of Arenavirus Infections. New York: Springer-Verlag, 2002:221–238.

6

Cerebral Malaria

Nicholas Day

Director, Wellcome Trust, Oxford Tropical Medicine Research Programme, Faculty of Tropical Medicine, Mahidol University, Mahidol, Thailand; and Honorary Consultant Physician, Nuffield Department of Clinical Medicine, University of Oxford, John Radcliffe Hospital, Headington, Oxford, U.K.

1. INTRODUCTION

Malaria caused by the mosquito-borne protozoan parasite *Plasmodium falciparum* is the most important parasitic disease of man, infecting between 300 and 400 million people annually, and causing an estimated 1.1 million deaths in sub-Saharan Africa alone. Most of these deaths are in children, many of whom succumb to the severe "cerebral" form of the disease, which has a mortality of 15–20%. Thus falciparum malaria is the commonest and potentially the most serious parasitic infection of the human central nervous system (CNS), and cerebral malaria is arguably the most common non-traumatic encephalopathy worldwide.

The coma that defines cerebral malaria is only one of a number of neurological manifestations of severe malaria, although it is undoubtedly the most important. Convulsions, the neurological consequences of hypoglycemia, and late post-malaria cerebellar syndromes and psychoses are all features of the disease. Nor is severe malaria solely a neurological condition. The clinical manifestations of falciparum malaria infection range from asymptomatic parasitemia to devastating multisystem failure encompassing coma, acute renal failure (ARF), jaundice, severe acidosis, and hemodynamic shock. The factors responsible for this diversity are not fully understood, but include the intensity of transmission in an area and the consequent level of immunity to infection.

Although this review will concentrate on the neurological aspects of falciparum malaria infection, it will also cover briefly the diagnosis, pathophysiology, and treatment of the non-neurological complications of the disease. "Pure" cerebral disease is rare, particularly in non-immune adults, and severe malaria must be thought of, investigated, and treated as a life-threatening multisystem disorder.

The burden of severe malaria falls overwhelmingly on developing countries which are ill-equipped to cope with the human and economic costs of the disease. The range of malaria has also extended in recent years, with severe malaria cases now commonplace in parts of India and Bangladesh from which malaria had previously been largely eradicated. With increasingly cheap international travel and the rise of "eco-tourism," cases of imported severe malaria are also seen more and more frequently in intensive care units in the developed world. Diagnosis in this setting may be dangerously delayed by failure of both primary care and hospital physicians to recognize this unfamiliar disease. Raising awareness of the clinical presentation of severe malaria, and of the ways in which cerebral malaria differs from other encephalopathies in both its pathophysiology, complications and treatment, will lead to earlier diagnosis, appropriate treatment and improvements in prognosis.

2. EPIDEMIOLOGY AND RISK FACTORS FOR SEVERE DISEASE

2.1. Malaria Transmission

Malaria transmission occurs through much of the tropical and parts of the subtropical world. To support transmission adequate densities of both the human host and vector have to be present, along with climatic conditions enabling sporogony to take place within the lifespan of the mosquito. If the temperature is too low sporogony is prolonged and the mosquitoes die before transmission can take place. For this reason transmission does not occur in temperate or cold climates or at altitudes greater than 2000 m.

Malaria transmission also depends on the ecology and habits of the vector. There are nearly 500 species in the genus *Anopheles*; around 70 are capable of transmitting malaria, though with greatly varying efficiency (1,2).

Behavior and response to infection of the human host plays a major role as well. In low transmission areas it is relatively non-immune adults venturing into scrubland or forest for economic purposes who are mainly responsible for the human part of the cycle, whereas in high transmission areas children have higher parasitemias and gametocytemias than the relatively immune adult population (3). They also bear the largest burden of disease, with one estimate from the Gambia that malaria causes around 25% of deaths in 1–4-year-olds (4). This may be an underestimate; in one study insecticide-impregnated bednets aimed at reducing malaria transmission were associated with 50% reduction of all-cause childhood mortality (5). However if children survive their early years in high transmission areas, they develop a degree of immunity to malaria, termed premonition. Premonition does not prevent infection, but controls it, such that with the notable exception of pregnant women adults in high transmission areas rarely suffer from severe disease (6).

2.2. Clinical Epidemiology

The most striking feature of the clinical epidemiology of severe malaria is the degree to which the clinical presentations change with age and geography. The geographical variation is probably due to a combination of transmission, human immunity and parasite factors. In Africa, in areas with moderate levels of transmission (ca. one infected mosquito bite per year), the predominant syndromes are cerebral malaria occurring in 3–7-year-old children, and severe anemia in slightly younger children (7). In high transmission areas in the same continent, with individuals receiving as many as one or two infected bites per day, the predominant syndrome is severe anemia in 1–3-year-olds and cerebral malaria is rare (8,9). However, one study of severe malaria in five different areas showed an inverse relationship between transmission intensity and the incidence of severe disease (10). In most of Africa severe malaria is absent in adults, and most infections are asymptomatic. Exceptions occur in areas where transmission is sporadic (11), and in cases where individuals leave a high transmission area and return several years later. In areas of low transmission, such as most of Asia, immunity is low or absent, and individuals of any age may develop a severe multisystem disease which may or may not include cerebral manifestations (12). Tourists from temperate countries venturing into any malaria endemic area worldwide are usually non-immune and fall into this category, though in low transmission areas the main victims are young adult migrant workers venturing into endemic areas for economic reasons.

2.3. Genetic Factors

A large number of genetic polymorphisms have now been associated with either resistance or susceptibility to severe malaria. The best known and the first group to be described are the inherited red cell disorders. These polymorphisms were first linked with malaria because their geographical distributions matched that of the disease, and it was postulated by Haldane in 1949 that heterozygote selection was responsible for their maintenance in the population (13). Heterozygotes for the variant hemoglobin S of sickle cell disease, Hb C, Hb E, and of the various α- and β- thalassemias have since been shown to protect against severe disease or death (14–17). The mechanisms behind these protective effects are currently under investigation.

Polymorphisms in genes involved in the host defense against malaria have also been implicated in determining susceptibility, suggesting that the immune response plays an important role in the pathogenesis of severe disease. At least three tumor necrosis factor (TNF-α) promotor polymorphisms have been associated with various types of severe disease in African children: the *TNF2* allele at the −308 position and the *TNF-376A* genotype have been associated with increased susceptibility to cerebral malaria (18,19), and the *TNF-238A* allele was associated with low TNF-α levels and severe anemia (20). Polymorphisms in HLA-B, HLA-DR, CD36 and ICAM-1 (both endothelial receptors mediating parasitized erythrocyte sequestration), CD40L, NOS type 2, the interferon gamma and alpha receptors, and the Fc gamma receptor CD32 have all been associated with variations in severe disease incidence (21–28). This large number of associations is a cause for concern, particularly as few have been repeatable in other populations. This lack of reproducibility may at least partly be caused by geographical differences in parasite-encoded virulence determinants, and by variation between human populations in genetic background, and hence through epistatic effects in susceptibility gene expression and penetrance. Linkage between apparent susceptibility loci may also partly explain the sheer number of associations described (29). That notwithstanding, it is clear that malaria has over the past 10,000 years or so exerted considerable selective pressure on the human populations it afflicts.

2.4. Acquired Risk Factors

2.4.1. Acquired Immunity

The immunological basis for the clinical phenomenon of premunition, described above, remains incompletely understood. In experimental systems it is clear that both antibody-dependent and antibody-independent (T-cell) immunity to the preerythrocytic stage can be induced by irradiated sporozoite challenge, and these are protective over short periods of time (30). In natural populations antisporozoite antibodies only appear around the age of 10 years (31), and immune adults have specific cytotoxic CD8$^+$ T cells in their peripheral blood (32,33).

The development of immunity to the asexual, erythrocytic, stage is complex and multifactorial. As clinical immunity develops a diverse repertoire of antibodies to parasitized erythrocyte surface antigens is built up (34). Most of these antibodies are generated against variants of *P. falciparum* erythrocyte membrane protein 1 (PfEMP1), a parasite-derived antigen on the surface of parasitized erythrocytes, which is involved in parasitized erythrocyte sequestration and in the pathogenesis of severe malaria (35,36). Antibodies are generated to specific PfEMP1 variants as they are encountered, and as the host repertoire increases the number of variants compatible with parasite survival in the semi-immune host is increasingly restricted (34). It has been hypothesized that by limiting the use by parasites of the most effective (and maybe the most virulent) PfEMP1 variants, the chance of severe disease, including cerebral malaria, is lessened (37,38). The acquired humoral immune response also includes the development of anti-merozoite antibodies, which cause agglutination of merozoites and inhibit erythrocyte invasion (39).

Although the asexual erythrocytic stage of the infection is not vulnerable to direct cytotoxic T-cell attack, as erythrocytes do not express HLA molecules, it has been hypothesized that T-cell priming by malaria infections in young children in endemic areas may substantially modify the immunopathology of subsequent infections, increasing their severity (40). The proposed mechanism involves priming of $\alpha\beta$ T cells leading to excessive production of interferon-γ (IFN-γ) and subsequent overproduction of TNF-α (41).

2.4.2. HIV

HIV infection and malaria coexist in many parts of the world, and given evidence that cellular immunity plays some role in protection against severe malaria (HLA associations at the population level, along with evidence of T-cell cytotoxicity against the liver stage of infection), there are theoretical grounds for believing that HIV co-infection will worsen the severity of malaria. Conversely malaria could hasten HIV progression. Conclusive evidence has been hard to come by, though recent studies do suggest a small but significant effect of HIV on malaria severity (42,43).

2.4.3. Parasite Factors

An increasing number of parasite virulence phenotypes are now being recognized as risk factors for severe malaria. The type of PfEMP1 antigen expressed by the parasite appears to play an important role; in one study expression a particular *var* gene product was associated with severe disease in West Africa (44), and in another PfEMP1 types from patients with cerebral malaria or severe anemia were found to be rare but commonly recognized by immune sera (37). The phenomenon of aggregation, in which parasitized red cells clump together in ex vivo cultures mediated by platelet CD36, is associated with severe malaria in African children (45).

3. CLINICAL FEATURES

3.1. General

Severe malaria occurs as part of spectrum of severity, with so-called uncomplicated malaria at one end and multiorgan failure at the other. In immune adults infection with malaria can be entirely asymptomatic. The proportion of acute malaria infections that progress to severe disease varies between areas and populations, and is greatly influenced by the availability of antimalarial treatment. In the Gambia it has been estimated that around one in 100 acute infections in children develop complications (46), and in adult malaria in Thailand the mortality is about one per 1000 (47,48).

As noted above the clinical presentation of severe disease also varies with age and geography, most notably between the two most studied groups, African children and Southeast Asian adults. The major differences between these two groups are outlined in Table 1. Multiorgan failure is much commoner in non-immune adults, and

Table 1   Severe Malaria: Differences Between African Children and Southeast Asian Adults

Feature	African children	Southeast Asian adults
Symptom duration before onset of complications	Typically 1–2 days	Often 4–5 days
Convulsions	Common; may occur without cerebral malaria	Uncommon. ; Usually usually a feature of cerebral malaria
Raised opening pressure on lumbar puncture	Common, and associated with poor outcome	Conflicting reports
Clinical syndrome of brainstem herniation	Well described	Rare
Renal failure	Very rare	Common (~30%), with ~10% requiring dialysis
Jaundice	Rare	Very common (~50%)
Hypoglycaemia	~40%, usually disease-related	~20%, often quinine-related
Coma duration in cerebral malaria following treatment	Usually 1 to –2 days	Usually 2–5 days
Rate of neurological sequelae post post-cerebral malaria	~10%	~1–2%

convulsions and neurological sequelae occur more frequently in children. Cerebral malaria, severe anemia and acidosis are features of both groups, though each form of the disease may vary in its presentation between the groups, possibly reflecting underlying differences in pathophysiology. Severe malaria tends not to occur in immune African adults from high transmission areas, and severe disease in Asian children has not been studied to the same extent as other groups. There is some evidence that as relatively young non-immune individuals they develop a syndrome midway between those seen in African children and Asian adults (49). As an example, dialysis-requiring renal failure occurs at an incidence of around 5%, compared with 0% in African children and 11% in non-immune adults (12,50) (D. Bethell, personal communication). "Cerebral malaria" appears to be systematically overdiagnosed clinically in both African adults and African children in endemic areas, probably because of the poor availability of blood film examination and the diagnostic means to exclude other causes of encephalitis (51,52).

3.2.   Cerebral Malaria and Other Neurological Manifestations

Cerebral malaria usually presents as a diffuse bilateral encephalitis, the major features of which are coma and convulsions. The causes of impairment of consciousness in severe malaria include "pure" cerebral malaria, convulsions and post-ictal states, hypoglycemia, uremia, severe acidosis, and hemodynamic shock). Although the "non-cerebral" causes of coma complicate any strict definition of cerebral malaria, in practice any patient with proven *P. falciparum* infection and impairment of consciousness, or other signs of cerebral dysfunction is severely ill, requiring intensive care monitoring, and parenteral anti-malarial therapy.

3.2.1. General Features of Cerebral Malaria

A strict definition of cerebral malaria requires the presence of asexual forms of *P. falciparum* on the peripheral blood film, unrousable coma which persists for at least 1 hr following a seizure, and exclusion of any other cause of encephalopathy (including bacterial meningitis and viral encephalopathies, common in much of the tropics) (53,54). Hypoglycemia should also be excluded. "Unrousable coma" in adults requires a best motor response on the Glasgow Coma Scale (GCS) of ≤3 (i.e., non-localizing) and best verbal response of ≤2 (at best incomprehensible sounds) (55). The eye opening part of the GCS is of limited value, as in cerebral malaria the eyes may remain open despite deep coma. In children a strict definition of cerebral malaria includes an inability to localize painful stimuli, which is difficult to assess in the very young. The Blantyre Coma Scale (Table 2), developed in Malawi specifically for cerebral malaria patients, is commonly used (cut-off score for defining cerebral malaria ≤2/5) though this is subject to a number of intrinsic inaccuracies (56,57). Older children can be assessed as adults using the GCS.

Focal neurological signs are unusual, though they are commoner in children, and when they occur hypoglycemia should be excluded as a cause. In cerebral malaria the time from the onset of febrile symptoms to onset of coma in African children is typically around 48 hr, considerably shorter than commonly seen in non-immune adults (56,58). They also regain consciousness more quickly, usually within 1–3 days (50,56). In adults coma usually resolves after 1–5 days (median ~2 days), but may occasionally continue for up to 2 weeks (12).

In profound coma conjugate gaze abnormalities, hypotonia, hypertonia, decorticate and decerebrate posturing (59), and opisthotonus may all occur

Table 2 Blantyre Coma Scale for Use in Children

Verbal	0:	No cry
	1:	Inappropriate cry or moan
	2:	Appropriate cry
Motor	0:	Non-specific or no response
	1:	Withdrawal from pain
	2:	Localises pain
Eye	0:	Not directed
	1:	Directed eye movements

(60,61). In true cerebral malaria abdominal reflexes are invariably absent. Death may be preceded by brainstem signs consistent with (but not necessarily caused by) brainstem herniation (62,63).

The marked meningism characteristic of bacterial meningitis with photophobia and board-like neck rigidity is rarely seen in adults with cerebral malaria (though mild neck stiffness can occur). In children assessment is difficult, and meningitis can easily be mistaken for cerebral malaria. Cerebrospinal fluid (CSF) examination is the gold standard, though worries about the risk of lumbar puncture (LP) in children with malaria have led some to recommend empirical antibiotic therapy in the comatose child. One feature of severe malaria which may help in the differential diagnosis is the frequent presence of retinal hemorrhages, which occur in both adults and children. These are usually flame shaped, often with a central pale area, and spare the macula. They are of both diagnostic and prognostic significance (52,64).

3.2.2. Convulsions

Convulsions are the commonest neurological manifestations of malaria in African children, and can occur either as part of cerebral malaria or as an independent entity. Over 70% of children with cerebral malaria have convulsions, and in one study 25% of those with seizures following admission had electroencephalographic (EEG) evidence of covert status epilepticus (65). In these children the clinical manifestations of seizure activity between overt fits was minimal and easily overlooked. The overall clinical condition of these children often improved dramatically with anticonvulsants treatment, suggesting that seizure activity may contribute significantly to the syndrome of "cerebral malaria." Poor outcome has been associated with initial EEG recordings showing very low frequency waves (0.5–3 Hz), background asymmetry, burst suppression, or interictal discharges (66).

In children infected with falciparum malaria without background impairment of consciousness seizures are also common, and although some of these may represent childhood febrile convulsions one study of Kenyan children presenting to hospital with convulsions and malaria 54% had rectal temperatures less than 38°C (67).

In non-immune adults convulsions are much less common than in children, occurring in around 20% of cases of cerebral malaria (12). Convulsions in the absence of impairment of consciousness are rare, and are not associated with episodes of hypoglycemia (12,67).

3.2.3. Hypoglycemia

Hypoglycemia is associated with severe malaria in both adults and children, and carries a poor prognosis (68,69). It can occur as a consequence of the severe anaerobic glycolysis, impaired gluconeogenesis, and high glucose turnover associated with severe malaria (68–73). It can also occur as a side effect of treatment, related to hyperinsulinemia caused by quinine or quinidine (68). Hypoglycemia of both etiologies is particularly common and refractory to treatment in pregnant women. The classical signs of hypoglycemia are often either absent or mistaken for clinical features of severe malaria itself (sweating, anxiety, confusion, and coma). If there is doubt and blood glucose measurement is not instantly available a therapeutic trial of 50% glucose should be administered immediately; if hypoglycemia is present this will often lead to a dramatic improvement in symptoms.

3.2.4. Neurological Sequelae

A proportion of African children who survive cerebral malaria develop long-term neurological complications. These include ataxia, cortical blindness, and hemiparesis, and represent a massive human and social burden. Sequelae have been clinically associated with protracted and deep coma, repeated convulsions, and hypoglycemia (74–77). The incidence of these complications has been underestimated but is probably over 20%, though this falls to <5% 6 months post-illness (77). There is conflicting evidence regarding the presence of persistent minor neuropsychiatric sequelae (78,79), and whether there is any long-term effect of cerebral malaria on the psychosocial and intellectual development of children is unknown. The vast majority of adults who survive cerebral malaria emerge from coma with no discernible residual neurological abnormalities.

3.2.5. Post-malaria Neurological Syndrome

Coma, seizures and neurological sequelae are not the only neurological manifestations of falciparum malaria. In Vietnamese adults a self-limiting "post-malaria neurological syndrome" has been described (80), in which patients presented with an acute confusional state, psychosis, seizures, or tremor a median (range) of 96 hr (6 hr to 60 days) after parasite clearance. In the Vietnam study it occurred in 0.12% of all falciparum malaria patients, but was 300 times more common following severe rather than uncomplicated malaria. In addition, in a randomized trial, it was significantly more likely to occur in patients given mefloquine to complete antimalarial treatment as opposed to the combination of quinine and sulfadoxine/pyrimethamine (80).

A syndrome of delayed cerebellar ataxia has been described following falciparum malaria in Sri Lanka and more recently in the Sudan (81,82). The ataxia is usually truncal, suggesting that midline cerebellar structures are predominantly affected. There is no impairment of consciousness, and symptoms resolve spontaneously a median (range) of 10 weeks (3–16) after their onset. In a recent prospective study of 441 Indian adults with cerebral malaria psychosis and cerebellar ataxia both occurred as post-malaria neurological syndromes in around 5% of patients (83).

Little is known about the pathophysiology of these post-infectious neurological conditions. Mefloquine appears to be associated with post-malaria psychosis and convulsions, and there is some evidence of an immunological mechanism for cerebellar ataxia. Compared with appropriate controls Sri Lankan patients with ataxia had significantly raised tumor necrosis factor and interleukin (IL)-6 in both serum and CSF (84). Radiological evidence of demyelination has also been associated with post-malaria cerebellar ataxia (85). What is clear from the literature is that the syndromes are invariably self-limiting, and the only treatment required is symptomatic and supportive.

3.3. Non-neurological Manifestations of Severe Malaria

3.3.1. Acidosis

In the past decade metabolic acidosis has been recognized as being of central pathophysiological and prognostic importance in both adult and childhood severe malaria. The clinical syndrome of respiratory distress in African children, previously either unrecognized or incorrectly attributed to heart failure secondary to severe anemia, is now thought to be caused chiefly by acidosis (7,86,87). Metabolic acidosis can occur with or without cerebral involvement, and in one study of adults with cerebral malaria CSF lactate was a powerful predictor of fatal outcome (88). Metabolic acidosis per se is strongly associated with death in both adults and children (12,89–91), and appears to be caused by a combination of lactic acidosis and renal failure. The latter is particularly true in non-immune adults in whom renal failure is common, but is also true in African children, where severe renal impairment never occurs (87). Hypovolemia and anemia are associated with lactic acidosis in the same population (92), with volume resuscitation associated with a reduction in acidosis (93). In a pilot study the antioxidant *N*-acetylcysteine was associated with an increased rate of clearance of lactate, though the mechanisms behind this have not been fully elucidated (94).

3.3.2. Renal Failure and Blackwater Fever

Acute renal failure is an important cause of morbidity and mortality in non-immune individuals, where it may occur in over 40% of cases of severe malaria (12,95,96). In African children any renal dysfunction is generally subclinical and the need for dialysis extremely rare (50,97). The ARF in severe malaria, which is clinically similar to the "acute tubular necrosis" seen in other intensive care settings, may present either acutely as part of a fulminant multisystem disorder, or develop over several days in patients recovering from the initial acute phase of severe disease. Patients developing renal failure acutely tend to be oliguric or anuric, frequently have jaundice and coexisting lactic acidosis, and usually require immediate dialysis.

Blackwater fever, an enigmatic condition once the scourge of tropical colonial administrations, is characterized by fever, massive intravascular hemolysis and hemoglobinuria, which in severe cases leads to ARF. Its etiology is unclear, though it occurs only in areas of the tropics endemic for malaria, and has been associated with malaria infection, quinine ingestion, and glucose-6-phosphate dehydrogenase deficiency (98). Once a major cause of renal failure and malaria-associated mortality, it is now relatively uncommon and rarely leads to severe ARF (98,99).

3.3.3. Hemodynamic Shock (Algid Malaria)

The hemodynamics of severe hypotension in severe malaria are similar to those observed in bacterial septic shock, with a very low systemic vascular resistance and normal or raised cardiac output (100,101). Hypovolemia may also make a major contribution to the etiology, particularly in African children (93). Shock in non-immune adults usually occurs on the background of other severe complications of malaria, and is associated with metabolic acidosis. Coexisting bacterial septicemia has been implicated in some cases, though it cannot explain the majority of cases (95,102). In hypotension refractory to fluid resuscitation the prognosis is poor despite inotropic support.

3.3.4. Pulmonary Edema

Clinically this serious complication of severe malaria resembles the adult respiratory distress syndrome (103–105), and though it can be precipitated by fluid overload it is usually associated with normal central venous and pulmonary artery occlusion pressures (106,107). It is particularly common in pregnant women, and is usually fatal if mechanical ventilation facilities are not on hand (which almost always they are not).

3.3.5. Jaundice

Jaundice is a feature of severe malaria in non-immune individuals (occurring in up to 60%), and is usually associated with other features of multisystem disease such as ARF, cerebral malaria and severe acidosis (12). Serious hepatic dysfunction with asterixis and hepatic encephalopathy never occurs, and jaundice is not independently associated with mortality. For these reasons jaundice is regarded as a marker of severe disease rather than a defining criterion (54). Its cause is a combination of hemolysis and mild hepatic dysfunction. However, low hepatic blood flow and a low splanchnic lactate extraction ratio are both positively associated with raised plasma lactate concentrations, suggesting that reduced hepatic function may contribute to lactic acidosis (91,108).

4. PATHOPHYSIOLOGY

4.1.   The Parasite Life Cycle

4.1.1.   Asexual Cycle

Pre-erythrocytic (Hepatic) Phase: The human host is inoculated with small motile sporozoites by an infected mosquito during feeding. They quickly invade hepatocytes through specific receptor-mediated binding between the parasite's circumsporozoite protein and glycosaminoglycans on the cell surface (109). The putative hepatitis C virus receptor, the tetraspanin CD81, has been shown to be essential for entry of the sporozoite into the hepatocyte and for its further differentiation into exo-erythrocytic forms (110). After a median of 6 days of parasite multiplication within the hepatocyte, the "hepatic schizont" ruptures releasing tens of thousands of merozoites into the bloodstream.

Erythrocytic Phase: In the blood stream the motile, ovoid, merozoites rapidly attach to erythrocytes via a combination of sialic acid-dependent and - independent mechanisms. The sialic acid-dependent pathways include binding of the merozoite ligands erythrocyte binding antigen-175 (EBA-175) and erythrocyte binding protein-2 (EBP-2) to the sialic acid moieties on erythrocyte glycophorin A and glycophorin C, respectively (111,112). A *P. falciparum* homolog of *Plasmodium vivax* reticulocyte binding protein (PfRh1), and *P. falciparum* JESEBL (also known as EBA-181), have also been implicated in sialic acid-dependent binding mechanisms (113,114). This apparent built-in redundancy is further extended by sialic acid-independent pathways involving EBA-175 (115), and involving the binding of merozoite surface proteins (MSP) 1 and 9 to regions of erythrocyte band 3 (116). Once attached internalization itself is effected by active "boring" of the wriggling merozoite into the red cell, causing invagination of the erythrocyte membrane. Once inside the erythrocyte the young ring form begins eating the contents of the red cell, which is mainly hemoglobin. Malaria pigment or hemozoin is a by-product of the detoxification of heme, and consists of a polymer of hemoglobin-derived hemin groups (protoporphyrin IX chelated to ferric iron) dimerized by iron-oxygen bonds, and then linked in chains by hydrogen bonding (117). The structure of this parasite-derived hemozoin is identical to that of the synthetic chemical β-hematin. The appearance of visible dirty dark brown crystals of pigment within the digestive vacuole of the developing parasite marks the transition to the trophozoite stage of the erythrocytic cycle. As the parasite grows it inserts transporter proteins into the erythrocyte membrane, making it more permeable. The cytoskeleton of the cell is altered, such that the erythrocyte becomes progressively less deformable and more ovoid in shape (118). This loss of deformability is in contrast with the increased deformability demonstrated by erythrocytes parasitized by *P. vivax* (119).

About midway through this 48-hr cycle the parasitized erythrocytes develop increased adhesiveness, mediated by parasite-derived ligands localized at protein-dense "knobs" on the erythrocyte cell surface (Fig. 1). The erythrocytes bind to endothelial cells (sequestration within blood vessels), uninfected red cells (rosetting), and other parasitized erythrocytes (aggregation). The parasite undergoes fur-

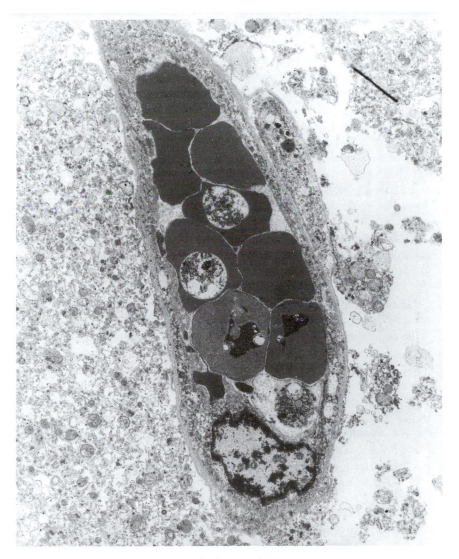

Figure 1 Electron micrograph demonstrating cytoadherence of a parasitized erythrocyte to a microvessel in the cerebral cortex of a Vietnamese cerebral malaria patient.

ther development and nuclear division, and at schizogony (merogony) the mature sequestered parasite bursts releasing a new generation of merozoites into the blood stream to invade new erythrocytes. Each schizont can release up to 32 merozoites, of which in a non-immune patient 10–20 successfully reinvade. This logarithmic increase in the parasitemias continues through several 2-day cycles before the parasites are detectable in the blood (usually around 11 days post-infection at a parasitemia of about 50/μL).

4.1.2. Sexual Cycle

Host Phase: After several asexual erythrocytic cycles some of the parasites differentiate into sexual gametes (gametocytogony), which can live for weeks within the blood stream waiting to be taken up by a female anopheline mosquito taking a blood feed.

Mosquito Phase: Within the mosquito the male gametes divide, develop flagella, and enters meiotic fusion with the activated female macrogamete. The zygote thus formed becomes motile (the ookinete) and encysts in the midgut. Here the oocyst (as it is now termed) rapidly enlarges as thousands of sporozoites develop. The oocyst ruptures and the sporozoites make their way to the salivary glands, from where they are injected into the next human host when the mosquito feeds. This process of sporogony takes at least 8 days, the exact time depending on the ambient temperature and the species of mosquito.

4.2. Pathophysiology of Cerebral Malaria

This section will concentrate on the pathophysiology of cerebral malaria, though it will also cover aspects of the pathogenesis of other complications of severe malaria, particularly as many patients with cerebral malaria will die of these complications rather than brain involvement itself.

The main clinical feature of cerebral malaria is coma, and the cause of this is unknown. A major feature of the coma is that, if the patient survives, it is usually completely reversible. This is particularly true in non-immune adults, where the neurological sequelae rate is <1%. Any theory of pathogenesis must therefore explain both the coma and its reversibility. The main contenders are (i) mechanical obstruction causing local hypoxia (the "mechanical hypothesis"), (ii) increased permeability of the blood–brain barrier leading to raised intracranial pressure, cerebral edema, and neuronal damage (the "permeability hypothesis"), (iii) immunopathology leading to the release locally of short-lived molecules such as cytokines and nitric oxide (NO), causing in turn transient neuronal damage or disturbance in neuronal function, and (iv) a combination of (i)–(iii).

4.2.1. Pathological Findings in Cerebral Malaria

Sequestration of Parasitized Erythrocytes: The central feature of falciparum malaria, not seen to any major degree in the other human malarias, is the sequestration of trophozoite and schizont-infected erythocytes in the deep microvasculature. This probably evolved as a strategy to avoid clearance of the stiff parasitized cells by the spleen, a hypothesis supported by the recent discovery that erythrocytes parasitized by *P. vivax*, which does not sequester, are hyperdeformable, presumably also to avoid splenic clearance (119). Sequestration occurs in all falciparum malaria infections, as mature parasites are very rarely seen on the peripheral blood film, and then only in the most severe cases (120).

Histological and electron micrograph examinations of autopsy specimens from patients who died of cerebral malaria have shown cerebral microvessels packed with both parasitized and unparasitized erythrocytes (Fig. 2). The parasitized erythrocytes are often found attached to the endothelial cell surface by electron dense "knobs." This is the clinical and pathological correlate of the in vitro phenomenon of cytoadherence.

Although sequestration is universally present in falciparum malaria, the pathological evidence is that in fatal cases at least it occurs to a greater degree in the brain than in other organs, and in cerebral malaria than non-cerebral severe malaria (121,122). In a recent ultrastructural study the parasite count in cerebral microvessels in cerebral malaria was more than 50 times that in the immediately pre-mortem peripheral blood (the sequestration index), compared with a median of 6.9 times in non-cerebral cases (123). This significantly greater sequestration was present in all parts of the brain compared with non-cerebral malaria, though it was more marked in the cerebrum and cerebellum than in the brainstem.

Although there is clearly a central role for sequestration in the pathophysiology of cerebral malaria, the mechanism by which it causes coma is unknown. The degree to which sequestration causes the other manifestations of severe malaria, along with any underlying mechanisms, is also unclear. Sequestration does cause microvascular obstruction, though phenomena described in vitro such as reduced unparasitized erythrocyte deformability, rosetting, and aggregation may also play a role in this (see below).

Pigment Deposition: After schizogony red cell "ghosts" are left attached to endothelial cells. These contain parasite remnants such as pigment, or hemozoin, produced by the parasite as a breakdown product of hemoglobin digestion. In histopathological studies this pigment can often be seen lining cerebral microvessels, and is a marker of previous sequestration. Circulating monocytes and neutrophils phagocytose ghost erythrocyte membranes and pigment. Pigment is known to have toxic effects on monocytes in vivo, including stimulation of the release of TNF-α and other cytokines, production via free radicals of lipoperoxides, inhibition of further phagocytosis, and impaired antigen presentation (124–126). Pigment has recently been shown to increase IFN-γ-inducible

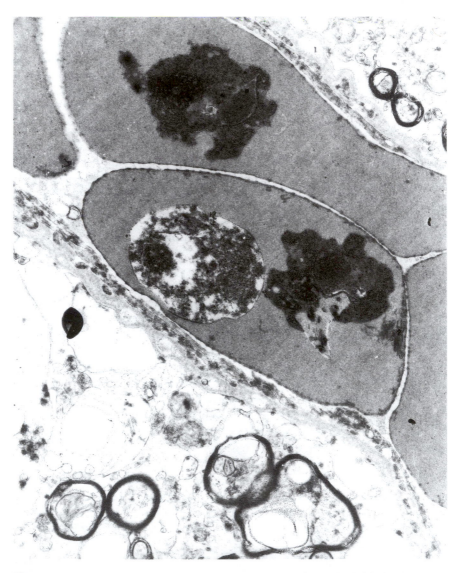

Figure 2 Electron micrograph showing a cerebral microvessel completely blocked by a combination of unparasitized and cytoadherent parasitized erythrocytes. This post-mortem specimen is from the temporal cortex of a Vietnamese adult patient who died of cerebral malaria.

macrophage NO generation, and may also have a direct immunomodulatory effect on cerebral endothelial cells (127,128).

Local Inflammatory Response: Although the intravascular sequestration of leukocytes is a major feature of the murine model of cerebral malaria, and may play a major role in its pathophysiology, the cellular inflammatory response in human cerebral malaria is much less marked.

In Vietnamese cerebral malaria patients there was activation of the cerebral endothelial cells, along with local disruption of the blood–brain barrier and associated activation of perivascular macrophages (129,130).

Hemorrhages: On macroscopic examination of the fresh brain from a case of cerebral malaria two features frequently stand out: the discoloration caused by pigment deposition; and the presence of multiple small petechial hemorrhages, often within the immediate subcortical rim of white matter. On histological examination these are of three types: simple petechial hemorrhages; ring hemorrhages (necrotic vessel surrounded by an inner ring of uninfected erythrocytes and an outer ring of parasitized erythrocytes and leucocytes); and Dürck's granulomata, a classical cell reaction typical of advanced disease involving reactive macrophages/microglial cells (131). The extent to which agonal processes are involved, particularly in the case of petechial hemorrhages, is unclear.

Disruption of Axonal Transport: Although there is little evidence of major neuron loss in cerebral malaria, more subtle forms of neurotoxicity and neuronal damage do occur. β-amyloid precursor protein (β-APP) immunocytochemistry has been used extensively in neuropathology as a marker of impaired axonal transport, allowing visualization of axonal damage in cases of head injury and multiple sclerosis (132). In a series of 54 adult Vietnamese severe malaria autopsy cases, β-APP immunocytochemistry was performed on brain sections from the cortex, internal capsule, pons, and cerebellum (133). The extent and intensity of β-APP staining was greater in patients with cerebral malaria than in those with no clinical cerebral involvement, and was inversely proportional to the Glascow Coma Score (Fig. 3). Impairment of axonal transport could adversely affect neurological function and cause coma, and in mild cases may be reversible. Axonal damage was sometimes but not always associated with areas of demyelination or hemorrhages, and it is probable that it results from a range of as yet undefined insults. It is certainly a candidate for a "final common pathway" leading to potentially reversible neurological impairment and coma in cerebral malaria.

4.2.2. Cytoadherence

Parasitized erythrocytes infected with *P. falciparum* bind to endothelial cells in culture. Other cytoadherent properties include binding to uninfected erythrocytes (rosetting), leucocytes, platelets and to each other (aggregation or auto-agglutination). These phenotypes are mediated by complex receptor–ligand interactions which are only just beginning to be understood (Fig. 4).

Host Receptors: A number of different host molecules have been shown to bind parasitized erythrocytes in vitro, though the extent to which they are all

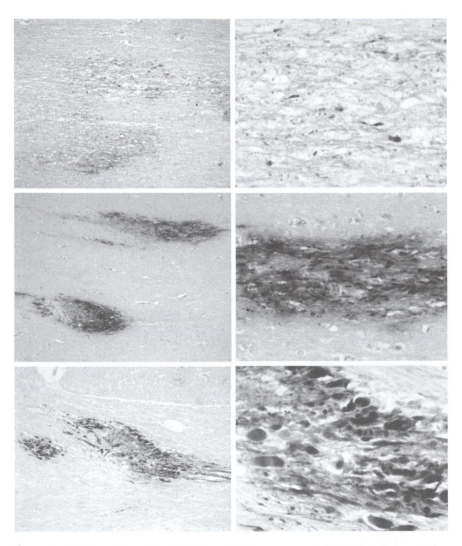

Figure 3 Brain sections stained for β-amyloid precursor protein (βAPP) demonstrating accumulation of βAPP due to interruption of axonal transport secondary to axonal injury in a Vietnamese patient with cerebral malaria.

involved in vivo is unclear. They include the constitutively expressed molecules CD36, thrombospondin (TSP), the $\alpha_v\beta_3$ integrin, hyaluronic acid (HA), chondroitin sulphate A (CSA), and PECAM-1 (CD31). Receptors with inducible expression include ICAM-1, VCAM-1, P-selectin, and E-selectin.

CD36 is widely expressed on endothelial cells, and binds to the vast majority of clinical isolates of *P. falciparum* (134). A nonsense mutation in CD36 was asso-

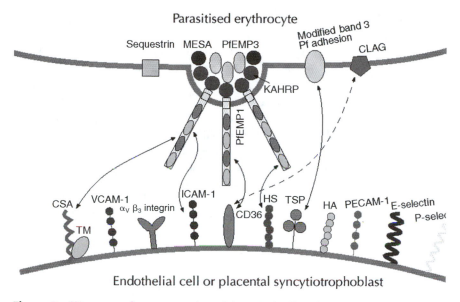

Figure 4 Diagrammatic representation of the parasite ligands and host receptors putatively involved in cytoadherence. Solid arrows represent well-established ligand–receptor interactions thought to be important in vivo. There is evidence from gene knockout studies that the CD36–CLAG interaction (dotted arrow) is essential for cytoadherence in vitro, but its importance in vivo is not known. For details of other putative interactions see text. Abbreviations: CSA, chondroitin sulfate A; TM, thrombomodulin; HS, heparan sulfate; TSP, thrombospondin; HA, hyaluronic acid; PS, phosphatidyl serine; MESA, mature parasite-infected erythrocyte surface antigen; KAHRP, knob-associated histidine rich protein; CLAG, cytoadherence-linked asexual gene.

ciated with protection from severe malaria, although not specifically cerebral malaria (135). Although it is expressed on cerebral microvascular endothelium, it is not upregulatable by cytokines (129), and probably acts synergistically with the inducible ICAM-1 (136). CD36 expressed on platelets has recently been shown to mediate cytoadherence of parasitized erythrocytes to endothelium lacking CD36, presumably by allowing the platelets to act as a "bridge" to the endothelial surface (137). Platelet CD36 may also worsen the mechanical obstructive effects of sequestration by mediating the aggregation (auto-agglutination) of infected erythrocytes (138).

A recent study has suggested that cytoadherence under flow conditions may be modulated through a signaling pathway involving CD36, Src-family kinases, and an ectoalkaline phosphatase (139). The authors suggest the possibility of novel treatments for severe malaria involving the targeting of endothelial ectoalkaline phosphatases (with an alkaline phosphatase inhibitor such as levamisole), or signaling molecules.

ICAM-1, a member of the immunoglobulin superfamily, is thought to play a central role in mediating sequestration in the brain. Its expression on endothelial cells is up-regulated by the cytokine TNF-α, the concentration of which is proportional to the severity of malaria, and on immunohistological studies of post-mortem cerebral malaria brains. ICAM-1 was co-localized with sequestered parasitized erythrocytes. In addition, a mutation in the ICAM-1 gene (ICAM-1[kilifi]) was associated with susceptibility to cerebral malaria in Kenya (23), but not in Thailand (140).

Although there is mounting evidence that CD36 and ICAM-1 are the major host receptors involved in cytoadherence, the other possible receptors mentioned above may still contribute to parasitized erythrocyte binding.

Thrombospondin, a trimeric glycoprotein, binds to a large number of putative ligands in vitro including the host molecules CD36, $\alpha_v\beta_3$ integrin, heparin, fibrinogen, fibronectin, plasminogen, and LDL receptor-related protein. On the parasitized red cell it has been reported to bind PfEMP1, pfalhesin (modified band 3) and phosphatidyl serine (a membrane phospholipid reportedly exposed on the parasitized erythrocyte surface) (141). TSP was the first protein to be identified as a putative host parasitized erythrocyte receptor. However in recent years attention has moved away from TSP and onto CD36 and ICAM-1, partly because TSP-mediated binding to parasitized erythrocytes appears not to be stable under physiological flow conditions (though this remains controversial) (141,142).

Other putative host receptors which may play a role in cytoadherence include P-selectin, PECAM (CD31), $\alpha_v\beta_3$ integrin, VCAM, and E-selectin. The contributions of these molecules in clinical disease are either in doubt or have not been fully determined (142).

Severe malaria in pregnancy is found in highly endemic areas where severe disease is otherwise very unusual. In keeping with this clinical deviation from the norm the host receptors involved in placental malaria constitute a special case. Current evidence points to a CSA-containing glycosaminoglycan, thrombomodulin, being the main parasitized erythrocyte receptor on the syncytiotrophoblast (143). Parasitized erythrocytes from the placenta bind CSA but not CD36, whereas the converse is true for parasitized erythrocytes recovered from the peripheral blood of non-pregnant women. Antibodies to parasitized erythrocytes which bind CSA develop in women who survive their first pregnancy, an observation consistent with the relative resistance to placental malaria seen clinically in multigravida (144).

PfEMP1 and *var* Genes: Since 1995, when three laboratories reported simultaneously that the parasite variant antigen PfEMP1 was the product of a gene family termed *var*, there have been huge advances in our understanding of the parasitized erythrocyte side of the cytoadherence equatrion (145–147). PfEMP1 molecules are encoded by approximately 60 *var* genes (59 in the genome sequence strain 3D7). These appear to undergo frequent non-homologous recombination leading to heterologous expression of antigenic variants both within and between different parasite lines. Only one PfEMP1 type is expressed on the surface of the erythrocyte during each 48 hr parasite erythrocytic cycle, and the type expressed switches at a rate of approximately 2% per cycle (145,148,149). The mechanism underlying this is not fully understood (38).

Each PfEMP1 molecule consists of an extracellular region consisting of several Duffy binding-like (DBL) domains interspersed with cysteine-rich inter-domain regions (CIDR), a transmembrane region (TM), and an intracellular acidic terminal segment (150). DBL and CIDR domains are labeled according to position (1–5 in the case of DBL and 1–2 for CIDR) and homology type groups $\alpha(\alpha-\epsilon$ and $\alpha-\gamma$, respectively). Within the 3D7 genome the PfEMP1 molecules encoded by the *var* genes are highly polymorphic, though 38 (64%) share the same basic domain structure: DBL1α–CIDR1α–DBL2δ–CIDR2x–TM–ATS.

Most of the CIDR2α domains bind CD36, as do most clinical isolates of *P. falciparum*. The DBL1 domains are relatively conserved, and seem to have a broad receptor specificity including complement receptor 1 (CR1) on other erythrocytes and heparan sulfate (38,151). The DBL1–CIDR1 end of the molecule has been termed the "multiadhesive semi-conserved head structure," but in the rest of the PfEMP1 molecule the domain structure and order is more variable. Binding to ICAM-1 has been associated with a DBL2β–C2 domain complex, which appears to be relatively conserved between ICAM-1 binding isolates (36,152). The DBL3γ domain has been associated with placental malaria, a finding that has raised hopes of developing a vaccine against this very serious form of the disease (153).

Other Parasitized Erythrocyte Surface Proteins: There are two additional large families of variant genes in the *P. falciparum* genome, the exact function of which is currently unknown. The stevor (subteloremic variant open reading frame) multigene family gene product is associated with Maurer's clefts (154), though whether or not it is actually expressed on the surface is unclear.

The rifins (repetitive interspersed family of genes, *rif*) are a very large multigene family encoding a group of proteins (RIFINS) that have been shown to co-traffic to the erythrocyte surface with PfEMP1 and to induce a host antibody response (155). Their function is unknown.

Two other parasite-derived surface proteins deserve mention as possibly having a role in cytoadherence. The clag (cytoadherence-linked asexual gene) family produces a protein transcribed in mature stage parasites which is thought to be exposed on the erythrocyte surface, and in vitro appears to be necessary for cytoadherence (142,156). Sequestrin is a 270-kDa surface protein which appears to mediate cytoadherence via CD36. However unlike PfEMP1 it is not a variant antigen, being conserved between isolates (157).

A further class of molecules involved in cytoadherence is host-derived, but aberrantly exposed on the surface of infected erythrocytes. These include pfalhesin, a usually cryptic part of the band 3 protein which is exposed during parasite growth. The main ligand for pfalhesin is TSP (158).

Phosphatidylserine (PS) is a membrane phospholipid usually confined to the inner part of the lipid bilayer, and like pfalhesin is exposed on the parasitized erythrocyte surface. PS has been implicated in binding to both TSP and CD36, but not ICAM-1, though the importance of these interactions in vivo has not been established (159).

4.2.3. Rosetting and Aggregation

The formation of "rosettes" of unparasitized erythrocytes adhering to mature parasite-containing erythrocytes may also contribute to microvascular obstruction. Like cytoadherence the ability to rosette develops around 16 hr into asexual parasite development, but unlike cytoadherence its role in the pathogenesis of severe disease is controversial (160–162). Not all field isolates of *P. falciparum* rosette, whereas they all cytoadhere, and malaria species which do not cytoadhere or cause severe disease (*P. ovale* and *P. vivax*) have the ability to form rosettes (163,164). In *P. falciparum* rosetting is thought to occur following interaction between PfEMP1 and the C3b binding site of CR1 on the surface of uninfected erythrocytes (165). Rosetting could contribute to microvascular obstruction by impairing flow in the venules, which in turn might promote cytoadherence.

The ability of infected erythrocytes to clump together is termed auto-agglutination or aggregation. It is mediated by platelet CD36 binding to PfEMP1, and as an in vitro phenotype has been associated with severe malaria in African children (138).

4.2.4. Erythrocyte Deformability

It has been known since 1984 that the development of the parasite inside an infected erythrocyte leads to a progressive loss of red cell deformability, with the usually biconcave erythrocyte becoming increasingly rigid and spherical (118). What has only recently been recognized is that in falciparum malaria there is a reduction in the deformability of *uninfected* erythrocytes, which may make a major contribution to microvascular obstruction in capillaries and venules (166). In support of this hypothesis clinical studies have shown that the degree of loss of deformability is highly predictive of poor outcome in both African children and Southeast Asian adults (167,168). In addition to this role in the microvasculature, reductions in deformability measured at shear stresses typical of the arterial side of the circulation have been correlated with anemia (169). The mechanism for the reduction in uninfected erythrocyte deformability has not been fully elucidated, though it appears that oxidative stress to the erythrocyte membrane is responsible, possibly related to release of parasite pigment at schizogeny (170). One of the major practical clinical implications of these findings is that they provide a rationale for the use of partial exchange transfusion in the treatment of severe malaria, a therapy that so far has not been subject to controlled clinical trial (169).

4.2.5. Cerebral Edema, Brain Swelling, and Raised Intracranial Pressure

There is evidence from radiological studies (171,172) that brain swelling plays a role in some cases of cerebral malaria. However, cerebral edema is not a common feature in post-mortem studies (173) (author's unpublished observations).

The intracranial pressure can be estimated from the CSF opening pressure at LP, or by intracranial pressure monitoring. Raised intracranial pressures have been associated with fatal outcome in African children, though any association is less clear in Southeast Asian adults (174–176). A raised intracranial pressure could reduce the cerebral perfusion pressure and cause hypoxia and secondary cytotoxic edema. Such a scenario may be responsible for the syndrome of brainstem herniation described in African children (62), which is rarely seen in Southeast Asian adults. Thus the contribution of raised intracranial pressures to the pathophysiology of cerebral malaria may vary between patient groups.

4.2.6. The Blood–Brain Barrier

Autopsy studies of severe malaria in both Asian adults and African children have shown that sequestration in the cerebral vasculature is associated with endothelial cell activation (129,177). As leukocyte binding to cerebral endothelial cells in culture induces intracellular signaling via ICAM-1, it is plausible that parasitized red blood cells binding to receptors on cerebral endothelial cells may cause changes in the structure and function of the blood–brain barrier. In an immunohistochemistry study examining the blood–brain barrier in human cerebral malaria in Vietnamese adults, the distribution of the cell junction proteins occludin, vinculin, and ZO-1 were altered in cases compared to controls (130). However, measurement of IgG and albumin in matched CSF and plasma samples has demonstrated that in terms of permeability there are only subtle changes in the functional integrity of the blood–brain barrier (177,178). The permeability hypothesis for the pathophysiology of cerebral malaria receives mixed support from these findings; there clearly are subtle changes in the structure and function of the blood–brain barrier in cerebral malaria, but this is probably insufficient to explain the degree of cerebral edema seen in some cases of cerebral malaria.

4.2.7. Soluble Neuroactive Mediators

The rapidly reversible nature of coma in cerebral malaria has raised interest in the possibility that soluble rapidly diffusible mediators might cause the symptoms of CM. Candidates include parasite toxins, host cytokine release induced by infection, or local release of neuroactive mediators within the CNS which could have an "anesthetic"-like action (179). Cerebral symptoms might also be caused by excitotoxins released following activation of microglia and astrocytes in the brain parenchyma.

Cytokines: Severe malaria has been associated with high circulating levels of proinflammatory cytokines such as TNF-α, IL-1, and IL-6. Raised levels of plasma TNF-α, measured by immunoassay, have been associated with disease severity in African children and Vietnamese adults (180–182). However the recent demonstration that it is lymphotoxin-α (LT-α), not TNF-α, which is over-expressed in experimental cerebral malaria, has cast some doubt on these observations, as these cytokines cannot be distinguished using the commonly used kits (183). By analogy with severe sepsis TNF-α is a strong candidate for causing the multisystem organ failure and hypotension seen in cases of severe malaria. However many other diseases, including *P. vivax* infection, are associated with high circulating TNF-α levels and yet do not have coma as a clinical feature; hence raised systemic TNF-α alone is unlikely to be the sole mediator of cerebral symptoms.

IFN-γ is increasingly recognized as playing a central role in the immunopathology of severe malaria, both in mice and humans (41). In mice, IFN-γ and TNF-α act synergistically to promote NO production, which is directly involved in parasite killing (184), and in humans IFN-γ production is associated with resistance to reinfection with *P. falciparum* and protection from fever and clinical malaria (185,186). In malaria infection IFN-γ is produced (i) as part of the early innate immune response by natural killer (NK) cells exposed directly to live parasitized erythrocytes, and (ii) by the adaptive immune response via parasite-specific CD8 cells, a process dependent on IL-12 and NK cells (187,188). Furthermore, parasite pigment (hemozoin) increases IFN-γ-inducible macrophage NO output, tying in parasitized erythrocyte sequestration and schizogony with local NO production (127).

Relative deficiency in the production of counterbalancing anti-inflammatory cytokines such as IL-10 and tumor growth factor-β has been associated with disease severity (182,186), though the full nature of the balancing act between pro- and anti-inflammatory responses to malaria remains poorly understood.

Nitric Oxide: The local release of NO within the brain has been suggested as a possible explanation for the coma of cerebral malaria. Clark and Cowden have hypothesized that a synergistic combination of IFN-γ release and hypoxia leads to the induction of inducible nitric oxide synthase (iNOS), resulting in NO release, which in turn may have an anesthetic-like effect via inhibition of neuronal NMDA calcium ion channels (186). Studies of serum and CSF NO metabolites (reactive nitrogen intermediates, or RNI) have provided conflicting results, and probably represent too blunt a tool. Some studies have found a positive correlation between plasma RNI and severity of disease (189–192). Others have shown either no association (193,194) or even an inverse association (195), suggesting that NO may play a protective role. CSF levels have also been uninformative (167,193). If NO plays a role in the pathogenesis of cerebral malaria, it is likely that it does so at a very local level.

Excitotoxins: Interferon-γ and hypoxia are potent inducers of the enzyme indoleamine 2,3-dioxygenase, which is the first step in the catabolism of tryptophan, a pathway which produces the excitotoxin quinolinic acid (QA) and the neuroprotective kynurenic acid (196). Quinolinic acid has been implicated in the pathogenesis of convulsions in murine cerebral malaria (197), and was found in increased concentrations in the CSF of Kenyan children with cerebral malaria (198). Although QA levels were raised in the CSF of adults with severe malaria, there was no association with convulsions or depth of coma, and multivariate analysis suggested that the elevated concentrations were a consequence of impaired renal function (199). However in a recent study in Malawian children with cerebral malaria, who did not have serious renal impairment, QA levels were associated with mortality (200). Malawian children also had higher mean levels of KA than Vietnamese adults, suggesting a greater neuroprotective response.

The past decade has seen major advances in our understanding of the pathophysiology of cerebral malaria, particularly at the molecular level, yet still the cause of coma remains unknown. Evidence exists to partially vindicate all three of the hypotheses outlined at the beginning of this section, but none offers a full and adequate explanation for the clinical syndrome. With the joint publication in 2002 of the genomes of the *P. falciparum* parasite and its most efficient vector, *An. gambiae*, we can hope that the pace of discovery will accelerate in the coming years and a breakthrough achieved (201).

5. TREATMENT

In 2000, a working party under the auspices of WHO produced detailed guidelines and recommendations for the treatment of severe malaria (54). These represent an extensive update of the successful and widely applied 1990 recommendations, and are an invaluable resource for anyone involved in the management of cases of severe malaria. Below I have reviewed the salient features of the principles of management of severe malaria, emphasizing any recent exciting developments where these have occurred.

5.1. Initial Assessment

An initial rapid clinical assessment of patients with suspected cerebral malaria should include assessment of conscious level (formally using either the Glasgow or Blantyre coma scales), hemodynamic and respiratory status, and state of hydration. Hypoglycemia should be excluded at the bedside or treated. A close examination for any continuous seizure activity should be made, and pharmacological causes of coma considered. Intravenous rehydration should be commenced if indicated, oxygen given if there is clinical or blood gas evidence of respiratory distress or hypoxia, and an appropriate antimalarial drug administered. If the presence of severe malaria is suspected the patient should be transferred to the highest level of care available (preferably an intensive care unit).

An LP should be performed to exclude meningitis. If this is felt to be contraindicated because of fears of brain swelling, appropriate anti-meningitis cover must be given. An LP can then be performed either after a CT scan has excluded significant brain swelling or after ~48 hr following neurological improvement. In adults there is little evidence for a major role for raised intracranial pressure, and an LP is generally considered safe.

Overzealous rehydration can lead to pulmonary edema, particularly in adults, whereas underhydration may cause hemodynamic shock, worsen acidosis, and precipitate renal failure. For these reasons monitoring of right-sided venous pressures via a central venous line should be carried out wherever possible, and used to guide fluid resuscitation.

5.2. Antimalarial Treatment

5.2.1. Quinine and Quinidine

The cinchona alkaloids (quinine and quinidine), derived from the bark of the cinchona tree, have been used for the treatment of severe malaria since the 1630s. They remained the mainstay of antimalarial therapy for severe malaria until the 1950s, when they were supplanted by the synthetic 4-aminoquinoline antimalarial chloroquine. With the inexorable worldwide rise of chloroquine resistance this drug can no longer be used to treat severe malaria, and quinine has returned to widespread use. Because of its cardiotoxicity intravenous infusion should be carried out for 4 hr, ideally with ECG monitoring. Where intravenous infusion is not practical it can be given by deep intramuscular injection (12,202). It is important that adequate parasitocidal drug levels are obtained rapidly, so in patients who have not received previous recent doses of quinine an initial loading dose of 20 mk/kg should be given (203,204).

Quinine commonly causes a complex of minor side effects collectively known as cinchonism (tinnitus, high-frequency hearing loss, and nausea), which although reversible is responsible for poor compliance with oral courses. Serious side effects of quinine include hyperinsulinemic hypoglycemia, which is particularly common in pregnant women and impossible to diagnose clinically in the already unconscious patient (68). Intramuscular quinine can cause sterile abscesses, and in Vietnam tetanus following quinine injection is almost invariably fatal (205). There is an epidemiological and clinical association between quinine and blackwater fever, though the pathophysiology underlying this is not understood (98,99).

5.2.2. The Artemisinin Derivatives

Artemisinin (Qinghaosu) is an endoperoxide-containing compound extracted from the leaves of the plant *Artemisia annua* (sweet wormwood), and along with its derivatives artemether, dihydroartemisinin, and artesunate are the most rapidly acting antimalarial drugs in terms of clearance of parasitemia. They represent one of the most exciting advances in malariology in recent years, though they are far from new to medicine. The use of *Artemisia annua* as a remedy for fever was mentioned in the Chinese medical literature almost 2000 years ago (206), and the active ingredient (Qinghaosu) was extracted by Chinese scientists in the 1970s. Since the late 1980s and early 1990s artemisinin and its derivatives have been used extensively in Southeast Asia and increasingly in Africa. Animal studies have raised concerns about possible neurotoxicity with high doses of these drugs, but so far this has not been reported in man (207,208). In fact the artemisinin derivatives are very well tolerated, with no significant side effects reported despite their use in several million patients with uncomplicated malaria.

In the late 1980s and early 1990s great hope surrounded the use of artemisinin derivatives for the treatment of severe malaria, with some early studies demonstrating dramatic advantages over conventional therapies such as quinine. In an attempt to gather unequivocal evidence of this superiority, if it existed, a series of studies comparing artemether with quinine were conducted under WHO oversight in both Africa and Asia. The individual results were largely inconclusive, with no one trial sufficiently powered to show a moderate but clinically important effect on primary outcomes such as mortality and sequelae. Although the trials in the Gambia and in Vietnam were the largest randomized trials ever conducted in severe childhood and adult malaria, respectively (12,209), they were small by the standards of other disciplines such as cardiology and diabetology; they would have been able to detect only a 50% reduction in mortality (16% vs. 8%). For this reason a meta-analysis of the results of all the artemether–quinine trials was carried out using individual patient data provided by the original investigators (210). Original individual patient data on 1919 patients were obtained from seven studies. Overall there was no significant difference in mortality between the two groups [14% vs. 17%, odds ratio (95% confidence interval) 0.8 (0.62–1.02), $p = 0.08$], nor were there significant differences in coma recovery or fever clearance times, or the development of neurological sequelae. However, the combined "adverse outcome" of either death or neurological sequelae was significantly less common in the artemether group [odds ratio (95% CI) 0.77 (0.62–0.96), $p = 0.02$]. In addition, on subgroup analyses, artemether was associated with a significantly lower mortality than quinine in adults with multisystem failure, suggesting a more marked treatment advantage with artemether in non-immune individuals.

Although the results of this meta-analysis were encouraging, and suggest that artemether is at least as good as if not better than quinine for the treatment of severe malaria, they were not dramatic. However, there are reasons to suspect that artemether may not be the ideal parenteral artemisinin derivative. Artemether is oil soluble and can only be given by intramuscular depot injection. There is evidence that it may be poorly absorbed in patients who are in hemodynamic shock or peripherally shut down, arguably the most severe patients in whom the need to achieve therapeutic levels quickly is most crucial (211). The water-soluble hemisuccinate of artemisinin, artesunate, has not been as well studied as artemether, chiefly because there has not been a GMP formulation of the drug. As it can be given intravenously it does not suffer from the distribution problems of artemether, and in an animal model is less neurotoxic (although neurotoxicity has not been a clinical problem for any artemisisin derivative in man) (212). A large (~3000 patients) comparison of artesunate and quinine is underway, and will hopefully define definitively the role of parenteral artemisinin derivatives in the treatment of severe malaria.

The use of suppositories containing artemisinin or one of its derivatives for the treatment of severe malaria in both adults and children was pioneered in Vietnam in the early 1990s (49,213). The suppositories used in these studies contained Vietnamese-grown artemisinin, and were not manufactured to GMP standards. Subsequently, the World Health Organization has sponsored the development of GMP-manufactured rectal artesunate capsules which have now undergone clinical trial in Thailand, Malawi, and South Africa (214,215), and appear likely to obtain US FDA registration in the near future. By delaying disease progression and buying time in which to reach health centers, home or village-based deployment of rectal artesunate in rural areas of Africa and Asia may play an important role in reducing malaria-associated morbidity and mortality.

5.3. Supportive Therapy

Good nursing care is essential in the management of severe malaria, with particular attention to fluid balance, management of the unconscious patient, and detection of potentially lethal complications such as hypoglycemia. All severe malaria patients should, if possible, be nursed on an intensive care unit.

Mechanical ventilation is often used in the unconscious cerebral malaria patient, particularly in Western ICUs, though its efficacy in terms of prevention of mortality and sequelae has not been proved. In Western settings severe malaria may have a better prognosis than in developing countries, though there may be many reasons for this.

5.3.1. Anticonvulsants

Seizures in cerebral malaria can be treated with diazepam and other standard anticonvulsants. Prophylactic phenobarbitone has been shown to reduce seizure incidence in adult cerebral malaria (216), but a recent study in children has raised concerns over the safety of this approach; a single prophylactic intramuscular dose of 20 mg/kg reduced seizures but increased mortality, possibly through respiratory depression induced by an interaction with diazepam (217).

5.3.2. Blood Transfusion and Exchange Transfusion

Severe malaria is associated with anemia, and severely anemic patients should be transfused if blood is available. However transfusion is not a risk-free practice, particularly in the developing world. The blood has to be cross-matched and screened for blood-borne pathogens such as hepatitis B and HIV, and medical and nursing care must be of a sufficient standard to minimize the risks of over- or under-transfusion.

The role of partial exchange blood transfusion has been controversial for many years, though recent observations that poor deformability of unparasitized erythrocytes is associated with severe malaria has added a theoretical justification for its use (168). Exchange transfusion is still recommended by some, particularly in non-immune patients with very high parasitemias (>30%). No adequately powered randomized controlled trial has yet been conducted, and as such this rather dramatic treatment cannot be routinely recommended (218).

5.3.3. Fluid Balance, Dialysis, and Inotropic Support

Hypovolemia is associated with acidosis and shock in severe malaria, and fluid overload is associated with pulmonary edema. The judgment about how much fluid to transfuse is a fine one, particularly in the absence of mechanical ventilation, though the balance of evidence is tilting toward ensuring adequate hydration despite the risks (93).

Malaria-associated ARF in adults has an untreated mortality of over 70%, and should be treated with adequate renal replacement therapy (219). Hemofiltration has been shown recently to be superior in terms of mortality and cost-effectiveness to peritoneal dialysis (220). If patients survive the acute illness, the renal prognosis is good, with few if any patients left dialysis-dependent.

Hemodynamic shock should be treated with oxygen and volume expansion. Massive hemorrhage (from gastrointestinal tract or rarely a ruptured spleen) should be sought and excluded. When necessary a dopamine or norepinephrine infusion for inotropic support should be started (100,101). Epinephrine should be avoided as it is associated with lactic acidosis (100).

In any patient with malaria developing shock or undergoing any sudden deterioration in condition, a septic screen including blood cultures should be carried out and appropriate broad spectrum antibiotics started to cover the possibility of bacterial sepsis.

5.4. Other Adjunctive Therapies

A wide range of adjuvant therapies have been proposed for the treatment of cerebral and other forms of severe malaria. Most have been suggested on theoretical grounds, often on the basis of unproven pathophysiological hypotheses. For some, encouraging preliminary results in pilot studies were not confirmed in larger trials [e.g., corticosteroids (55,221), iron chelators (222), anti-TNF antibodies (223)]. Others though promising remain largely unstudied and have failed to find a place in standard clinical practice [e.g. osmotic anticerebral edema agents such as mannitol (175), dichloracetate (224), and the antioxidant *N*-acetylcysteine (94)]. At the time of writing no properly powered randomized drug trial of a study drug (antimalarial or otherwise) in severe malaria has ever shown a significant improvement in mortality over existing standard treatment.

6. CONCLUSION

Cerebral malaria is a major cause of morbidity and mortality in developing countries, and increasingly affects travelers returning from the tropics to developed countries in more temperate climes. The pathophysiology of the condition remains incompletely understood, though major advances have occurred in recent years, particularly in our knowledge of the mechanisms behind sequestration. In particular the *P. falciparum* variant antigen story, though complex and still unfolding, promises to dramatically improve our understanding of the pathophysiology of severe malaria, providing useful leads for the development of new treatments and vaccines.

The development of effective clinical management strategies lags behind the scientific understanding of the disease, though it is possible this will change with the results of clinical trials planned or currently underway of artemisinin derivatives and of adjuvant therapies such as the antioxidant *N*-acetylcysteine. Progress toward the holy grail of scientific malaria research, an effective and deployable vaccine, remains slow. Control of uncomplicated malaria may be the best strategy for reducing the morbidity and mortality of severe malaria. This can be achieved through disease prevention (through vector control, and hopefully in the future through vaccination), and by making effective oral antimalarial treatment both affordable and widely available.

ACKNOWLEDGMENTS

I would like to thank David Ferguson and Emsri Pongponratn for use of the electron micrographs in Figs 1 and 2, and Isabelle Medana for allowing me to use the photographs of -APP brain sections in Fig. 3. I am very grateful to Dr Gareth Turner for his helpful ideas and support.

REFERENCES

1. Krzywinski J, Besansky NJ. Molecular systematics of *Anopheles*: from subgenera to subpopulations. Annu Rev Entomol 2003; 48:111–139.

2. Phillips RS. Current status of malaria and potential for control. Clin Microbiol Rev 2001; 14(1):208–226.
3. Akim NI, Drakeley C, Kingo T, Simon B, Senkoro K, Sauerwein RW. Dynamics of *P. falciparum* gametocytemia in symptomatic patients in an area of intense perennial transmission in Tanzania. Am J Trop Med Hyg 2000; 63(3/4):199–203.
4. Greenwood B, Bradley A, Greenwood A, et al. Mortality and morbidity from malaria among children in a rural area of the Gambia, West Africa. Trans R Soc Trop Med Hyg 1987; 81:478–486.
5. Alonso PL, Lindsay SW, Armstrong JR, et al. The effect of insecticide-treated bed nets on mortality of Gambian children. Lancet 1991; 337(8756):1499–1502.
6. Brabin BJ. An analysis of malaria in pregnancy in Africa. Bull World Health Organ 1983; 61(6):1005–1016.
7. Marsh K, Forster D, Waruiru C, et al. Indicators of life-threatening malaria in African children. N Engl J Med 1995; 332(21):1399–1404.
8. Brewster DR, Greenwood BM. Seasonal variation of paediatric diseases in The Gambia, West Africa. Ann Trop Paediatr 1993; 13(2):133–146.
9. Snow RW, Bastos de Azevedo I, Lowe BS, et al. Severe childhood malaria in two areas of markedly different falciparum transmission in east Africa. Acta Trop 1994; 57(4):289–300.
10. Snow RW, Omumbo JA, Lowe B, et al. Relation between severe malaria morbidity in children and level of *Plasmodium falciparum* transmission in Africa. Lancet 1997; 349(9066):1650–1654.
11. Endeshaw Y, Assefa D. Cerebral malaria. Factors affecting outcome of treatment in a suboptimal clinical setting. J Trop Med Hyg 1990; 93(1):44–47.
12. Hien TT, Day NPJ, Phu NH, et al. A controlled trial of artemether or quinine in Vietnamese adults with severe falciparum malaria. N Engl J Med 1996; 335:76–83.
13. Haldane J. Disease and evolution. Ric Sci 1949; A(suppl):68–76.
14. Allison A. Protection afforded by sickle cell trait against subtertian malarial infection. BMJ 1954; 1:290–294.
15. Modiano D, Luoni G, Sirima BS, et al. Haemoglobin C protects against clinical *Plasmodium falciparum* malaria. Nature 2001; 414(6861):305–308.
16. Hutagalung R, Wilairatana P, Looareesuwan S, Brittenham GM, Aikawa M, Gordeuk VR. Influence of hemoglobin E trait on the severity of falciparum malaria. J Infect Dis 1999; 179(1):283–286.
17. Flint J, Hill AV, Bowden DK, et al. High frequencies of alpha-thalassaemia are the result of natural selection by malaria. Nature 1986; 321(6072):744–750.
18. McGuire W, Hill AV, Allsopp CE, Greenwood BM, Kwiatkowski D. Variation in the TNF-alpha promoter region associated with susceptibility to cerebral malaria. Nature 1994; 371(6497):508–510.
19. Knight JC, Udalova I, Hill AV, et al. A polymorphism that affects OCT-1 binding to the TNF promoter region is associated with severe malaria. Nat Genet 1999; 22(2):145–150.
20. McGuire W, Knight JC, Hill AV, Allsopp CE, Greenwood BM, Kwiatkowski D. Severe malarial anemia and cerebral malaria are associated with different tumor necrosis factor promoter alleles. J Infect Dis 1999; 179(1):287–290.
21. Hill A, Allsop C, Kwiatkowski D, et al. Common West African HLA antigens are associated with protection from severe malaria. Nature 1991; 352:595–600.
22. Aitman TJ, Cooper LD, Norsworthy PJ, et al. Malaria susceptibility and CD36 mutation. Nature 2000; 405(6790):1015–1016.

23. Fernandez-Reyes D, Craig AG, Kyes SA, et al. A high frequency African coding polymorphism in the N-terminal domain of ICAM-1 predisposing to cerebral malaria in Kenya. Hum Mol Genet 1997; 6(8):1357–1360.

24. Sabeti P, Usen S, Farhadian S, et al. CD40L association with protection from severe malaria. Genes Immun 2002; 3(5):286–291.

25. Burgner D, Usen S, Rockett K, et al. Nucleotide and haplotypic diversity of the NOS2A promoter region and its relationship to cerebral malaria. Hum Genet 2003; 112(4):379–386.

26. Aucan C, Walley AJ, Hennig BJ, et al. Interferon-alpha receptor-1 (IFNAR1) variants are associated with protection against cerebral malaria in The Gambia. Genes Immun 2003; 4(4):275–282.

27. Koch O, Awomoyi A, Usen S, et al. IFNGR1 gene promoter polymorphisms and susceptibility to cerebral malaria. J Infect Dis 2002; 185(11):1684–1687.

28. Cooke GS, Aucan C, Walley AJ, et al. Association of Fcgamma receptor IIa (CD32) polymorphism with severe malaria in West Africa. Am J Trop Med Hyg 2003; 69(6):565–568.

29. Kwiatkowski D. Genetic susceptibility to malaria getting complex. Curr Opin Genet Dev 2000; 10(3):320–324.

30. Clyde DF. Immunity to falciparum and vivax malaria induced by irradiated sporozoites: a review of the University of Maryland studies, 1971–75. Bull World Health Organ 1990; 68(suppl):9–12.

31. Nardin EH, Nussenzweig RS, McGregor IA, Bryan JH. Antibodies to sporozoites: their frequent occurrence in individuals living in an area of hyperendemic malaria. Science 1979; 206(4418):597–599.

32. Nardin EH, Nussenzweig RS. T cell responses to pre-erythrocytic stages of malaria: role in protection and vaccine development against pre-erythrocytic stages. Annu Rev Immunol 1993; 11:687–727.

33. Doolan DL, Hoffman SL. Pre-erythrocytic-stage immune effector mechanisms in *Plasmodium* spp. infections. Philos Trans R Soc Lond B Biol Sci 1997; 352(1359):1361–1367.

34. Bull PC, Marsh K. The role of antibodies to *Plasmodium falciparum*-infected-erythrocyte surface antigens in naturally acquired immunity to malaria. Trends Microbiol 2002; 10(2):55–58.

35. Yipp BG, Anand S, Schollaardt T, Patel KD, Looareesuwan S, Ho M. Synergism of multiple adhesion molecules in mediating cytoadherence of *Plasmodium falciparum*-infected erythrocytes to microvascular endothelial cells under flow. Blood 2000; 96(6):2292–2298.

36. Smith JD, Craig AG, Kriek N, et al. Identification of a *Plasmodium falciparum* intercellular adhesion molecule-1 binding domain: a parasite adhesion trait implicated in cerebral malaria. Proc Natl Acad Sci U S A 2000; 97(4):1766–1771.

37. Nielsen MA, Staalsoe T, Kurtzhals JA, et al. *Plasmodium falciparum* variant surface antigen expression varies between isolates causing severe and nonsevere malaria and is modified by acquired immunity. J Immunol 2002; 168(7):3444–3450.

38. Flick K, Chen Q. var genes, PfEMP1 and the human host. Mol Biochem Parasitol 2004; 134(1):3–9.

39. Guevara Patino JA, Holder AA, McBride JS, Blackman MJ. Antibodies that inhibit malaria merozoite surface protein-1 processing and erythrocyte invasion are

blocked by naturally acquired human antibodies. J Exp Med 1997; 186(10):1689–1699.

40. Riley EM. Is T-cell priming required for initiation of pathology in malaria infections? Immunol Today 1999; 20(5):228–233.

41. Artavanis-Tsakonas K, Tongren JE, Riley EM. The war between the malaria parasite and the immune system: immunity, immunoregulation and immunopathology. Clin Exp Immunol 2003; 133(2):145–152.

42. Chirenda J, Siziya S, Tshimanga M. Association of HIV infection with the development of severe and complicated malaria cases at a rural hospital in Zimbabwe. Cent Afr J Med 2000; 46(1):5–9.

43. Grimwade K, French N, Mbatha DD, Zungu DD, Dedicoat M, Gilks CF. Childhood malaria in a region of unstable transmission and high human immunodeficiency virus prevalence. Pediatr Infect Dis J 2003; 22(12):1057–1063.

44. Ariey F, Hommel D, Le Scanf C, et al. Association of severe malaria with a specific *Plasmodium falciparum* genotype in French Guiana. J Infect Dis 2001; 184(2):237–241.

45. Roberts DJ, Pain A, Kai O, Kortok M, Marsh K. Autoagglutination of malaria-infected red blood cells and malaria severity. Lancet 2000; 355(9213):1427–1428.

46. Greenwood B, Marsh K, Snow R. Why do some African children develop severe malaria? Acta Anaesth Scand 1991; 7:277–281.

47. Meek SR. Epidemiology of malaria in displaced Khmers on the Thai-Kampuchean border. Southeast Asian J Trop Med Public Health 1988; 19(2):243–252.

48. Luxemburger C, Ricci F, Nosten F, Raimond D, Bathet S, White NJ. The epidemiology of severe malaria in an area of low transmission in Thailand. Trans R Soc Trop Med Hyg 1997; 91(3):256–262.

49. Cao XT, Bethell DB, Pham TP, et al. Comparison of artemisinin suppositories, intramuscular artesunate and intravenous quinine for the treatment of severe childhood malaria. Trans R Soc Trop Med Hyg 1997; 91(3):335–342.

50. Waller D, Krishna S, Crawley J, et al. Clinical features and outcome of severe malaria in Gambian children. Clin Infect Dis 1995; 21(3):577–587.

51. Makani J, Matuja W, Liyombo E, Snow RW, Marsh K, Warrell DA. Admission diagnosis of cerebral malaria in adults in an endemic area of Tanzania: implications and clinical description. QJM 2003; 96(5):355–362.

52. Taylor TE, Fu WJ, Carr RA, et al. Differentiating the pathologies of cerebral malaria by postmortem parasite counts. Nat Med 2004; 10(2):143–145.

53. World Health Organization. Severe and complicated malaria. Trans R Soc Trop Med Hyg 1990; 84(suppl 2):1–65.

54. World Health Organization. Severe falciparum malaria. Trans R Soc Trop Med Hyg 2000; 94(suppl 1):S1–S90.

55. Warrell D, Looareesuwan S, Warrell M, et al. Dexamethasone proves deleterious in cerebral malaria: a double-blind trial in 100 comatose patients. N Engl J Med 1982; 306:313–319.

56. Molyneux ME, Taylor TE, Wirima JJ, Borgstein A. Clinical features and prognostic indicators in paediatric cerebral malaria: a study of 131 comatose Malawian children. QJM 1989; 71(265):441–459.

57. Newton CR, Chokwe T, Schellenberg JA, et al. Coma scales for children with severe falciparum malaria. Trans R Soc Trop Med Hyg 1997; 91(2):161–165.

58. Mabeza GF, Moyo VM, Thuma PE, et al. Predictors of severity of illness on presentation in children with cerebral malaria. Ann Trop Med Parasitol 1995; 89(3):221–228.

59. Plum F, Posner J. The Diagnosis of Stupor and Coma. 3rd ed. Philadelphia: FA Davis Company, 1980.

60. Warrell DA. Cerebral malaria: clinical features, pathophysiology and treatment. Ann Trop Med Parasitol 1997; 91(7):875–884.

61. Newton CR, Hien TT, White N. Cerebral malaria. J Neurol Neurosurg Psychiatry 2000; 69(4):433–441.

62. Newton CR, Kirkham FJ, Winstanley PA, et al. Intracranial pressure in African children with cerebral malaria. Lancet 1991; 337(8741):573–576.

63. Newton CR, Marsh K, Peshu N, Kirkham FJ. Perturbations of cerebral hemodynamics in Kenyans with cerebral malaria. Pediatr Neurol 1996; 15(1):41–49.

64. Looareesuwan S, Warrell DA, White NJ, et al. Retinal hemorrhage, a common sign of prognostic significance in cerebral malaria. Am J Trop Med Hyg 1983; 32(5):911–915.

65. Crawley J, Smith S, Kirkham F, Muthinji P, Waruiru C, Marsh K. Seizures and status epilepticus in childhood cerebral malaria. QJM 1996; 89(8):591–597.

66. Crawley J, Smith S, Muthinji P, Marsh K, Kirkham F. Electroencephalographic and clinical features of cerebral malaria. Arch Dis Child 2001; 84(3):247–253.

67. Waruiru CM, Newton CR, Forster D, et al. Epileptic seizures and malaria in Kenyan children. Trans R Soc Trop Med Hyg 1996; 90(2):152–155.

68. White NJ, Warrell DA, Chanthavanich P, et al. Severe hypoglycemia and hyperinsulinemia in falciparum malaria. N Engl J Med 1983; 309(2):61–66.

69. White NJ, Marsh K, Turner RC, et al. Hypoglycaemia in African children with severe malaria. Lancet 1987:708–711.

70. Looareesuwan S, White N, Karbwang J, et al. Quinine and severe falciparum malaria in late pregnancy. Lancet 1985; II:4–8.

71. Taylor TE, Molyneux ME. Blood glucose levels in Malawian children before and during administration of intravenous quinine for severe malaria. N Engl J Med 1988; 319:1040–1047.

72. English M, Wale S, Binns G, Mwangi I, Sauerwein H, Marsh K. Hypoglycaemia on and after admission in Kenyan children with severe malaria. QJM 1998; 91(3):191–197.

73. Davis TM, Looareesuwan S, Pukrittayakamee S, Levy JC, Nagachinta B, White NJ. Glucose turnover in severe falciparum malaria. Metabolism 1993; 42(3):334–340.

74. Bondi FS. The incidence and outcome of neurological abnormalities in childhood cerebral malaria: a long-term follow-up of 62 survivors. Trans R Soc Trop Med Hyg 1992; 86(1):17–19.

75. Brewster DR, Kwiatkowski D, White NJ. Neurological sequelae of cerebral malaria in children. Lancet 1990; 336(8722):1039–1043.

76. Bajiya HN, Kochar DK. Incidence and outcome of neurological sequelae in survivors of cerebral malaria. J Assoc Physicians India 1996; 44(10):679–681.

77. van Hensbroek MB, Palmer A, Jaffar S, Schneider G, Kwiatkowski D. Residual neurologic sequelae after childhood cerebral malaria. J Pediatr 1997; 131(1 Pt 1):125–129.

78. Muntendam AH, Jaffar S, Bleichrodt N, van Hensbroek MB. Absence of neuropsychological sequelae following cerebral malaria in Gambian children. Trans R Soc Trop Med Hyg 1996; 90(4):391–394.

79. Varney NR, Roberts RJ, Springer JA, Connell SK, Wood PS. Neuropsychiatric sequelae of cerebral malaria in Vietnam veterans. J Nerv Ment Dis 1997; 185(11):695–703.

80. Nguyen TH, Day NP, Ly VC, et al. Post-malaria neurological syndrome. Lancet 1996; 348(9032):917–921.

81. Senanayake N, de Silva HJ. Delayed cerebellar ataxia complicating falciparum malaria: a clinical study of 74 patients. J Neurol 1994; 241(7):456–459.

82. Abdulla MN, Sokrab TE, Zaidan ZA, Siddig HE, Ali ME. Post-malarial cerebellar ataxia in adult Sudanese patients. East Afr Med J 1997; 74(9):570–572.

83. Kochar DK, Shubhakaran, Kumawat BL, et al. Cerebral malaria in Indian adults: a prospective study of 441 patients from Bikaner, north-west India. J Assoc Physicians India 2002; 50:234–241.

84. de Silva HJ, Hoang P, Dalton H, de Silva NR, Jewell DP, Peiris JB. Immune activation during cerebellar dysfunction following *Plasmodium falciparum* malaria. Trans R Soc Trop Med Hyg 1992; 86(2):129–131.

85. Dey AB, Trikha I, Banerjee M, Jain R, Nagarkar KM. Acute disseminated encephalomyelitis—another cause of post malaria cerebellar ataxia. J Assoc Physicians India 2001; 49:756–758.

86. English M, Waruiru C, Marsh K. Transfusion for respiratory distress in life-threatening childhood malaria. Am J Trop Med Hyg 1996; 55(5):525–530.

87. English M, Sauerwein R, Waruiru C, et al. Acidosis in severe childhood malaria. QJM 1997; 90(4):263–270.

88. White NJ, Warrell DA, Looareesuwan S, Chanthavanich P, Phillips RE, Pongpaew P. Pathophysiological and prognostic significance of cerebrospinal-fluid lactate in cerebral malaria. Lancet 1985; 1(8432):776–778.

89. Taylor TE, Borgstein A, Molyneux ME. Acid–base status in paediatric *Plasmodium falciparum* malaria. QJM 1993; 86(2):99–109.

90. Krishna S, Waller DW, ter Kuile F, et al. Lactic acidosis and hypoglycaemia in children with severe malaria: pathophysiological and prognostic significance. Trans R Soc Trop Med Hyg 1994; 88(1):67–73.

91. Day NP, Phu NH, Mai NT, et al. The pathophysiologic and prognostic significance of acidosis in severe adult malaria. Crit Care Med 2000; 28(6):1833–1840.

92. Maitland K, Levin M, English M, et al. Severe *P. falciparum* malaria in Kenyan children: evidence for hypovolaemia. QJM 2003; 96(6):427–434.

93. Maitland K, Pamba A, Newton CR, Levin M. Response to volume resuscitation in children with severe malaria. Pediatr Crit Care Med 2003; 4(4):426–431.

94. Watt G, Jongsakul K, Ruangvirayuth R. A pilot study of N-acetylcysteine as adjunctive therapy for severe malaria. QJM 2002; 95(5):285–290.

95. Bruneel F, Hocqueloux L, Alberti C, et al. The clinical spectrum of severe imported falciparum malaria in the intensive care unit: report of 188 cases in adults. Am J Respir Crit Care Med 2003; 167(5):684–689.

96. Naqvi R, Ahmad E, Akhtar F, Naqvi A, Rizvi A. Outcome in severe acute renal failure associated with malaria. Nephrol Dial Transplant 2003; 18(9):1820–1823.

97. Burchard GD, Ehrhardt S, Mockenhaupt FP, et al. Renal dysfunction in children with uncomplicated, *Plasmodium falciparum* malaria in Tamale, Ghana. Ann Trop Med Parasitol 2003; 97(4):345–350.

98. Tran TH, Day NP, Ly VC, et al. Blackwater fever in southern Vietnam: a prospective descriptive study of 50 cases. Clin Infect Dis 1996; 23(6):1274–1281.

99. Bruneel F, Gachot B, Wolff M, Regnier B, Danis M, Vachon F. Resurgence of blackwater fever in long-term European expatriates in Africa: report of 21 cases and review. Clin Infect Dis 2001; 32(8):1133–1140.

100. Day NP, Phu NH, Bethell DP, et al. The effects of dopamine and adrenaline infusions on acid–base balance and systemic haemodynamics in severe infection [published erratum appears in Lancet 1996 Sep 28; 348(9031):902]. Lancet 1996; 348(9022):219–223.

101. Bruneel F, Gachot B, Timsit JF, et al. Shock complicating severe falciparum malaria in European adults. Intensive Care Med 1997; 23(6):698–701.

102. Bygbjerg I, Lanng C. Septicaemia as a complication of falciparum malaria (letter). Trans R Soc Trop Med Hyg 1982; 76:705.

103. Fein IA, Rackow E, Shapiro L. Acute pulmonary edema in *Plasmodium falciparum* malaria. Am Rev Respir Dis 1978; 118:425–429.

104. Martell R, Kallenbach J, Zwi S. Pulmonary oedema in falciparum malaria. BMJ 1979; i:1763–1764.

105. Taylor WR, White NJ. Malaria and the lung. Clin Chest Med 2002; 23(2):457–468.

106. James M. Pulmonary damage associated with falciparum malaria: a report of ten patients. Ann Trop Med Parasitol 1985; 79:123–138.

107. Blanloeil Y, Baron D, de Lajartre AY, Nicolas F. Acute respiratory distress syndrome (ARDS) in cerebral malaria (author's transl). Sem Hop 1980; 56(21–24):1088–1090.

108. Pukrittayakamee S, White NJ, Davis TM, et al. Hepatic blood flow and metabolism in severe falciparum malaria: clearance of intravenously administered galactose. Clin Sci (Colch) 1992; 82(1):63–70.

109. Cerami C, Frevert U, Sinnis P, et al. The basolateral domain of the hepatocyte plasma membrane bears receptors for the circumsporozoite protein of *Plasmodium falciparum* sporozoites. Cell 1992; 70(6):1021–1033.

110. Silvie O, Rubinstein E, Franetich JF, et al. Hepatocyte CD81 is required for *Plasmodium falciparum* and *Plasmodium yoelii* sporozoite infectivity. Nat Med 2003; 9(1):93–96.

111. Narum DL, Fuhrmann SR, Luu T, Sim BK. A novel *Plasmodium falciparum* erythrocyte binding protein-2 (EBP2/BAEBL) involved in erythrocyte receptor binding. Mol Biochem Parasitol 2002; 119(2):159–168.

112. Jakobsen PH, Heegaard PM, Koch C, et al. Identification of an erythrocyte binding peptide from the erythrocyte binding antigen, EBA-175, which blocks parasite multiplication and induces peptide-blocking antibodies. Infect Immun 1998; 66(9):4203–4207.

113. Rayner JC, Vargas-Serrato E, Huber CS, Galinski MR, Barnwell JW. A *Plasmodium falciparum* homologue of *Plasmodium vivax* reticulocyte binding protein (PvRBP1) defines a trypsin-resistant erythrocyte invasion pathway. J Exp Med 2001; 194(11):1571–1581.

114. Gilberger TW, Thompson JK, Triglia T, Good RT, Duraisingh MT, Cowman AF. A novel erythrocyte binding antigen-175 paralogue from *Plasmodium falciparum* defines a new trypsin-resistant receptor on human erythrocytes. J Biol Chem 2003; 278(16):14,480–14,486.

115. Duraisingh MT, Maier AG, Triglia T, Cowman AF. Erythrocyte-binding antigen 175 mediates invasion in *Plasmodium falciparum* utilizing sialic acid-dependent and independent pathways. Proc Natl Acad Sci U S A 2003; 100(8):4796–4801.

116. Li X, Chen H, Oo TH, et al. A co-ligand complex anchors *Plasmodium falciparum* merozoites to the erythrocyte invasion receptor band 3. J Biol Chem 2003.

117. Bohle DS, Kosar AD, Stephens PW. Phase homogeneity and crystal morphology of the malaria pigment beta-hematin. Acta Crystallogr D Biol Crystallogr 2002; 58(Pt 10 Pt 1):1752–1756.

118. Cranston HA, Boylan CW, Carroll GL, et al. *Plasmodium falciparum* maturation abolishes physiologic red cell deformability. Science 1984; 223(4634):400–403.

119. Suwanarusk R, Cooke BM, Dondorp AM, et al. The deformability of red blood C cells parasitized by *Plasmodium falciparum* and *P. vivax*. J Infect Dis 2004; 189(2):190–194.

120. Silamut K, White NJ. Relation of the stage of parasite development in the peripheral blood to prognosis in severe falciparum malaria. Trans R Soc Trop Med Hyg 1993; 87(4):436–443.

121. Macperson GG, Warrell MJ, White NJ, Looareesuwan S, Warrell DA. Human cerebral malaria: a quantitative ultrastructural analysis of parasitized erythrocyte sequestration. Am J Pathol 1985; 119:385–401.

122. Pongponratn E, Riganti M, Punpoowong B, Aikawa M. Microvascular sequestration of parasitized erythrocytes in human falciparum malaria: a pathological study. Am J Trop Med Hyg 1991; 44(2):168–175.

123. Pongponratn E, Turner GD, Day NP, et al. An ultrastructural study of the brain in fatal *Plasmodium falciparum* malaria. Am J Trop Med Hyg 2003; 69(4):345–359.

124. Taverne J, Bate CA, Kwiatkowski D, Jakobsen PH, Playfair JH. Two soluble antigens of *Plasmodium falciparum* induce tumor necrosis factor release from macrophages. Infect Immun 1990; 58(9):2923–2928.

125. Arese P, Schwarzer E. Malarial pigment (haemozoin): a very active "inert" substance. Ann Trop Med Parasitol 1997; 91(5):501–516.

126. Schwarzer E, Alessio M, Ulliers D, Arese P. Phagocytosis of the malarial pigment, hemozoin, impairs expression of major histocompatibility complex class II antigen, CD54, and CD11c in human monocytes. Infect immun 1998; 66(4):1601–1606.

127. Jaramillo M, Gowda DC, Radzioch D, Olivier M. Hemozoin increases IFN-gamma-inducible macrophage nitric oxide generation through extracellular signal-regulated kinase- and NF-kappa B-dependent pathways. J Immunol 2003; 171(8):4243–4253.

128. Taramelli D, Basilico N, De Palma AM, et al. The effect of synthetic malaria pigment (beta-haematin) on adhesion molecule expression and interleukin-6 production by human endothelial cells. Trans R Soc Trop Med Hyg 1998; 92(1):57–62.

129. Turner GD, Morrison H, Jones M, et al. An immunohistochemical study of the pathology of fatal malaria. Evidence for widespread endothelial activation and a potential role for intercellular adhesion molecule-1 in cerebral sequestration. Am J Pathol 1994; 145(5):1057–1069.

130. Brown H, Hien TT, Day N, et al. Evidence of blood–brain barrier dysfunction in human cerebral malaria. Neuropathol Appl Neurobiol 1999; 25(4):331–340.

131. Turner G. Cerebral malaria. Brain Pathol 1997; 7(1):569–582.

132. Medana IM, Esiri MM. Axonal damage: a key predictor of outcome in human CNS diseases. Brain 2003; 126(Pt 3):515–530.

133. Medana IM, Day NP, Hien TT, et al. Axonal injury in cerebral malaria. Am J Pathol 2002; 160(2):655–666.

134. Ockenhouse CF, Ho M, Tandon NN, et al. Molecular basis of sequestration in severe and uncomplicated *Plasmodium falciparum* malaria: differential adhesion of infected erythrocytes to CD36 and ICAM-1. J Infect Dis 1991; 164(1):163–169.

135. Pain A, Urban BC, Kai O, et al. A non-sense mutation in Cd36 gene is associated with protection from severe malaria. Lancet 2001; 357(9267):1502–1503.

136. McCormick CJ, Craig A, Roberts D, Newbold CI, Berendt AR. Intercellular adhesion molecule-1 and CD36 synergize to mediate adherence of *Plasmodium falciparum*-infected erythrocytes to cultured human microvascular endothelial cells. J Clin Invest 1997; 100(10):2521–2529.

137. Wassmer SC, Combes V, Grau GE. Pathophysiology of cerebral malaria: role of host cells in the modulation of cytoadhesion. Ann N Y Acad Sci 2003; 992:30–38.

138. Pain A, Ferguson DJ, Kai O, et al. Platelet-mediated clumping of *Plasmodium falciparum*-infected erythrocytes is a common adhesive phenotype and is associated with severe malaria. Proc Natl Acad Sci U S A 2001; 98(4):1805–1810.

139. Yipp BG, Robbins SM, Resek ME, Baruch DI, Looareesuwan S, Ho M. Src-family kinase signaling modulates the adhesion of *Plasmodium falciparum* on human microvascular endothelium under flow. Blood 2003; 101(7):2850–2857.

140. Ohashi J, Naka I, Patarapotikul J, Hananantachai H, Looareesuwan S, Tokunaga K. Absence of association between the allele coding methionine at position 29 in the N-terminal domain of ICAM-1 (ICAM-1(Kilifi)) and severe malaria in the northwest of Thailand. Jpn J Infect Dis 2001; 54(3):114–116.

141. Baruch DI, Rogerson SJ, Cooke BM. Asexual blood stages of malaria antigens: cytoadherence. Chem Immunol 2002; 80:144–162.

142. Sherman IW, Eda S, Winograd E. Cytoadherence and sequestration in *Plasmodium falciparum*: defining the ties that bind. Microbes Infect 2003; 5(10):897–909.

143. Rogerson SJ, Novakovic S, Cooke BM, Brown GV. *Plasmodium falciparum*-infected erythrocytes adhere to the proteoglycan thrombomodulin in static and flow-based systems. Exp Parasitol 1997; 86(1):8–18.

144. Maubert B, Fievet N, Tami G, Cot M, Boudin C, Deloron P. Development of antibodies against chondroitin sulfate A-adherent *Plasmodium falciparum* in pregnant women. Infect immun 1999; 67(10):5367–5371.

145. Smith JD, Chitnis CE, Craig AG, et al. Switches in expression of *Plasmodium falciparum* var genes correlate with changes in antigenic and cytoadherent phenotypes of infected erythrocytes. Cell 1995; 82(1):101–110.

146. Borst P, Bitter W, McCulloch R, Van Leeuwen F, Rudenko G. Antigenic variation in malaria. Cell 1995; 82(1):1–4.

147. Su XZ, Heatwole VM, Wertheimer SP, et al. The large diverse gene family var encodes proteins involved in cytoadherence and antigenic variation of *Plasmodium falciparum*-infected erythrocytes. Cell 1995; 82(1):89–100.

148. Roberts DJ, Craig AG, Berendt AR, et al. Rapid switching to multiple antigenic and adhesive phenotypes in malaria. Nature 1992; 357(6380):689–692.

149. Chen Q, Fernandez V, Sundstrom A, et al. Developmental selection of var gene expression in *Plasmodium falciparum*. Nature 1998; 394(6691):392–395.

150. Robinson BA, Welch TL, Smith JD. Widespread functional specialization of *Plasmodium falciparum* erythrocyte membrane protein 1 family members to bind CD36 analysed across a parasite genome. Mol Microbiol 2003; 47(5):1265–1278.

151. Chen Q, Heddini A, Barragan A, Fernandez V, Pearce SF, Wahlgren M. The semi-conserved head structure of *Plasmodium falciparum* erythrocyte membrane protein

1 mediates binding to multiple independent host receptors. J Exp Med 2000; 192(1):1–10.

152. Chattopadhyay R, Taneja T, Chakrabarti K, Pillai CR, Chitnis CE. Molecular analysis of the cytoadherence phenotype of a *Plasmodium falciparum* field isolate that binds intercellular adhesion molecule-1. Mol Biochem Parasitol 2004; 133(2):255–265.

153. Lekana Douki JB, Traore B, Costa FT, et al. Sequestration of *Plasmodium falciparum*-infected erythrocytes to chondroitin sulfate A, a receptor for maternal malaria: monoclonal antibodies against the native parasite ligand reveal pan-reactive epitopes in placental isolates. Blood 2002; 100(4):1478–1483.

154. Kaviratne M, Khan SM, Jarra W, Preiser PR. Small variant STEVOR antigen is uniquely located within Maurer's clefts in *Plasmodium falciparum*-infected red blood cells. Eukaryot Cell 2002; 1(6):926–935.

155. Haeggstrom M, Kironde F, Berzins K, Chen Q, Wahlgren M, Fernandez V. Common trafficking pathway for variant antigens destined for the surface of the *Plasmodium falciparum*-infected erythrocyte. Mol Biochem Parasitol 2004; 133(1):1–14.

156. Holt DC, Gardiner DL, Thomas EA, et al. The cytoadherence linked asexual gene family of *Plasmodium falciparum*: are there roles other than cytoadherence? Int J Parasitol 1999; 29(6):939–944.

157. Ockenhouse CF, Klotz FW, Tandon NN, Jamieson GA. Sequestrin, a CD36 recognition protein on *Plasmodium falciparum* malaria-infected erythrocytes identified by anti-idiotype antibodies. Proc Natl Acad Sci U S A 1991; 88(8):3175–3179.

158. Eda S, Lawler J, Sherman IW. *Plasmodium falciparum*-infected erythrocyte adhesion to the type 3 repeat domain of thrombospondin-1 is mediated by a modified band 3 protein. Mol Biochem Parasitol 1999; 100(2):195–205.

159. Eda S, Sherman IW. Cytoadherence of malaria-infected red blood cells involves exposure of phosphatidylserine. Cell Physiol Biochem 2002; 12(5/6):373–384.

160. Carlson J, Helmby H, Hill AV, Brewster D, Greenwood BM, Wahlgren M. Human cerebral malaria: association with erythrocyte rosetting and lack of anti-rosetting antibodies. Lancet 1990; 336(8729):1457–1460.

161. Rowe A, Obeiro J, Newbold CI, Marsh K. *Plasmodium falciparum* rosetting is associated with malaria severity in Kenya. Infect immun 1995; 63(6):2323–2326.

162. al-Yaman F, Genton B, Mokela D, et al. Human cerebral malaria: lack of significant association between erythrocyte rosetting and disease severity. Trans R Soc Trop Med Hyg 1995; 89(1):55–58.

163. Udomsanpetch R, Thanikkul K, Pukrittayakamee S, White NJ. Rosette formation by *Plasmodium vivax*. Trans R Soc Trop Med Hyg 1995; 89(6):635–637.

164. Angus BJ, Thanikkul K, Silamut K, White NJ, Udomsangpetch R. Short report: Rosette formation in *Plasmodium ovale* infection. Am J Trop Med Hyg 1996; 55(5):560–561.

165. Rowe JA, Rogerson SJ, Raza A, et al. Mapping of the region of complement receptor (CR) 1 required for *Plasmodium falciparum* rosetting and demonstration of the importance of CR1 in rosetting in field isolates. J Immunol 2000; 165(11):6341–6346.

166. Dondorp AM, Pongponratn E, White NJ. Reduced microcirculatory flow in severe falciparum malaria: pathophysiology and electron-microscopic pathology. Acta Trop 2004; 89(3):309–317.

167. Dondorp A, Angus B, Hardeman M, et al. Prognostic significance of reduced red cell deformability in severe falciparum malaria. Am J Trop Med Hyg 1997; 57:507–511.

168. Dondorp AM, Nyanoti M, Kager PA, Mithwani S, Vreeken J, Marsh K. The role of reduced red cell deformability in the pathogenesis of severe falciparum malaria and its restoration by blood transfusion. Trans R Soc Trop Med Hyg 2002; 96(3):282–286.

169. Dondorp AM, Angus BJ, Chotivanich K, et al. Red blood cell deformability as a predictor of anemia in severe falciparum malaria. Am J Trop Med Hyg 1999; 60(5):733–737.

170. Dondorp AM, Omodeo-Sale F, Chotivanich K, Taramelli D, White NJ. Oxidative stress and rheology in severe malaria. Redox Rep 2003; 8(5):292–294.

171. Looareesuwan S, Wilairatana P, Krishna S, et al. Magnetic resonance imaging of the brain in patients with cerebral malaria. Clin Infect Dis 1995; 21(2):300–309.

172. Patankar TF, Karnad DR, Shetty PG, Desai AP, Prasad SR. Adult cerebral malaria: prognostic importance of imaging findings and correlation with postmortem findings. Radiology 2002; 224(3):811–816.

173. Lucas S, Hounnou A, Bell J, et al. Severe cerebral swelling is not observed in children dying with malaria. QJM 1996; 89:351–353.

174. Waller D, Crawley J, Nosten F, et al. Intracranial pressure in childhood cerebral malaria. Trans R Soc Trop Med Hyg 1991; 85:362–364.

175. Newton CR, Crawley J, Sowumni A, et al. Intracranial hypertension in Africans with cerebral malaria. Arch Dis Child 1997; 76(3):219–226.

176. White NJ. Lumbar puncture in cerebral malaria. Lancet 1991; 338(8767):640–641.

177. Brown H, Rogerson S, Taylor T, et al. Blood–brain barrier function in cerebral malaria in Malawian children. Am J Trop Med Hyg 2001; 64(3/4):207–213.

178. Brown HC, Chau TT, Mai NT, et al. Blood–brain barrier function in cerebral malaria and CNS infections in Vietnam. Neurology 2000; 55(1):104–111.

179. Clark I, Rockett K. The cytokine theory of human cerebral malaria. Parasitol Today 1994; 10:410–412.

180. Grau GE, Taylor TE, Molyneux ME, et al. Tumor necrosis factor and disease severity in children with falciparum malaria. N Engl J Med 1989; 320(24):1586–1591.

181. Kwiatkowski D, Hill AV, Sambou I, et al. TNF concentration in fatal cerebral, non-fatal cerebral, and uncomplicated *Plasmodium falciparum* malaria. Lancet 1990; 336(8725):1201–1204.

182. Day NP, Hien TT, Schollaardt T, et al. The prognostic and pathophysiologic role of pro- and anti-inflammatory cytokines in severe malaria. J Infect Dis 1999; 180(4):1288–1297.

183. Engwerda CR, Mynott TL, Sawhney S, De Souza JB, Bickle QD, Kaye PM. Locally up-regulated lymphotoxin alpha, not systemic tumor necrosis factor alpha, is the principle mediator of murine cerebral malaria. J Exp Med 2002; 195(10):1371–1377.

184. Jacobs P, Radzioch D, Stevenson MM. In vivo regulation of nitric oxide production by tumor necrosis factor alpha and gamma interferon, but not by interleukin-4, during blood stage malaria in mice. Infect Immun 1996; 64(1):44–49.

185. Luty AJ, Lell B, Schmidt-Ott R, et al. Interferon-gamma responses are associated with resistance to reinfection with *Plasmodium falciparum* in young African children. J Infect Dis 1999; 179(4):980–988.

186. Dodoo D, Omer FM, Todd J, Akanmori BD, Koram KA, Riley EM. Absolute levels and ratios of proinflammatory and anti-inflammatory cytokine production in vitro predict clinical immunity to *Plasmodium falciparum* malaria. J Infect Dis 2002; 185(7):971–979.

187. Artavanis-Tsakonas K, Riley EM. Innate immune response to malaria: rapid induction of IFN-gamma from human NK cells by live *Plasmodium falciparum*-infected erythrocytes. J Immunol 2002; 169(6):2956–2963.

188. Doolan DL, Hoffman SL. IL-12 and NK cells are required for antigen-specific adaptive immunity against malaria initiated by CD8+ T cells in the *Plasmodium yoelii* model. J Immunol 1999; 163(2):884–892.

189. Cot S, Ringwald P, Mulder B, et al. Nitric oxide in cerebral malaria. J Infect Dis 1994; 169(6):1417–1418.

190. Nussler A, Eling W, Kremsner P. Patients with *Plasmodium falciparum* malaria and *Plasmodium vivax* malaria show increased nitrite and nitrate plasma levels. J Infect Dis 1994; 169:1418–1419.

191. Kremsner P, Winkler S, Wildling E, et al. High plasma levels of nitrogen oxides are associated with severe disease and correlate with rapid parasitological and clinical cure in *Plasmodium falciparum* malaria. Trans R Soc Trop Med Hyg 1996; 90:44–47.

192. al-Yaman F, Awburn MM, Clark IA. Serum creatinine levels and reactive nitrogen intermediates in children with cerebral malaria in Papua New Guinea. Trans R Soc Trop Med Hyg 1997; 91(3):303–305.

193. Agbenyega T, Angus B, Bedu-Addo G, et al. Plasma nitrogen oxides and blood lactate concentrations in Ghanaian children with malaria. Trans R Soc Trop Med Hyg 1997; 91(3):298–302.

194. Taylor AM, Day NP, Sinh DX, et al. Reactive nitrogen intermediates and outcome in severe adult malaria. Trans R Soc Trop Med Hyg 1998; 92(2):170–175.

195. Anstey NM, Weinberg JB, Hassanali MY, et al. Nitric oxide in Tanzanian children with malaria: inverse relationship between malaria severity and nitric oxide production/nitric oxide synthase type 2 expression. J Exp Med 1996; 184(2):557–567.

196. Sanni LA. The role of cerebral oedema in the pathogenesis of cerebral malaria. Redox Rep 2001; 6(3):137–142.

197. Sanni LA, Thomas SR, Tattam BN, et al. Dramatic changes in oxidative tryptophan metabolism along the kynurenine pathway in experimental cerebral and noncerebral malaria. Am J Pathol 1998; 152(2):611–619.

198. Dobbie M, Crawley J, Waruiru C, Marsh K, Surtees R. Cerebrospinal fluid studies in children with cerebral malaria: an excitotoxic mechanism? Am J Trop Med Hyg 2000; 62(2):284–290.

199. Medana IM, Hien TT, Day NP, et al. The clinical significance of cerebrospinal fluid levels of kynurenine pathway metabolites and lactate in severe malaria. J Infect Dis 2002; 185(5):650–656.

200. Medana IM, Day NP, Salahifar-Sabet H, et al. Metabolites of the kynurenine pathway of tryptophan metabolism in the cerebrospinal fluid of Malawian children with malaria. J Infect Dis 2003; 188(6):844–849.

201. Gardner MJ, Hall N, Fung E, et al. Genome sequence of the human malaria parasite *Plasmodium falciparum*. Nature 2002; 419(6906):498–511.

202. Waller D, Krishna S, Craddock C, et al. The pharmacokinetic properties of intramuscular quinine in Gambian children with severe falciparum malaria. Trans R Soc Trop Med Hyg 1990; 84:488–491.

203. White NJ, Looareesuwan S, Warrell DA, et al. Quinine loading dose in cerebral malaria. Am J Trop Med Hyg 1983; 32(1):1–5.

204. White N. The treatment of malaria. N Engl J Med 1996; 335:800–806.

205. Yen LM, Dao LM, Day NP, et al. Role of quinine in the high mortality of intramuscular injection tetanus. Lancet 1994; 344(8925):786–787.

206. Hong G. Handbook of Emergency Treatments; AD 340.

207. Brewer TG, Peggins JO, Grate SJ, et al. Neurotoxicity in animals due to arteether and artemether. Trans R Soc Trop Med Hyg 1994; 88(suppl 1):S33–S36.

208. Hien TT, Turner GD, Mai NT, et al. Neuropathological assessment of artemether-treated severe malaria. Lancet 2003; 362(9380):295–296.

209. van Hensbroek MB, Onyiorah E, Jaffar S, et al. A trial of artemether or quinine in children with cerebral malaria. N Engl J Med 1996; 335(2):69–75.

210. Artemether–Quinine Meta-analysis Study Group. A meta-analysis using individual patient data of trials comparing artemether with quinine in the treatment of severe falciparum malaria. Trans R Soc Trop Med Hyg 2001; 95(6):637–650.

211. Murphy SA, Mberu E, Muhia D, et al. The disposition of intramuscular artemether in children with cerebral malaria; a preliminary study. Trans R Soc Trop Med Hyg 1997; 91(3):331–334.

212. Nontprasert A, Nosten-Bertrand M, Pukrittayakamee S, Vanijanonta S, Angus BJ, White NJ. Assessment of the neurotoxicity of parenteral artemisinin derivatives in mice. Am J Trop Med Hyg 1998; 59(4):519–522.

213. Hien TT, Arnold K, Vinh H, et al. Comparison of artemisinin suppositories with intravenous artesunate and intravenous quinine in the treatment of cerebral malaria. Trans R Soc Trop Med Hyg 1992; 86(6):582–583.

214. Sabchareon A, Attanath P, Chanthavanich P, et al. Comparative clinical trial of artesunate suppositories and oral artesunate in combination with mefloquine in the treatment of children with acute falciparum malaria. Am J Trop Med Hyg 1998; 58(1):11–16.

215. Gomez M. Briefing document: artesunate rectal capsules. In: FDA Division of Anti-infective Drug Products Advisory Committee, Gaithersburg, MD, USA, July 10, 2002.

216. White NJ, Looareesuwan S, Phillips RE, Chanthavanich P, Warrell DA. Single dose phenobarbitone prevents convulsions in cerebral malaria. Lancet 1988; 2(8602):64–66.

217. Crawley J, Waruiru C, Mithwani S, et al. Effect of phenobarbital on seizure frequency and mortality in childhood cerebral malaria: a randomised, controlled intervention study [In Process Citation]. Lancet 2000; 355(9205):701–706.

218. Riddle MS, Jackson JL, Sanders JW, Blazes DL. Exchange transfusion as an adjunct therapy in severe *Plasmodium falciparum* malaria: a meta-analysis. Clin Infect Dis 2002; 34(9):1192–1198.

219. Trang TT, Phu NH, Vinh H, et al. Acute renal failure in patients with severe falciparum malaria. Clin Infect Dis 1992; 15(5):874–880.

220. Phu NH, Hien TT, Mai NT, et al. Hemofiltration and peritoneal dialysis in infection-associated acute renal failure in Vietnam. N Engl J Med 2002; 347(12):895–902.

221. Hoffman SL, Rustama D, Punjabi NH, et al. High-dose dexamethasone in quinine-treated patients with cerebral malaria: a double-blind, placebo-controlled trial. J Infect Dis 1988; 158(2):325–331.

222. Thuma PE, Mabeza GF, Biemba G, et al. Effect of iron chelation therapy on mortality in Zambian children with cerebral malaria [In Process Citation]. Trans R Soc Trop Med Hyg 1998; 92(2):214–218.

223. van Hensbroek MB, Palmer A, Onyiorah E, et al. The effect of a monoclonal antibody to tumor necrosis factor on survival from childhood cerebral malaria. J Infect Dis 1996; 174(5):1091–1097.

224. Krishna S, Supanaranond W, Pukrittayakamee S, et al. Dichloroacetate for lactic acidosis in severe malaria: a pharmacokinetic and pharmacodynamic assessment. Metabolism 1994; 43(8):974–981.

7

Rabies

Alan C. Jackson

Departments of Medicine and Microbiology and Immunology,
Queen's University, Kingston, Ontario, Canada

1. INTRODUCTION

Rabies can be prevented with appropriate therapy after a recognized exposure (1), but rabies in humans is normally fatal even despite aggressive therapeutic attempts (2). Worldwide, human rabies continues to be an important public health problem in geographical areas where canine rabies is endemic with over 30,000 reported deaths per year (3). Dog-to-dog transmission of rabies virus occurs in many developing countries due to adverse economic factors and inadequate infrastructure, resulting in a continuing threat to human health in these areas. Asia and Africa continue to be problem areas with human and canine rabies. However, efforts have led to marked improvement in the control of canine rabies and a resulting reduction in human deaths in Latin America. Rabies virus has continued to emerge over many years by adaptation to novel hosts, and there are now multiple sylvatic vectors in the United States. The number of human rabies cases has increased during the 1990s in the United States and Australia. Most human rabies cases in the United States are transmitted by insect-eating bats, and a rabies virus variant isolated in silver-haired and eastern pipistrelle bats is responsible for the majority of human cases. Usually patients are not aware that they have been bitten by a bat, although some of the victims have a history of contact with bats. Recently, there have been foci with sustained transmission of bat rabies virus variants, which illustrate the process by which new variants naturally emerge. Five rabies-related lyssaviruses have caused rare cases of human rabies in Europe (European bat lyssaviruses type 1 and type 2), Africa (Duvenhage virus and Mokola virus), and Australia (Australian bat lyssavirus). Australian bat lyssavirus is endemic in bats and recently caused two fatal human cases. Rabies virus infection without recognized disease or mortality has been observed in spotted hyenas in the Serengeti, and other unusual infections may occur in animals under natural conditions.

2.   RABIES IN THE UNITED STATES

Dog rabies came under control in the United States during the 1950s, which was associated with a marked reduction in the number of human cases of rabies. During the 1970s and 1980s there were only about one to two human rabies cases per year. Although rabies in wildlife was prevalent during this period, transmission occurred uncommonly to humans. During the 1990s there was an increase in the number of human cases of rabies in the United States with up to three to six cases occurring per year (4); five cases occurred in 2000 (5) and three cases in 2002. Of the 46 cases of human rabies in the United States that have occurred during the period 1980–2002, 14 (30%) were imported (all transmitted from dogs) and 32 (70%) were acquired indigenously (within the United States). Bats, raccoons, skunks, foxes, and coyotes are the important rabies vectors in the United States (Figs 1 and 2) (6). Rabies virus variants associated with these vectors can be characterized by reverse transcriptase-polymerase chain reaction (RT-PCR) amplification and sequencing or monoclonal antibody analyses, and these tech-

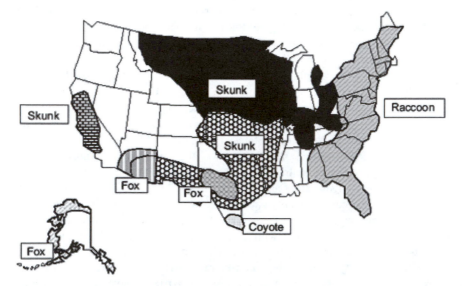

Figure 1   Geographic distribution of terrestrial vectors of rabies in the United States. (From, Ref. 6; Centers for Disease Control and Prevention.)

niques have provided much important information about enzootic maintenance cycles of specific rabies virus variants in the United States (4). Although our understanding of the pathogenesis of rabies has increased in recent years (7), the biologic factors that limit transmission of specific variants within a species have not yet been adequately studied.

2.1. Raccoon Rabies

Raccoon rabies emerged in Florida in the late 1940s, and was not associated with rabies in other species of wildlife. Although the origin of the raccoon rabies virus variant is uncertain, genetic analyses of the glycoprotein gene indicate that host switching from an insectivorous bat variant is a likely possibility (8). By 1977 the outbreak of raccoon rabies had extended north into Georgia, Alabama, and South Carolina and was moving northward at a rate of about 40 km per year (9). In 1977 and 1978 rabid raccoons were identified in adjoining counties of West Virginia and Virginia and subsequently spread to produce a focus in the mid-Atlantic states. The virus variant was similar to that found in southeastern states and distinct from variants found elsewhere in the United States. Many raccoons were translocated from Florida into Virginia by the Virginia Game Commission from 1971 to 1977 for restocking of hunting preserves (9), and rabies was documented in translocated raccoons (10). The raccoon epizootic spread up the entire eastern coast of the United States into New England, spread to Ohio in the west, and spread across the Canadian border from New York into southeast Ontario during 1999 (11), and also from Maine into southwest New Brunswick during 2000 (12). There are consistent declines in the size and interepizootic period in successive epizootics in affected counties in the United States, and these findings are consistent with the development of low levels of immunity within raccoon populations (13). In 2001 there were 2767 reported cases of rabies in raccoons in the United States (6), although this was determined using a passive surveillance system that greatly underestimates the actual number of cases. Raccoon exposures accounted for only about 0.5% of animal exposures in a study of patients presenting to university-affiliated emergency departments during the period 1996–1998 (14). However, interaction of raccoons with cats and dogs results in many human exposures. There has been documentation of only a single human case of rabies due to a raccoon rabies virus variant in 2003 and there was no known exposure (15).

Control of rabies in wildlife is an important challenge for government officials. Oral vaccination programs have been highly successful in the control of fox rabies in the United States, Canada, and Europe (16,17). Vaccination programs have been deployed against raccoon rabies, including oral vaccination projects using a vaccinia-rabies virus glycoprotein recombinant virus vaccine (16). To date, a program has been effective in preventing the spread of raccoon rabies into Cape Cod, Massachusetts (18). However, it remains to be seen how effective oral vaccines will be in containing and controlling the raccoon rabies epizootic in the eastern United States and Canada. The cost-effectiveness of this approach will also need to be demonstrated (19).

2.2.   Bat Rabies

Bat rabies is widely distributed in every state in the United States except Hawaii (Fig. 2) (6). Rabies virus variants in bats are responsible for the majority of recent human rabies cases in the United States and Canada (4,20,21), although bats constitute only about 17% of all reported rabies cases (6) and bats accounted for only about 0.2% of animal exposures in a study of patients presenting to emergency departments (14). During the period 1980–2002, 29 of the 32 (91%) indigenous cases of human rabies in the United States were caused by bat rabies virus variants. Characterization of the bat rabies virus variants has indicated that the majority are caused by a virus found in silver-haired bats (*Lasionycterius noctivigans*) (Fig. 3) and eastern pipistrelle bats (*Pipestrelle subflavus* species) (4,22,23). Only two of the 32 patients infected by rabies virus

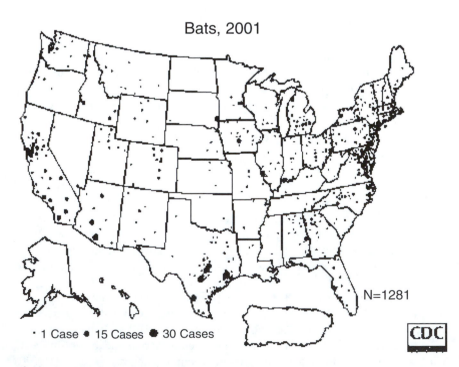

Figure 2   Distribution of bat rabies cases in the United States during 2001. (From Ref. 6; Centers for Disease Control and Prevention.)

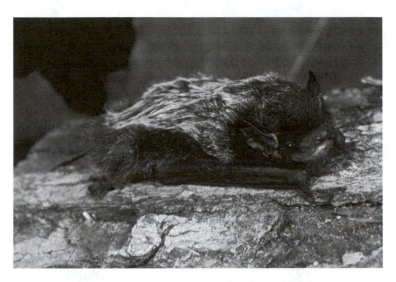

Figure 3   A silver-haired bat (*Lasionycteris noctivagans*), which is an important vector for transmission of rabies virus to humans in the United States. The rabies bat virus variant in silver-haired bats is also present in eastern pipistrelle bats (*Pipistrellus subflavus*). Both of these species of bats are present in the United States and Canada. (Courtesy of Dr. M. Brock Fenton, University of Western Ontario, Lundon, Ontario, Canada.)

variants had a history of an actual bat bite, although several had a history of some contact with bats without a recognized bite. Silver-haired bats and eastern pipistrelle bats are typically found in trees (only rarely in houses) and they normally have little contact with humans. They are only infrequently submitted for diagnostic testing for rabies. Bat bites, including bites from silver-haired bats, may be very small and may not exhibit characteristic features (Fig. 4) (24). The only plausible explanation for human cases of rabies caused by bat rabies virus variants is that they occur as a result of unrecognized bat bites. The silver-haired bat rabies virus variant may have undergone successful biological adaptation that allows it to replicate well at relative low temperatures of the skin and infect cell types that are present in the dermis, and this has been demonstrated in a laboratory study comparing the virus with another wild-type (street) strain (25). Post-exposure rabies prophylaxis, including wound cleansing and administration of five doses of rabies vaccine and human rabies immune globulin, is likely responsible for the prevention of rabies after recognized bat exposures. In 1999, new rabies prevention guidelines recommend initiation of post-exposure prophylaxis in circumstances when there is a reasonable probability that a bite exposure may have occurred (26). Hence, if a sleeping person awakes with a bat found in the same room or a bat is found in the room with an infant or mentally challenged or intoxicated person, then initiation of preventive measures should be strongly considered.

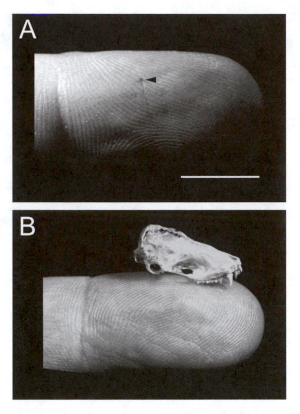

Figure 4   Small puncture wound (arrowhead) involving the right ring finger of a bat biol-
ogist (A) caused by a defensive bite from a canine tooth of a silver-haired bat
(*Lasionycteris noctivagans*) (Bar = 10 mm). Skull of a silver-haired bat (B) (length of 17.1
mm) is resting on a distal phalanx, which demonstrates the small size of the bat and its
teeth. (Reproduced from Jackson AC, Fenton MB. *Lancet* 2001; 357:1714.)

2.3.   Coyote Rabies

In the early 1990s, the number of cases of coyote rabies gradually increased in an
area of southern Texas bordering Mexico. The coyote was a novel rabies vector, and
the rabies virus variant identified in coyotes was the same as that in dogs along the
United States–Mexico border, indicating that transmission of rabies virus from dogs
to coyotes initiated the enzootic cycle within coyotes (27,28). Translocation of
infected coyotes for sport hunting from the Texas focus was also responsible for
transmission of this variant to a small number of dogs in Florida and Alabama (29).
An oral vaccination program involving aerial bait distribution has been highly effective in controlling coyote rabies in south Texas (30), and currently only rare cases of
coyote rabies are recognized in Texas, including only a single cases in 2001 (6).

2.4. Gray Fox Rabies

Gray fox rabies was a problem in southeastern United States beginning at least in the 1940s (31). In recent years gray fox rabies has been known to be present in small areas of Arizona and west Texas. An oral vaccination program with aerial bait distribution has been quite successful in controlling rabies in gray foxes in west Texas (32), and there were only 20 cases in Texas in 2001 (6).

3. RABIES IN EUROPE

3.1. Fox Rabies

Although fox rabies was prevalent during the nineteenth century, it essentially disappeared in the early twentieth century (33). A rabies epizootic in red foxes emerged in Europe in the area of the Poland–Russia border in about 1939, and then spread to the rest of Europe moving south and west and reached France in 1982 (34). Oral immunization programs have been successful in controlling rabies in Europe with the first field trial in Switzerland in 1978 (35). Finland, the Netherlands, Italy, Switzerland, France, and Belgium are now considered free of rabies, at least in terrestrial animals, due to the efforts of oral immunization programs (36).

3.2. European Bat Lyssavirus Type 1

Between 1958 and 2000 there was a total of 641 rabies positive bats reported in Europe due to European bat lyssaviruses, including European bat lyssavirus type 1 (EBLV-1) and European bat lyssavirus type 2 (EBLV-2), with a peak of 279 cases found between 1985 and 1987 (37). In 1985 an 11-year-old girl from Belgorod, Russia was bitten on the lower lip by an unidentified bat and died with signs of rabies (38). The viral isolate was called Yuli virus and classified as EBLV-1 (39). An earlier similar case occurred in the Ukraine in 1977 (40). In Denmark in 1998 three sheep were reported to be infected with EBLV-1, which was the first observed spillover infection of EBLV-1 from insectivorous bats to a terrestrial animal species (37); an additional sheep developed rabies due to EBLV-1 in Denmark in 2002 (41). In 2001 a rabid stone martin was reported from Germany due to EBLV-1 infection, which was the first documented transmission of EBLV-1 infection to a wildlife species and this resulted in intensification of surveillance measures in the area (37).

3.3. European Bat Lyssavirus Type 2

In 1985 a 30-year-old zoologist from Finland developed numbness in his right arm and neck with leg weakness (42). His cerebrospinal fluid (CSF) was normal without a pleocytosis. Subsequently, he developed myoclonus of his legs, agitation, hyper-excitability, inspiratory spasms, dysarthria, dysphagia, and hypersalivation. He had a delirium that progressed to coma. He died 23 days after the onset of the illness. He had never been vaccinated against rabies and had been bitten by bats in several countries over the previous 5-year period, including an exposure in southern Finland 51 days prior to the onset of his symptoms. EBLV-2 was isolated (39). This patient also had a clinical illness that was indistinguishable from that caused by rabies virus.

In November 2002, a 56-year-old male died of rabies in Dundee, Scotland due to EBLV-2 infection (43). He had apparently been bitten by bats, most recently by what he believed was a Daubenton bat (*Myotis daubentonii*) about 19 weeks earlier in Angus, Scotland, and he did not receive post-exposure rabies prophylaxis. This was the first case of human rabies acquired indigenously in the United Kingdom since 1902. EBLV-2 had been previously identified in two Daubenton bats in the United Kingdom (44,45).

4. RABIES IN AUSTRALIA

For many years Australia had been considered free of rabies. In November 1996, a 39-year-old female from Rockhampton, who had cared for fruit bats and had been scratched or bitten by a yellow-bellied sheathtail bat (an insectivorous bat), developed a clinical illness suggestive of rabies and typical pathologic changes of rabies were observed at autopsy (46). RT-PCR amplification of nucleic acids extracted from brain tissue and CSF indicated that she was infected with a virus identical to Australian bat lyssavirus (ABLV), which had previously been identified in flying foxes (fruit-eating bats) only a few months earlier in June 1996 (47). In 1998 a 37-year-old female, who was bitten at the base of her little finger by a flying fox 27 months earlier, developed a fatal illness typical of rabies and RT-PCR analyses on multiple tissues and saliva identified ABLV (48). The distribution of ABLV is now believed to be widespread in a variety of species of Australian bats, but much is unknown about exactly when and how this virus obtained a foothold in Australian bats (49). A recent report of active surveillance in the Philippines showed that 22 of 231 (9.5%) bat sera had neutralizing antibodies against ABLV, including four of 11 *Miniopterus schreibersi* (Schreiber's long-fingered bats) (50). Hence, lyssavirus infections of bats are not restricted to the Australian continent, but a determination of their full geographic distribution requires further study.

5. RABIES IN DEVELOPING COUNTRIES

5.1. Canine Rabies

Worldwide, domestic animals are by far the major threat for transmission of rabies virus to humans. Canine rabies is endemic in much of the developing world, including many countries in Latin America, eastern Europe, Africa, and Asia. Most human rabies cases in the world occur as a result of untreated dog bites in rabies endemic areas. Males and children are frequent victims of both dog bites and rabies. Canine rabies virus strains have been shown to be quite similar throughout the world, which may be due to the effect of European colonization with translocation of dogs with rabies worldwide (51). The world dog population is large and there are many stray dogs in developing countries. Inadequate programs involving vaccination and stray animal control are employed for management of dog rabies in many areas. Mass destruction of dogs is not thought to have a significant impact on dog population densities or on the spread of rabies because the high population turnover of dogs can easily compensate for even the highest recorded removal rate (52,53). In contrast, mass vaccination programs are key to the control of dog rabies and regular vaccination campaigns are necessary. In the future oral vaccination of dogs may become an adjunct to parenteral vaccination, although at this point only early field trials of oral vaccines for dogs have been completed (54,55).

Dog bites are common in developing countries, and guidelines for post-exposure rabies prophylaxis are frequently not followed for a variety of reasons, including lack of knowledge by patients or health care workers, large travel distances for therapy, and the unavailability or high cost of biologics (vaccine and rabies immune globulin), which may be of inferior quality and cause adverse effects. Certain travelers to rabies endemic areas and also residents of rabies endemic areas should consider pre-exposure rabies immunization.

5.2. Vampire Bat Rabies

Nine miners died of paralytic rabies transmitted by vampire bats in British Guiana (presently Guyana) in 1953 (56), and an unusual human outbreak of paralytic rabies affecting over 70 people occurred in Trinidad between 1929 and 1937 with transmission of the virus from vampire bats (57). Vampire bat rabies continues to be a problem in Latin America with a threat to humans and also to cattle, resulting in important economic losses (58). Current approaches for the prevention of rabies in cattle transmitted by vampire bats using anticoagulants have shown moderate success (59,60).

5.3. Rabies in Marmosets

Between 1991 and 1998 eight human deaths in the state of Ceará, Brazil were caused by a rabies virus variant transmitted by white-tufted-ear marmosets (*Callithrix jacchus jacchus*) (61). Marmosets are small primates that feed on insects, fruits, and tree exudates, and are highly adaptable to different habitats. The origin of this new variant is unknown and it is the only rabies virus variant that has been recognized to potentially have its reservoir in non-human primates.

5.4. Duvenhage Virus

In 1970, a 31-year-old male from rural South Africa died of rabies (62). He had been bitten on the lip by a bat while sleeping about 4 weeks earlier. The virus isolated from the patient's brain was a new virus and was characterized and named Duvenhage virus. Subsequently, isolates of Duvenhage virus have been obtained from bats in South Africa and Zimbabwe (31,63), but no further human isolates have been identified.

5.5. Mokola Virus

Little is known about the epidemiology and natural history of Mokola virus infections (31). Mokola virus was first isolated from shrews in Nigeria (64). In 1968, a three-and-a-half-year-old girl from Nigeria presented with febrile convulsions (65). Although Mokola virus was isolated from her CSF, the shrew isolate of Mokola virus was handled in the same laboratory during the same time period and cross-contamination of specimens in the laboratory remains a possible explanation for this viral isolation (57). A 6-year-old girl died in Nigeria in 1971 after a 6-day illness (66). She presented with drowsiness, confusion, and extremity weakness, and there was progression to coma. Shrews were plentiful around the house where she lived, although it was unknown whether she had actually been bitten. At autopsy there were large eosinophilic inclusion bodies in the cytoplasm of neurons and Mokola virus was isolated from her brain. Mokola virus can cause a fatal illness in cats and dogs (31), and it is uncertain if other human rabies cases due to Mokola virus in Africa have gone unrecognized.

6. HOST SWITCHING FROM BATS TO TERRESTRIAL MAMMALS

Genetic analyses of the glycoprotein sequences of 17 variants from bats and 36 variants from terrestrial mammals provided evidence that point mutations are the main force in the evolution of rabies viruses; a phylogenetic reconstruction indicated that host switching likely occurred from bats to terrestrial mammals about 888–1459 years ago, probably due to spillover from bats (8). Furthermore, partial glycoprotein gene sequencing indicated that the raccoon rabies virus variant and the south central skunk variant in the United States likely both originated from insectivorous bat variants (8).

Spillover of a rabies virus variant into another species is normally a dead-end event without sustained transmission. However, there have been recent examples of sustained transmission of variants from insectivorous bats to terrestrial animals. In Dutchess County, New York separate incidents in 1984 and 1987 each involved rabies of bat origin in three gray foxes (67), and there was also a cluster of fox cases in Nevada in 1995–1996 (68). In 1993 three foxes were infected by a bat virus variant in Prince Edward Island, Canada (69). The most remarkable example of sustained transmission from an insectivorous bat virus variant, found commonly in *Eptesicus fuscus* and *Myotis* bats, was transmission of an insectivorous bat variant to 19 skunks in Flagstaff, Arizona in 2001 (6,68).

7. NON-FATAL OUTCOME OF RABIES VIRUS INFECTIONS

Although rabies is usually considered a uniformly fatal disease, it has been recognized that animals may sometimes recover from rabies. An important issue is whether a "carrier state" can occur where a rabies vector is able to secrete virulent infectious virus in the saliva and remain healthy.

7.1. Dogs

In a series of reports from the Pasteur Institute of Southern India, the unusual case of a chronically infected dog was described (57). A 14-year-old boy died with hydrophobia 48 days after he was bitten in November 1965 (70). The dog was observed at the Pasteur Institute until it died in February 1969 (71). During that period, rabies virus was isolated from multiple saliva samples taken from the dog between January 1966 and January 1967. Rabies virus was not isolated postmortem from the dog's brain, spinal cord, or salivary glands, although fluorescent antibody staining showed rabies virus antigen in its brain and spinal cord (71). Anti-rabies virus antibodies were not found in the dog's blood at any time. It is unlikely that this seronegative dog excreted a virulent rabies virus that was responsible for the boy's death. The boy may have become infected from an undocumented rabies exposure months or even years earlier. Because of a number of inconsistencies in these reports that there remains uncertainty about the validity of this series of reports (57).

Fekadu reported five dogs in Ethiopia that secreted rabies virus for up to 72 months, but these viruses had not caused human disease (72,73). Excretion of rabies virus was also documented in the saliva of a dog experimentally infected with an Ethiopian strain of dog rabies virus for up to 6 months after its recovery from rabies (74).

7.2. Bats

A carrier state for rabies was initially reported in vampire bats in the 1930s in Trinidad, but the methods were inadequate (75). A study of Brazilian free-tailed bats from a dense cave population in New Mexico revealed that 69% of the bats had neutralizing rabies virus antibodies, but only 0.5% had active infection as assessed by direct fluorescent antibody testing of the brain (76). Hence, seroconversion likely occurs in many naturally infected bats, although it is unknown whether any central nervous system involvement normally occurs in this setting, and fatal infections may be relatively infrequent. In Spain serotine bats (*Eptesicus serotinus*), in which EBLV-1 infection has been recognized, were recently studied with RT-PCR amplification of oropharyngeal swabs and simultaneous brain samples. Of 33 bats, a positive RT-PCR result was found in 13 (39%) oropharyngeal swabs and five (15%) brains, and the positive brains were usually associated with clinical disease (77). Unless the infection was associated with a previously unrecognized pattern of viral spread in the host, then there was clearance of viral RNA from the brain but not from extraneural tissues in many of these bats. Of course, a positive RT-PCR result does not indicate the presence of infectious virus at a site and it may be a marker of remote infection in some cases.

7.3. Spotted Hyenas

A recent study of rabies virus infection in spotted hyenas in the Serengeti changes our perspective about naturally occurring variations in rabies pathogenesis (78). In this study spotted hyenas were monitored in three social groups for periods of 9–13 years. Clinical rabies was never observed. On the basis of rabies virus neutralization antibody (VNA) titers, 37% (37 of 100) were found to be seropositive and repeat studies in six indicated that half of the seropositives became seronegative. High-ranking hyenas had high VNA titers. They also had high oral (open mouths licked by clan members at rates of over twice an hour) and bite contact rates, and they lived to a mature age of over 4 years. Although infectious rabies virus was not isolated from saliva, almost half of the seropositive hyenas demonstrated saliva positive for rabies virus RNA by RT-PCR. Rabies virus RNA was also detected in three of 23 hyena brain samples in which the hyenas were killed by motor vehicles or other causes. Sequence analysis showed sequence divergence with strains found in the Serengeti in African wild dogs, bat-eared foxes, and the white-tailed mongoose, and the sequence in the spotted hyenas more closely resembled that found in dogs in the Middle East and Europe. This excellent report really changes our perspective on the ecology of less virulent viral variants and is an exception to the old dogma that rabies virus kills the great majority of exposed individuals. It is likely that in the future we will learn that under some circumstances the situation is similar in other species, including bats. Much more research is needed in order to gain a better understanding of the full spectrum of the ecology of rabies virus infection.

8. SUMMARY

Although rabies is an ancient disease, rabies viruses continue to emerge in new hosts throughout the world and cause disease in humans and animals. The full scope of infections caused by lyssaviruses is probably well obscured in developing countries by disease caused by canine rabies virus variants. All rabies viruses may have evolved from bat rabies viruses. In recent years bats have become the most important vector of rabies virus or lyssaviruses in the United States, United Kingdom, and Australia. Surveillance with molecular characterization of variants will be necessary in order to have an understanding of the epidemiology of the infections, which is needed for initiation and maintenance of appropriate rabies control measures. The success of rabies virus is related to its ability to change through mutations and there is certainty that the virus will continue to emerge and re-emerge in the future in new hosts and in places where it is not expected.

REFERENCES

1. Jackson AC. Rabies. Curr Treat Options Infect Dis 2003; 5:35–40.
2. Jackson AC, Warrell MJ, Rupprecht CE, Ertl HCJ, Dietzschold B, O'Reilly M, Leach RP, Fu ZF, Wunner WH, Bleck TP, Wilde H. Management of rabies in humans. Clin Infect Dis 2003; 36:60–63.
3. World Health Organization. World Survey of Rabies no. 34 for the Year 1998. Geneva: World Health Organization, 2000.
4. Noah DL, Drenzek CL, Smith JS, Krebs JW, Orciari L, Shaddock J, Sanderlin D, Whitfield S, Fekadu M, Olson JG, Rupprecht CE, Childs JE. Epidemiology of human rabies in the United States, 1980 to 1996. Ann Intern Med 1998; 128:922–930.
5. Van Fossan D, Jagoda L, LeSage A, Hartmann R, Johl J, Sharman J, Jay M, Schnurr D, Crawford-Miksza L, Glaser C, Vugia D, et al. Human rabies—California, Georgia, Minnesota, New York, and Wisconsin, 2000. MMWR Morb Mortal Wkly Rep 2000; 49:1111–1115.
6. Krebs JW, Noll HR, Rupprecht CE, Childs JE. Rabies surveillance in the United States during 2001. J Am Vet Med Assoc 2002; 221:1690–1701.
7. Jackson AC. Pathogenesis. In: Jackson AC, Wunner WH, eds. Rabies. San Diego, CA: Academic Press, 2002:245–282.
8. Badrane H, Tordo N. Host switching in lyssavirus history from the chiroptera to the carnivora orders. J Virol 2001; 75:8096–8104.
9. Rupprecht CE, Smith JS. Raccoon rabies: the re-emergence of an epizootic in a densely populated area. Semin Virol 1994; 5:155–164.
10. Nettles VF, Shaddock JH, Sikes RK, Reyes CR. Rabies in translocated raccoons. Am J Public Health 1979; 69:601–602.
11. Wandeler AI, Rosatte RC, Williams D, Lee TK, Gensheimer KF, Montero JT, Trimarchi CV, Morse DL, Eidson M, Smith PF, Hunter JL, Smith KA, Johnson RH,

Jenkins SR, Berryman C. Update: raccoon rabies epizootic—United States and Canada, 1999. MMWR Morb Mortal Wkly Rep 2000; 49:31–35.

12. Buchanan T. Rabies control in New Brunswick in 2001. Rabies Rep 2001; 12:4–8.

13. Childs JE, Curns AT, Dey ME, Real LA, Feinstein L, Bjornstad ON, Krebs JW. Predicting the local dynamics of epizootic rabies among raccoons in the United States. Proc Natl Acad Sci U S A 2000; 97:13,666–13,671.

14. Moran GJ, Talan DA, Mower W, Newdow M, Ong S, Nakase JY, Pinner RW, Childs JE. Appropriateness of rabies postexposure prophylaxis treatment for animal exposures. JAMA 2000; 284:1001–1007.

15. Silverstein MA, Salgado CD, Bassin S, Bleck TP, Lopes MB, Farr BM, Jenkins SR, Sockwell DC, Marr JS, Miller GB. First human death associated with raccoon rabies—Virginia, 2003. MMWR Morb Mortal Wkly Rep 2003; 52:1102–1103.

16. Hanlon CA, Childs JE, Nettles VF. Article III: rabies in wildlife. The National Working Group on Rabies Prevention and Control. J Am Vet Med Assoc 1999; 215:1612–1619.

17. MacInnes CD, Smith SM, Tinline RR, Ayers NR, Bachmann P, Ball DG, Calder LA, Crosgrey SJ, Fielding C, Hauschildt P, Honig JM, Johnston DH, Lawson KF, Nunan CP, Pedde MA, Pond B, Stewart RB, Voigt DR. Elimination of rabies from red foxes in eastern Ontario. J Wildl Dis 2001; 37:119–132.

18. Robbins A, Moore B, Niezgoda M, Buchanan R, Algeo T, Rupprecht C, Rowell S. Skunk to skunk transmission of mid-Atlantic strain racoon rabies in Massachusetts, USA, and the implications for oral rabies vaccination. Presented at the XIIIth International Meeting on Research Advances and Rabies Control in the Americas in Oaxaca, Mexico November 4, 2002.

19. Meltzer MI. Assessing the costs and benefits of an oral vaccine for raccoon rabies: a possible model. Emerg Infect Dis 1996; 2:343–349.

20. Varughese P. Human rabies in Canada—1924–2000. Can Commun Dis Rep 2000; 26:210–211.

21. Messenger SL, Smith JS, Rupprecht CE. Emerging epidemiology of bat-associated cryptic cases of rabies in humans in the United States. Clin Infect Dis 2002; 35:738–747.

22. Kunz TH. *Lasionycteris noctivagans*. Mamm Species 1982; 172:1–5.

23. Fujita MS, Kunz TH. *Pipistrellus subflavus*. Mamm Species 1984; 228:1–6.

24. Jackson AC, Fenton MB. Human rabies and bat bites (Letter). Lancet 2001; 357:1714.

25. Morimoto K, Patel M, Corisdeo S, Hooper DC, Fu ZF, Rupprecht CE, Koprowski H, Dietzschold B. Characterization of a unique variant of bat rabies virus responsible for newly emerging human cases in North America. Proc Natl Acad Sci U S A 1996; 93:5653–5658.

26. Centers for Disease Control and Prevention. Human rabies prevention—United States, 1999: recommendations of the Advisory Committee on Immunization Practices (ACIP). MMWR Morb Mortal Wkly Rep 1999; 48(RR-1):1–21.

27. Clark KA, Neill SU, Smith JS, Wilson PJ, Whadford VW, McKirahan GW. Epizootic canine rabies transmitted by coyotes in south Texas. J Am Vet Med Assoc 1994; 204:536–540.

28. Rohde RE, Neill SU, Clark KA, Smith JS. Molecular epidemiology of rabies epizootics in Texas. Clin Diagn Virol 1997; 8:209–217.

29. Belcuore T, Conti L, Hlady G, Crockett L, Hopkins R, Dunbar M. Translocation of coyote rabies—Florida, 1994. MMWR Morb Mortal Wkly Rep 1995; 44:580–587.
30. Fearneyhough MG, Wilson PJ, Clark KA, Smith DR, Johnston DH, Hicks BN, Moore GM. Results of an oral rabies vaccination program for coyotes. J Am Vet Med Assoc 1998; 212:498–502.
31. Childs JE. Epidemiology. In: Jackson AC, Wunner WH, eds. Rabies. San Diego, CA: Academic Press, 2002:113–162.
32. Moore GM. A summary of the Texas Oral Rabies Vaccination Program (ORVP) for gray foxes 1996–2002. Presented at the XIIIth International Meeting on Research Advances and Rabies Control in the Americas in Oaxaca, Mexico, November 6, 2002.
33. Niezgoda M, Hanlon CA, Rupprecht CE. Animal rabies. In: Jackson AC, Wunner WH, eds. Rabies. San Diego, CA: Academic Press, 2002:163–218.
34. Müller WW. Review of reported rabies case data in Europe to the WHO Collaborating Centre Tübingen from 1977 to 2000. Rabies Bull Europe 2000; 24:11–19.
35. Steck F, Wandeler A, Bichsel P, Capt S, Schneider L. Oral immunisation of foxes against rabies: a field study. Zentralblatt fur Veterinarmedizin. Reihe B 1982; 29:372–396.
36. Pötzsch CJ. Summarizing the rabies situation in Europe 1990–2002 from the Rabies Bulletin Europe. Rabies Bull Europe 2002; 26:11–17.
37. Müller T, Cox J, Peter W, Schäfer R, Bodamer P, Wulle U, Burow J, Müller W. Infection of a stone martin with European bat lyssa virus (EBL1). Rabies Bull Europe 2001; 25.
38. Selimov MA, Tatarov AG, Botvinkin AD, Klueva EV, Kulikova LG, Khismatullina NA. Rabies-related Yuli virus; identification with a panel of monoclonal antibodies. Acta Virol 1989; 33:542–546.
39. Bourhy H, Kissi B, Lafon M, Sacramento D, Tordo N. Antigenic and molecular characterization of bat rabies virus in Europe. J Clin Microbiol 1992; 30:2419–2426.
40. Anonymous. Possible rabies-like infection in Scotland. Commun Dis Rep Wkly 2002; 12.
41. Ronsholt L. A new case of European bat lyssavirus (EBL) infection in Danish sheep. Rabies Bull Europe 2002; 26.
42. Roine RO, Hillbom M, Valle M, Haltia M, Ketonen L, Neuvonen E, Lumio J, Lahdevirta J. Fatal encephalitis caused by a bat-borne rabies-related virus: clinical findings. Brain 1988; 111:1505–1516.
43. Nathwani D, McIntyre PG, White K, Shearer AJ, Reynolds N, Walker D, Orange GV, Fooks AR. Fatal human rabies caused by European bat lyssavirus type 2a infection in Scotland. Clin Infect Dis 2003; 37:598–601.
44. Whitby JE, Heaton PR, Black EM, Wooldridge M, McElhinney LM, Johnstone P. First isolation of a rabies-related virus from a Daubenton's bat in the United Kingdom. Vet Rec 2000; 147:385–388.
45. Johnson N, Selden D, Parsons G, Fooks AR. European bat lyssavirus type 2 in a bat found in Lancashire (Letter). Vet Rec 2002; 151:455–456.
46. Samaratunga H, Searle JW, Hudson N. Non-rabies lyssavirus human encephalitis from fruit bats: Australian bat lyssavirus (pteropid lyssavirus) infection. Neuropathol Appl Neurobiol 1998; 24:331–335.

47. Fraser GC, Hooper PT, Lunt RA, Gould AR, Gleeson LJ, Hyatt AD, Russell GM, Kattenbelt JA. Encephalitis caused by a lyssavirus in fruit bats in Australia. Emerg Infect Dis 1996; 2:327–331.

48. Hanna JN, Carney IK, Smith GA, Tannenberg AEG, Deverill JE, Botha JA, Serafin IL, Harrower BJ, Fitzpatrick PF, Searle JW. Australian bat lyssavius infection: a second human case, with a long incubation period. Med J Aust 2000; 172:597–599.

49. Scott JG. Australian bat lyssavirus: the public health response to an emerging infection (Editorial). Med J Aust 2000; 172:573–574.

50. Arguin PM, Murray-Lillibridge K, Miranda ME, Smith JS, Calaor AB, Rupprecht CE. Serologic evidence of *Lyssavirus* infections among bats, the Philippines. Emerg Infect Dis 2002; 8:258–262.

51. Smith JS, Seidel HD. Rabies: a new look at an old disease. Prog Med Virol 1993; 40:82–106.

52. Bögel K. Control of dog rabies. In: Jackson AC, Wunner WH, eds. Rabies. San Diego, CA: Academic Press, 2002:429–443.

53. World Health Organization. WHO Expert Committee on Rabies. 8th Report ed. Geneva: World Health Organization, 1992.

54. Knobel DL, du Toit JT, Bingham J. Development of a bait and baiting system for delivery of oral rabies vaccine to free-ranging African wild dogs (*Lycaon pictus*). J Wildl Dis 2002; 38:352–362.

55. World Health Organization. Oral Immunization of Dogs Against Rabies: Report of the Sixth WHO Consultation Organized with the Participation of the Office International des Epizooties (OIE), Geneva, Switzerland, July 24–25, 1995. WHO/EMC/ZDI/98.13. Geneva: World Health Organization, 1998:1–28.

56. Nehaul BBG. Rabies transmitted by bats in British Guiana. Am J Trop Med Hyg 1955; 4:550–553.

57. Jackson AC. Human disease. In: Jackson AC, Wunner WH, eds. Rabies. San Diego, CA: Academic Press, 2002:219–244.

58. McColl KA, Tordo N, Aguilar Setien AA. Bat lyssavirus infections. Rev Sci Tech 2000; 19:177–196.

59. Linhart SB, Flores Crespo R, Mitchell GC. Control of vampire bats by means of an anticoagulant (Spanish). Bol Oficina Sanit Panam 1972; 73:100–109.

60. Thompson RD, Mitchell GC, Burns RJ. Vampire bat control by systemic treatment of livestock with an anticoagulant. Science 1972; 177:806–808.

61. Favoretto SR, de Mattos CC, Morais NB, Alves Araujo FA, de Mattos CA. Rabies in marmosets (*Callithrix jacchus*), Ceara, Brazil. Emerg Infect Dis 2001; 7:1062–1065.

62. Meredith CD, Rossouw AP, Koch HvP. An unusual case of human rabies thought to be of chiropteran origin. S Afr Med J 1971; 45:767–769.

63. Bingham J, Javangwe S, Sabeta CT, Wandeler AI, Nel LH. Report of isolations of unusual lyssaviruses (rabies and Mokola virus) identified retrospectively from Zimbabwe. J S Afr Vet Assoc 2001; 72:92–94.

64. Shope RE, Murphy FA, Harrison AK, Causey OR, Kemp GE, Simpson DIH, Moore DL. Two African viruses serologically and morphologically related to rabies virus. J Virol 1970; 6:690–692.

65. Familusi JB, Moore DL. Isolation of a rabies related virus from the cerebrospinal fluid of a child with "aseptic meningitis." Afr J Med Sci 1972; 3:93–96.

66. Familusi JB, Osunkoya BO, Moore DL, Kemp GE, Fabiyi A. A fatal human infection with Mokola virus. Am J Trop Med Hyg 1972; 21:959–963.

67. Smith JS, Baer GM. Epizootiology of rabies: the Americas. In: Campbell JB, Charlton KM, eds. Rabies. Boston, MA: Kluwer Academic Publishers, 1988:267–299.

68. Smith J, Rohde R, Mayes B, Parmely C, Leslie MJ. Molecular evidence for sustained transmission of a bat variant of rabies virus in skunks in Arizona. Presented at the 12th International Meeting on Research Advances and Rabies Control in the Americas in Peterborough, Ontario, November 13, 2001.

69. Daoust PY, Wandeler AI, Casey GA. Cluster of rabies cases of probable bat origin among red foxes in Prince Edward Island, Canada. J Wildl Dis 1996; 32:403–406.

70. Veeraraghavan N, Gajanana A, Rangasami R. Hydrophobia among persons bitten by apparently healthy animals. The Pasteur Institute of Southern India, Coonoor: Annual Report of the Director 1965 and Scientific Report 1966. Chennai: Diocesan Press, 1967:90–91.

71. Veeraraghavan N, Gajanana A, Rangasami R, Oonnunni PT, Saraswathi KC, Devaraj R, Hallan KM. Studies on the salivary excretion of rabies virus by the dog from Surandai. The Pasteur Institute of Southern India, Coonoor: Annual Report of the Director 1968 and Scientific Report 1969. Chennai: Diocesan Press, 1970:66.

72. Fekadu M. Atypical rabies in dogs in Ethiopia. Ethiop Med J 1972; 10:79–86.

73. Fekadu M. Asymptomatic non-fatal canine rabies (Letter). Lancet 1975; 1:569.

74. Fekadu M, Shaddock JH, Baer GM. Intermittent excretion of rabies virus in the saliva of a dog two and six months after it had recovered from experimental rabies. Am J Trop Med Hyg 1981; 30:1113–1115.

75. Pawan JL. Rabies in the vampire bat of Trinidad, with special reference to the clinical course and the latency of infection. Ann Trop Med Parasitol 1936; 30:401–422.

76. Steece R, Altenbach JS. Prevalence of rabies specific antibodies in the Mexican free-tailed bat (*Tadarida brasiliensis mexicana*) at Lava Cave, New Mexico. J Wildl Dis 1989; 25:490–496.

77. Echevarria JE, Avellon A, Juste J, Vera M, Ibanez C. Screening of active lyssavirus infection in wild bat populations by viral RNA detection on oropharyngeal swabs. J Clin Microbiol 2001; 39:3678–3683.

78. East ML, Hofer H, Cox JH, Wulle U, Wiik H, Pitra C. Regular exposure to rabies virus and lack of symptomatic disease in Serengeti spotted hyenas. Proc Natl Acad Sci U S A 2001; 98:15,026–15,031.

8

Lyme Disease

Patricia K. Coyle, Mustafa A. Hammad, and Firas G. Saleh

Department of Neurology, School of Medicine, Health Sciences Center, Stony Brook State University of New York, Stony Brook, New York, U.S.A.

1. INTRODUCTION

Lyme disease is a tick-borne infection caused by bacterial spirochetes of the *Borrelia burgdorferi sensu lato* group. Except for rare congenital cases, all documented transmissions involve the bite of *Ixodes* species ticks. Clinical manifestations encompass suggestive syndromes of skin, musculoskeletal, heart, and nervous systems, often accompanied by multiple nonspecific systemic complaints. Rare cases may show ocular, lymphatic, liver, renal, or even pulmonary disease (1).

The term Lyme disease was first used in 1977 to explain a geographic cluster of juvenile rheumatoid arthritis in the town of Old Lyme, CT, USA. However, the disease had been recognized in Europe for more than a century (2). In 1883 Buchwald, a German physician, described acrodermatitis chronica atrophicans (ACA), a late infection skin manifestation of Lyme disease. In 1910 the Swedish physician Afzelius recognized erythema migrans (EM) following tick bite, but attempts to isolate an organism failed (3). In 1922 two French physicians, Garin and Bujadoux, described meningoradiculoneuritis after tick bite. Two years later Bannwarth, a German physician, described a series of patients (including children) with painful lymphocytic meningoradiculoneuritis and facial nerve palsy. This disorder was subsequently referred to as Bannwarth's syndrome. The first case of meningoencephalitis with EM was described in 1930 by the Swedish physician Hellerström.

The Old Lyme, Connecticut outbreak occurred between 1972 and 1976. Fifty-two individuals developed episodic arthritis initially misdiagnosed as juvenile rheumatoid arthritis (4). Thirteen reported preceding rash, very similar to the EM described from Europe. Initially called Lyme arthritis, this new disorder was renamed Lyme disease once its multiorgan involvement was appreciated.

In 1982 Willy Burgdorfer discovered a new spirochete in an *Ixodes scapularis* tick from Shelter Island, Long Island (5). The spirochete, named *Borrelia burgdorferi* after its discoverer, was later cultured from blood, cerebrospinal fluid (CSF), and skin of Lyme disease patients (6,7). Subsequent studies confirmed *B. burgdorferi* isolates in European patients with skin and neurologic syndromes.

Although initially considered a recent import from Europe, later studies indicated a long presence of *B. burgdorferi* in North America. There is a case of EM in a Wisconsin physician from 1969 (8). Montauk knee, a painless monoarticular arthritis, was described in the 1940s on the eastern tip of Long Island. Archival data, using polymerase chain reaction (PCR), has revealed *B. burgdorferi* DNA in U.S. specimens dating back to the late 1800s (9,10).

Lyme disease is a major issue. It accounts for 96% of all vector-borne infections in the United States, and is the most commonly reported arthropod infection in the United States and Europe (11). Controversies remain surrounding diagnosis, management, and medical economic issues. *Borrelia burgdorferi* infection is a useful model to study an emerging pathogen with neurologic consequences. This chapter will review current information and expected advances for this unique infection.

2. EPIDEMIOLOGY

Lyme disease occurs worldwide in at least 50 countries of North America, Europe, and Asia (12,13) (Table 1). It is restricted to regions containing the tick vector. These areas are expanding due to key host populations (deer and mice),

Table 1 Lyme Disease Epidemiology

- Reported from over 50 nations on three main continents (North America, Europe, Asia)
  —Major arthropod-borne infection in North America and Europe
- Restricted to regions inhabited by *Ixodes ricinus* tick family
- United States has three main foci:
  —Northeast (Maine to Maryland)
  —Midwest (Wisconsin, Upper Minnesota)
  —West (Northern California, Oregon)
- European forested areas
  —Central Europe (Germany, Austria, Slovenia)
  —Scandinavia (Sweden)
- Asia (China, Japan, Asian parts of Russia)

---

and possibly geographic movements of unusual hosts such as migrating birds, lizards, and race horses.

In the United States Lyme disease is endemic in more than 15 states, and reported from 49 states. Three major foci are the northeastern seaboard (Maine to Maryland), the upper midwest (Wisconsin, Minnesota), and the west (northern California, Oregon). More than 90% of cases come from nine states (Connecticut, Rhode Island, New York, Pennsylvania, Delaware, New Jersey, Maryland, Massachusetts and Wisconsin). In Europe Lyme Disease is concentrated in forested areas. Possible cases have been reported from South America, Africa, Australia, and Mexico.

In 1982 the Centers for Disease Control and Prevention (CDC) made Lyme disease reportable. At least 15,000 new cases occur each year (14), for an estimated prevalence rate of six cases per 100,000 population. In highly endemic areas the attack rate may reach 3%, with a 20% asymptomatic infection rate (11). Lyme disease is markedly underreported, with estimates of sevenfold more cases than formally reported (15).

In temperate climates infection occurs between May and September, with more than half of cases in June and July. There is no sex preference. Although all ages are affected major peaks occur at ages 10–19 and 50–59 years of age (11, 168). The major epidemiologic risk factor is time spent out-of-doors within endemic areas, particularly when the ixodid tick population has a high infection rate. Clearly Lyme disease can also occur with brief exposure, and possibly from ticks brought into the home on domestic pets.

3. ORGANISM

Borrelia burgdorferi is a motile, thin, gram-negative spirochete 10–30 µm in length and 0.2–0.25 µm in width. It has a protoplasmic cylinder, periplasm with motile flagella, and an outer membrane. There is great genetic variation and multiple strains. The strain B31 genome has been completely sequenced (16). It contains 1.5 Mb, with a 950-kb linear chromosome and 21 (12 linear, nine circular) plasmids that make up 40% of the DNA. The plasmids encode 535 open reading frames (ORFs), most of which are unrelated to any known bacterial sequences. These genes likely contribute to the spirochete's ability to survive, as it alternates between warm-blooded mammals and cold-blooded ticks. *Borrelia burgdorferi* has a remarkable 137 unique or shared lipoproteins (16,17). The outer cell membrane contains outer surface proteins (Osps) encoded by plasmid genes, such as OspA through OspF and VlsE. Some of these proteins are differentially expressed, and VlsE undergoes extensive antigenic variation (18). In particular, there is differential expression of Osp genes during transmission, but the exact role these proteins play in infection is not known (19). *Borrelia burgdorferi* has limited biosynthetic activity and depends on its host for nutrition. It does not require iron for growth in vitro, a very unusual finding (20). Known virulence factors involve surface attachment proteins. Gene expression is influenced by environmental factors such as temperature, and will differ for spirochetes in the vector, host, or test tube (21,22).

There are at least 11 distinct genospecies within the *B. burgdorferi sensu lato* complex. Human pathogens are limited to *B. burgdorferi sensu stricto, B. afzelii, B. garinii,* and possibly *B. bissettii* (1,23). *Borrelia burgdorferi sensu stricto* is the only genospecies recognized in North America. In contrast, all three pathologic genospecies are found in Europe (Table 2).

The other human spirochetal pathogens are *Treponema pallidum* (syphilis), *Leptospira interrogans* (leptospirosis), and the multiple *Borrelia* species which produce relapsing fever. All these pathogens produce some degree of vasculopathy and cause distinct syndromes associated with local, early disseminated, and late-stage infection. They are all capable of producing a latent infection, with periodic reactivations and clinical disease.

3.1. Vectors and Host

Ixodes ticks are hard bodied and very small. They have a 2-year life cycle encompassing three stages (larva, nymph, and adult). Ticks engage in only three blood meals (one per stage), and feed painlessly to repletion. There is little transovarial transmission of *B. burgdorferi,* so that most ticks become infected by feeding on spirochetemic hosts (14,24). Spirochetes reside in the tick gut. As the tick is exposed to blood, there is an explosion in spirochete numbers, and they migrate to the tick mouthpiece and salivary glands. Saliva fluid transmits organism into the bite site.

The white-footed mouse (*Peromyscus leucopus*) is the natural host and reservoir for *B. burgdorferi*. Deer, chipmunks, voles, birds, lizards, and other strains of mice are other major spirochete reservoirs. Ticks prefer to feed on white-footed mice in the larval and nymphal stages, and on white-tailed deer in the adult stage. Humans are accidental hosts, and are most likely to be bitten by

Table 2 Geographic and Clinical Correlates of Pathogenic Genospecies

Genospecies	Geographic regionsr	Disease features
B. burgdorferi sensu stricto	North America, Europe	Linked to all cases in North America Causes virulent disease
B. afzelii	Europe, Asia	Causes mild disease Associated with dermatologic involvement
B. garinii	Europe, Asia	Associated with neurologic involvement

questing nymphs. Nymphal ticks are quite small and their painless bite is easily missed. They feed during spring and early summer.

In the United States, the tick vector is *Ixodes scapularis* (formerly known as *Ixodes dammini*) in the northeast and midwest, and *Ixodes pacificus* in the west. Tick infection rates are relatively low in the south and west. A major host in the south is the lizard, which does not support spirochetemia. *Ixodes pacificus* is a poor reservoir for *B. burgdorferi* due to complement-mediated killing (25). Its infection rate is 1–3%, compared to 10–20% for *I. scapularis* nymphs, and 20–40% for adult ticks (26). The vector ecology in the west involves two intersecting cycles which include a nonhuman biting ixodid tick (27). *Ixodes ricinus* is the major vector in Europe, while *Ixodes persulcatus* is the vector in Asia and eastern Europe (28).

Studies suggest that infected ticks must feed for at least 24–48 hr to transmit *B. burgdorferi* (19,29). This emphasizes the value of daily whole-body tick checks to prevent Lyme disease.

3.2. Clinical Disease Characteristics

Up to 20% of *B. burgdorferi* infections are asymptomatic. This could reflect nonpathogenic strains, too small an inoculum, or an effective host immune response. Similar to other human spirochetal infections, Lyme disease occurs in stages with distinct early local, early disseminated, and late-stage clinical syndromes (Table 3) (30).

The most common presentation of Lyme disease is EM. This early local infection syndrome is the only clinical pathognomonic disease marker (31,32). Other skin manifestations are borrelial lymphocytoma (which involves the earlobe, nipple, or scrotum) and ACA (12,30,33). Lymphocytoma and ACA basically do not occur in the United States, since they reflect *B. afzelii* infection. However, in exceptional cases *B. burgdorferi sensu stricto* has been isolated from both of these skin lesions (34, 169).

Once spirochetes are inoculated into the skin via tick bite, they multiply locally in an explosive fashion. EM forms at the bite site as a slowly expanding painless erythematous macule (or papule), with frequent central clearing. The classic picture is a bull's-eye lesion, with a diameter that typically enlarges over days to many inches. The EM accounts for up to 90% of Lyme disease cases. It occurs at the bite site within 7–10 (mean 1–30) days after inoculation (35). Lesions that occur within 24 hr are not EM, but an allergic reaction to the tick bite. The EM often occurs on the legs and feet in adults, and on the upper body in children (30,36). Unusual cases may note pain, pruritis, diffuse urticarial eruptions, and even erythema multiforme (37). The EM lesions may be small and irregular, so a high index of suspicion is required.

Punch biopsy of the leading edge of the EM lesion shows spirochetes by silver stain, with positive PCR. Skin culture is positive in up to 80–90% of

Table 3 Lyme Disease Infection Stages

Stage	Infection duration	Organ involvement

I. Early local infection	≤30 days	• Skin
		  – EM
		• Systemic
		  – Flu-like illness
		• Nervous system (pre-meningitic CNS seeding)

II. Early disseminated infection	≤3 months	• Skin
		  – Multifocal EM
		  – Lymphocytoma cutis (plasma cell nodules; seen in Europe)
		• Heart
		  – High-grade AV nodal block
		  – Myo/pericarditis
		  – Mild LV dysfunction
		  – Dilated cardiomyopathy (mainly in Europe)
		  – Pancarditis (fatal)
		• Musculoskeletal
		  – Migratory arthralgias
		  – Myalgias
		  – Tenosynovitis
		• Ocular
		  – Conjunctivitis
		• Nervous system

III. Late-stage infection	>3 months	• Skin
		  – Acrodermatitis chronica atrophicans (dermatitis on sun-exposed surfaces; associated with sensory polyneuropathy; seen in Europe)
		• Musculoskeletal
		  – Oligoarticular arthritis
		  – Chronic arthritis
		• Eye
		  – Uveitis
		• Nervous system

patients, although organisms take several weeks to grow out in specialized media. Up to 68% of EM patients experience constitutional symptoms (fatigue, arthralgias, myalgias, headache, fever, chills, stiff neck), while up to 42% show examination abnormalities (localized lymphadenopathy, fever, malar rash, meningismus, joint tenderness, joint swelling, facial nerve palsy) (38). This probably reflects disseminated infection. Liver enzymes are elevated in up to 37%, and may suggest viral hepatitis. In contrast, only 10% of patients complain of gastrointestinal symptoms.

Lymphocytoma is a solitary bluish-red swelling made up of plasma cells and lymphocytes with a diameter of up to a few centimeters (33,39–41). This early dissemination lesion often involves the earlobe, nipple, or scrotum (33,39–41). Most arise in the vicinity of a previous or concurrent EM (39,40), which aids in diagnosis (33,39,40).

Acrodermatitis chronica atrophicans is a late-stage manifestation. It is most common in elderly women, and can be misdiagnosed as vascular insufficiency (30,33). Like other late infection syndromes, it does not resolve spontaneously. Acrodermatitis chronica atrophicans typically involves extensor surfaces of the distal legs and occasionally distal arms. Lymphocytes and plasma cells infiltrate the dermis, with slow lesion expansion over months to years. Associated edema slowly disappears with time and atrophy becomes prominent, leaving thin and sclerotic skin over the infected area (33,42). Virtually all ACA patients are seropositive (30,33,42).

In addition to these three characteristic skin lesions, there are suggested associations between *B. burgdorferi* infection and cases of eosinophilic fasciitis, lichen sclerosis, morphea, progressive hemifacial atrophy, and panniculitis.

When the EM rash appears spirochetes have already disseminated in up to half of cases. Multiple EM lesions clearly document dissemination (43). After initial growth at the bite site organisms spread via blood, and possibly lymphatics and skin, to seed target organs. At the height of spirochetemia there are 1000 organisms per milliliter of blood. In addition to multifocal EM, syndromes of early disseminated infection involve migratory musculoskeletal pains, cardiac involvement (heart block), ocular involvement (conjunctivitis), and specific neurologic syndromes (see below).

Late-stage infection syndromes occur months to years after tick bite and also involve suggestive target organ abnormalities. Arthritis (60% of cases) is the most common late manifestation of Lyme disease. The classic picture is oligoarticular or monoarticular large joint involvement, a tenosynovitis with joint swelling (Steere, 1997). The knee is most often involved, followed by the elbow, ankle, and sometimes shoulder or hip. Temporomandibular joint involvement occurs in a minority of patients, but is a highly suggestive feature. Onset of arthritis is acute, with effusion and warmth without redness (12). Swelling usually lasts days to weeks, but sometimes persists over months (44). Knee swelling can be associated with Baker cyst formation. Joint involvement may be painful, but often involves pronounced swelling with little pain. At least half of Lyme arthritis patients have a laboratory disturbances such as elevated erythrocyte sedimentation rate, leukocytosis, increased serum IgM, positive cryoglobulins, or elevated circulating immune complexes. In contrast, C-reactive protein is usually within normal range. Most patients are not positive for rheumatoid factor or antinuclear antibodies, although low titers are occasionally seen (12). Synovial fluid leukocyte counts range from 0.5 to 110 million cells per mL, with a predominance of polymorphonuclear leukocytes (44–46). Pathological changes within the joint involve cell infiltration, vascular proliferation, and synovial hypertrophy. Lyme arthritis shows a variable course. Typically there are recurrent attacks over several years, which become less severe and infrequent. Some 10% of patients develop a chronic antibiotic-refractory arthritis (44,45).

Cardiac involvement can occur during dissemination, but this is now infrequent (5% or less of patients). Women are more likely affected by a ratio of three to one (47). The characteristic syndrome is high-degree atrioventricular block. With or without treatment, heart-related symptoms and electrocardiogram abnormalities usually disappear within 3–6 weeks (48,49). However, arrhythmias may be life-threatening, and patients who develop complete heart block may require temporary pacing. Other rare cardiac complications include acute myo/pericarditis, mild left ventricular dysfunction, dilated cardiomyopathy (mainly seen in Europe), and fatal pancarditis.

Ocular involvement due to Lyme disease is very rare and usually associated with other organ system involvement (50,51). Syndromes include conjunctivitis, keratitis, iridocyclitis, retinal vasculitis, choroiditis, and even optic neuropathy, with rare cases of episcleritis, panuveitis, and panophthalmitis. Ocular manifestations may also involve cranial nerve palsy and orbital myositis (50–52).

3.3. Neurologic Manifestations

Lyme disease can involve both the central (CNS) and peripheral (PNS) nervous systems, and neurologic involvement can occur at any stage (53–55) (Table 4). EM patients may already have disseminated infection, with positive blood and CSF cultures. In one study, 10% of EM patients had CNS seeding without overt neurologic problems (56). It is always a concern that EM patients with prominent headache and meningismus have early meningitis. Early dissemination and late infection stages are associated with distinct neurologic syndromes. Characteristic early dissemination syndromes are meningitis, meningoencephalitis, cranial nerve palsy, and acute painful radiculoneuritis (57,58).

Lyme meningitis can be quite subtle. It mimics an aseptic process rather than the typical acute bacterial meningitis. In Germany, Lyme meningitis accounts for 12–40% of childhood aseptic meningitis cases (59). Headache is the most common symptom with features suggestive of a vascular or muscle contraction problems (60). Pain ranges from very mild to quite severe, is typically frontal or occipital, and may be accompanied by meningismus, nausea, vomiting, low-grade fever, and photophobia. If present, meningeal signs are mild (53,61). Untreated, Lyme meningitis lasts 4–8 weeks and spontaneously resolves. In rare instances it can become chronic.

Table 4   Neurologic Lyme Disease Syndromes

Early local infection
- EM with CNS seeding, either asymptomatic or symptomatic (headache, stiff neck, cognitive difficulties, etc.)
- Flu-like syndrome with CNS seeding (headache, stiff neck, cognitive difficulties, etc.)

Early disseminated infection
- Aseptic meningitis
- Meningoencephalomyelitis (includes acute cerebellar ataxia, acute myelitis)
- Cranial nerve palsy (especially facial nerve palsy)
- Acute painful radiculoneuritis (Bannworth's syndrome, lymphocytic meningo-radiculitis)

Late persistent infection
- Encephalopathy
- Chronic axonal polyradiculoneuropathy
- Chronic encephalomyelitis (predominantly European, esp. *B. garinii)*
- Stroke-like syndromes
- CNS vasculitis
- Multifocal encephalitis

Important clues for Lyme meningitis are associated facial nerve and spinal nerve root involvement. CSF shows a mononuclear pleocytosis of about 100–200 WBC/mm^3 (range 5–4000 WBC/mm^3), which may include plasma cells and occasional atypical plasmocytoid cells. CSF protein is increased, while CSF glucose is normal. Opening pressure is generally normal. Intrathecal anti-*B. burgdorferi* antibody production is found in all European neurologic patients (by definition), but only in 50–60% of North American cases. In Europe oligoclonal IgG and IgM, and intrathecal nonspecific IgG production, are reported in virtually all cases. In contrast, in North America oligoclonal bands and intrathecal IgG production occur in 20% or less of cases. At the more severe end of this meningitis spectrum are patients who present with a prominent parenchymal component. Patients may show acute confusional states, movement disorders, cerebellar syndrome, or transverse myelitis. Milder manifestations include cognitive, mood, and behavioral changes. CSF is almost always inflammatory, even when there is no obvious headache or meningismus.

Cranial nerve palsy is another early dissemination syndrome. Although in theory any nerve can be affected, the vast majority of cases involve the facial nerve. Up to 35% of patients show bilateral involvement, which is usually asymmetric, and the second facial nerve palsy may occur during therapy as the patient is improving. Important clues for Lyme-related facial nerve palsy are occurrence during summer and fall (in endemic areas with a winter), and concurrent multi-symptom complex (headache, stiff neck, arthralgias, myalgias, fatigue, concentration difficulties). Patients often have mononuclear pleocytosis, despite lack of meningeal features (53,61,62). This occult meningitis indicates CNS seeding even with a peripheral pattern for facial nerve involvement (63). Other cranial nerve involvement (optic nerve, nerves three through eight, and least often nine through twelve) is occasionally seen. As expected, most patients make a good recovery from Lyme-related facial nerve palsy, even without treatment (30,53,58).

Acute painful radiculoneuritis, also called Bannwarth's syndrome or lymphocytic meningoradiculitis, is another early dissemination syndrome (64). It often starts with severe pain between the scapulae, which radiates down the spine or into the extremities. There may also be belt-like pain, most pronounced at night. The pain is associated with asymmetric focal or multifocal dermatomal and myotomal abnormalities. This syndrome shows the most inflammatory CSF changes. Painful radiculoneuritis is more common with European *B. burgdorferi* infection, and generally is more frequent and more pronounced in adults rather than children (30,58,61). Motor nerve involvement may result in asymmetric paresis or scapular winging (53,61).

Late-stage infection also has three characteristic neurologic syndromes. Unlike early disseminated syndromes, they do not spontaneously improve (65). The most common late infection syndrome in North America is a subtle encephalopathy involving memory, concentration, and mental processing abnormalities. Patients show low-grade CSF abnormalities, disturbed cerebral blood flow on brain SPECT, and abnormal cognitive function testing. These laboratory abnormalities improve with antibiotic treatment. Lyme encephalopathy likely reflects CNS infection.

The most unusual late-stage neurologic syndrome is a chronic progressive encephalomyelitis, which can mimic brain tumor, multiple sclerosis (MS), or neurodegenerative disease. Most cases have occurred in Europe.

The third late-stage neurologic syndrome is a chronic axonal radiculoneuropathy (66). The CSF is typically normal, unless patients also have encephalopathy. Unlike acute radiculoneuritis, pain is not prominent. It may be absent, or confined to occasional brief shock-like sensation in the extremities. Patients often note intermittent paresthesias, and may complain of extremity numbness or restless legs. In Europe, symmetric distal sensory polyneuropathy often accompanies the late infection ACA skin lesion (67).

In addition to the above suggestive neurologic syndromes, in unusual cases Lyme disease is associated with a variety of other problems (2). Vascular syndromes include transient ischemic attack, ischemic infarction, intracranial aneurysm, and subarachnoid hemorrhage (68). An important diagnostic clue is accompanying inflammatory CSF changes. There is an apparent age-restricted intracranial hypertension syndrome, noted in children and adolescents. Important clues are lack of obesity and abnormal CSF. Lyme disease can involve skeletal muscle, most often following EM. Patients show single or multiple muscle involvement in limb, orbital, or oropharyngeal muscles. Psychiatric, dementia, and motor neuron disease-like syndromes have also been attributed to Lyme disease (69,70). Psychiatric and dementia syndromes probably represent manifestations of encephalitis, while the motor neuron disease syndrome may represent CNS or PNS (motor nerve) involvement. Psychiatric disease is unusual. In one prospective serosurvey of patients admitted to a psychiatric hospital in Westchester County in New York, all 517 patients evaluated over 16 months were seronegative (71). It can be difficult to provide convincing proof that *B. burgdorferi* infection is responsible for an unusual neurologic disorder. To support causality, one would like to document seropositivity, consistent CSF abnormalities, and a convincing response to antibiotics.

3.4. Pediatric Lyme Disease

Age may influence disease expression. Children have the highest rate of *B. burgdorferi* infection. Most (90%) present with EM or multifocal EM, while the most common neurologic syndrome is facial nerve palsy (72–74). In contrast to adults PNS involvement is unusual, and as noted above there is an intracranial hypertension syndrome basically limited to children and adolescents (74). Compared to adults, children show more sleep disturbances but have less fatigue complaints. Children have an excellent prognosis, and recover faster and with less sequelae than adults. In a recent study of 201 consecutive children (66% EM, 23% multifocal EM, 6% arthritis, 3% facial nerve palsy, 2% meningitis, 0.5% carditis), 94% were completely asymptomatic at 1 month (75). At extended follow up (on average 25 months) none had late or recurrent disease.

3.5. Congenital Infection

There is no recognized congenital Lyme disease syndrome (76). Although autopsy and clinical studies implicate gestational Lyme disease in a variety of medical problems (fetal death, hydrocephalus, cardiovascular anomalies, neonatal respiratory distress, hyperbilirubinemia, intrauterine growth retardation, cortical blindness, sudden infant death syndrome, maternal toxemia of pregnancy), epidemiologic studies indicate a very low rate of congenital infection. One study of 19 maternal infections showed a zero transmission rate, even though only 13 of the women received antibiotics (77). In a European study of pregnant women with EM treated with ceftriaxone or penicillin, no adverse fetal effects were noted (78). Serologic surveys find no difference in fetal outcomes for seropositive and seronegative mothers. For infection during pregnancy, oral amoxicillin or parenteral ceftriaxone can be used. Cefotaxime is preferred to ceftriaxone for term pregnancies, since it does not involve biliary excretion and does not carry risk of jaundice for the newborn.

3.6. Pathology

The limited neuropathologic studies of Lyme disease suggest that neurologic manifestations reflect indirect damage mechanisms (Table 5). There is little tis-

Table 5   Lyme Disease Neuropathology.

General features
- Vasculopathy (mild)
- Inflammatory changes (mild)
- Rare extracellular organisms
- Limited tissue destruction

CNS
- Microglial inflammatory nodules (predominance of lymphocytes, plasma cells)
- Meningeal inflammation
- Scattered perivascular mononuclear (CD4+ T cells) infiltrates
- Focal microgliosis
- Mild spongiform changes
- Rare pathologic changes
  - Demyelinating lesions
  - Extracellular spirochetes
  - Granulomatous changes
  - Vasculitis

PNS

Nerve
- Variable perivascular mononuclear (CD4+ T cells, macrophage) infiltrates in epineurium, perineurium
- Axon damage
- Vasa nervorum angiopathy

Muscle
- Focal myositis, interstitial inflammation, occasional focal necrosis
- Rare spirochetes

sue destruction, and pathologic changes are generally confined to focal inflammation, mild vasculopathy, and modest parenchymal changes. Obliterative vasculopathy has been seen in late infection, and there are rare reports of prominent demyelination and granulomatous tissue (79,80). Occasional spirochetes are seen in brain and muscle, but never in peripheral nerve. In a single patient *B. burgdorferi* DNA was detected in sural nerve biopsy tissue (81). Peripheral nerve changes involve axon damage and perivascular inflammation (82). In vitro, *B. burgdorferi* causes injury to both astrocytes and oligodendrocytes (83).

3.7. Pathogenesis

Lyme disease is a complex entity, and involves multiple organism and host factors which influence disease expression. *Borrelia burgdorferi* genospecies and strains show distinct organotropisms. The spirochete activates the immune system to produce inflammation out of proportion to organism numbers. *Borrelia burgdorferi* stimulates production of matrix metalloproteinases, and expression of plasminogen activator suppressor. These factors contribute to dissemination (84,85). Spirochetes are always found extracellularly in the host, associated with matrix collagen fibers. In vivo, they never produce intracellular infection.

At lease 132 genes of *B. burgdorferi* encode putative lipoproteins. These genes make up 5% of the chromosomal ORFs, and 14.5–17% of the functionally complex ORFs on plasmids. Lipoproteins are important for pathogenesis. They activate a variety of cells (macrophages, endothelial cells, neutrophils, B cells), induce chemokine production (86), and cause aggregation of monocytes. Lipoproteins bind to CD14, toll-like receptors on macrophages (87). They provoke a strong cytokine and antibody response. One of the most important lipoproteins is outer surface protein A (Osp A). Osp A is a major surface lipoprotein with 257 amino acids. It has a molecular weight of 29 kDa, but actually migrates as a 31-kDa protein. It binds to a plasminogen receptor, and is implicated in dissemination (88). The crystal structure Osp A has been identified. It is lipidated at the n-terminus, with three fatty acid chains added during translocation into the periplasm. Osp A shows several amino acid variations in *B. burgdorferi sensu stricto* isolates. Expression of Osp A is locally regulated. The antigen causes B-cell proliferation, and interleukin-6 (IL-6) production by macrophages and endothelial cells. Epitopes from amino acids 165 to 173 show molecular mimicry with the lymphocyte functional antigen (LFA-1) adhesion molecule.

It is unclear what role antigenic variation plays in *B. burgdorferi* infection. This mechanism is important for *Borrelia* species which cause relapsing fever, and contributes to immune evasion. *Borrelia burgdorferi* does show segmental recombination within a plasmid-borne locus named the variable-major-protein (Vmp)-like sequence or VES (89), situated on linear plasmid lp28-1.

Only selected *B. burgdorferi* strains appear to be neurotropic and able to invade the CNS (90). Of the more than 20 distinct expressions of Osp C (an early immunodominant protein), in different strains, only four are associated with disseminated CNS disease (89).

Spirochetes shed pieces of outer surface membrane (so-called "blebs"), which contain DNA and Osp proteins. These blebs induce inflammation. In the rat, Osp A-containing spirochetal fractions provoke antigen-induced arthritis.

Strain differences in binding ability play a role in pathogenesis. *Borrelia burgdorferi* shows strong tissue tropism. Spirochetes adhere to most mammalian cells by way of glycosaminoglycans, and to endothelium and platelets by way of integrins (91). *Borrelia burgdorferi* also binds to red blood cells, plasminogen, and glycosphingolipids on the surface of neurons, astrocytes, oligodendrocytes, and Schwann cells. Decorin-binding proteins A and B of the spirochete are key binding factors (92,93). Spread of spirochetes through tissue may be facilitated by surface binding to plasminogen and its activators (Goleman et al., 1997).

Borrelia spirochetes are highly motile and invasive, and will spread to and localize in selected tissues. They cross blood vessels through intercellular openings, or can directly transcytose endothelial layers by binding to host-derived plasmin (94). Spirochetes can persist undetected for years only to cause late clinical illness.

Once *B. burgdorferi* disseminates in tissue spirochetes may be absent, present in very low numbers, or present as fragments (e.g., DNA) rather than whole organisms. All of the major and characteristic neurologic Lyme disease syndromes reflect active infection. Among the early dissemination syndromes, meningitis and acute radiculoneuritis clearly have CNS invasion. Since facial nerve palsy is often associated with occult meningitis, it also likely reflects CNS invasion. In the minority of facial nerve palsy patients with normal CSF and electrophysiologic changes consistent with PNS involvement, it is not possible to rule out CNS infection. Late-stage infection syndromes also represent nervous system infection, and patients stabilize or improve with antibiotic treatment.

Not all Lyme disease syndromes are due to active infection. Chronic arthritis (10% of Lyme arthritis) is an immune-mediated/inflammatory process (44). It is associated with HLA-DR4 (DRB1*0401) positivity (95). Patients show enhanced humoral and cellular immune responses to Osp A (96). The arthritis does not respond to antibiotics, and synovial fluid is PCR negative (97). Involved joint compartments contain high levels of anti-Osp A antibodies, CD4 Th1 lymphocytes reactive to Osp A, and elevated levels of proinflammatory cytokines. There is marked upregulation of synovial adhesion molecule expression (98). Arthritis severity parallels the synovial fluid Th1:Th2 ratio.

Another important pathogenesis factor is antigen expression, as influenced by the microenvironment. Certain antigens such as p21, Erp, and decorin-binding proteins are upregulated in the host. From a diagnostic point of view, they would serve as useful targets in future serologic assays.

Multiple studies implicate cytokines in the pathogenesis of Lyme disease. *Borrelia burgdorferi* induces proinflammatory cytokines such as IL-1, IL-6, and tumor necrosis factor (TNF-α). All are elevated in the synovial fluid of Lyme arthritis patients (99). Cloned T-cell lines from synovial fluid and blood of Lyme arthritis patients secrete interferon-γ (IFN-γ) when exposed to *B. burgdorferi*. The ratio of synovial fluid IL-1 to IL-1 receptor correlates with prognosis in Lyme arthritis (98). Of note, *B. burgdorferi* preferentially activates the IL-1 gene over the antagonist IL-1 receptor gene. Mononuclear cells collected from neurologic patients preferentially secrete IFN-γ when exposed to *B. burgdorferi* Osp proteins (100).

A number of pathogenetic factors may play a role in neurologic Lyme disease syndromes (Table 6). With regard to the intrathecal compartment, CSF cells show a striking preferential IFN-γ synthesis compared to peripheral blood cells, while an antagonistic anti-inflammatory/regulatory cytokine IL-4 is downregulated. Neurologic Lyme disease patients show increased CSF levels of IL-1 and TNF-α. Soluble IL-2 receptors are increased in both CSF and blood in active disease, and decrease after treatment (101). Longstanding Lyme disease shows increased lymphocyte production of IL-12, a cytokine which favors production of Th1 cells (102). Overall, the cytokine data suggests Lyme disease patients have an imbalance in the CD4+ Th1 to Th2 cell ratio, with Th1 cells predominant in late infection. This favors cell-mediated immunity and proinflammatory cytokine production. In contrast, humoral immunity appears to be protective in *B. burgdorferi* infection. Both complement activation and serum resistance may also have a role in disease pathogenesis (103–105).

There is evidence that toxic factors play some role. *Borrelia burgdorferi* induces nitric oxide production by CNS cells, which leads to production of toxic peroxynitrate. Quinolinic acid, a NMDA receptor antagonist and excitotoxin, is elevated in the CSF of neurologic Lyme disease patients. Both peroxynitrate and NMDA are neurotoxins which disrupt cell function.

Although humoral immunity (presumably cytotoxic antibodies) appears to protect against infection, there is some evidence that antibodies and immune complexes may also have a pathologic role. *Borrelia burgdorferi* and its bleb material are B-cell mitogenic. Infection can produce autoreactive antibodies to acidic gangliosides (GM1, asialo-GM1), anticardiolipin IgM, anti-axonal IgM, antibodies to myelin and myelin components, antineuronal antibodies, antibodies to heat shock protein, and antibodies to a 46-kDa protein which cross-reacts with myosin (79,106,107). *Borrelia burgdorferi*-specific immune complexes have been reported in both serum and CSF, and may correlate with disease activity (108,109).

Animal models of Lyme disease are diverse and offer excellent opportunities to study disease pathogenesis. The best studied is the mouse model, where *B. burgdorferi* infection produces arthritis and carditis. In this model disease is multifactorial with severity determined not only by the number of organisms and

---

Table 6 Pathogenic Factors Implicated in Neurologic Lyme Disease

- Blood vessel disruption
- Cytokine disturbances
    - Induction of proinflammatory cytokines and chemokines
    - Change in cytokine receptor expression
    - Change in Th1 to Th2 cytokine ratio
- Induction of toxins
    - Nitric oxide
    - Quinolinic acid
- Humoral immunity
    - B-cell mitogenic activity
    - Molecular mimicry involving generation of autoreactive antibodies
    - Immune complex formation
    - Bystander damage (antibody, complement-mediated)
- Cellular immunity
    - Molecular mimicry involving generation of cross reactive cell-mediated immune response
    - Cell-mediated bystander damage

strain virulence, but also by host genotype and immune responses. The best animal model for neurologic disease is the primate. Rhesus monkeys can be infected by tick bite or needle inoculum, and show histopathological evidence of CNS and PNS involvement both in acute and chronic stages of infection (110). Immunocompromised primates develop a higher spirochete burden, with organisms in leptomeninges, spinal nerve roots, and peripheral nerve perineurium and perimysium (111). Unlike cardiac or skeletal muscle tissue, CNS tissue shows relatively limited inflammation despite presence of spirochetes (112). Similar to human disease, culture is rarely positive, and PCR is often used to document active infection.

4. DIAGNOSIS

Lyme disease is a clinical diagnosis, ideally supported by laboratory data. The only exception is EM, a pathognomonic clinical marker. Clues for diagnosis of neurologic Lyme disease are outlined in Table 7 (2,113). Formalized diagnostic criteria and consensus guidelines are available. The CDC surveillance definition

Table 7 Clues to the Diagnosis of Neurologic Lyme Disease

- Historical clues
  - Endemic area exposure (time spent out-of-doors)
  - Ixodid tick exposure or bite (small tick)
  - Engorged attached tick
  - Geographic origin of tick (hyperendemic regions)
  - EM, or rash suspicious for EM, preceding onset of neurologic syndrome
  - Suggestive flu-like illness, prior to onset of neurologic syndrome
  - Suggestive neurologic syndrome
  - Neurologic syndrome with associated multi-symptom complex (fatigue, arthralgias, myalgias, palpitations)
- Examination clues
  - Extraneural involvement (skin, musculoskeletal, cardiovascular, ocular disease)
  - Unilateral/bilateral facial nerve palsy
  - Radicular abnormalities
- Laboratory clues
  - Detectable anti-*B. burgdorferi* antibodies (seropositivity)
  - Elevated acute phase reactants, liver enzymes (early infection)
  - Anticardiolipin IgM antibodies (early infection)
  - CSF abnormalities (intrathecal anti-*B. burgdorferi* antibody production, mononuclear pleocytosis, increased protein)
  - Electrophysiologic studies consistent with multifocal radiculoneuropathy
  - Abnormal brain SPECT
  - Abnormal neurocognitive function tests
  - Abnormal electrocardiogram (conduction block)

for Lyme disease is quite strict, and should be reserved for epidemiologic studies. The American Academy of Neurology (AAN) has a Practice Parameter for diagnosis of neurologic Lyme disease. They specify acceptable neurologic manifestations, supportive laboratory data or skin manifestations, and require that other diseases be ruled out (Table 8) (114). Definitive diagnosis of neurologic Lyme disease requires intrathecal organism-specific antibody production, demonstration of apirochetes by culture or histology, or detection of *B. burgdorferi* nucleic acid by PCR. In contrast to the CDC case definition, the AAN Practice Parameter recognizes encephalopathy and peripheral neuropathy syndromes, does not require intrathecal antibody production for encephalomyelitis, and acknowledges that cranial neuropathy often occurs in the setting of meningitis.

The most valuable laboratory diagnostic test is serology, which involves a two-tier test system. Antibody testing has become a controversial issue. Seropositivity documents historical exposure and not necessarily active infection. Test costs in the United States are staggering, with the test ordered much more often than is indicated (115,116). Guidelines for testing have been established based on diagnostic probability and cost-efficiency studies (117,118). Patients with a high probability of infection (EM-like skin lesion with endemic area exposure) can be diagnosed and treated without laboratory testing. Patients with a suggestive syndrome and reasonable probability of infection are tested, while those with a low probability (nonspecific symptoms) are tested only if there are other supportive clinical features.

First-generation enzyme-linked immunosorbent assays (ELISA) and immunofluorescent assays (IFA) have false-positive rate of 5–50%. They are based on reactivity to whole spirochete or sonicate components. Many immuno-

Table 8 American Academy of Neurology Practice Guidelines for Diagnosis of Neurologic Lyme Disease

- Possible exposure to appropriate ticks in Lyme-endemic region
- One or more of the following:
  - Skin manifestation (EM, or histologically proven lymphocytoma cutis acrodermatitis chronica atrophicans)
  - Immunologic evidence of *B. burgdorferi* exposure (positive serology)
  - Detection of *B. burgdorferi* (by culture, histology, or PCR)
- One or more specified disorders, with other etiologies excluded; possible additional testing needed (such as CSF evaluation for suspected CNS infection)
  - Causally related disease
    - Lymphocytic meningitis, with or without cranial neuropathy, painful radiculoneuritis, or both
    - Encephalomyelitis
    - Peripheral neuropathy
  - Causally related syndrome
    - Encephalopathy

(From Ref. 114.)

dominant antigens are not unique to *B. burgdorferi*. In particular, strong humoral responses to the p41 flagellin, and a variety of P58–66 heat shock proteins, may be induced by many processes. Other spirochetal infections, and even autoimmune diseases, can produce a false-positive Lyme serology. *Treponema denticola* is a common mouth flora spirochete. Gum disease, even recent dental work, can also give a false-positive serology. In one study, up to one-third of healthy and other neurologic disease subjects from an endemic area had a positive Lyme ELISA (119). Important clues to a false-positive serology are low or inconsistently positive titer.

At the current time, immunoblot confirmation of positive ELISA or IFA provides greater specificity. Some difficulties with immunoblot are the qualitative nature of the interpretation, and lack of standardization by using recombinant proteins and monoclonal antibodies. It is a more costly and time-consuming assay. Although unusual, it is possible to have negative screening ELISA and positive immunoblot. There are also Lyme disease cases with high-positive ELISA, and an equivocal immunoblot which does not meet CDC criteria for positivity. These patients most likely have true infections, so it becomes problematic to be too rigid about serologic criteria when exposure is clear, and the clinical picture is supportive.

There are several new second-generation antibody tests which are not widely adopted, but should improve diagnosis by decreasing false-positives. Several groups have also investigating detection of antibody within circulating immune complexes as a possible active infection serology assay (89,120,121).

Most Lyme disease cases have a positive ELISA. However, seronegative patients do exist and may account for up to 10% of infections. Early antibiotics (generally within roughly 2 weeks of tick bite) interfere with the humoral response, and may lead to seronegativity. Approximately half of EM cases are seropositive, while another 20–30% never seroconvert after therapy. Antibodies take a finite period of time to develop. The earliest detectable antibody response is typically on IgM immunoblot, some 2 weeks after spirochete inoculation.

There are a number of other useful diagnostic laboratory tests. *Borrelia burgdorferi* culture is rarely positive and not routinely performed. It requires special media and a dedicated laboratory, and organisms take weeks to grow out. CSF studies are useful to confirm CNS involvement. However, North American Lyme disease patients do not show the marked inflammatory changes reported from Europe. The most helpful CSF test is intrathecal anti-*B. burgdorferi* antibody production, which provides indirect evidence of CNS seeding. Paired CSF and serum samples must be examined. Positive PCR in CSF is direct evidence of infection, but unfortunately has a low yield. It is positive in less than 40% of meningitis cases (122). This low sensitivity reflects the fact that spirochetes are tissue tropic, and do not typically float free in CSF. PCR positivity is increased when a centrifuged pellet is examined. The PCR assay requires a reliable laboratory, since controls must be used to avoid false-positives contaminant so it is most useful for skin-punched biopsies and synovial fluid (46). Nonspecific (but supportive) CSF abnormalities are mononuclear pleocytosis, increased protein, normal glucose, negative VDRL, and negative cytology. Oligoclonal bands and elevated IGG index are found in less than 20% of North American cases. An unusual CSF matrix metalloproteinase (MMP) pattern (130 kDa MMP, without the 92 kDa MMP-9) was reported in neurologic patients, but awaits confirmation (123).

4.1. Differential Diagnosis

Neurologic Lyme disease encompasses so many syndromes that the differential diagnosis is broad. Lyme meningitis mimics an aseptic meningitis, which can be due to many different pathogens (mainly viruses), as well as noninfectious causes. The differential diagnosis of Lyme-related facial nerve palsy includes idiopathic Bell's palsy as well as other disorders which can affect the seventh cranial nerve. Bilateral involvement supports Lyme disease rather than idiopathic Bell's palsy. However, Guillain–Barre syndrome, neurosarcoidosis, Epstein–Barr virus (EBV) infection, Tangier disease, and human immunodeficiency virus type I infection can also affect both facial nerves. Acute radiculoneuritis occurs with herpes virus infections (varicella zoster virus, cytomegalovirus, EBV) as well as neurosarcoidosis, vasculitic neuropathies, and proximal diabetic radiculoneuropathy. Late Lyme encephalopathy is typically subtle. It can be confused with toxic and metabolic causes of encephalopathy, as well as chronic fatigue, and fibromyalgia syndromes. Differential diagnosis of the late-stage PNS syndrome involves all the disorders that can produce a polyradiculoneuropathy syndrome. Lyme encephalomyelitis can be confused with MS, brain tumor, other structural CNS lesions, or degenerative neurologic disorders. MS is not associated with extraneural features or PNS involvement, is more likely to have abnormal brain MRI and CSF oligoclonal bands/intrathecal IgG production, and is less likely to have CSF pleocytosis, increased protein, or detectable *B. burgdorferi* antibodies (124).

4.2. Treatment

Patients with early local or disseminated infection syndromes will spontaneously recover without treatment, but are at risk for late infection syndromes. With antibiotics, they typically recover faster. The best results are seen with early treatment. Most patients who receive adequate antibiotics have an excellent prognosis (125). The Infectious Disease Society of America published treatment guidelines in 2000 (Table 9) (126). They recommend intravenous antibiotics for neurologic involvement. Although some experts believe that oral antibiotics may be sufficient for treatment of isolated facial nerve palsy or very mild neurologic symptoms, this is based on European rather than North American data. There have been North American patients

Table 9 Treatment Guidelines for Lyme Disease (Infectious Disease Society of America)

Stage	Antibiotic
Early infection (local or disseminated)	Doxycycline, 100 mg bid orally for 14–21 days Amoxicillin, 500 mg tid, orally If allergic: cefuroxime axetil, 500 mg bid, or erythromycin, 250 mg qid orally Children: amoxicillin, 250 mg orally tid or 50 mg/kg/day divided tid (erythromycin, 30 mg/kg/day divided tid)
Neurologic disease	Ceftriaxone, 2 g IV qd for 14–28 days Cefotaxime, 2 g IV q 8 hr Penicillin G, 3.3 million U IV q 4 hr (20 million U/day) If allergic: doxycycline 100 mg tid for 30 days Children: ceftriaxone, 75–100 mg/kg/day (maximum 2 g); cefotaxime, 150 mg/kg/day divided tid and qid; penicillin G sodium, 200,000 to –400,000 U/kg/d in six divided doses
Isolated facial nerve palsy	Oral regimens possibly adequate
Arthritis	Oral regimens 30–60 days or IV regimens for 14–28 days
Carditis	
First-degree AV block	Oral regimens for 14–21 days
High-degree AV block	IV regimens plus cardiac monitoring

bid: two times a day; tid: three times a day; qid: four times a day; IV: intravenous; qd: every day; q: every; AV: atrioventricular.

who developed neurologic disease following weeks of oral antibiotics (amoxicillin or doxycyclline). In addition, CSF is often abnormal in facial nerve palsy patients who otherwise appear to have peripheral disease (127). Table 10 shows recommended antibiotic therapies for neurologic Lyme disease. Ceftriaxone, a third-generation cephalosporin, is first-line treatment for neurologic Lyme disease because of excellent organ penetration and in vitro activity against *B. burgdorferi* (128). The usual treatment course is 2 g once a day (half of the acute meningitis dose) for 4 weeks (up to 6 weeks when there is late parenchymal involvement (129). Patients treated with such a broad spectrum antibiotic are at risk for pseudomembranous colitis; this risk is lessened by concomitant use of acidophilus (lactobacillus). In rare cases, ceftriaxone therapy is associated with biliary cholelithiasis, especially in young women and children treated for prolonged periods. Intravenous cefotaxime, penicillin G or doxycycline can be used as alternatives to ceftriaxone.

Table 10 Current Treatment Practice for Neurologic Lyme Disease

IV ceftriaxone, 2 g qd for 4 weeks (may extend to 6–8 weeks for significant late-stage infection parenchymal involvement)
Alternative therapies
– IV cefotaxime, 2 g tid
– IV or oral doxycycline, 200 mg bid (not empty stomach)
– IV penicillin G, 3–4 million units q 4 hr

Doxycycline is the first-line agent for EM. It is preferred to amoxicillin because it is also effective against *Ehrlichia* infections. Use should be avoided in children under age 8 because of dental and bone complications. It is also avoided in pregnant or breastfeeding patients. If used to treat neurologic involvement, it is generally given at twice the regular dose (200 mg twice daily), because this provides superior CSF drug levels. There are some physicians who treat Lyme disease patients for prolonged periods, or who use combination antimicrobial therapy. No clinical trials support such unusual treatment regimens (130,131). It is important not to base a diagnosis of Lyme disease strictly on serology (125,132). In addition, patients who sustain ixodid tick bite may have another tick-born infection. Patients with neurologic complaints commonly do well after treatment, although some individuals have mild residual pain, cognitive, and fatigue symptoms (65,133).

4.3. Prevention

Lyme disease can be prevented by avoiding tick contact. Regular skin inspection is encouraged. If attached ticks are found early and removed, they will not transmit infection. Prophylactic antibiotics after tick bite lower disease risk. In a landmark study, a single dose (200 mg) of doxycycline given within 72 hr of tick bite prevented Lyme disease in 87% of cases (134). In appropriate settings (high risk area, *Ixodes* tick bite engorgement), prophylactic antibiotics are indicated (135).

Effective immunoprophylaxis is the optimal preventive measure. Unfortunately, the LYMErix vaccine, after being approved for use in 1998, was withdrawn from the U.S. market in early 2002. The market never reached expected numbers, and a small minority of vaccinees developed severe pain syndromes with multisystem complaints. This vaccine consisted of recombinant Osp-A lipoprotein, given in three doses intramuscularly at 0, 1, and 12 months. It showed a protection rate of 49% after two doses and 76% after three doses (136). Immunity developed based on formation of specific anti-Osp A antibodies that killed spirochetes within the feeding tick. Because these antibodies were transient, it was likely that regular booster vaccination would have been required to maintain immunity.

Despite failure of LYMErix™ vaccine in the market place, other (particularly multivalent) Lyme disease vaccines are under development. An anti-tick vaccine has also been proposed.

4.4. Prognosis

Overall Lyme disease patients have a very good prognosis. Except for severe cardiac disease there is virtually no mortality. Early dissemination syndromes spontaneously recover, and will typically improve within 3–5 days of starting antibiotics. Radicular pain can improve within hours of starting therapy. Excellent treatment responses occur in 90% of EM and multifocal EM cases, and 70–80% of disseminated syndromes other than multifocal EM. Some 7% of patients appear not to respond or even worsen during therapy. Facial nerve palsy which occurs during antibiotic therapy does not reflect treatment failure, and patients typically do well. Lyme disease-related facial nerve palsy improves in 85% of patients, with 70% showing complete recovery (137).

Late-stage infection neurologic syndromes do not improve or remit spontaneously. Encephalopathy patients seem to have better outcome after antibiotics than encephalomyelitis cases. Three to 6 months after intravenous ceftriaxone, encephalopathy patients show improvements in neuropsychiatric symptoms, cognitive measures, CSF abnormalities, and brain SPECT disturbances. Improvement may continue for months after antibiotics are stopped. Although rare, patients who truly relapse following treatment may benefit from a second course of antibiotics. Patients who relapse after 2 weeks of treatment have responded to more extended treatment (4 weeks of antibiotics).

4.5. Tick Copathogens

Ixodid ticks can carry multiple pathogens (bacteria, parasites, viruses) other than *B. burgdorferi*, and patients may be coinfected with two or more pathogens following tick bite (138–141). Coinfection with a parasite (babesia) or a rickettsia-like bacterium (ehrlichia) are estimated to occur in 4–30% of Lyme disease patients. In a recent prospective study of EM, 4% had a coinfection (142). Within endemic areas in the northeast, it is increasingly common to screen for babesiosis and human granulocytic ehrlichiosis (HGE) in any patient with possible Lyme disease. Coinfection results in a more prolonged spirochetemia, more severe clinical illness, and poorer therapeutic response (143,144). Acute babesiosis is a malaria-like illness, while chronic infection manifest as persistent fatigue, with episodic fevers and chills (145). Patients with coinfection are more likely to experience fatigue, headache, sweats, chills, anorexia, emotional lability, nausea, conjunctivitis, and splenomegaly (143). They are 13 times more likely to experience months of symptoms. They are three times more likely to be PCR positive in blood for circulating *B. burgdorferi* DNA. Coinfection has important therapeutic implications, since antimicrobials for babesia infection are entirely different than those for *B. burgdorferi*.

Ehrlichiae are obligate intracellular gram-negative-like bacteria which resemble rickettesiae. They were originally recognized to cause diseases in animals. Ehrlichiae show a marked tropism for leukocytes, and can cause chronic infection. The HGE, *Anaphylasta phagocyctophila*, infects ixodid ticks (146,147). Ehrlichia infection responds well to tetracycline agents such as doxycycline. Patients with dual infections may experience more severe clinical syndromes.

Clues to coinfection are an increase in alanine aminotransferase, and thrombocytopenia. Both are unusual in Lyme disease. Babesia and Ehrlichia infections produce a degree of immunosuppression, which may explain in part more severe clinical illness. In endemic areas it is reasonable to check for tick copathogen exposure when evaluating Lyme disease. Serology (IFA) is the simplest way to screen for exposure, but both PCR and culture are available for these agents.

4.6. Post-Lyme Syndrome (Chronic Lyme Disease Syndrome)

Perhaps half or more of Lyme disease patients (especially those treated after dissemination) note persistent symptoms 6 months or longer after antibiotic therapy (148–151). Post-treatment symptoms include fatigue, arthralgias, myalgias, headache, cognitive problems, sleep disturbance, and depression or other mood disturbances (152,153). There are many possible explanations for persistent post-treatment problems in addition to persistent infection.

Post Lyme disease syndrome (also referred to as chronic Lyme disease syndrome) is a controversial diagnosis without accepted criteria. Patients are quite heterogeneous. In fact, both seropositive and seronegative patients with nonspecific symptoms of fatigue, arthralgias, myalgias, and other complaints are given this diagnosis. There is no convincing data that such patients show a consistent response to antibiotics (154,155). In particular, patients with nonspecific symptoms and without laboratory evidence of *B. burgdorferi* exposure should not be considered to have Lyme disease (156). Chronic Lyme disease syndrome patients are often treated with extended and combination antibiotics. No data supports a response to such treatment. In fact, recent studies suggest most chronic Lyme disease patients do not have any substantive response to antibiotics (157–159).

5. SUMMARY

Lyme disease is a fascinating and complex infection which has become a focus of public interest and controversy. It provides a model for a pathogen which causes broad spectrum neurologic disease. Current studies are focusing on better understanding of neurotropism, pathogenicity, the role of strain heterogeneity, and host immune and inflammatory response in disease manifestation. Diagnosis should improve with the introduction of second-generation antibody tests. Future challenges involve the paradigm of chronic Lyme disease syndrome, delineating the role of dual infection, and development of a viable and effective vaccine.

REFERENCES

1. Stanek G, Strle F. Lyme borreliosis. Lancet 2003; 362:1639–1647.
2. Coyle PK. Lyme disease. In: Roos KL, ed. Central Nervous System Infectious Diseases and Therapy. New York: Marcel Dekker, 1997:213–236.
3. Dammin GJ. Erythema migrans: a chronicle. Rev Infect Dis 1989; 11:142–151.
4. Steere AC, Malawista SE, Snydman DR. Lyme arthritis: an epidemic of oligoarticular arthritis in children and adults in three Connecticut communities. Arthritis Rheum 1977; 20:7–17.
5. Burgdorfer W. Discovery of the Lyme disease spirochete and its relation to tick vectors. Yale J Biol Med 1984; 57:515–520.
6. Steere AC, Grodzicki RL, Kornblatt JP, et al. The spirochetal etiology of Lyme disease. N Engl J Med 1983; 308:733–740.
7. Benach JL, Bosler EM, Hanrahan JP, et al. Spirochetes isolated from the blood of two patients with Lyme disease. N Engl J Med 1983; 308:740–742.
8. Burgdorfer W. How the discovery of *Borrelia burgdorferi* came about. Clin Dermatol 1993; 11(3):335–338.
9. Marshall WF III, Telford SR III, Rys PN, Rutledge BJ, Mathiesen D, et al. Detection of *Borrelia burgdorferi* DNA in museum specimens of *Peromyscus leucopus*. J Infect Dis 1994; 170:1027–1032.
10. Matuschka FR, Ohlenbush A, Eiffert H, Richter D, Spielman A. Characteristics of Lyme disease spirochetes in archived European ticks. J Infect Dis 1996; 174:424–426.
11. Coyle PK. Lyme disease. Curr Neurol Neurosci Rep 2002; 2(6):479–487.
12. Steere AC. Lyme disease. N Engl J Med 2001; 345:115–125.
13. Shapiro ED, Gerber MA. Lyme disease. Clin Infect Dis 2000; 31:533–542.
14. Orloski KA, Hayes EB, Campbell GL, et al. Surveillance for Lyme disease— United States, 1992–1998. MMWR Morb Mortal Wkly Rep 2000; 49(SS03):1–11.
15. Campbell GL, Fritz CL, Fish D, Nowakowski J, Nadelman RB, Wormser GP. Estimation of the incidence of Lyme disease. Am J Epidemiol 1998; 148:1018–1026.
16. Fraser CM, Casjens S, Huang WM, et al. Genomic sequence of a Lyme disease spirochaete, *Borrelia burgdorferi*. Nature 1997; 390(6660):580–586.
17. Liang FT, Nelson FK, Fikrig E. DNA microarray assessment of putative *Borrelia burgdorferi* lipoprotein genes. Infect Immun 2002; 70(6):3300–3303.
18. Zhang, JR, Norris, SJ. Genetic variation of the *Borrelia burgdorferi* gene vlsE involves cassette-specific, segmental gene conversation. Infect Immun 1998; 66:3698–3704.
19. Ohnishi J, Piesman J, de Silva AM. Antigenic and genetic heterogeneity of *Borrelia burgdorferi* populations transmitted by ticks. Proc Natl Acad Sci U S A 2001; 98(2):670–675.

20. Posey JE, Gherardini FC. Lack of a role for iron in the Lyme disease pathogen. Science 2000; 288:1651–1653.
21. Revel AT, Talaat AM, Norgard MV. DNA microarray analysis of differential gene expression in *Borrelia burgdorferi*, the Lyme disease spirochete. Proc Natl Acad Sci U S A 2002; 99(3):1562–1567.
22. Babb K, El-Hage N, Miller JC, et al. Distinct regulatory pathways control expression of *Borrelia burgdorferi* infection-associated OspC and Erp surface proteins. Infect Immun 2001; 69:4146–4153.
23. Picken RN, Cheng Y, Strle F, Picken MM. Patients isolates of *Borrelia burgdorferi sensu lato* with genotypic and phenotypic similarities to strain 25015. J Infect Dis 1996; 174:1112–1115.
24. Lane RS, Loye JE. Lyme disease in California: interrelationship of ixodid ticks (Acari), rodents, and *Borrelia burgdorferi*. J Med Entomol 1991; 28(5):719–725.
25. Kuo MM, Lane RS, Giclas, PC. A comparative study of mammalian and reptilian alternative pathway of complement-mediated killing of the Lyme disease spirochete *Borrelia burgdorferi*. J Parasitol 2000; 86:1223–1228.
26. Hengge UR, Tannapfel A, Tyring SK, Erbel R, Arendt G, Ruzicka T. Lyme borreliosis. Lancet Infect Dis 2003; 3(8):489–500 [Review. Erratum in: Lancet Infect Dis 2003; 3(12):815].
27. Steere AC, Coburn J, Glickstein L. The emergence of Lyme disease. J Clin Invest 2004; 113(8):1093–1101.
28. Stanek G, Strle F. Lyme borreliosis and emerging tick-borne diseases in Europe. Wien Klin Wochenschr 1998; 110(24):847–849.
29. Piesman J. Dynamics of *Borrelia burgdorferi* transmission by nymphal *Ixodes dammini* ticks. J Infect Dis 1993; 167(5):1082–1085.
30. Steere AC. Lyme disease. N Engl J Med 1989; 321:586–596.
31. Feder HM Jr, Whitaker DL. Misdiagnosis of erythema migrans. Am J Med 1995; 99:412–419.
32. Nadelman RB, Wormser GP. Erythema migrans and early Lyme disease. Am J Med 1995; 98:15S–24S.
33. Asbrink E, Hovmark A. Early and late cutaneous manifestations in *Ixodes*-borne borreliosis (Erythema migrans borreliosis, Lyme borreliosis). Ann N Y Acad Sci 1988; 539:4–15.
34. Picken RN, Strle F, Picken MM, et al. Identification of three species of *Borrelia burgdorferi sensu lato* (*B. burgdorferi sensu stricto*, *B. garinii*, and *B. afzelii*) among isolates from acrodermatitis chronica atrophicans lesions. J Invest Dermatol 1998; 110:211–214.
35. Berger BW. Current aspects of Lyme disease and other *Borrelia burgdorferi* infections. Dermatol Clin 1997; 15:247–255.
36. Straubinger RK, Summers BA, Chang YF, Appel MJG. Persistence of *Borrelia burgdorferi* in experimentally infected dogs after antibiotic treatment. J Clin Microbiol 1997; 35:111–116.
37. Schuttelaar ML, Laeijendecker R, Heinhuis RJ, Van Joost T. Erythema multiforme and persistent erythema as early cutaneous manifestations of Lyme disease. J Am Acad Dermatol 1997; 37:873–875.
38. Nadelman RB, Nowakowski J, Forseter G, Goldberg NS, et al. The clinical spectrum of early Lyme disease in patients with culture-confirmed erythema migranes. Am J Med 1996; 100:502–508.

39. Strle F, Pleterski-Rigler D, Stanek G, Pejovnik-Pustinek A, Ruzic E, Cimperman J. Solitary borrelial lymphocytoma: report of 36 cases. Infection 1992; 20:201–206.

40. Strle F, Nelson JA, Ruzic-Sabljic E, et al. European Lyme borreliosis: 231 culture-confirmed cases involving patients with erythema migrans. Clin Infect Dis 1996; 23:61–65.

41. Maraspin V, Cimperman J, Lotric-Furlan S, et al. Solitary borrelial lymphocytoma in adult patients. Wien Klin Wochenschr 2002; 114:515–523.

42. Asbrink E, Hovmark A, Olsson I. Clinical manifestations of acrodermatitis chronica atrophicans in 50 Swedish patients. Zbl Bakt Hyg A 1986; 263:253–261.

43. Goodman JL, Bradley JF, Ross AE, et al. Bloodstream invasion in early Lyme disease: results from a prospective, controlled, blinded study using the polymerase chain reaction. Am J Med 1995; 99:6–12.

44. Steere AC, Schoen RT, Taylor E. The clinical evolution of Lyme arthritis. Ann Intern Med 1987; 107:725–731.

45. Rees DH, Axford JS. Lyme arthritis. Ann Rheum Dis 1994; 53:553–556.

46. Nocton JJ, Dressler F, Rutledge BJ, et al. Detection of *Borrelia burgdorferi* DNA by polymerase chain reaction in synovial fluid from patients with Lyme arthritis. N Engl J Med 1994; 330:229–234.

47. Nagi KS, Joshi R, Thakur RK. Cardiac manifestations of Lyme disease: a review. Can J Cardiol 1996; 12:503–506.

48. Steere AC, Batsford WP, Weinberg M, et al. Lyme carditis: cardiac abnormalities of Lyme disease. Ann Intern Med 1980; 93:8–16.

49. van der Linde MR. Lyme carditis: clinical characteristics of 105 cases. Scand J Infect Dis Suppl 1997; 77:81–84.

50. Strle F. Ocular manifestations of Lyme borreliosis. Acta Derm Venereol APA 1994; 1/2:71–76.

51. Mikkila HO, Seppala IJ, Viljanen MK, Peltomaa MP, Karma A, The expanding clinical spectrum of ocular Lyme borreliosis. Ophthalmology 2000; 107:581–587.

52. Schonherr U, Strle F. Ocular manifestations. In: Weber K, Burgdorfer W, eds. Aspects of Lyme Borreliosis. 1st ed. Berlin: Springer-Verlag, 1993:131–151.

53. Hansen K. Lyme neuroborreliosis: improvements of the laboratory diagnosis and a survey of epidemiological and clinical features in Denmark 1985–1990. Acta Neurol Scand 1994; 89(suppl 151):7–44.

54. Haass A. Lyme neuroborreliosis. Curr Opin Neurol 1998; 11:253–258.

55. Garcia-Monco JC, Benach JL. Lyme neuroborreliosis. Ann Neurol 1995; 37:691–702.

56. Kuiper H, de Jongh BM, van Dam AP, Dodge DE, et al. Evaluation of central nervous system involvement in Lyme borreliosis patients with a solitary erythema migrans lesion. Eur J Clin Microbiol Infect Dis 1994; 13:379–387.

57. Kristoferitsch W, Spiel G, Wessely P. Meningopolyneuritis (Garin-Bujadoux, Bannwarth). Clinical aspects and laboratory findings. Nervenarzt 1983; 54:640–646.

58. Pachner AR, Steere AC. The triad of neurologic manifestations of Lyme disease: meningitis, cranial neuritis, and radiculoneuritis. Neurology 1985; 111:47–53.

59. Christen HJ. Lyme disease in children. Ann Med 1996; 28:235–240.

60. Scelsa S, Lipton R, Sander H, et al. Headache characteristics in hospitalized patients with Lyme disease. Headache 1995; 35:125–130.

61. Kristoferitsch W. Neurological manifestations of Lyme borreliosis: clinical definition and differential diagnosis. Scand J Infect Dis Suppl 1991; 77:64–73.

62. Lotric-Furlan S, Cimperman J, Maraspin V, et al. Lyme borreliosis and peripheral facial palsy. Wien Klin Wochenschr 1999; 111:970–975.

63. Belman AL, Reynolds L, Preston T, et al. Cerebrospinal fluid findings in children with Lyme disease-associated facial nerve palsy. Arch Pediatr Adolesc Med 1997; 151:1224–1228.

64. Hansen K, Lebech A-M. The clinical and epidemiological profile of Lyme neurologic Lyme disease in Denmark 1985–1990. Brain 1992; 115:399–423.

65. Logigian EL, Kaplan RF, Steere AC. Chronic neurologic manifestations of Lyme disease. N Engl J Med 1990; 323:1438–1444.

66. Halperin JJ, Luft BJ, Volkman DJ, Dattwyler RJ. Lyme neurologic Lyme disease: peripheral nervous system abnormalities. Brain 1990; 113:1207–1221.

67. Kindstrand E, Nilsson BY, Hovmark A, Pirskanen R, Asbrink E. Peripheral neuropathy in acrodermitis chronica atrophicans—a late *Borrelia* manifestation. Acta Neurol Scand 1997; 95:338–345.

68. Chehrenama M, Zagardo MT, Koski CL. Subarachnoid hemorrhage in a patient with Lyme disease. Neurology 1997; 48(2):520–523.

69. Danek A, Uttner I, Yoursry T, Pfister HW. Lyme neuroborreliosis disguised as normal pressure hydrocephalus. Neurology 1996; 46:1743–1745.

70. Fallon H, Nields A. Lyme disease: a neuropsychiatric illness. Am J Psychiatry 1994; 151:1571–1583.

71. Nadelman RB, Horowitz HW, Hsieh TC, et al. Simultaneous human granulocytic ehrlichiosis and Lyme borreliosis. N Engl J Med 1997; 337:27–30.

72. Cook SP, Macartney KK, Rose CD, Hunt PG, et al. Lyme disease and seventh nerve paralysis in children. Am J Otolaryngol 1997; 18:320–323.

73. Shapiro ED, Seltzer EG. Lyme disease in children. Semin Neurol 1997; 17:39–44.

74. Belman AL, Iyer M, Coyle PK, Dattwyler R. Neurologic manifestations in children with North American Lyme disease. Neurology 1993; 43:2609–2614.

75. Gerber MA, Shapiro ED, Burke GS, Parcells VJ, Bell GL. Lyme disease in children in southeastern Connecticut. Pediatric Lyme Disease Study Group. N Engl J Med 1996; 335:1270–1274.

76. Silver HM. Lyme disease during pregnancy. Infect Dis Clin N Am 1997; 11:93–97.

77. Markowitz LE, Steere AC, Benach JL, et al. Lyme disease during pregnancy. J Am Med Assoc 1986; 225:3394–3396.

78. Maraspin V, Cimperman J, Lotric-Furlan S, et al. Treatment of erythema migrans in pregnancy. Clin Infect Dis 1996; 22:788–793.

79. Coyle PK. *Borrelia burgdorferi* infection: clinical diagnostic techniques. Immunol Invest 1997; 26:117–128.

80. Oksi J, Kalimo H, Marttila RJ, Marjamaki M, et al. Inflammatory brain changes in Lyme borreliosis. A report on three patients and review of the literature. Brain 1996; 119:2143–2154.

81. Maimone D, Villanova M, Stanta G, et al. Detection of *Borrelia burgdorferi* DNA and complement membrane attack complex deposits in the sural nerve of a patient with chronic polyneuropathy and tertiary Lyme disease. Muscle Nerve 1997; 20:969–975.

82. Vallat JM, Hugon J, Lubeau M, Leboutet MJ, Dumas M, Desproges-Gotteron R. Tick-bite meningoradiculoneuritis: clinical, electrophysiologic, and histologic findings in 10 cases. Neurology 1987; 37:749–753.

83. Benach JL. *Borrelia burgdorferi* in the central nervous system. JAMA 1992; 268(7):872.

84. Coleman JL, Gebbia JA, Benach JL. *Borrelia burgdorferi* and other bacterial products induce expression and release of the urokinase receptor (CD87). J Immunol 2001; 166:473–480.

85. Gebbia JA, Coleman JL, Benach JL. *Borrelia* spirochetes upregulate release and activation of matrix metalloproteinase gelatinase B (MMP-9) and collagenase 1 (MMP-1) in human cells. Infect Immun 2001; 69:456–462.

86. Sprenger H, Krause A, Kaufmann A, Priem S, et al. *Borrelia burgdorferi* induces chemokines in human monocytes. Infect Immunol 1997; 65:4384–4388.

87. Hirschfeld M, Kirschning CJ, Schwandner R, et al. Cutting edge: inflammatory signaling by *Borrelia burgdorferi* lipoproteins is mediated by toll-like receptor 2. J Immunol 1999; 163:2382–2386.

88. Coleman JL, Gebbia JA, Piesman J, et al. Plasminogen is required for efficient dissemination of *B. burgdorferi* in ticks and for enhancement of spirochetemia in mice. Cell 1997; 89:1111–1119.

89. Seinost G, Dykhuizen DE, Dattwyler RJ, et al. Four clones of *Borrelia burgdorferi sensu stricto* cause invasive infection in humans. Infect Immun 1999; 67:3518–3524.

90. Wilske B, Busch U, Eiffert H, Fingerle V, et al. Diversity of OspA and OspC among cerebrospinal fluid isolates of *Borrelia burgdorferi sensu lato* from patients with neuroborreliosis in Germany. Med Microbiol Immunol 1996; 184:195–201.

91. Coburn J, Magoun L, Bodary SC, Leong JM. Integrins alpha(v)beta3 and alpha5beta1 mediate attachment of Lyme disease spirochetes to human cells. Infect Immun 1998; 66:1946–1952.

92. Brown EL, Wooten RM, Johnson BJ, et al. Resistance to Lyme disease in decorin-deficient mice. J Clin Invest 2001; 107:845–852.

93. Guo BP, Brown EL, Dorward DW, et al. Decorin-binding adhesions from *Borrelia burgdorferi*. Mol Microbiol 1998; 30:711–723.

94. Wooten RM, Weis JJ. Host–pathogen interactions promoting inflammatory Lyme arthritis: use of mouse models for dissection of disease processes. Curr Opin Microbiol 2001; 4:274–279.

95. Steere AC, Dwyer E, Winchester R. Association of chronic Lyme arthritis with HLA-DR4 and HLA-DR2 alleles. N Engl J Med 1990; 323:219–223.

96. Gross DM, Forsthuber T, Tary-Lehmann M, Etling C, et al. Identification of LFA-1 as a candidate autoantigen in treatment-resistant Lyme arthritis. Science 1998; 281:703–706.

97. Gross DM, Steere AC, Huber BT. T helper 1 response is dominant and localized to the synovial fluid in patients with Lyme arthritis. J Immunol 1998; 160:1022–1028.

98. Akin E, Aversa J, Steere AC. Expression of adhesion molecules in synovia of patients with treatment-resistant lyme arthritis. Infect Immun 2001; 69(3):1774–1780.

99. Yin Z, Braun J, Neure L, Wu P, et al. T cell cytokine pattern in the joints of patients with Lyme arthritis and its regulation by cytokines and anticytokines. Arthr Rheum 1997; 40:69–79.

100. Ekerfelt C, Ernerudh J, Bunikis J, Vrethem M, et al. Compartmentalization of antigen specific cytokine responses to the central nervous system in CNS borreliosis: secretion of IFN-gamma predominates over IL-4 secretion in response to outer surface proteins of Lyme disease *Borrelia* spirochetes. J Neuroimmunol 1997; 79:155–162.

101. Nilsson I, Alves M, Nässberger L. Response of soluble IL-2 receptor, interleukin-2 and interleukin-6 in patients with positive and negative *Borrelia burgdorferi* serology. Infection 1994; 22:316–320.
102. Pohl-Koppe A, Balashov KE, Steere AC, Logigian EL, Hafler DA. Identification of a T cell subset capable of both IFN-gamma and IL-10 secretion in patients with chronic *Borrelia burgdorferi* infection. J Immunol 1998; 160:1804–1810.
103. Brade V, Kleber I, Acker G. Differences of two *Borrelia burgdorferi* strains in complement activation and serum resistance. Immunobiology 1992; 185:453–465.
104. Kraiczy P, Skerka C, Zipfel PF, Brade V. Complement regulator-acquiring surface proteins of *Borrelia burgdorferi*: a new protein family involved in complement resistance. Wien Klin Wochensch 2002; 114:568–573.
105. Kraiczy P, Hellwage J, Skerka C, et al. Immune evasion of *Borrelia burgdorferi*: mapping of a complement-inhibitor factor H-binding site of BbCRASP-3, a novel member of the Erp protein family. Eur J Immunol 2003; 33:697–707.
106. Yu Z, Tu J, Chu YH. Confirmation of cross-reactivity between Lyme antibody H9724 and human heat shock protein 60 by a combinatorial approach. Anal Chem 1997; 69:4515–4518.
107. Sigal LH. Lyme disease: a review of aspects of its immunology and immunopathogenesis. Ann Rev Immunol 1997; 15:63–92.
108. Coyle PK, Schutzer SE, Belman AL, et al. CSF immune complexes in patients exposed to *Borrelia burgdorferi*: detection of *Borrelia* specific and nonspecific complexes. Ann Neurol 1990; 28:739–744.
109. Schutzer SE, Coyle PK, Reid P, Holland B. *Borrelia burgdorferi*-specific immune complexes in acute Lyme disease. JAMA 1999; 282:1942–1946.
110. Roberts ED, Bohm RP Jr, Lowrie RC Jr, et al. Pathogenesis of Lyme neuroborreliosis in the rhesus monkey: the early disseminated and chronic phases of disease in the peripheral nervous system. J Infect Dis 1998; 178:722–732.
111. Cadavid D, O'Neill T, Schaefer H, Pachner AR. Localization of *Borrelia burgdorferi* in the nervous system and other organs in a nonhuman primate model of lyme disease. Lab Invest 2000; 80:1043–1054.
112. Pachner AR, Cadavid D, Shu G, et al. Central and peripheral nervous system infection, immunity, and inflammation in the NHP model of Lyme borreliosis. Ann Neurol 2001; 50:330–338.
113. Sigal LH, Zahradnik JM, Lavin P, et al. A vaccine consisting of recombinant *Borrelia burgdorferi* outer-surface protein A to prevent Lyme disease. N Engl J Med 1998; 339:216–222.
114. AAN Quality Standards Subcommittee, Halperin JJ, Logigian EL, Finkel MF, Pearl RA. Practice parameters for the diagnosis of patients with nervous system Lyme borreliosis (Lyme disease).Quality Standards Subcommittee of the American Academy of Neurology. Neurology 1996; 46:619–627.
115. Fix AD, Strickland T, Grant J. Tick bites and Lyme disease in an endemic setting: problematic use of serologic testing and prophylactic antibiotic therapy. JAMA 1998; 279:206–210.
116. Strickland GT, Karp AC, Mathews A, Pena CA. Utilization and cost of serologic tests for Lyme disease in Maryland. J Infect Dis 1997; 176:819–821.
117. Nichol G, Dennis DT, Steere AC, Lightfoot R, et al. Test-treatment strategies for patients suspected of having Lyme disease: a cost-effectiveness analysis. Ann Int Med 1998; 128:37–48.

118. Tugwell P, Dennis DT, Weinstein A, Wells G, et al. Clinical guideline, Part 2. Laboratory evaluation in the diagnosis of Lyme disease. Ann Int Med 1997; 127:1109–1123.

119. Beitinjaneh F, Rizvi S, Coyle PK, Krupp LB. Diagnostic accuracy of serologic testing for Lyme disease. Neurology 2001; 56:A479.

120. Brunner M, Sigal LH. Use of serum immune complexes in a new test that accurately confirms early Lyme disease and active infection with *Borrelia burgdorferi*. J Clin Microbiol 2001; 39:3213–3221.

121. Schutzer SE, Coyle PK, Belman AL, Golightly MG, Drulle J. Sequestration of antibody to *Borrelia burgdorferi* in immune complexes in seronegative Lyme disease. Lancet 1999; 335:312–315.

122. Nocton JJ, Bloom BJ, Rutledge BJ, et al. Detection of *Borrelia burgdorferi* DNA by polymerase chain reaction in cerebrospinal fluid in Lyme neuroborreliosis. J Infect Dis 1996; 174:623–627.

123. Perides G, Charness ME, Tanner LM, et al. Matrix metalloproteinases in the cerebrospinal fluid of patients with Lyme neuroborreliosis. J Infect Dis 1998; 177:401–408.

124. Coyle PK. *Borrelia burgdorferi* antibodies in multiple sclerosis patients. Neurology 1989; 39:760–761.

125. Strle F. Principles of the diagnosis and antibiotic treatment of Lyme borreliosis. Wien Klin Wochenschr 1999; 111:911–915.

126. Wormser GP, Nadelman RB, Dattwyler RJ, et al. Practice guidelines for the treatment of Lyme disease. The Infectious Diseases Society of America. Clin Infect Dis 2000; 31(suppl 1):1–14.

127. Steere AC, Levin RE, Molloy PJ, Kalish RA, Abraham JH 3rd, Liu NY, Schmid CH. Treatment of Lyme arthritis. Arthritis Rheum 1994; 37(6):878–888.

128. Dattwyler RJ, Halperin JJ, Volkman DJ, Luft BJ. Treatment of late Lyme borreliosis—randomised comparison of ceftriaxone and penicillin. Lancet 1988; 1:1191–1194.

129. Coyle PK. In: Johnson RT, Griffin JW and McArthur JC, eds. Neurologic Lyme Disease. Current Therapy and Neurologic Disease, 6th ed. St Louis, MO: Mosby, 2001:159–164.

130. Wormser GP, Nowakowski J, Nadelman RB. Duration of treatment for Lyme borreliosis: time for a critical reappraisal. Wien Klin Wochenschr 2002; 114:613–615.

131. Wormser GP, Ramanathan R, Nowakowski J, et al. Duration of antibiotic therapy for early Lyme disease. A randomized, double-blind, placebo-controlled trial. Ann Intern Med 2003; 138:697–704.

132. Wormser GP. Controversies in the use of antimicrobials for the prevention and treatment of Lyme disease. Infection 1996; 24:178–181.

133. Krüger H, Kohlehepp W, König S. Follow-up of antibiotically treated and untreated neuroborreliosis. Acta Neurol Scand 1990; 82:59–67.

134. Nadelman RB, Nowakowski J, Fish D, et al. Prophylaxis with single-dose doxycycline for the prevention of Lyme disease after an *Ixodes scapularis* tick bite. N Engl J Med 2001; 345:79–84.

135. Hayes EB, Piesman J. How can we prevent Lyme disease? N Engl J Med 2003; 348:2424–2430.

136. Steere AC, Sikand VK, Meurice F, et al. Vaccination against Lyme disease with recombinant *Borrelia burgdorferi* outer-surface lipoprotein A with adjuvant. Lyme Disease Vaccine Study Group. N Engl J Med 1998; 339:209–215.

137. Smouha EE, Coyle PK, Shukri S. Facial nerve palsy in Lyme disease: evaluation of clinical diagnostic criteria. Am J Otolaryngol 1997; 18:257–261.

138. Thompson C, Spielman A, Krause PJ. Coinfecting deer-associated zoonoses: Lyme disease, babesiosis, and ehrlichiosis. Clin Infect Dis 2001; 33:676–685.

139. Mitchell PD, Reed KD, Hofkes JM. Immunoserologic evidence of coinfection with *Borrelia burgdorferi*, *Babesia microti*, and human granulocytic *Ehrlichia* species in residents of Wisconsin and Minnesota. J Clin Microbiol 1996; 34:724–727.

140. Persing DH. The cold zone: a curious convergence of tick-transmitted diseases. Clin Infect Dis 1997; 25:S35–S42.

141. Walker DH, Barbour AG, Oliver JH, et al. Emerging bacterial zoonotic and vector-borne diseases. Ecological and epidemiological factors. JAMA 1996; 275:463–469.

142. Steere AC, et al. Prospective study of coinfection in patients with erythema migranes. Clin Infect Dis 2003; 36:1078–1081.

143. Krause PJ, Telford SR, Spielman A, et al. Concurrent Lyme disease and babesiosis. Evidence for increased severity and duration of illness. JAMA 1996; 275:1657–1660.

144. Thomas V, Anguita J, Barthold SW, Fikrig E. Coinfection with *Borrelia burgdorferi* and the agent of human granulocytic ehrlichiosis alters murine immune responses, pathogen burden, and severity of Lyme arthritis. Infect Immun 2001; 69:3359–3371.

145. Krause PJ, Spielman A, Telford SR, et al. Persistent parasitemia after acute babesiosis. N Engl J Med 1998; 339:160–165.

146. Dumler JS. Is human granulocytic ehrlichiosis a new Lyme disease? Review and comparison of clinical, laboratory, epidemiological, and some biological features. Clin Inf Dis 1997; 25:S43–S47.

147. Walls JJ, Asanovich KM, Bakken JS, Dumler JS. Serologic evidence of a natural infection of white-tailed deer with the agent of human granulocytic ehrlichiosis in Wisconsin and Maryland. Clin Diagn Lab Immunol 1998; 5(6):762–765.

148. Asch ES, Bujak DI, Weiss M, et al. Lyme disease: an infectious and postinfectious syndrome. J Rheumatol 1994; 21:454–461.

149. Benke TH, Gasse TH, Hittmair-Delazer M, Schmutzhard E. Lyme encephalopathy: long term neuropsychological deficits years after acute neuroborreliosis. Acta Neurol Scand 1995; 91:353–357.

150. Shadick NA, Phillips CB, Logigian EL, et al. The long-term clinical outcomes of Lyme disease. A population-based retrospective cohort study. Ann Intern Med 1994; 121:560–567.

151. Treib J, Fernandez A, Haass A, Grauer MT, et al. Clinical and serologic follow-up in patients with neuroborreliosis. Neurology 1998; 51:1489–1491.

152. Bujak DI, Weinstein A, Dornbush RI. Clinical and neurocognitive features of the post Lyme syndrome. J Rheumatol 1996; 23:1392–1397.

153. Gaudino EA, Coyle PK, Krupp LB. Post Lyme syndrome and chronic fatigue syndrome. Neuropsychiatric similarities and differences. Arch Neurol 1997; 54:1372–1376.

154. Fawcett PT, Rose CD, Gibney KM, Doughty RA. Correlation of seroreactivity with response to antibiotics in pediatric Lyme borreliosis. Clin Diagn Lab Immunol 1997; 4:85–88.
155. Svenungsson B, Lindh G. Lyme borreliosis—an overdiagnosed disease? Infection 1997; 25:2140–2143.
156. Reid MC, Schoen RT, Evans J, et al. The consequences of overdiagnosis and overtreatment of Lyme disease: an observational study. Ann Intern Med 1998; 128:354–362.
157. Klempner MS, Hu LT, Evans J, et al. Two controlled trials of antibiotic treatment in patients with persistent symptoms and a history of Lyme disease. N Engl J Med 2001; 345:85–92.
158. Klempner MS, Schmid CH, Hu L, et al. Intralaboratory reliability of serologic and urine testing for Lyme disease. Am J Med 2001; 110:217–219.
159. Krupp LB, Hyman LG, Grimson R, et al. Study and treatment of post Lyme disease (STOP-LD): a randomized double masked clinical trial. Neurology 2003; 60(12):1923–1930.
160. Gomes-Solecki MJ, Wormser GP, Persing D, et al. A first-tier rapid assay for the serodiagnosis of *Borrelia burgdorferi* infection. Arch Intern Med 2001; 161:2015–2020.
161. Halperin JJ. Nervous system Lyme disease. J Neurol Sci 1998; 153:182–191.
162. Horowitz HW, Dworkin B, Forseter G, Nadelman RB, et al. Liver function in early Lyme disease. Hepatology 1996; 23:1412–1417.
163. Logigian EL, Steere AC. Clinical and electrophysiologic findings in chronic neuropathy of Lyme disease. Neurology 1992; 42:303–311.
164. Logigian EL, Johnson KA, Kijewski MF, Kaplan RF, et al. Reversible cerebral hypoperfusion in Lyme encephalopathy. Neurology 1997; 49:1661–1670.
165. Marques AR, Martin DS, Philipp MT. Evaluation of the C6 peptide enzyme-linked immunosorbent assay for individuals vaccinated with the recombinant OspA vaccine. J Clin Microbiol 2002; 40(7):2591–2593.
166. Mokry M, Flaschka G, Kleinert G, et al. Chronic Lyme disease with an expansive gratulomatous lesion in the cerebellopontine angle. Neurosurgery 1990; 27:446–451.
167. Sumiya H, Kobayashi K, Mizukoshi C, et al. Brain perfusion SPECT in Lyme Neuroborreliosis. J Nucl Med 1997; 38:1120–1122.
168. Pena, et al. Incidence rates of Lyme disease in Maryland: 1993 through 1996. Md Med J 1999; (Mar-Apr) 48 (2): 68–73.
169. Picken RN, Strle F, Picken MM, et al. Indentification of three species of *Borrelca burgdorferi Sensu Lato* (*B. burgdorferi Sensu Stricto*, *B. Garinu*, and *B. afzelü*) among isolates from acrodermatitis chronica atrophicans lesions. J Invest Desonatol 1998; 110: 211–214.

9

Flaviviridae

Deborah S. Asnis and Robert Crupi

Flushing Hospital Medical Center, Flushing, New York, U.S.A.

1. INTRODUCTION

Nearly 100 years ago, it was discovered that yellow fever, the protype flavivirus disease, was caused by a filterable virus and transmitted to humans by mosquitoes. It was the first member to be isolated in the flaviviridae family in 1927. The Flaviviridae obtain their name from "yellow" (flavus, Latin) fever. The Flaviviridae consist of positive-sense, single-stranded RNA viruses that are spherical in shape with a diameter of 40–60 nm (1). The flavivirus virion has a spherical nucleocapsid surrounded by a lipid bilayer envelope with small projections from the surface. The envelope proteins, E (envelope) and M (membrane) are embedded in the lipid layer. The E-protein is the most immunologically important structural protein, is the viral hemagglutinin and mediates virus–host cell binding. It causes most of the virus-neutralizing antibodies.

The flavivirus genus includes greater than 68 members separated into three groups: 1) flaviviruses, 2) pestiviruses, and 3) hepatitis C viruses by their serological interrelatedness (2). Most flaviviruses are arthropod-borne and transmit infection to vertebrates by infected mosquito or tick vectors. Isolates from bats and rodents have also been identified. Flaviviruses have been classified into at least eight antigenic complexes by a neutralization test and include: tick-borne encephalitis, Japanese encephalitis (JE), Uganda S, Dengue, Rio Bravo, Modoc, Tyulenly, Ntaya and Ungrouped of which only six cause human disease (2). The viruses within tick-borne, dengue, and JE serocomplexes share up to 77% of amino acid sequences whereas there is only 40–45% homology across all serocomplexes (1).

West Nile virus (WNV) and Japanese encephalitis virus (JEV) belong to the JE complex along with St. Louis encephalitis, Murray Valley encephalitis, Kunjin, and other pathogens. Members of the JE complex are closely related and often require additional testing to distinguish the specific flavivirus. There is a high subclinical: clinical infection ratio in both diseases. They can cause zoonotic infections and cycles of transmission will occur in wild vertebrate hosts through the bite of an arthropod. In the case of WNV, wild birds can serve as intermediary host in comparison with JE where both pigs and wild birds can play a role in viral amplification. Clinical hosts like humans and horses are incidental in both WNV and JE and are not involved in the transmission cycle (1). Arbovirus infection generally causes three clinical syndromes: febrile illness, hemorrhagic fever, and meningoencephalitis. Arbovirus encephalitis cannot be differentiated from other causes of central nervous system infections on a clinical basis. Headache, confusion, nausea and vomiting can be presenting complaints. Fever, meningismus, cranial nerve palsies, sensory deficits, convulsions, and coma are some of the initial signs. Once established, the treatment in arboviral infections is limited but studies are ongoing. Both of these agents will be discussed separately as far as epidemiology, transmission, clinical presentation, laboratory, outcome, treatment, and prevention. Comparisons between these two flaviviruses viruses may be found in Table 1.

2. WEST NILE VIRUS

2.1. Epidemiology

West Nile virus was first isolated and identified in 1937 from the blood of a febrile asymptomatic woman in the West Nile district of Uganda (3). It was later isolated from the blood of three patients in Egypt (4), a sick child in Israel (5), and 40 patients in an Israeli outbreak (6). WNV is found throughout Africa, the Middle East, Europe, Russia, India, and Indonesia (7). Since its discovery in 1937, human outbreaks have been infrequent causing only mild febrile illnesses up until the 1990s.

During the 1950s, studies performed on children attending a medical clinic in Egypt found that most WNV infections presented with mild acute febrile episodes without any central nervous involvement. It was clear that most either had mild or no symptoms (8). In 1951, the first proved epidemic occurred in an agricultural community in Israel with 123 clinical cases in both children and adults mainly less than 30 years of age. There were no fatalities and no neurologic illness or sequelae. Recovery occurred faster in the pediatric group (9). In 1957, a large epidemic occurred in Israel and data was collected in three separate groups: soldiers in army camps, children and adults in Hadera, and elderly persons residing in nursing homes. The first two groups presented with symptoms similar to previous outbreaks. In the latter group, 16 of 49 nursing home patients greater than 65 years old developed meningoencephalitis and four died. Autopsy of three brains showed basal ganglia cells in

Table 1 Comparison of West Nile Virus (WNV) and Japanese Encephalitis Virus (JEV)

	WNV	JEV
Incubation	3–15 days	1–2 weeks
Vector transmission	*Culex* mosquito	*Culex* mosquito
Host	Birds	Birds, pigs
Asymptomatic:		
symptomatic ratio	1:150–1:300	1:300
Clinically infected	>50 years old	3–10 years old
Muscle weakness and/or flaccid paralysis	+	+
Seizures	Rare	85% Children;10% adults
Flaccid paralysis	+	+
White blood cells	Normal or elevated (lymphocytopenia)	Leukocytosis
EMG/NCV	Axonal neuropathy, anterior horn disease	Anterior horn disease
CT scan	Non-specific; age-related	Non-enhancing low density
MRI	Enhancement of leptomeninges and/or periventricular area	High-intensity signal thalamus, cerebrum, cerebellum
Treatment	Supportive	Supportive
Prevention	None	Vaccine
Mortality	10%	30%
Sequelae	+	+

varying stages of necrosis, perivascular cuffing, hemorrhages, and edema although serological tests were not done. This outbreak demonstrated that WNV infection was more severe in the elderly and was responsible for fatalities (10). Sporadic fatalities due to WNV infection have occurred in children with encephalitis in India (11) and young adults with hepatitis in the Central African Republic (12).

In 1974, a large outbreak of thousands of clinical cases occurred in the Cape Province of South Africa following unusually heavy rains and high summer temperatures (13). In 1999, WNV first entered the Western hemisphere and has spread throughout the United States into Canada and the Cayman Islands. During 1999–2002, there was exponential spread of WNV throughout the United States. The number of human cases seen in the 4-year period has been documented (62 persons from one state in 1999, 21 persons from three states in 2000, 66 persons from 10 states in 2001 and 4156 persons from 39 states in 2002) according to the ArboNET surveillance program (see Table 2) (14).

It was not until the 1990s that three new epidemiological trends emerged for WNV infections (15): 1) an increase in frequency of outbreaks in humans and

Table 2 West Nile Virus Outbreaks in the United States (1999–2002)

Year	Human WNV cases	States with human WNV	Deaths	States with avian or mosquito WNV activity
1999	62	1	7	4
2000	21	3	2	12 and Washington, D.C.
2001	61	10	9	27 and Washington, D.C.
2002	4156	39	284	44 and Washington, D.C.

(CDC website as of August 14, 2003.)

horses (Algeria 1994; Roumania 1996; Morocco 1996; Tunisia 1997; Italy 1998; Israel 1998–2000; Russia 1999, United States 1999–2002, and France 2000) (16–26); 2) an increase in severe human presentations (21–29); and 3) high avian death rates concurrent with human outbreaks (30,31). The exact reason for this change in frequency and presentation is unexplained but may be due to differences in the virulence of the virus, age structure affected, background herd immunity, or prevalence of chronic conditions in the population (32).

West Nile virus can be divided genetically into two lineages. Viruses in lineage 1 are primarily from West African, Middle Eastern, Eastern European, and Australian origin (33). Only members from lineage 1 have been associated with clinical human encephalitis (WNV lineage type is unresolved from South Africa 1974 outbreak). Lineage 2 is exclusively from the African continent and has not been involved in either human or equine outbreaks but rather enzootic cycles. The WNV responsible for the U.S. outbreak (NY99) is >99.8% homologous to a strain of WN isolated from an Israeli goose in 1998. Only the United States and Israel have reported illness and mortality in humans and animals with this particular strain. The genotype of the NY99 WNV has remained stable with very few genomic modifications (34).

2.2. Transmission

West Nile virus like other arboviruses have two separate transmission cycles: a primary enzootic or amplification cycle with one set of vectors and avian hosts and a secondary cycle with possibly different arthropods and transmission to different hosts like humans and domestic animals (35). In the primary cycle, ornithophagic mosquitoes like *Culex pipiens*, feed on viremic birds (amplification hosts) get infected and spread WNV to other amplification hosts. This cycle is usually silent and unrecognized in nature. If certain conditions exist (temperature, mosquito species, mosquito population density, number of susceptible hosts) an epizootic cycle will occur in the bird population. If there is significant amplification, there will be large numbers of bridge vector mosquitoes that bite both humans and birds, and thus cause human infections. These general feeders are not as efficient amplification vectors but pose more of a risk to humans, horses, and other mammals (35). Epidemics/epizootics in humans and domestic animals can then occur in the secondary cycle but they are dead-end hosts since viremia is not sufficient to infect another arthropod and continue the transmission cycle.

WNV has been isolated from 43 mosquito species primarily of the genus *Culex*. In Africa and the Middle East, *Culex univittatus* and *Culex pipiens molestus* and in Asia, *Culex tritaeniorhynchus* are the major vectors. In the United States, different *Culex* spp. mosquitoes are responsible for maintenance: *Cx. pipiens pipiens* and *Cx. restuans* in the northeast, *Cx. pipiens quinquefasciatus* in the south and *Cx. tarsalis* in the west. It is still not elucidated which mosquito is responsible for human infection. WNV has been isolated in overwintering mosquitoes (36). WNV has been recovered in ticks (both ixodid and argasid) in Russia but no clear role has been found in transmission (37).

Birds are the primary reservoir hosts. Dramatic avian mortality rates have occurred in the Israeli and the U.S. outbreaks. The highest mortality rates were recorded among American crows (*Corvus brachyrhynchos*) and North American corvids (ravens, jays and other crows) and preceded human illness (38). Surveillance systems recording dead birds, sentinel chickens, and ill horses have recorded the geographic expanse of this disease in the United States: 1999 (four states), 2000 (12 states and the District of Columbia), 2001 (27 states and D.C.), and 2002 (44 states and D.C.) (see Table 1) (38,39).

Camels, sheep, goats, dogs, and cats can also become infected but the virus is not maintained as well as with birds due to a lower population density and slower reproductive rate. WNV has been isolated in horses with encephalitis in Egypt, Portugal, Morocco, and Italy but this was uncommon until the more recent outbreaks (40).

Laboratory exposure has been documented by both the aerosolized route (41) and by percutaneous means (42). In 2002, WNV was transmitted by transfusion (43), organ transplant (44), and possibly breastfeeding (45). It is recommended to test a person for WNV infection within 3–21 days after the receipt of blood transfusion, organ transplantation or breast milk if they become ill. In 2002, a baby was born with WNV who contracted it from an infected mother during her 27th week of her pregnancy (46).

2.3. Clinical Presentation

The incubation period of West Nile fever is 3–14 days (38). Illness is often asymptomatic. In the Nile Delta region of Egypt where it is endemic, WNV seroprevalence ranged from 6% in schoolchildren to 40% in young adults (47 in earlier outbreaks, symptoms typically include fever, headache, backache, and myalgia lasting 3–6 days). Pharyngitis, conjunctival injection, nausea, vomiting, diarrhea, and abdominal pain are also reported. About 50% develop a non-pruritic, roseolar, or maculopapular rash on the chest, back, and arms which lasts 1 week (1). Rash was only seen in 20% of recent cases recently (21,27). Diffuse lymphadenopathy was reported to be common in earlier studies (1) although in more recent reports can range from less than 2% (27) to 4% of cases (21).

In the United States, it was determined that about 20% of infected persons with WNV developed WNV fever and only 50% sought medical help (48). Previously, neurological infection was rarely seen but can present as aseptic meningitis, meningoencephalitis, myelitis, optic neuritis, or polyradiculitis (1,49). In a study done on cancer patients inoculated with WNV, 89% of the patients had no clinical illness other than fever. Eleven percent had signs of diffuse encephalitis with twitching, mental confusion and one of the patients had flaccid paralysis of the extremities. The neurological signs were transient and recovery was complete (50).

Severe muscle weakness (50%) in hospitalized patients, and acute flaccid paralysis (10%) were reported recently (27,28). A Guillain–Barre syndrome was attributed to WNV (51) and muscle weakness was so severe in a few patients that they were treated for Guillain–Barre despite inconclusive electromyography and nerve conduction velocities that showed a sensory and motor polyneuropathy (25). A poliomyelitis-like syndrome can occur with asymmetric flaccid paralysis, fever, areflexia, and intact sensation. Electrodiagnostic tests confirmed anterior horn cell or motor axon involvement (52,53). Extraneurologic sites can include myocarditis, pancreatitis, and hepatitis.

In two serosurveys in New York City (1999 and 2000) about one in 150 infections resulted in meningitis or encephalitis. Advanced age was a marker for severe neurological illness. The attack rate was highest for those above 80 and this was not based simply on exposure (27) since a household survey showed uniform incidence of WNV infection across ages (48).

2.4. Laboratory Features

Laboratory findings include leukopenia and, in neurological cases, CSF pleocytosis and elevated protein (1). A relative lymphocytopenia (54) has been reported which can last up to 52 days (55). The virus can be recovered from the blood of an immunocompetent febrile patient for up to 10 days. In the immunocompromised patient it has been found up to 22–28 days after infection (50). Peak viremia is seen between 4 and 8 days (50) but the titer is usually low at 103/mL (40). Standard precautions should be followed with handling specimens. Virus could not be isolated in feces, urine, or throat washings (50).

The diagnosis is made by serology, PCR, or viral isolation. IgM detection by antibody capture enzyme immunosorbent assay (EIA) in the serum is one of the preferred methods. The presence of IgM in CSF reflects intrathecal production. Cross-reactions with other flaviviruses occur, therefore, other endemic viruses must be excluded by the plaque reduction neutralization test (PRNT) antibody to WNV (40). Serial rising antibody titers can by demonstrated by EIA, complement fixation, neutralization or hemagglutination inhibition tests (40). In patients with meningoencephalitis, virus can be isolated from blood, CSF, and autopsied brains either by detection of gene sequences by PCR or viral antigens by IHC stain (24). In 1999, the yield of WNV PCR in CSF was 57% but only 14% in the serum. Whereas the PCR technique is specific for WNV, the IHC stain will detect flaviviral antigens in the JE complex. IHC staining can be performed on formalin fixed, biopsy and necropsy material. The virus may be grown in the laboratory by intracranial inoculation into suckling mice or on continuous cell lines of mosquito or mammalian origin (40).

WNV is classified as a biosafety level 3 agent. Ninety percent of serum IgM antibody will be positive within 8 days of symptoms (38). A case is confirmed by a fourfold rise in the serum antibody titer, isolation of virus or demonstration of viral antigen or genomic sequences in tissue, blood, CSF, or other body fluid, or specific IgM antibody by enzyme immunoassay (EIA) antibody captured in CSF. Serum IgM antibodies alone should be confirmed by demonstration of immunoglobulin G antibodies by another serologic assay such as neutralization or hemagglutination inhibition (56).

People recently vaccinated with either yellow fever or JE vaccines or people recently infected with a related flavivirus (St. Louis encephalitis or dengue) may have a positive IgM antibody test with WNV. The PRNT may help to distinguish cross-reactions between these closely related flaviviruses (57). Also people infected can produce IgM antibody for longer than 6 months and some even beyond 1 year. Therefore, diagnosis based solely on one IgM capture enzyme-linked immunosorbent assay (ELISA) antibody may be misleading especially among those with no or mild symptoms. Confirmatory testing with acute and convalescent titer, using PRNT will help clarify a new vs. old infection (58).

In 2003, blood collection agencies in the United States began to screen all donations with WNV nucleic acid-amplification tests (NATS) so as to reduce transfusion spread of WNV. Blood donors who are infected with WNV are often asymptomatic and their serology is negative. Therefore, these tests will hopefully detect early WNV and eliminate infectious blood components (59).

Computed tomographic scans of the brain have not shown substantial abnormalities. Magnetic resonance imaging of the brain can show enhancement of the leptomeninges, the periventricular areas or both (27). Electroencephalogram (EEG) was consistent with encephalitis (80%) but no specific pattern for WNV infection was found (21).

On autopsy, there is mononuclear inflammation, formation of microglial nodules and perivascular clusters in both white and gray matter in the brain, consistent with encephalitis. The brain stem, especially the medulla has been shown to be involved. Cranial nerve root inflammation can also be seen (59,60). The spinal cord can have variable involvement with the lumbar cord most affected. A loss of anterior-horn neurons in conjunction with gliosis, macrophages, neuronophagia, and perivascular lymphocytes can be seen. Focal microglial nodules and chronic perivascular inflammation with leptomeningitis and infiltration of the anterior nerve roots by lymphocytes have been described (61).

2.5. Clinical Outcome and Sequelae

The attack rate of clinical infection climbs with age; the rate found in people 50 years or older was 20 times higher than those younger than 50 years of age (27). The case-fatality rate (CFR) ranged from 4% (Romania-1996) to 12% (New York, USA-1999) to 14% (Israel-2000) (21,22,27). The CFR was highest in the oldest patients. Persons 75 years of age and older were nine times more likely to die than younger patients (27). Patients admitted with a diagnosis of encephalitis and muscle weakness did worse than those with encephalitis without muscle weakness or meningitis. The presence of diabetes mellitus or immunosuppression may be a risk factor for death (27). In a review of the 59 patients in New York City (1999), there were eight immunosuppressed patients (14%): cancer (5/8), HIV (1/8), prednisone for asthma (1/8) and alcoholism (1/8) (27). In an Israeli study of 233 patients (2000), there were 16 who were immunosuppressed (organ transplantation, malignancy and chemotherapy) and mortality was higher in this group (5/16) in contrast to non-immunosuppressed patients (28/217) (21).

There are few studies examining long-term sequelae secondary to WNV infection. In 2000, among hospitalized patients in New York and New Jersey, more than half did not return to their functional level by discharge, and only 37% were fully ambulatory (28). The New York City Department of Health conducted a 1-year follow-up study on survivors from the 1999 outbreak and found persistent complaints: fatigue (67%), memory loss (50%), difficulty walking (49%), had muscle weakness (44%),and depression (38%) (58). In 2002, 16 patients (five meningitis, eight encephalitis and three acute flaccid paralysis with one death) were followed over time. At an 8-month follow-up, fatigue, headache, and myalgias were persistent symptoms. Gait and movement disorders continued in six patients. Those with WNV meningitis or encephalitis had favorable outcomes. Two of the three with acute flaccid paralysis had no improvement of limb strength and EMG data showed permanent motor neuron loss suggesting poor recovery in the future (62).

2.6. Treatment

The treatment is largely supportive. In vitro, ribavirin and interferon-alpha-2b were effective but clinical trials have not been done (63). A comatose patient who was administered ribavirin and interferon alpha did not improve (28). In Israel, patients treated with ribavirin had a higher mortality rate than those who did not receive it (21).

Intravenous gammaglobulin enriched with WNV antibodies in Israel was given to a patient with chronic lymphocytic leukemia (CLL) in Israel with success and a clinical trial has begun in the United States (64). A vaccine is being developed using either the yellow fever backbone (65) or dengue but is several years away from clinical trials in humans (66).

2.7. Prevention

Until human vaccines are developed, the best prevention will continue to rely on reducing the number of vector mosquitoes by public or authorities and prevention of mosquitoes from biting humans by means of mosquito repellants, avoiding locations with high activity and use of barrier methods (window screens and long sleeved clothing).

Homeowners must drain water from their properties and eliminate stagnant water by cleaning gutters, pools, and birdbaths. Larvicides can be applied to stagnant water. *Bacillus thuringiensis* var. *israelensis* and *B. sphavericus* are two larvicides with a biological organism as the active ingredient. Organophosphates or pyrethroid formulations are used in small amounts for ground or aerial spraying for adult mosquito control. Mosquito repellants with DEET (*N,N*-diethyl-3-methylbenzamide) is available in many strengths. Repellants should have less than 10% DEET if used on children. Repellants containing 10–50% DEET are sufficient in most situations and instructions must be followed closely (38).

3. JAPANESE ENCEPHALITIS

3.1. Introduction

Japanese encephalitis is a common mosquito-borne encephalitis that occurs across eastern and southern Asia and the Pacific Rim. Epidemics of JE were first described in Japan in the 1870s. The term type B encephalitis was originally used to differentiate it from type A encephalitis (von Economo encephalitis or encephalitis lethargica). Type B encephalitis was known to occur in summer epidemics whereas type A encephalitis occurred during winter months with a different clinical presentation. The term "type B" encephalitis has since been abandoned.

Japanese encephalitis virus was first isolated from the brain of a fatal case in 1935. Japanese encephalitis is now recognized throughout much of Asia, and is considered the most important mosquito-borne viral encephalitis worldwide, with an estimated 50,000 cases and 15,000 deaths annually (67,68). Survivors commonly suffer from permanent neuropsychiatric sequelae. From a public health perspective, the burden of illness from JE is enormous for a disease that often occurs in somewhat predictable epidemics and is vaccine preventable.

3.2. Transmission

JEV is transmitted by the bites of zoophilic mosquitoes of the *Culex vishnui* complex. The *Culex tritaeniorhynchus* mosquito is the principal vector to humans in China and many endemic areas of Asia. The individual vector species differs in specific geographic regions. Typical high-risk regions are those in which there is a combination of rice cultivation, pigs, and birds (69). Mosquito larvae can be found in flooded rice fields, marshes and stagnant pools of water around cultivated fields. The mosquito typically breeds in water collections some distance from human dwellings and flies to peridomestic areas for blood meals. Wild and domesticated animals are the principal hosts. Pigs are considered to be an important source of viremic blood for mosquitoes (70,71). Bird–mosquito cycles are felt to play an important role in maintaining and amplifying JEV in the environment (72). Man is thought to be a dead-end host for this virus considering the short duration and low titer of viremia in man. In addition, the vector mosquitoes have a relative preference for animals over man even though they bite with enough frequency to account for transmission of the virus.

In the tropics, transmission of JE may occur year round (73). Although seasonal epidemics may occur, they usually begin during the rainy seasons when mosquito populations are greatest in number. In temperate zones, mosquito vectors are most abundant from June through September and are inactive during the winter. The virus is thought to survive the cool season of temperate and subtropical climates by overwintering of the virus in hibernating mosquitoes, mosquito eggs, and reptiles, or through reintroduction of the virus by migrating birds (69).

Despite the occurrence of fatal encephalitis in horses and fetal wastage in infected sows, animals infected with JEV generally remain asymptomatic (74). Likewise, most human infections are asymptomatic. The age distribution of disease differs according to the region (69). In endemic areas, the highest age-specific attack rates are usually seen in children between 3 and 6 years of age. The higher morbidity among children of this age group is consistent with a greater risk for increased exposure due to behavioral factors such as increased outdoor play, especially after dusk (75,76). Tapering off of age-specific attack rates after age 14 years is associated with an increased prevalence of neutralizing antibody. This suggests that the reduction in attack rates seen in heavily affected populations is due to immunity resulting from natural exposure or subclinical infection. Where all age groups are affected, it is most likely that the virus was recently introduced into a relatively non-immune population (73).

3.3. Clinical Presentation

Japanese encephalitis is thought to have an incubation period between 1 and 2 weeks (69). Patients usually present after several days of non-specific febrile illness. The patient's history may include complaints of coryza, diarrhea, and rigors (69,77). These symptoms are often followed by a history of headache of 1–3 days duration, frequently associated with nausea or vomiting, and a depressed level of consciousness. The latter symptoms are often heralded by a seizure. Coma often follows which, in non-fatal cases, may resolve in 1–2 weeks (69). Patients are almost always febrile. Particularly in older children and adults, abnormal behavior may be the only presenting feature and may be confused with psychiatric illness. Aseptic meningitis may occur without encephalitis.

Generalized seizures are often seen in JE, especially in children. Seizures have been reported in up to 85% of children and 10% of adults (78,79).

In children, a single seizure may be followed by a rapid normalization of consciousness leading to a mistaken diagnosis of a febrile seizure (77). Generalized tonic–clonic seizures are seen more frequently than focal motor seizures. Multiple or prolonged seizures and status epilepticus are reported to be associated with poor outcomes (77). A severely depressed level of consciousness on initial presentation is also associated with poor outcomes (75,80,81).

Japanese encephalitis is often accompanied by the classic findings of a dull flat mask-like facies with wide unblinking eyes, tremor, generalized hypertonia, and cogwheel rigidity (77). Between 70% and 80% of afflicted American service personnel, and 20–40% of Indian children were reported to show these features (82,83). Opisthotonus and rigidity spasms seen in about 15% of patients are associated with a poor prognosis (82,83). Extrapyramidal findings may include head nodding, athetoid movements, opsoclonus myoclonus, choreoathetosis, bizarre facial grimacing, and lip smacking (82–84). About 10% of children develop upper motor neuron facial palsies that are sometimes subtle or intermittent (77). Abnormalities of respiratory pattern, pupillary and oculocephalic reflexes and flexor/extensor posturing indicate a poor outcome (75,82,83) and may result from either encephalitis of the brainstem or transtentorial herniation (77,85).

A poliomyelitis-like acute flaccid paralysis has been described in a subgroup of patients infected with JEV (86). A short febrile illness is followed by a rapid onset of flaccid paralysis in one or more limbs without an alteration in consciousness. Weakness was usually asymmetric (86). The legs were more often found to have weakness than the arms. Thirty percent of such patients later developed encephalitis, but most had acute flaccid paralysis as the only feature (86). Persistent weakness and marked wasting in the affected limbs were observed on follow-up 1–2 years later (86). Anterior horn cell damage was suggested by the demonstration of markedly reduced motor amplitudes on nerve conduction studies and chronic partial denervation on EMG (86). About 5–20% of patients with JE and coma have also been reported to have flaccid paralysis (78,87). Electrophysiological studies have confirmed anterior horn cell damage (86). MRI of the spinal cord revealed abnormal signal intensity on T2-weighted images (88). Although uncommon, respiratory muscle paralysis may be the presenting symptom in JE (89).

JEV infection usually does not manifest an apparent illness (90,91). For every identifiable clinical case, between 50 and 300 infections occurs. Data on the ratio of apparent to unapparent infections is limited and may be different in specific populations. The low ratio of symptomatic to asymptomatic cases has been explained according to viral factors, host factors or preexisting immunity (69).

3.4. Laboratory Features

Most patients show evidence of a peripheral neutrophil leukocytosis. Hyponatremia is known to occur as a consequence of inappropriate antidiuretic hormone secretion (SIADH) (77). About 50% of patients have an increased CSF opening pressure on lumbar puncture. Elevated CSF pressure (>250 mm) is associated with a poor outcome (77). A moderate CSF pleocytosis of 10–100 cells/mm3 is usually seen with a predominance of lymphocytes. Polymorphonuclear cells sometimes predominate early in the illness. On occasion, there may be no CSF pleocytosis (80). Typically, CSF protein is mildly increased (50–200 mg%) with a normal glucose ratio (77).

CT shows bilateral non-enhancing low-density areas in about 50% of patients. In such cases, these low-density areas are seen in one or more areas of the thalamus, basal ganglia, midbrain, pons, and medulla (92,93). However, MRI imaging is more sensitive and usually demonstrates more extensive lesions (typically high signal intensity on T2-weighted images) of the thalamus, cerebral hemispheres, and cerebellum (88,93). Mixed intensity signals of the thalamus on T1- and T2-weighted images suggesting hemorrhage may be seen (84,88). The utility of imaging studies is greatest in distinguishing JE from herpes simplex encephalitis, where the latter characteristically shows frontotemporal changes (94). However, the diagnostic value of scans performed early is unknown since most reports are of scans performed late in the course of JE (77).

Electroencephalographic abnormalities have been reported in JE but are non-specific (77,92). Diffuse slowing may help in distinguishing JE from herpes simplex virus in which characteristic frontotemporal changes are seen (94). Delays in central motor conduction times on measurement of evoked potentials indicate widespread involvement at the cortical and subcortical levels (92). In cases involving acute flaccid paralysis, nerve conduction studies and EMG findings are consistent with anterior horn cell damage as previously described (86).

Isolation of JEV from clinical specimens is rarely successful (95). The reasons are most likely attributable to low viral titers and rapid production of neutralizing antibodies (95). Viral isolates obtained from CSF are associated with a failure of antibody production and a high mortality rate (81,95). Immunohistochemical staining of CSF cells with anti-JEV polyclonal antibodies is sometimes positive (80,96). For many years, the hemagglutination inhibition test was used for diagnosis but could not provide early diagnosis and had many limitations including the need for paired serum (77,97). At the present time, JE is diagnosed serologically (77). Since the 1980s, IgM and IgG capture ELISA have become the diagnostic procedure of choice (98,99). Anti-JEV IgM appears in the CSF after the first few days of illness (100). Earlier testing may yield a false-negative result. The presence of virus-specific IgM has a sensitivity and specificity of greater than 95% for CNS infection with the JEV (100). Unfortunately, ELISA testing is neither practical nor available in rural areas where JE is most likely to occur. However, the IgM ELISA was recently modified to a simple nitrocellulose-based format that allows for rapid diagnosis by detection of a change in color (101). Since the test is simple to perform and does not require specialized equipment, it should prove useful for diagnosis in rural hospitals. Lastly, JEV RNA has been detected in human CSF samples using the reverse transcriptase-polymerase chain reaction (102,103). Its reliability as a routine diagnostic test has not been demonstrated. It would also be impractical for use in the rural setting.

3.5. Clinical Outcome and Sequelae

The CFR for JE has been reported to be as high as 30%. About 50% of survivors develop severe neurological sequelae (77). Mortality rates are reduced with better hospital facilities, but with a concomitant increase in sequelae (68,77). Frank motor deficits are seen in about 30% of survivors (67). A mixture of upper and lower motor neuron weakness, and cerebellar and extrapyramidal signs may occur (104,105). Fixed flexion deformities of the arms and hyperextension of the legs with "equine feet" are common findings (77). Severe cognitive and language impairment is seen in 20% of survivors, usually in association with motor deficits (106,107). Additional seizure activity is seen in 20% of patients (106,107). Overall, children are reported to have a higher rate of sequelae than adults (108). Among patients considered to have a good recovery, studies have shown that about 50% have subtle sequelae such as learning difficulties, behavioral problems, and subtle neurological findings (106). Infection with JEV during pregnancy has been shown to infect the fetus transplacentally and may result in fetal malformations or spontaneous abortion (109,110).

3.6. Treatment

The treatment of JE is primarily supportive. Seizures need to be controlled. Elevated intracranial pressure must be identified and treated to prevent transtentorial herniation (77). Corticosteroids are no longer recommended. A double-blind randomized placebo-controlled trial of dexamethasone failed to demonstrate any benefit (75). Reduction in the risk of bed sores, malnutrition, and contractures must be sought through meticulous nursing care and aggressive physiotherapy (77). Aspiration pneumonia due to an impaired gag reflex is common and appropriate precautions must be taken (77). Although no specific treatment is available for JE, there are promising areas of research. Isoquinolone compounds have been shown to be effective in vitro (111). Monoclonal antibodies have demonstrated effectiveness in animal models (112,113). At the moment, interferon-alpha appears to be the most promising potential treatment. It is produced naturally in the CSF in response to infection with JEV (114). Interferon-alpha has been shown to have activity against the virus in vitro (115). Recombinant interferon-alpha has shown encouraging results in open trials involving a few patients (116). Its prospects as a future treatment await the results of a placebo-controlled double-blind trial.

3.7. Prevention

Strategies to control JE include vector control, vector avoidance, immunization of susceptible persons, and immunization of amplifying hosts. All of these methods are intended to either interfere with the enzootic cycle of the virus or prevent disease in the human host. Measures intended to control breeding of *Culex* mosquitoes have been demonstrated to be ineffective (85). Such efforts include the application of larvicides to rice fields and insecticide spraying. Widespread vaccination to protect swine against the virus is not feasible in most settings (77). Residents and travelers to endemic areas need to exercise personal protection to reduce the risk of *Culex* bites. Minimizing outdoor exposure at dusk and dawn, wearing sufficient clothing to lessen skin exposure, using insect repellents containing at least 30% DEET (*N,N*-diethyl-3-methylbenzamide) and sleeping under bed nets are all useful measures for the short-term visitor. Unfortunately, these measures are not practical for residents of endemic areas.

Japanese encephalitis vaccine is recommended for native and expatriate residents of endemic areas and for travelers spending 30 days or more in endemic areas (117,118). Short-term travelers (>30 days) areas are advised to receive the vaccine if there will be extensive outdoor activity in rural, farming areas, or during known epidemics (117,118). Laboratory workers who may be potentially exposed to the virus should be vaccinated. Because of the variable incidence of JE and the unreliability of some epidemiological data, it is often difficult to identify areas of epidemic transmission (77). In view of the devastating impact of acquiring JE, the benefit of immunization exceeds the risk of vaccine-related adverse events (85). The report of two cases of the disease in short-term travelers (>2 weeks) supports the argument that all travelers to endemic areas should be vaccinated (116,119,120).

The recommended primary immunization series is three doses administered subcutaneously on days 0, 7 and 30 (118). About 20% of recipients experience local reactions or mild systemic effects such as fever, headache, myalgias, and malaise. Serious allergic reactions occur in about 0.6% of recipients and can be aborted by standard drug therapy. Hypersensitivity reactions may occur within minutes or up to 1 week after immunization. A past history of urticaria carries the greatest risk for a serious allergic reaction. A known allergy to the JE vaccine or other mouse-derived vaccines is a contraindication to immunization.

3.8. West Nile Virus and Japanese Encephalitis: Future Implications

A dramatic emergence and resurgence of vector-borne diseases has been witnessed worldwide. The expanding geographic distribution for both vectors and viruses has coincided with more frequent and intense epidemics. Improved transportation and increased mobility have brought humans, animals and commodities into different regions of the world along with the pathogens that accompany them. Genetic variations among pathogens may have contributed to an increased virulence and spread of these diseases (121).

Weather and climate conditions may affect mosquito populations and ultimately, outbreaks. For WNV, a mild winter followed by a dry spring and hot summer is thought to enhance the amplification of its life cycle. The urban-dwelling mosquito, *Culex pipiens*, breeds favorably in stagnant water typically found in city drains and catch basins. Drought conditions result in organic material being concentrated in water where mosquitoes are even more capable of thriving. Reduced rainfall has the effect of decreasing the size of frog and dragonfly populations, the natural predators of the *Culex* mosquitoes. Droughts also cause birds to congregate at fewer areas leading to increased circulation of virus. Finally, high temperatures are known to speed WNV viral production within mosquitoes (122).

Over the past 50 years, JE has extended its reach beyond East Asia and is now more commonly seen in Southeast Asia and Southern Asia. The reasons for its change in distribution are not entirely understood. Population growth may have been a significant force as a consequence of unmonitored urbanization into underdeveloped areas. Contributing factors may include agricultural practices such as the increased use of irrigation and animal husbandry. Deforestation might also play a role (121). At the same time, developed countries such as Japan, Taiwan and South Korea have seen in a decline in JE cases, most likely as a result of their improved standard of living and effective public health measures (85). However, even this success has been met with new challenges. In South Korea, the widespread vaccination of children has led to a higher incidence of JE infection for those over 15 years of age (123).

The WNV and JEV will remain important public health problems for the indefinite future. Because of the enzootic nature of these viruses, there is no possibility of global eradication in the same way as smallpox and polio. For both viruses, disease prevention and containment relies on public health infrastructures and vector surveillance. Less-developed countries with limited resources may require international assistance to address their needs. In order to reverse the trend of increased arboviral outbreaks, public health systems will need to improve early detection. Greater emphasis must be placed on monitoring, and limiting mosquito populations where feasible. Prevention strategies such as vaccination, as in the case of JEV, must be implemented in selected populations as appropriate. Funding for research to develop treatments will remain a necessity even where effective disease prevention measures can be employed (121). Lastly, despite the lack of scientific proof that changes in climate or weather has been responsible for the recent emergence and resurgence of vector-borne diseases, further investigation into environmental and ecological factors merits serious attention.

REFERENCES

1. Monath TP, Tsai TF. Flaviviruses. In: Richman DD, Whitley RJ, Hayden FG, eds. Clinical Virology. New York: Churchill Livingstone, 1997:1133–1185.
2. Rice CM. Flaviviridae: the viruses and their replication. In: Fields BN, Knipe DM, Howley PM, eds. Fields Virology. Philadelphia: Lippincott, 1985:931–959.
3. Smithburn KC, Hughes TP, Burke AW, Paul JH. A neurotropic virus isolated from the blood of a native of Uganda. Am J Trop Med 1940; 20:471–492.
4. Melnick JL, et al. Isolation from human sera in Egypt of virus apparently identical to West Nile virus. Proc Soc Exp Biol Med 1951; 77:661–665.
5. Benkopf H, Levine S. Isolation of a virus closely related to West Nile virus from the blood of a sick child during an epidemic in Maayan Zvi. Bull Res Counc Isr 1952; 2:209.
6. Goldblum N, Sterk VV, Jasinska-Klingberg W. The natural history of West Nile fever. II. Virological findings and the development of homologous and heterologous antibodies in West Nile infection in man. Am J Hyg 1957; 66:363–380.
7. Monath TP. Flaviviruses. In: Fields BN, Knipe DM, Chanock RM, Melnick JL, Roizman B, Shope RE, eds. Virology. New York: Raven Press, 1985:955–1004.
8. Taylor RM, Work TH, Hurlbu HS, Rizk F. A study of the ecology of West Nile virus in Egypt. Am J Trop Med Hyg 1956; 5:579–620.
9. Bernkopf H, Levine S, Nerson R. Isolation of West Nile virus in Israel. J Infect Dis 1953; 93:207–218.
10. Spigland W, Jasinska-Klingberg W, Hofshi E, et al. Clinical and laboratory observations in an outbreak of West Nile fever in Israel. Harefuah 1958; 54:275–281 (in Hebrew with English abstract).
11. George S, Gourie-Devi M, Rao JA, Prasad SR, Pavri KM. Isolation of West Nile virus from the brains of children who had died of encephalitis. Bull World Health Organ 1984; 62(6):879–882.
12. Georges AJ, Lesbordes JL, Georges-Courbot MC, et al. Fatal hepatitis from West Nile virus. Ann Inst Pasteur/Virol 1987; 138:237–244.
13. McIntosh BM, Jupp PG, Dos Santos I, et al. Epidemics of West Nile and Sindbis viruses in South Africa with *Culex univittatus theobold* as a vector encephalitis. S Afr J Sci 1970.

14. Centers for Disease Control West Nile Virus Information Website. 1999–2002; *http://www.cec.gov/od/oc/media/wncount.htm.*

15. Petersen LR, Roehrig JT. West Nile virus: a reemerging global pathogen. Emerg Infect Dis 2001; 7:611–614.

16. Le Guenno F, Bougermouh A, Azzam T, Bouakaz R. West Nile: a deadly virus? Lancet 1996; 348:1315.

17. Tber, Abdelhaz A. West Nile fever in horses in Morocco. Bull OIE 1996; 11:867–869.

18. Triki H. Epidemie de menigo-encephalite a virus West Nile en Tunisie. Submitted to Trop Med. Date of application: March 2001.

19. Cantile C, et al. Clinical and neuropathological features of west Nile virus equine encephalomyelitis in Italy. Equine Vet J 2000; 32:31–35.

20. Murgue B, et al. West Nile outbreak in horses in Southern France (2000): the return 35 years later. Emerg Infect Dis 2001; 7:692–696.

21. Chowers M, Lang R, Nassar F, Ben-David D, Giladi M, Rubinshtein E, Itzhaki A, Mishal J, Siegman-Igra Y, Kitzes R, Pick N, Landau Z, Wolf D, Bin H, Mendelson E, Pitlik SD, Weinberger M. Clinical characteristics of the West Nile fever outbreak, Israel, 2000. Emerg Infect Dis 2001; 7:675–678.

22. Tsai TF, Popovivi F, Cernescu C, Campbell GL, Nedelcu NI. West Nile encephalitis epidemic in southeastern Romania. Lancet 1998; 352:767–771.

23. Platanov AE, Shipulin GA, Shipulina OY, Tyutyunnik EN, Frolochkina TI, Lanciotti RS, et al. Outbreak of West Nile Virus Infection, Volgograd Region, Russia, 1999. Emerg Infect Dis 2001; 7:128–132.

24. Centers for Disease Control and Prevention. Outbreak of West Nile-like viral encephalitis: New York, 1999. MMWR Morb Mortal Wkly Rep 1999; 48:845–849.

25. Asnis DS, Conetta R, Teixeira AA, Waldman G, Sampson BA. The West Nile virus outbreak of 1999 in New York: the flushing hospital experience. Clin Infect Dis 2000; 30:413–418.

26. Asnis DA. West Nile virus infection in the United States: a review and update. Infect Med 2002; 19:266–278.

27. Nash D, Mostashari F, Fine A, Miller J, O'Leary D, Murray K, Huang A, Rosenberg A, Greenberg A, Sherman M, Wong S, Layton M for the 1999 West Nile Outbreak Response Working Group. The outbreak of West Nile virus infection, New York City area, 1999. N Engl J Med 2001; 344:1807–1814.

28. Weiss D, Carr D, Kellachan J, Tan C, Phillips M, Bresnitz E, Layton M, for the West Nile Virus Outbreak Response Working Group. Clinical findings of West Nile virus infection in hospitalized patients, New York and New Jersey, 2000. Emerg Infect Dis 2001; 7:654–658.

29. Cernescu C, Ruta SM, Tardei G, Grancea C, Moldoveanu L, Spulbar E, Tsai T. A high number of severe neurologic clinical forms during an epidemic of West Nile virus infection. Rom J Virol 1997; 48:13–25.

30. Eidson M, Komar N, Sorhage F, Nelson R, Talbot T, Mostashari F, McLean R and the West Nile Virus Avian Mortality Surveillance Group. Crow deaths as a sentinel surveillance system for West Nile virus in the northeastern United States, 1999. Emerg Infect Dis 2001; 7:615–620.

31. Bin H, Grossman Z, Pokamunski S, Malkinson M, Weiss L, Duvdevani P, Banet C, Weisman Y, Annis E, Gandaku D, Yahalom V, Hindyieh M, Shulman L, Mendelson

E. West Nile fever in Israel 1999–2000 from Geese to Humans. Ann N Y Acad Sci 2001; 951:127–142.

32.   Hubalek Z. Comparative symptomatology of West Nile fever. Lancet 2001; 358:254–255.

33.   Lanciotti RS, Roehrig JT, Deubel V, et al. Origin of the West Nile virus responsible for an outbreak of encephalitis in the northeastern United States. Science 1999; 286:2333–2337.

34.   Ebel GD, Dupuis AO II, Ngo K, Nicholas D, et al. Partial genetic characterization of West Nile virus strains, New York State, 2000. Emerg Infect Dis 2001; 7:650–653.

35.   Turell MJ, Sardelis MR, Dohm DJ, O'Guinn MJ. Potential North American vectors of West Nile virus. Ann N Y Acad Sci 2001; 951:317–324.

36.   Centers for Disease Control and Prevention. Update: surveillance for West Nile virus in overwintering mosquitoes—New York, 2000. MMWR Morb Mortal Wkly Rep 2000; 49:178–179.

37.   Hubalek A, Halouzka J. West Nile fever—a reemerging mosquito-borne viral disease in Europe. Emerg Infect Dis 1999; 5(5):643–650.

38.   Petersen LR, Marfin AA. West Nile virus: a primer for the clinician. Ann Intern Med 2002; 137:173–179.

39.   CDC. West Nile virus—United States, November 14–20, 2002, and Missouri, January 1–November 9, 2002. MMWR Morb Mortal Wkly Rep 2002; 51:1049–1051.

40.   Peiris JSM, Amerasinghe FP. West Nile fever. In: Beran GW, Steele JH, eds. Handbook of Zoonoses Section B. Viral. Boca Raton, FL: CRC Press, 1994:139–148.

41.   Nir YD. Airborne West Nile virus infection. Am J Trop Med Hyg 1959; 8:537–539.

42.   CDC. Laboratory-acquired West Nile virus infections—United States, 2002. MMWR Morb Mortal Wkly Rep 2002; 51:1133–1135.

43.   CDC. Investigations of West Nile virus infections in recipients of blood transfusions. MMWR Morb Mortal Wkly Rep 2002; 51:973–974.

44.   CDC. Update. Investigations of West Nile virus infections in recipients of organ transplantation and blood transfusion. MMWR Morb Mortal Wkly Rep 2002; 51:833–836.

45.   CDC. Possible West Nile virus transmission to an infant through breast-feeding—Michigan, 2002. MMWR Morb Mortal Wkly Rep 2002; 51:879–880.

46.   CDC. Intrauterine West Nile virus infection—New York, 2002. MMWR Morb Mortal Wkly Rep 2002; 51:1135–1136.

47.   Corwin A, Habib M, Watts D, Darwish M, Olson J, Botros B, Hibbs R, Kleinosky M, Lee HW, Shope R, Kilpatrick M. Community-based prevalence profile of arboviral, rickettsial, and Hantaan-like viral antibody in the Nile River Delta of Egypt. Am J Trop Med Hyg 1993; 48:776–783.

48.   Mostashari F, Bunning MI, Kitsutani PT, Singer DA, Nash D, Cooper M, Katz N, Kiljebjelke KA, Biggerstaff BJ, Fine AD, Layton MC, Mullin SM, Johnson AJ, Martin DA, Hayes EB, Campbell GL. Epidemic West Nile encephalitis, New York, 1999: results of a household-based seroepidemiological survey. Lancet 2001; 358:261–264.

49.   Gadoth N, Weltzman S, Lehmann EE. Acute anterior myelitis complicating West Nile Fever. Arch Neurol 1979; 36:172–173.

50. Southam CM, Moore AE. Induced virus infections in man by the Egypt isolates of West Nile virus. Am J Trop Med Hyg 1954; 3:19–50.

51. Ahmed S, Libman R, Wesson K, Ahmed F, Einberg K. Guillain–Barre syndrome: an unusual presentation of West Nile virus infection. Neurology 2000; 55:144–146.

52. Leis AA, Stokic DS, Polk JL, Dostrow V, Winkelmann M. A poliomyelitis-like syndrome from West Nile virus infection. N Eng J Med 2002; 347:1279–1280.

53. Glass JD, Samuels O, Rich MM. Poliomyelitis due to West Nile virus. N Engl J Med 2002; 347:1280–1281.

54. Asnis DA, Conetta R, Waldman G, Teixeira A. The West Nile virus encephalitis outbreak in the United States (1999–2000) from flushing, New York, to beyond its borders. Ann N Y Acad Sci 2001; 161–171.

55. Cunha BA, Minnaganti V, Johnson DJ. Klein N. Profound and profounded lymphocytopenia with West Nile encephalitis. Clin Infect Dis 2000; 31:1116–1117.

56. CDC. Case definitions for infectious conditions under public health surveillance. MMWR Morb Mortal Wkly Rep 1997; 46(rr-10):1–55.

57. Martin DA, Biggerstaff BJ, Allen B, Johnson AJ, Lanciotti RS, Roehrig JT. Use of immunoglobulin M cross-reactions in differential diagnosis of human flaviviral encephalitis infections in the United States. Clin Diagn Lab Immunol 2002; 9:544–549.

58. The New York City Department of Health. West Nile virus surveillance and control: an update for healthcare providers in New York City. City Health Inf 2001; 20:1–7.

59. CDC. Detection of West Nile virus in blood donations—United States, 2003. MMWR Morb Mortal Wkly Rep 2003; 52(32):769–772.

60. Sampson BA, Ambrosi C, Charlot A, Reiber K, Veress JF, Armbrustmacher V. The pathology of human West Nile virus infection. Hum Pathol 2000; 31:527–531.

61. Kelly TW, Prayson RA, Isada CM. Spinal cord disease in West Nile virus infection. N Eng J Med 2003; 348(6):564–566.

62. Sejvar JJ, Haddad MB, Tierney BC, Campbell GL, Marfin AA, Gerpen JAV, Fleischauer A, Leis AA, Stokic DS, Petersen LR. Neurologic manifestations and outcome of West Nile virus infection. JAMA 2003; 290; 511–515.

63. Anderson JF, Rahal JJ. Efficacy of interferon alpha-2b and ribavirin against West Nile virus in vitro [Letter]. Emerg Infect Dis 2002; 8:107–108.

64. Shimoni Z, Niven MJ, Pitlick S, Bulvik S. Treatment of West Nile virus encephalitis with intravenous gammaglobulin. Emerg Infect Dis 2001; 7:759.

65. Monath TP. Prospects for development of a vaccine against the West Nile virus. Ann N Y Acad Sci 2001; 951:1–12.

66. Pletnev AG, Putnak R, Speicher J, et al. West Nile virus/dengue type 4 virus chimeras that are reduced in neurovirulence and peripheral virulence without loss of immunogenicity or protective efficacy. Proc Natl Acad Sci U S A 2002; 99:3036–3041.

67. Tsai TF. Factors in the changing epidemiology of Japanese encephalitis and West Nile fever. In: Saluzzo JF, Dodet B, eds. Factors in the Emergence of Arbovirus Diseases. Paris: Elsevier, 1997:179–189.

68. Solomon T. Viral encephalitis in southeast Asia. Neurol Infect Epidemiol 1997; 2:191–199.

69. Vaughn DW, Charles H, Hoke Jr. The epidemiology of Japanese encephalitis: prospects for prevention. Epidemiol Rev 1992; 14:197–220.

70.   Scherer WF, Moyer JT, Izumi T, et al. Ecologic studies in Japanese encephalitis virus in Japan. VI. Swine infection. Am J Trop Med Hyg 1959; 8:698–706.

71.   Scherer WF, Moyer JT, Izumi T. Immunologic studies of Japanese encephalitis in Japan. V. Maternal antibodies, antibody responses and viremia following infection of swine. J Immunol 1959; 83:620–706.

72.   Soman RS, Rodrigues FM, Guttikar SN, et al. Experimental viraemia and transmission of Japanese encephalitis by mosquitoes in ardeid birds. Indian J Med Res 1977; 66:709–718.

73.   Umenai T, Krzysko R, Bektimirov TA, et al. Japanese encephalitis: current worldwide status. Bull World Health Organ 1985; 63:625–631.

74.   Burke DS, Leake CJ. Japanese encephalitis. In: Monath TP, ed. The Arboviruses: Epidemiology and Ecology. Vol. III. Boca Raton, FL: CRC Press, 1988:63–92.

75.   Hoke CH, Vaughn DW, Nisalak A, et al. The effect of high dose dexamethasone on the outcome of acute encephalitis due to Japanese encephalitis virus. J Infect Dis 1992; 165:631–637.

76.   Huang CH. Studies of Japanese encephalitis in China. Adv Virus Res 1982; 27:71–101.

77.   Solomon T, Nguyen MD, et al. Neurological aspects of tropical disease: Japanese encephalitis. J Neurol Neurosurg Psychiatry 2000; 68:405–415.

78.   Dickerson RB, Newton JR, Hansen JE. Diagnosis and immediate prognosis of Japanese B encephalitis. Am J Med 1952; 12:277–288.

79.   Ponepraset B. Japanese encephalitis in children in northern Thailand. Southeast Asian J Trop Med Public Health 1989; 20:599–603.

80.   Mathur A, Kumar R, Sharma S, et al. Rapid diagnosis of Japanese encephalitis by immunofluorescent examination of cerebrospinal fluid. Indian J Med Res 1990; 91:1–4.

81.   Burke DS, Lorsomrudee W, Leake CJ, et al. Fatal outcome in Japanese encephalitis. Am J Trop Med Hyg 1985; 34:1203–1210.

82.   Solomon T, Thao LTT, Dung NM, et al. Clinical features of Japanese encephalitis: prognostic and pathophysiological significance in 50 patients. In: 7th International Congress of Infectious Diseases. Hong Kong: International Society for Infectious Diseases, 1996:132.

83.   Kumar R, Mathur A, Kumar A, et al. Clinical features and prognostic indicators of Japanese encephalitis in children in Lucknow (India). Indian J Med Res 1990; 91:321–327.

84.   Misra UK, Kalita J. Movement disorders in Japanese encephalitis. J Neurol 1997; 244:299–303.

85.   Innis BL. Japanese encephalitis. In: Porterfield JS, ed. Exotic Viral Infections. London: Chapman & Hall, 1995:147–174.

86.   Solomon T, Kneen R, Dung NM, et al. Poliomyelitis-like illness due to Japanese encephalitis virus. Lancet 1998; 351:1094–1097.

87.   Kumar S, Agarwal SP, Waklu I, et al. Japanese encephalitis: an encephalomyelitis. Indian Pediatr 1991; 23:1525–1533.

88.   Kumar R, Misra UK, Kalita J, et al. MRI in Japanese encephalitis. Neuroradiology 1997; 39:180–184.

89.   Tzeng SS. Respiratory paralysis as a presenting symptom in Japanese encephalitis: a case report. J Neurol 1989; 236:265–269.

90.   Brandt WE. Development of dengue and Japanese encephalitis vaccines. J Infect Dis 1990; 162:577–583.

91. Shoji H, Murakamo T, Murai I, et al. A follow-up study by CT and MRI in 3 cases of Japanese encephalitis. Neuroradiology 1990; 32:215–219.

92. Misra UK, Kalita J, Jain SK, et al. Radiological and neurophysiological changes in Japanese encephalitis. J Neurol Neurosurg Psychiatry 1994; 57:1484–1487.

93. Huang C-R, Chang W-N, Lui C-C, et al. Neuroimages of Japanese encephalitis: report of 3 patients. Chin Med J (Engl) 1997; 60:105–108.

94. Misra UK, Kalita J. A comparative study of Japanese and herpes simplex encephalitis. Electromyogr Clin Neurophysiol 1998; 38:41–46.

95. Leake CJ, Burke DS, Nisalak A, et al. Isolation of Japanese encephalitis virus from clinical specimens using a continuous mosquito cell line. Am J Trop Med Hyg 1986; 35:1045–1050.

96. Desai A, Shankar SK, Ravi V, et al. Japanese encephalitis virus antigen in the brain and its topographical distribution. Acta Neuropathol 1995; 89:368–373.

97. Clark CH, Casals J. Techniques for hemaglutination inhibition with arthropod viruses. Am J Trop Med Hyg 1958; 7:561–573.

98. Bundo K, Igarashi A. Antibody-capture ELISA for detection of immunoglobulin M antibodies in sera from Japanese encephalitis and dengue hemorrhagic fever patients. J Virol Methods 1985; 11:15–22.

99. Innis BL, Nisalak A, Nimmannitya S, et al. An enzyme-linked immunosorbent assay to characterize dengue infections where dengue and Japanese encephalitis co-circulate. Am J Trop Med Hyg 1989; 40:418–427.

100. Burke DS, Nisalak A, Ussery MA, et al. Kinetics of IgM and IgG responses to Japanese encephalitis virus in human serum and cerebrospinal fluid. J Infect Dis 1985; 151:1093–1099.

101. Solomon T, Thao LTT, Dung NM, et al. Rapid diagnosis of Japanese encephalitis by using an IgM dot enzyme immunoassay. J Clin Microbiol 1998; 36:2030–2034.

102. Igarashi A, Tanaka M, Morita K, et al. Detection of West Nile and Japanese encephalitis viral genome sequences in cerebrospinal fluid from acute encephalitis cases in Karachi, Pakistan. Microbiol Immunol 1994; 38:827–830.

103. Meiyu F, Huosheng C, Cuihua C, et al. Detection of flavivirus by reverse transcriptase-polymerase chain reaction with the universal primer set. Microbiol Immunol 1997; 41:209–213.

104. Richter RW, Shimojyo S. Neurologic sequelae of Japanese B encephalitis. Neurology 1961; 11:553–559.

105. Simpson TW, Meiklehohn G. Sequelae of Japanese B encephalitis. Am J Trop Med Hyg 1947; 27:727–731.

106. Kumar R, Mathur A, Singh YD, et al. Clinical sequelae of Japanese encephalitis in children. Indian J Med Res 1993; 97:9–13.

107. Huy BV, Tu HC, Luan TV, et al. Early mental and neurological sequelae after Japanese B encephalitis. Southeast Asian J Trop Med Public Health 1994; 25:549–553.

108. Schneider RJ, Firestone MH, Edelman R, et al. Clinical sequelae after Japanese encephalitis: a one year follow up study in Thailand. Southeast Asian J Trop Med Public Health 1974; 5:560–568.

109. Chaturvedi UC, Mathur A, Chandra A, et al. Transplacental infection with Japanese encephalitis virus. J Infect Dis 1980; 141:712–715.

110. Mathur A, Tandon HO, Mathur KR, et al. Japanese encephalitis virus infection during pregnancy. Indian J Med Res 1985; 81:9–12.

111. Takegami T, Simamura E, Hirai K-I, et al. Inhibitory effect of furanonaphtoquinone derivatives on the replication of Japanese encephalitis virus. Antiviral Res 1998; 37:37–45.

112. Kimura-Kuroda J, Yasui K. Protection of mice against Japanese encephalitis virus by passive administration with monoclonal antibodies. J Immunol 1988; 15:3606–3610.

113. Zhang M, Wang M, Jiang S, et al. Passive Protection of mice, goats and monkeys against Japanese encephalitis with monoclonal antibodies. J Med Virol 1989; 29:133–138.

114. Burke DS, Morill JC. Levels of interferon in the plasma and cerebrospinal fluid of patients with acute Japanese encephalitis. J Infect Dis 1987; 155:797–799.

115. Harinasuta C, Wasi C, Vithanomsat S. The effect of interferon on Japanese encephalitis virus vitro. Southeast Asian J Trop Med Public Health 1984; 15:564–568.

116. Harinasatu C, Nimmanitya S, Titsyakorn U. The effect of interferon alpha on two cases of Japanese encephalitis in Thailand. Southeast Asian J Trop Med Public Health 1985; 16:332–336.

117. Anonymous. Inactivated Japanese encephalitis virus vaccine. Recommendations of the Advisory Committee on Immunization Practices (ACIP). MMWR Morb Mortal Wkly Rep 1993; 42:1–15.

118. Anonymous. www.cdc.gov/travel/jencph.htm 2002:1–7.

119. Tsai TF, Yu YX. Japanese encephalitis vaccines. In: Plotkin SA, Mortimer EAJ, eds. Vaccines. Philadelphia: WB Saunders, 1994:671–713.

120. Gambel JM, DeFraites RF, Hoke Jr CH, et al. Japanese encephalitis vaccine: persistence of antibody up to 3 years after a three dose primary series. J Infect Dis 1995; 171:1074.

121. Gubler DJ. Human Arbovirus infections worldwide. Ann N Y Acad Sci 2001; 951:13–24.

122. Epstein PR. West Nile virus and the climate. J Urban Health 2001; 78:367–371.

123. Vaughn DW, Hoke CH. The epidemiology of Japanese encephalitis: prospects for prevention. Epidemiol Rev 1992; 14:197–221.

10

Neurocysticercosis

Larry E. Davis

*Neurology Service, New Mexico VA Health Care System and Department of
Neurology, University of New Mexico School of Medicine,
Albuquerque, New Mexico, U.S.A.*

Worldwide, neurocysticercosis is the most common parasitic infection of the
brain. In Latin America alone, it is estimated that over 400,000 people have
symptomatic neurocysticercosis (1). The burden of neurocysticercosis is considerable. In Peru, about one in 2000 adults have seizures due this infection
and 25% of adult-onset epilepsy in Latin America is due to neurocysticercosis (1,2). Annual economic costs from neurocysticercosis have been estimated
to be about $85 million in Mexico and Brazil and $9 million in the United
States (3).

The term neurocysticercosis refers to the presence of cysticerci within
the human central nervous system (CNS) that belong to the parasite,
Cysticercus cellulosae. The parasite is highly endemic in Central and South
America (2,4–6), India (7), and parts of China and Korea (8). In rural Peru,
seroprevalence rates for *C. cellulosae* by the sensitive and specific antibody
immunoblot test ranged from 7% to 24% for humans and 13% to 67% for free-
ranging pigs in the same area (1). Similar studies for other Latin American
countries find human seroprevalence rates from 10% to 23% (1,9). In parts of
rural Mexico, cysticerci were found in the brains of 2% of routine autopsies
(9). The parasite is also endemic in areas of Central and South Africa,
Thailand, Indonesia, Portugal, Poland and Romania (10,11). Taeniasis is rare
in Muslim regions of Asia and Israel because the Koran and Torah prohibit the
consumption of pork.

In the United States, neurocysticercosis and taeniasis are rare due to high
sanitary conditions, lack of human feces used as fertilizer, and obligatory

inspection of pork meat for the presence of cysticercosis. However, in the past 30 years, neurocysticercosis has gone from being just an exotic disease to the most common CNS parasite found in the United States. The dramatic increase in prevalence stems from increased immigration of infected individuals from Central America (12). In the early 1980s, the patients were found mainly in states bordering Mexico. From 1973 to 1985, one hospital in Los Angeles treated over 497 patients (12). However, by the 1990s, the disease was found throughout the United States as Latin American immigrants moved in increasing numbers to every state (13). Americans who travel to endemic countries on vacation rarely develop neurocysticercosis unless they stay in rural areas with poor sanitation. Occasional Americans who never traveled abroad have developed neurocysticercosis. These individuals usually were infected through fecal contamination from other, often Hispanic, individuals who carried the pork tapeworm (12,14).

This chapter focuses on the pathogenesis, pathology, clinical features, and treatment of neurocysticercosis. To understand the pathogenesis and clinical features of neurocysticercosis, it is important to understand the life cycle of the pork tapeworm and the stages of neurocysticercosis.

1. LIFE CYCLE OF *TAENIA SOLIUM*

Taenia solium is a zoonotic cestode with two hosts—pig and man (Fig. 1). Humans may be the definitive host when infected with a tapeworm or the intermediate host when infected with the cysticercus. The pig only becomes the intermediate host and is infected with the cysticercus.

1.1. The Human as the Definitive Host

A human becomes the definitive host when they ingest insufficiently cooked pork that contains viable cysticercosis larvae, called *C. cellulosae*. Upon reaching the small intestine, the protoscolex of the cyst evaginates forming a scolex and attaches to the mucosa using its four lateral suckers and a rostellum located in the terminal portion of the scolex that has 25–50 hooklets (15). The tapeworm then grows to a length of 1–8 m usually causing few clinical symptoms. It is estimated by the World Health Organization that over 2 million people worldwide harbor the adult tapeworm. *Taenia solium* is a hermaphrodite and releases three to six terminal proglottids/day, bearing 30,000–70,000 eggs or ova per proglottid into the intestine. Nearly 250,000 eggs are passed daily into the stool (15,16). *Taenia solium* eggs are spherical and 30–40 mm in diameter.

If these ova contaminate food or water that is eaten by the pig, the life cycle continues and the pig becomes the intermediate host. Studies in Peru have

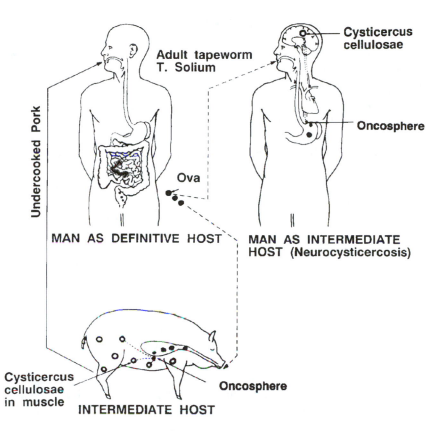

Figure 1 Life cycle of *Taenia solium* in humans and pigs. (Reproduced from Davis LE, Kornfeld M. Neurocysticercosis: neurologic, pathogenic, diagnostic and therapeutic aspects. Eur Neurol 1991; 31:229–240.)

found that *C. cellulosae* infections are highest in free-ranging pigs (1). If the swine are tethered or kept in closed quarters as in a pig farm, the infestation rate is low. Upon eating infected ova, the pig (or human) gastric and pancreatic enzymes liberate oncospheres or hexacant embryos. Aided by tiny hooklets, the 20-mm oncospheres penetrate the intestinal wall, circulate within the blood, and lodge primarily within muscle of the pig. Within 60–70 days, the oncosphere looses its hooklets, acquires a vesicular shape with a bladder wall, and undergoes gradual evagination of the protoscolex (invaginated scolex) to become a cysticercus. The mature cyst (*C. cellulosae*) is a transparent 5–15 mm diameter cyst that is the larval stage of *T. solium*. The cycle continues when humans eat under-cooked pork that contains the viable cysticercus. This pork is often called "mealy pork."

1.2. The Human as an Intermediate Host

When humans consume the ova released in human stools, they become intermediate hosts similar to the pig. Over 95% of the time, this infection occurs when the individual ingests food or water that is contaminated with *T. solium* ova. Use of human feces for fertilizer (night soil) is the most common situation but some infections are the result of food contamination by feces of restaurant workers or relatives who carry the *T. solium* tapeworm. Occasionally, individuals with an intestinal tapeworm can become self-infected via the fecal–oral route (17,18).

Similar to the pig, when a human ingests *T. solium* ova, the ova are partially digested in the stomach to release oncospheres that penetrate intestinal mucosa to reach the bloodstream. These oncospheres may lodge in any body tissue but show a predilection for the brain. The reason for oncospheres preferentially lodging in the brain in man and in muscle in swine is unknown. Less common sites of human infestation include the skeletal muscle, heart, eye, and subcutaneous tissue. In the brain, the oncospheres commonly lodge in small blood vessels located between the gray and white matter. The oncosphere then appears to move through the vessel wall into the adjacent brain or into the leptomeninges often deep within the sulcus (19). These brain oncospheres then develop into mature cysts causing neurocysticercosis. Occasional oncospheres lodge in the meninges, ependyma, or choroid plexus producing a chronic meningitis or ventriculitis.

In summary, human consumption of under-cooked infected pork results in infection with the tapeworm while human consumption of ova released in stools by humans infected with the tapeworm results in neurocysticercosis.

2. NATURAL HISTORY OF NEUROCYSTICERCOSIS

The signs and symptoms as well as the treatment of neurocysticercosis depend upon the stage of cysticerci in their life cycle (20,21). Thus, understanding the natural history of CNS cysts is important and the following discussion is broken into the major stages of neurocysticercosis (see Table 1). Various authors have attempted to classify cysticercosis into either four or five stages based on clinical, pathological, or neuroimaging observations (22,23). This chapter uses a system of four stages that is useful clinically and for determining treatment (20,21).

2.1. Stage 1: Immature Viable Vesicles

Within 1–2 weeks after the oncosphere lodges in the brain, it expands into a small edematous lesion. As a larva expands into a cyst, a protoscolex develops surrounded by a bladder wall of 1–3 mm in diameter. When the number of cysticerci is small,

Table 1 Major Stages of *Cysticercus cellulosae* in Brain Parenchyma

Stage	Time after ova ingestion	Pathology	CT/MRI scan	Common clinical features
1 (immature cyst)	1–4 weeks	Larval migration to brain with early cyst formation	Small non-contrast enhancing or homogenous contrast-enhancing lesions	Mainly asymptomatic, occasional flu-like illness, rare seizures, rare increased intracranial pressure from massive infestation
2 (vesicular or viable cyst)	2 months to 10+ years	Mature cyst with no or minimal surrounding inflammation or edema	3–18 mm non-contrast-enhancing cyst without adjacent edema	Mainly asymptomatic
3 (colloid or degenerating cyst)	2–10+ years	Degenerating cyst with thick cystic fluid, thickened capsule and adjacent inflammation	Ring-contrast enhancing cyst with adjacent edema	Seizures most common, occasional focal neurologic signs and increased intracranial pressure
4 (nodular, dead, calcified cyst)	3–10+ years	Collapsed fibrotic cyst with mineralization	Isodense or calcified nodule	Asymptomatic or persistent non-provoked seizures

CT = computed tomography, MRI = magnetic resonance imaging.
(Modified with permission from Davis LE. Neurocysticercosis: pathophysiology, diagnosis, and management, The Neurologist 1996; 2:356–364.)

they seldom produce clinical symptoms. Although treatment with praziquantel or albendazole would be effective in killing cysts, treatment is seldom given at this early stage as the diagnosis is rarely made. Occasionally, the individual has a massive brain infection of up to several hundred immature cysts that is called cysticercotic encephalitis (24). These patients experience deterioration of their mental status, seizures, and multiple focal neurologic signs, including papilledema from increased intracranial pressure (25,26). Neuroimaging with CT/MRI shows small non-contrast enhancing edematous lesions and later multiple small homogeneous contrast-enhancing lesions that are ill defined (27). High-dose corticosteroids are administered to reduce the cerebral edema (26) but antihelminthic drugs have been shown to be detrimental (25). Patients with these heavy *C. cellulosae* infestations often have a *T. solium* tapeworm in their intestine (28).

2.2. Stage 2: Vesicular (Viable) Cyst Stage

The *C. cellulosae* becomes mature about 2 months after egg ingestion. The mature cyst measures 3–18 mm in diameter (29). The bladder wall is a membranous structure composed of three layers: an outer or cuticular layer, middle or cellular layer with pseudoepithelial structure, and inner or reticular layer (15,29). The cyst has a protoscolex with clear fluid filling the cyst bladder and causes minimal or no surrounding inflammation (Fig. 2).

How the cysticercus down-regulates host cellular immunity is incompletely understood. There is evidence that the cyst produces proteins that block the local host immune response (30,31). Taeniaestatin, a parasite serine protease inhibitor, inhibits complement activation, down-regulates lymphocyte proliferation, blocks cytokine production, and interferes with neutrophil function (32). Paramyosin inhibits the function of the classical pathway of complement (33). Sulfated polysaccharides activate complement away from the parasite (34). Glutathione S-transerase and other molecules are produced that detoxify reactive oxygen intermediates (35). Finally cysts produce poorly characterized small molecules that suppress host inflammation (36,37). The net result of the cyst's locally block-

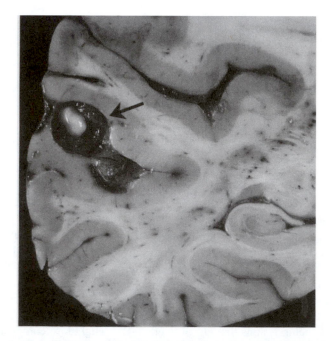

Figure 2 A 26-year-old man from Mexico who died of unrelated causes had a neurocysticercosis cyst in the cerebral cortex at autopsy. Note the protoscolex (arrow) within the cyst bladder. (Courtesy of Mark Becher, MD.)

ing the host immune response is that the cerebrospinal fluid (CSF) of patients with intraparenchymal cysts often does not reflect evidence of intrathecal antibody production. In one study before antihelminthic treatment, the CSF IgG index was elevated in only 29% and CSF oligoclonal bands were found in only 53% (38).

Neuroimaging at stage 2 usually demonstrates a non-contrast enhancing cyst. On CT, the cyst on CT has a thin wall and low-density fluid that appears almost identical to CSF (Fig. 3A). On T1-weighted MRI images, one can often detect a small nodule (protoscolex) within the bladder fluid because the protoscolex contains considerable lipid. On T2-weighted images, the bladder fluid appears hyperintense (Fig. 3B). Identification of the protoscolex usually establishes the cyst as being from cysticercosis. There is an absence of surrounding edema. Serial imaging shows once the typical cyst reaches 10–18 mm in diameter, it no longer expands. Thus, unless there are a large number of cysts they do not produce a mass effect. The majority of patients with viable cysts seldom experience any clinical signs or symptoms. One exception to this rule is when the cyst occasionally lodges in a critical site such as the brainstem, spinal cord or eye. The second exception is the occasional cyst that expands to become a "giant cyst" with a diameter reaching several centimeters (39). These "giant cysts" tend to be

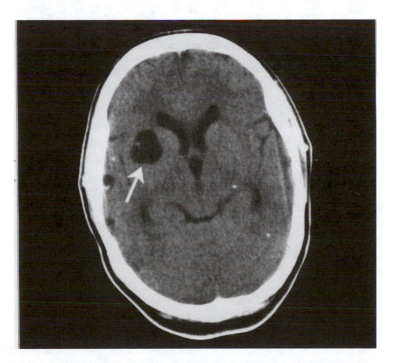

Figure 3A   A 25-year-old immigrant woman from Mexico presented with seizures. CT scan shows a stage 2 vesicular cyst with an apparent protoscolex (arrow).

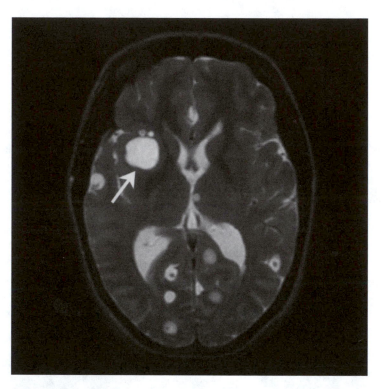

Figure 3B A 25-year-old immigrant woman from Mexico presented with seizures. T2-weighted MRI scan several days later demonstrating the same cyst with a protoscolex (arrow) plus additional cysts.

located in the Sylvian fissure and may become large enough to cause a mass effect sufficient to produce shifting of midline brain structures (Fig. 4). It is unclear whether the Sylvian fissure cysts always originate in the cerebral cortex or can develop in the adjacent meninges, allowing easy cyst expansion.

Because stage 2 cysts are usually asymptomatic, they are seldom discovered and thus not treated with antihelminthic drugs. However, both albendazole and praziquantel are effective in killing the viable cysts. There is currently disagreement as to whether a solitary stage 2 cyst should be treated if discovered on neuroimaging (see Sec. 2.9).

2.3. Stage 3: Colloid (Degenerating) Cyst Stage

Two to 10+ years after the intraparenchymal cyst becomes mature, it begins to die. At that time, the cyst fluid thickens, and becomes opaque. The bladder wall thickens and undergoes hyaline degeneration and early mineralization (29). The cyst no

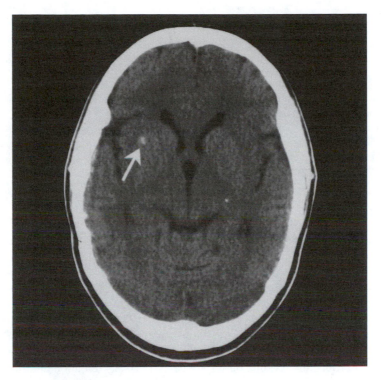

Figure 3C A 25-year-old immigrant woman from Mexico presented with seizures. CT scan 1-year later demonstrating disappearance of the original cyst and presence of a tiny calcified nodule (stage 4 cyst) (arrow). (Courtesy of Blaine Hart, MD, University of New Mexico School of Medicine.)

longer prevents a host immune response and *C. cellulosae* antigens appear to leak from the bladder wall. The intense inflammation developing around the degenerating cyst is mediated by both humoral and cellular immune responses (38,40). The inflammation has a predominance of Th1 lymphocytes along with some neutrophils and eosinophils (41). Gamma interferon and interleukin-2 are identified early in cyst degeneration (41). The inflammation triggers fibroblasts to form a capsule-like structure around the cyst. The colloid cyst stage can be as short as 3 months but can last over 24 months (42). If the patient has multiple cysts, they usually do not degenerate simultaneously. Thus, the patient's neuroimaging often shows both viable stage 2 cysts along with degenerating stage 3 cysts. If the individual has been repeatedly exposed to cysticercosis ova, there may also be calcified stage 4 cysts identified.

The colloid stage is the period when most patients develop clinical signs and symptoms most likely due to the surrounding inflammation causing irritation and dysfunction of the adjacent cerebral cortex. Table 2 lists the most common clinical signs seen in patients with neurocysticercosis in the United States. In

Table 2 Presenting Signs and Symptoms in Neurocysticercosis Commonly Seen in the United States

Signs and symptoms[a]	Percentage (%)
Seizures (focal or generalized)	75
Headaches, nausea, vomiting, lethargy, papilledema from increased intracranial pressure	10
Altered mental status (confusion, dementia, stupor, coma)	15
Focal neurologic signs (hemiparesis, visual loss, paraparesis, ataxia)	5
Asymptomatic and incidental	15

[a]Patients may present with more than one sign due to multiple intraparenchymal, meningeal and intraventricular cysts. Percentage is estimated from Refs (7,8,43–45) and the author's personal experience.

endemic countries patients often have more clinical signs that are more severe reflecting the higher CNS parasite load found in these patients (28). For patients with only intraparenchymal cysts, the most common symptom is seizures, either focal or generalized (46). If multiple cysts simultaneously degenerate, the resulting cerebral edema may produce signs of increased intracranial pressure.

The rare patient will have a cyst located in the spinal cord (usually thoracic) (7,47). The cyst may be intramedullary producing a progressive spastic paraparesis or quadraparesis or in the meninges and subarachnoid space (often lumbosacral) producing asymmetric leg weakness, urinary retention and impotence (48,49). It appears the myelopathy may begin in stage 2 but rapidly progress when the cyst begins to degenerate. Most patients also have other cysts located within the brain parenchyma or brain subarachnoid space. Surgical removal of the cyst is usually indicated along with albendazole treatment (50).

Neuroimaging in stage 3 intraparenchymal cysts usually demonstrates the cyst with adjacent mild to moderate cerebral edema (Fig. 5). Administration of a CT contrast agent or gadolinium for MRI demonstrates a thickened contrast enhancing cyst wall (51,52) (Fig. 6).

2.4. Stage 4: Nodular Calcified (Dead) Cyst Stage

At this stage, the cyst is dead either spontaneously or from antihelminthic drugs. The wall collapses and the cyst slowly becomes granulation tissue surrounded by a thick collagenous capsule. The surrounding inflammation subsides and Th2 lymphocytes secreting interleukin-4 predominate over Th1 lymphocytes (41). Over months to years, many of the collapsed nodules calcify. If the calcification becomes large enough, CT scans demonstrate tiny 3–5 mm nodules without surrounding edema (Fig. 3C). Stage 4 cysts may be missed by MRI since calcium is hypointense or by CT when the amount of calcification is tiny. Thus, the previously identified cyst appears to have disappeared on follow-up scans.

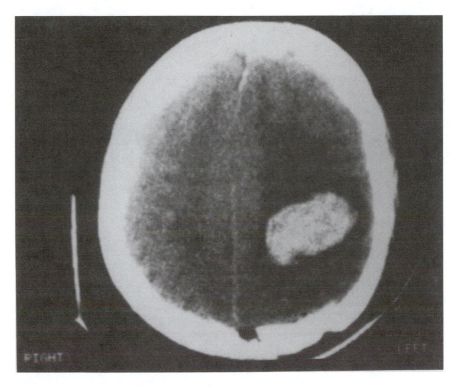

Figure 4 CT scan of 38-year-old man from Mexico with neurocysticercosis and a "giant cyst" located in the Sylvian fissure that was surgically proven. (Reproduced from Davis LE. Neurocysticercosis: pathophysiology, diagnosis and management. Neurologist 1996; 2:356–364.)

Since the dead cyst no longer produces foreign antigens, the host inflammatory reaction subsides. As such, provoked seizures disappear and the patient often becomes asymptomatic (53,54). Some patients experience a permanent seizure disorder (epilepsy) that may be coincidental or secondary to gray matter gliosis.

2.5. Meningeal Cysticercosis

Although the majority of oncospheres lodge within the brain parenchyma, about 15% lodge in the meninges, ependyma, or choroid plexus of the ventricles. Half of these patients also have parenchymal cysts. Under these circumstances, the meningeal cysticerci often do not develop into typical cysts and become racemose lacking a scolex and becoming lobulated with thin-walled bladders appearing like a bunch of grapes (55). These defective cysts slowly grow and frequently slowly leak *C. cellulosae* antigens into the subarachnoid CSF producing chronic low-

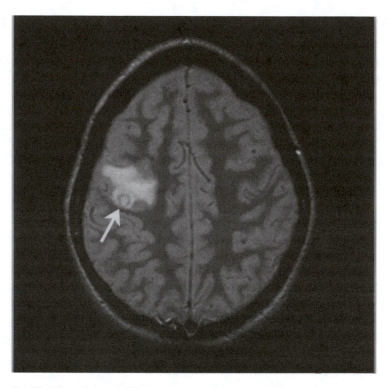

Figure 5 FLAIR-weighted MRI scan of a 21-year-old woman from Mexico with seizures. Scan demonstrates a stage 3 colloid cyst containing a protoscolex and adjacent edema (arrow). (Courtesy of Blaine Hart, MD, University of New Mexico School of Medicine.)

grade meningitis that often develops into arachnoiditis (56). The subarachnoid inflammation contains lymphocytes, multinucleated giant cells, eosinophils, parasite membranes, and collagen fibers. The arachnoiditis is most intense at the basal cisterns from the optochiasmatic region to the foramen magnum. The lumbar CSF has a cell count of 50–150 cells/mm3 (predominately lymphocytes), protein level of 100–400 mg/dL and normal glucose levels (57). The chronic CSF meningitis persists for at least 5–10 years but about 20% spontaneously resolve after several years, especially following albendazole treatment.

Patients with meningeal cysticercosis develop clinical signs and symptoms by two mechanisms. The arachnoiditis and racemose cysts can obstruct CSF pathways at the level of the basal cisterns and tentorium producing hydrocephalus (57). The arachnoiditis can also trap cranial nerves along the base of the brain. Patients with hydrocephalus experience subacute to chronic signs of increased intracranial pressure such as headaches, nausea, vomiting, altered mental status (confusion, dementia, stupor) cranial nerve palsies (esp. CN 3, 6, 7) and occasionally papilledema. If the patient does not undergo ventriculo-peritoneal or lumbar CSF shunting, coma and death from brain herniation may ensue (58).

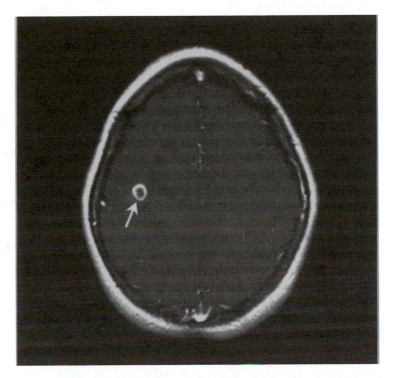

Figure 6 Gadolinium-enhanced T1-weighted MRI scan of a 28-year-old Hispanic man with seizures demonstrating ring enhancement of the stage 3 colloid cyst (arrow). (Courtesy of Blaine Hart, MD, University of New Mexico School of Medicine.)

The second mechanism of brain damage is from stroke. The persistent CSF inflammation, especially along the base of the brain, can cause sufficient arteritis of vessels traversing the meninges to cause thrombosis (50,59). In most cases the involved artery is of small diameter, often in the territory of the lenticulostriate arteries. The resulting strokes are usually lacunar involving the internal capsule or brainstem. Occasionally, a degenerating "giant" cyst in the Sylvian fissure has sufficient adjacent inflammation to cause thrombosis of the middle cerebral artery producing a large cortical stroke (60).

2.6. Intraventricular Cysticercosis

Intraventricular cysts can occur in the lateral, third, or fourth ventricles. These viable cysts are usually not racemose but contain a thin bladder wall, clear cyst fluid, and a protoscolex. They may be free floating in ventricular CSF or attached to ependyma or choroid plexus. In the viable vesicular cyst, the cyst contents match CSF on CT and are difficult to detect (61). If contrast media is introduced into the ventricle, however, CT allows the cyst to appear dark and is outlined by hyperdense CSF containing contrast media (62). T2-weighted MRI images likewise often do not detect viable intraventricular cysts but often they can be distinguished from CSF on proton density images (63). T1-weighted MRI images often, but not always, demonstrate the thin bladder wall with a protoscolex within the CSF-isointense cystic fluid. In the degenerating colloid cyst, the cystic fluid often becomes hyperintense or hyperdense to CSF on MRI and CT. The colloid cyst may leak *C. cellulosae* antigens into CSF causing a ventriculitis and ependymitis that can be seen on MRI as ependymal or choroid plexus enhancement after administration of gadolinium (62). Like meningeal cysts, patients with an intraventricular cyst often have intraparenchymal lesions.

Clinically, intraventricular cysts may be asymptomatic and identified coincidentally on MRI when a degenerating parenchymal cyst causes a seizure or symptoms appear with obstructive hydrocephalus caused by three mechanisms. First, a free-floating viable cyst may block CSF passage at the foramen of Monro, aqueduct of Sylvius, or outflow pathways of the fourth ventricle (64). Second, a degenerating cyst may swell to several times its former size and block a CSF pathway (64). Third, the degenerating cyst may release *C. cellulosae* antigens into the CSF producing an inflammatory response resulting in ventriculitis, ependymitis, and choroid plexitis. CSF inflammatory debris, the ependymitis or the swollen-inflamed choroid plexus can block CSF pathways (65). Patients with obstructive hydrocephalus develop symptoms and signs similar to those seen from obstructive hydrocephalus in meningeal cysticercosis (64,66). Sudden death may occur if the obstructed ventricle is not shunted or externally drained (64). Occasionally, free-floating cysts may migrate from one ventricle to another (67).

2.7. Ophthalmic Cysticercosis

Patients may develop ocular signs from *C. cellulosae* lodged in the extraocular muscles (most common site), globe (usually vitreous humor, occasionally in retina, subretinal, or anterior chamber) and subconjunctiva (68). Cysts in extraocular muscles may cause, proptosis, pain, diplopia, and decreased vision. Subconjunctival cysts produce pain, swelling and redness while cysts located in the eye cause visual loss. Visual loss can also result from obstructive hydrocephalus causing chronic papilledema or from meningeal cysticercosis causing arachnoiditis of the optic nerves. Orbital cysts can be identified on neuroimaging and ultrasound. Treatment is individualized based on cyst location. Cysts within the globe are usually surgically removed but many patients are left with poor vision (69). Cyst removal early in the clinical course carries a better prognosis for return of vision. Administration of antihelminthic drugs for cysts within the eye globe creates an inflammatory response that may permanently damage the retina. Extraorbital cysts usually are treated with antihelminthic drugs and corticosteroids (70) but may be surgically removed (71).

2.8. Diagnostic Workup

Neurocysticercosis should be considered in older children and adults from countries endemic for cysticercosis presenting with new seizures, unexplained chronic meningitis, obstructive hydrocephalus, strokes, or CNS cystic masses. The diagnosis of cysticercosis in the United States is often easier than in the endemic country because of more available neuroimaging and increased specificity of *C. cellulosae* antibody tests due to a lower prevalence of cysticercosis.

Neuroimaging with CT or MRI frequently is sufficient to establish the diagnosis, especially when the cysts are multiple or the protoscolex is seen. However, it is important not only to make the diagnosis but also to determine the cyst location (parenchymal, meningeal or intraventricular) and the stage of the cyst as these factors determine the type of treatment offered to the patient. Table 1 and the previous section describe the typical neuroimaging findings for each stage and location of the cyst. The diagnosis becomes somewhat more difficult when the cyst is solitary, larger than 20 mm in diameter, nodular, irregular in shape, surrounded by marked edema, has thick ring enhancement, or the entire cyst enhances when gadolinium or contrast media is administered. The differential diagnosis includes tuberculoma, pyogenic abscess, toxoplasma abscess, syphilitic gumma, primary brain tumor, metastatic tumor, arteriovenous malformation, cavernous malformation, and unusual CNS parasitic infections (echinococcus, schistosomiasis, and ameba). Tuberculomas, a major concern, tend to be larger than 20 mm in diameter, have irregular outline, cause more mass effect and produce a progressive focal neurologic deficit. In contrast, *C. cellulosae* cysts usually are less than 18 mm in diameter, have a smooth, regular outline and seldom cause focal neurologic deficits (72).

Blood hemograms are usually normal without increased eosinophils. The electroencephalogram may be abnormal and demonstrate focal sharp waves (from cortical irritation produced by a degenerating intraparenchymal cyst) or non-specific generalized slowing (as in obstructive hydrocephalus) (19,73).

The CSF, abnormal in 50% of patients, results from inflammatory cells leaking into the CSF from a superficial cortical degenerating cyst or from meningeal or ventricular cysticercosis. Table 3 lists the CSF findings most commonly seen in the United States. In patients living in endemic countries where the number of cysts in the brain is higher than that seen in patients in the United States, the percentage of abnormalities for all categories is somewhat higher. The most common abnormality is lymphocytic pleocytosis. In 15% of patients, eosinophils are seen on sediment stained with Wright's or Giemsa stain. CSF eosinophils are uncommon in bacterial or tuberculous meningitis and thus increase the probability of meningeal neurocysticercosis. However, eosinophils occasionally are present in CSF from other causes of meningitis such as fungi (*Coccidioides immitis, Histoplasma capsulatum*), parasites (*Echinococcus granulosus, Trichinella spiralis, Ascaris lumbricoides, Angiostrongylus canonensis,*

Table 3 Cerebrospinal Fluid in Neurocysticercosis Commonly Seen in the United States

CSF finding	Percentage (%)
Elevated opening pressure (>200 mm H2O)	25
Pleocytosis (>10 WBC/mm3)	45
Eosinophils	15
Elevated protein (>60 mg/dL)	40
Low glucose (>40 mg/dL)	15
Normal CSF	50
Positive immunoblot test for *C. cellulosae* antibody	
Pleocytosis and multiple stage 2 or 3 cysts seen on neuroimaging	~98
Normal CSF and solitary cyst or calcified cysts	~30

Gnathostoma spinigerum, Toxocara cati and *canis), Rickettsia rickettsii*, Hodgkin's lymphoma, leukemia, granulomatous meningitis, and idiopathic eosinophilic meningitis (74).

Serologic tests for cysticercosis have improved. Currently, the most sensitive and specific diagnostic test is an enzyme-linked immunoelectrotransfer blot assay (EITB) that was initially developed by the Centers for Disease Control and Prevention in Atlanta, GA (75,76). Studies have shown serum testing is highly sensitive (95%) and specific (98%) for patients with multiple cysts but less sensitive in detecting solitary cysts (28–70%) (76,77). After the cysticercus dies, the patient's cysticercus antibody titer may fall to undetectable levels. Thus, patients with only calcified cysts have a positive test ranging up to 88% for patients with multiple calcified cysts to as low as 10% for solitary calcified cysts. In general, most studies find the serum EITB test is as sensitive and specific as the test done on CSF but one study reported slightly higher sensitivity with CSF (75).

Older serologic tests that use unfractionated cysticercus antigens including the enzyme-linked immunosorbent assay (ELISA) and complement fixation (CF) assay are cheaper and easier to perform than the EITB assay but associated with high rates of false-positive and false-negative reactions giving the test a sensitivity of only 69% and specificity of 71% (78). Some of the false-positive reactions are due to cross-reactions with host antibodies produced in reaction to other helminthic infections, especially *Echinococcus granulosus*. The specificity of these tests improves when CSF rather than serum is assayed.

A monoclonal antibody-based antigen detection ELISA to detect cysticercus antigens in CSF and serum has been developed. This test is quite sensitive (86%) for detection of cysticercus antigens in the CSF of patients with multiple intraparenchymal or meningeal cysticercosis but not sensitive for detection of solitary parenchymal cysts (79). The test on serum had a sensitivity of 85% and specificity of 92% for detection of multiple viable cysts (80). The serum test was positive in 48% of patients with hydrocephalus from neurocysticercosis but negative in patients with only cerebral calcifications (81). Overall, the antigen test is most sensitive for patients with viable vesicular stage cysts, less sensitive for patients with only degenerating colloid stage cysts and negative in patients with only calcified cysts. Thus, the antigen test may be helpful in following response to antihelminthic drug treatment in patients with meningeal cysticercosis where neuroimaging assessment is difficult.

2.9. Management

The management of neurocysticercosis can be medical (antihelminthic drugs and corticosteroids) or surgical (removal of the cyst or placement of CSF shunt). Optimal management depends on the location and stage of the cysts. Albendazole and praziquantel are FDA approved for treatment of neurocysticercosis. Albendazole is moderately well absorbed by oral administration especially when given with a fatty meal. The drug is rapidly metabolized in first passage by the liver to its active sulfoxide metabolite (82), of which 70% is bound to protein. The sulfoxide plasma half-life is between 8 and 14 hr and it is eliminated in urine with an elimination half-life of 8.5 hr (82). The drug readily crosses the blood–brain and blood–CSF barriers to achieve concentrations in CSF that are higher than corresponding serum concentrations and higher than that achieved by praziquantel. However, the sulfoxide concentration in cyst fluid is lower than that of plasma levels but is sufficient to kill the cyst. Albendazole is well tolerated with minimal adverse effects that include dizziness, gastrointestinal distress, rashes, leucopenia, and elevated serum liver enzymes (83). Albendazole has been shown to cause teratogenic effects in rats and rabbits and should be avoided in pregnancy. The mechanism by which the cyst dies is incompletely understood but the drug seems to interfere with energy production in the parasite, in part by blocking the ability of the parasite to uptake glycogen in the gut, and interfering with cyst wall metabolism (82,84). The dose of albendazole is usually 15 mg/kg/day divided into two doses for 8–14 days (82) but other regiments have been published. Concomitant administration of corticosteroids has been shown to increase serum albendazole concentration by 50% (84). Administration of anticonvulsants or other medications does not affect the serum drug concentration.

Praziquantel is well absorbed orally and undergoes extensive first passage hepatic metabolism with the metabolites being inactive (82). Peak plasma levels occur 1.5–2 hr after administration. About 80% of praziquantel is bound to plasma but free praziquantel rapidly is distributed in body tissue due to its high lipid solubility. Praziquantel traverses the blood–brain and blood–CSF barriers to achieve therapeutic concentrations in CSF and within cyst fluid (82,84). Praziquantel has a plasma and elimination half-life of 1.5–2.5 hr. The drug is well tolerated with few side effects that include gastrointestinal distress, dizziness, fever, headache, and occasionally a diminished sense of well-being (85). Praziquantel has not been shown to be teratogenic in animals. The mechanism of action of praziquantel is poorly understood but the drug appears to kill the scolex and protoscolex (86). Thus, the racemose form of neurocysticercosis, which lacks a protoscolex, may not be killed by the drug. The usual dose of praziquantel is 50 mg/kg/day divided into three doses for 15 days (87). Unlike albendazole, concomitant administration of corticosteroids, phenytoin, or carbamazepine will decrease serum and CSF levels of praziquantel (87,88). Concomitant administration of praziquantel with cimetidine or a high fat or high carbohydrate diet elevates serum praziquantel levels (89).

Albendazole has become the drug of choice over praziquantel because it is less expensive and corticosteroids and anticonvulsants do not lower CSF and brain drug levels. Albendazole has also been shown effective in treating "giant," meningeal, and intraventricular cysts (39,90).

Corticosteroid administration along with the antihelminthic drug is often indicated to minimize transient worsening of clinical symptoms that may occur early in the treatment. Both antihelminthic drugs rapidly kill the viable cyst releasing antigenic material into the surrounding brain or CSF. As a consequence, there can be a marked increase in inflammation and cerebral edema that can produce new or increased clinical signs that include: increased intracranial pressure (with headaches, lethargy, nausea, and vomiting), seizures, and focal neurologic signs such as hemiparesis, ataxia, or visual loss. The symptoms often begin on day 2–3 of treatment and last 3–5 days (82). When albendazole is used, the corticosteroids should be given simultaneously and continued until day 5 or longer if there is a large parasite burden or a severe reaction develops. Dexamethasone, 8–24 mg/day in four divided doses orally, intramuscularly or intravenously or prednisone 1 mg/kg/day orally are usually given (82). When praziquantel is administered, the corticosteroids are often withheld for 1–2 days or longer if possible since steroids decrease serum praziquantel levels by 50% (88). If increased symptoms develop, steroids are then administered intramuscularly or intravenously for rapid effect and continued as long as necessary.

Table 4 gives an outline of treatment recommendations based on recent published recommendations (50) as modified by my experience. The most common presentation is an adult with seizures and one to three intraparenchymal cysts, some of which are degenerating. Controversy exists as to whether these patients require treatment with antihelminthic drugs. The argument for antihelminthic treatment is based on shortening the time to cyst disappearance on CT/MRI and killing all cysts simultaneously, preventing prolongation of brain inflammation due to multiple cysts degenerating at different times (91). The solution to this controversy is difficult. There is clinical evidence that viable cysts from a single exposure can persist in the brain for over a decade before becoming symptomatic, presumably from degeneration (7). Once one of several viable cysts begins to die, all cysts do not all degenerate simultaneously and some viable cysts may remain in the vesicular stage for years. In addition, the time to death for a degenerating cyst varies. In a study of 129 subjects presenting with a seizure

Table 4   Treatment Recommendations for *C. cellulosae* Cysts.

Type of neurocysticercosis	Recommendations[a]
Parenchymal cysts	Antihelminthic drugs +/- steroids or no anti-
Viable vesicular cysts	helminthic treatment
1–3 cysts on neuroimaging	Antihelminthic drugs + steroids
4+ cysts on neuroimaging	Antihelminthic drugs +/- steroidsor no anti-
Degenerating colloid cysts	helminthic treatment
1–3 cysts on neuroimaging	Antihelminthic drugs + steroids
4+ cysts on neuroimaging	No antihelminthic treatment
Dead calcified cysts	
Cysticercotic encephalitis	High dose steroids without antihelminthic drugs
Giant cysts	Albendazole with steroids, CSF shunting if hydro- cephalus develops
Meningeal cysts	
With hydrocephalus	CSF shunting, albendazole with steroids often in high dosage for years, careful monitoring of patient for shunt malfunction
Without hydrocephalus	Albendazole in 1to -2 courses with careful moni- toring of patient for possible hydrocephalus
Intraventricular cysts	
With hydrocephalus	CSF shunting, careful monitoring of patient for shunt malfunction, albendazole with steroids, surgical removal of cyst when possible
Without hydrocephalus	Surgical removal of cyst when possible with steroids, or albendazole with steroids
Spinal cysts	Surgical cyst removal when possible with steroids, or albendazole with steroids
Ophthalmic cysts	
Cysts in globe	Surgical cyst removal
Cysts outside globe	Antihelminthic drug with steroids, or surgical cyst removal when possible

[a]Patients should be given anticonvulsants as needed for seizures.

and MRI evidence of a solitary degenerating cyst, patients were followed without antihelminthic treatment for up to 2 years with serial MRI scans (42). At 6 months 36% of the cysts had resolved; by 12 months, 63% had resolved; and by 24 months, 89% had resolved. Thus, almost one-third the lesions were still active by MRI criteria at 1 year and 11% continued to be active past 2 years.

    Whether treatment with antihelminthic drugs shortens the time to death of the cyst is uncertain. Several non-randomized clinical studies reported a higher percentage of cyst disappearance by CT than in non-treated subjects but these studies had subjects with solitary and multiple vesicular and colloid cysts (53,88,92). Estimating the rate of cyst disappearance following antihelminthic treatment is difficult since each study tended to use only one follow-up CT. For example, after combining three studies of solitary colloid cysts treated with albendazole, 48% of the cysts had disappeared on CT at 3 months follow up (93–95). Another study of solitary "active" cysts treated with either albendazole or praziquantel reported a 44% cyst disappearance at 3–6 months and 62% by 9–12 months (96). Using these numbers, the disappearance rate following anti-helminthic treatment for a solitary cyst appears only slightly better than that reported for an untreated cyst. Finally, a Cochrane analysis of several randomized or quasi-randomized studies of antihelminthic vs. no treatment found only a trend that did not reach statistical significance for antihelminthic treatment to hasten the time to cyst disappearance (97).

It is also unclear whether antihelminthic drugs affect the course of seizures. The same Cochrane review of treatment trials did not find sufficient evidence to assess whether cysticidal therapy of neurocysticercosis was associated with ben-eficial effects on seizures (97). Since the Cochrane review, a double-blind placebo-controlled study of 120 Peruvian patients with seizures statistically sig-nificant 67% reduction in seizures with generalization following treatment with albendazole. A trend for reduction of partial seizures was also found (54).

The most recent evidence supports use of antihelminthic therapy in patients with seizures and viable or degenerating cysts identified on neuroimaging. This is particularly important in seizure patients with a moderate to large number of intraparenchymal cysts as these patients have a higher likelihood to have cysts degenerate over a prolonged period of time, some of which could be symptomatic in the future (50).

Anticonvulsants should be administered to all seizure patients. Anticonvulsants should be continued for 1–2 years or until the active cysts have disappeared on neuroimaging and the brain irritation has subsided (54). About 80% of patients do not subsequently develop seizures after the anticonvulsants are discontinued. Patients with subsequent seizures should be considered to have epilepsy from unprovoked seizures and restarted on long-term anticonvulsants (54).

For meningeal cysticercosis, treatment is more difficult since arachnoiditis often persists and causes obstructive hydrocephalus. Patients with hydrocephalus usually require ventriculoperitoneal shunting to relieve the increased intracranial pressure. Patients require corticosteroids along with the CSF shunt. After control of the elevated CSF pressure is achieved, albendazole is given. Following shunt placement, patients must be followed carefully due to a high incidence of shunt malfunction. The albendazole is administered for 3–4 weeks or the standard 14-day course is repeated 1 month later (50). Corticosteroids often must be given in higher doses for prolonged periods, such as prednisone 50 mg orally three times a week, for as long as the CSF inflammation persists. In one study the chronic arachnoiditis resolved in only 18% of patients (98).

Intraventricular cysticercosis usually presents with the signs and symptoms of obstructive hydrocephalus and increased intracranial pressure but occasionally is found incidentally. The mainstay of treatment for patients with marked obstructive hydrocephalus has been administration of albendazole and surgical therapy either to place a CSF shunt or remove the cyst (99). If the cyst is not producing marked hydrocephalus, albendazole, but not praziquantel, may eliminate the cyst without need of surgery (66,100). If the free-floating cyst is producing hydrocephalus, the cyst often can be removed via an open or endoscopic surgical approach. During endoscopic surgery the bladder wall is often punctured allowing the cyst to collapse. When this happens the surgeon irrigates the involved ventricle cavity repeatedly after cyst removal and adds corticosteroids to lessen the inflammation reaction from the leaking *C. cellulosae* antigens (101). It is important to note that free-floating intraventricular cysts may migrate down the CSF pathway and move from a lateral ventricle to the third, etc. As such, an MRI scan should be performed just prior to surgery. If the cyst is entirely removed, the obstructive hydrocephalus may resolve eliminating the need for a permanent CSF shunt (101).

In some patients with meningeal cysticercosis, the cysts may be racemose or degenerating producing a ventriculitis, ependymitis, and choroid plexitis. In these patients, the cyst is solidly attached to the ependyma or choroid plexus and difficult to surgically remove. Such patients require treatment with albendazole and CSF shunting. Shunt failures are common due to persistent CSF inflammation (62). One report that found the addition of prednisone 50 mg three times weekly lessened the ventriculitis and resulted in fewer shunt failures (102).

Antihelminthic drugs are seldom administered to patients with heavy enhancing cyst infestation (cysticercotic encephalitis) or patients with ocular cysticercosis as the sudden increase in inflammation and intracranial pressure from drug treatment can be detrimental (25,50).

2.10. Prognosis

Most patients with neurocysticercosis have an excellent prognosis. For many, the viable cysts eventually degenerate without causing any neurologic symptoms. In three-fourths of patients who develop seizures, the seizures subside after 1–2 years when the inflammation around the cysts subsides. In the remaining 25%, the epilepsy usually is easy to treat with anticonvulsants. For some, the etiology of the epilepsy is independent of the cysticercosis while in others it develops from permanent gliosis around the dead cyst. Patients who experience meningeal cysticercosis have a poorer prognosis. Up to 50% develop obstructive hydrocephalus, which requires CSF shunting. The shunts frequently become blocked from inflammatory debris due to the continuing arachnoiditis and require one or more shunt revisions. If the shunts are not revised, death or severe dementia can develop due to progressive hydrocephalus. Patients with ventricular cysts may become cured if the cyst is surgically removed or may develop obstructive hydrocephalus if the cyst blocks the ventricular CSF pathway. The hydrocephalus patients require CSF shunting and follow a similar course as those with meningeal cysticercosis.

2.11. Prevention

To prevent development of an intestinal tapeworm, all pork should be thoroughly cooked prior to eating (103). In addition, freezing pork to −20°C for several days kills *Cysticerci* (104). However, smoked or dried pork may still contain viable *Cysticerci*. There is now evidence that pigs can be vaccinated with recombinant *C. cellulosae* vaccines to prevent or minimize subsequent infestation by ova (105,106). These new vaccines may be of benefit to endemic countries to eradicate the disease and thus prevent neurocysticercosis in humans.

Prevention of neurocysticercosis is best accomplished by avoiding ova-contaminated food. In endemic areas, consumption of raw vegetables should be avoided as they may be contaminated. Heating food above 60°C or freezing below 30°C is usually sufficient to kill ova (16). Restaurant food workers from endemic areas should have their stools routinely checked for the presence of tapeworm ova. Stool assays to detect *C. cellulosae* antigens are more sensitive than microscopic inspection of one to three stool samples but are not widely available (107). It is encouraging to note, however, that American tourists visiting Mexico or Latin America seldom develop neurocysticercosis (13).

ACKNOWLEDGMENT

I thank Dr. Molly King for her suggestions and critical review of the manuscript.

REFERENCES

1.   Bern C, Garcia H, Evans C, et al. Magnitude of the disease burden from neurocysticercosis in a developing country. Clin Infect Dis 1999; 29:1203–1209.
2.   Medina MT, Roasa E, Rubio-Donnadieuy F, Sotelo J. Neurocysticercosis as the main cause of late-onset epilepsy in Mexico. Arch Intern Med 1990; 150:325–327.
3.   Roberts T, Murrell KD, Marks S. Economic losses caused by food borne parasitic diseases. Parasitol Today 1994; 11:419–423.
4.   Lombardo L, Mateos JH. Cerebral cysticercosis in Mexico. Neurology 1961; 11:824–828.
5.   Schenone H, Villarroel F, Rojas A, Ramirez R. Epidemiology of human cysticercosis in Latin America. In: Flisser A, Willms K, Laclette JP, Larralde C, Ridaura C, Beltran F, eds. Cysticercosis: Present State of Knowledge and Perspectives. New York, Academic Press, 1982:25–38.
6.   Schultz TS, Ascherl GF. Cerebral cysticercosis: occurrence in the immigrant population. Neurosurgery 1978; 3:164–169.

7. Dixon HBF, Lipscomb FM. Cysticercosis: An Analysis and Follow-Up of 450 Cases. Privy Council, Medical Research Council Special Report Series, No. 299. London: Her Majesty's Stationery Office, 1961:1–58.

8. Wei G-Z, Li C-J, Meng J-M, Ding, M-C. Cysticercosis of the central nervous system. Chin Med J 1988; 101:493–500.

9. Sarti E, Schantz PM, Plancarte A, et al. Prevalence and risk factors for *Taenia solium* taeniasis and cysticercosis in humans and pigs in a village in Morelos, Mexico. Am J Trop Med Hyg 1992; 46:677–685.

10. Stepien L. Cerebral cysticercosis in Poland: clinical symptoms and operative results in 132 cases. J Neurosurg 1962; 19:505–513.

11. Sorasuchart A, Khunadorn N, Edmeads J. Parasitic diseases of the nervous system in Thailand. Can Med Assoc J 1968; 98:859–867.

12. Richards FO, Schantz PM, Ruiz-Tiben E, Sorvillo FJ. Cysticercosis in Los Angeles county. JAMA 1985; 254:3444–3448.

13. Ong S, Talan DA, Moran GJ, et al. Neurocysticercosis in radiographically imaged seizure patients in U.S. emergency departments. Emerg Infect Dis 2002; 8:608–613.

14. Schantz PM, Moore AC, Munoz JL, et al. Neurocysticercosis in an orthodox Jewish community in New York City. N Engl J Med 1992; 327:692–695.

15. Pittella JEH. Neurocysticercosis. Brain Pathol 1997; 7:681–693.

16. Lawson Jr, Gremmell MA. Hydatidosis and cysticercosis: the dynamics of transmission. Adv Parasitol 1983; 22:261–308.

17. McCormick GF, Zee C-S, Heiden J. Cysticercosis cerebri: review of 127 cases. Arch Neurol 1982; 39:534–539.

18. Loo L, Braude A. Cerebral cysticercosis in San Diego: a review of 23 cases and a review of the literature. Medicine 1982; 61:341–359.

19. Thomas JA, Knoth R, Volk B. Disseminated human neurocysticercosis. Acta Neuropathol 1989; 78:594–604.

20. Davis LE, Kornfeld M. Neurocysticercosis: neurologic, pathogenic, diagnostic and therapeutic aspects. Eur Neurol 1991; 31:229–240.

21. Davis LE. Neurocysticercosis: pathology, diagnosis, and management. Neurologist 1996; 2:356–364.

22. Sotelo J, Guerrero V, Rubio F. Neurocysticercosis: a new classification based on active and inactive forms. Arch Intern Med 1985; 145:442–445.

23. Carpio A, Placencia M, Santillan F, Escobar A. A proposal for classification of neurocysticercosis. Can J Neurol Sci 1994; 21:43–47.

24. Thomas JA, Knoth R, Volk B. Disseminated human neurocysticercosis. Acta Neuropathol 1989; 78:594–604.

25. Wadia N, Sesai S, Bhatt M. Disseminated cysticercosis. Brain 1988; 111:597–614.

26. Rangel R, Torres B, Del Bruto O, Sotelo J. Cysticercotic encephalitis: a severe form in young females. Am J Trop Med Hyg 1987; 36:387–392.

27. Kramer LD, Locke GE, Byrd SE, Daryabagi J. Cerebral cysticercosis: documentation of natural history with CT. Radiology 1989; 171:459–462.

28. Gilman RH, Del Brutto OH, Garcia HH, Martinez M, Cysticercosis Working Group in Peru. Prevalence of taeniasis among patients with neurocysticercosis is related to severity of infection. Neurology 2000; 55:1062.

29. Escobar A. The pathology of neurocysticercosis. In: Palacios E, Rodriguez-Carbajal J, Taveras JM, eds. Cysticercosis of the Central Nervous System. Springfield: Thomas, 1983:27–59.

30. White AC Jr, Robinson P, Kuhn R. *Taenia solium* cysticercosis: host–parasite interactions and the immune response. Chem Immunol 1997; 66:209–230.

31. Leid RW, Suquet CM, Tanigoshi L. Parasite defense mechanisms for evasion of host attack: a review. Vet Parasitol 1987; 25:147–162.

32. Leid RW, Grant RF, Suquet CM. Inhibition of equine neutrophil chemotaxis and chemokinesis by a *Taenia taeniaeformis* proteinase inhibitor, taeniaestin. Parasite Immunol 1987; 9:195–204.

33. Larralde C, Montoya RM, Sotelo J, et al. Murine *T. crassiceps* antigens in immunodiagnosis of *T. solium* human neurocysticercosis, *T. saginata* bovine cysticercosis, and human E. Granulosus hydatidosis. Bull Soc Fr Parasitol 1990; 8:S8B.

34. Leid RW, Suquet CM, Tanigoshi L. Oxygen detoxifying enzymes in parasites: a review. Acta Leiden 1989; 57:107–114.

35. Leid RW, Suquet CM. A superoxide dismutase of metacestode of *Taenia taeniaformis*. Mol Biochem Parasitol 1986; 18:301–311.

36. Tato P. Castro AM, Rodriguez D, Soto R, Arachavaleta F, Molinari JL. Suppression of murine lymphocyte proliferation induced by a small RNA purified from the *Taenia solium* metacestode. Parasitol Res 1995; 81:181–187.

37. Arechavaleta F, Molinari LM, Tato P. A *Taenia solium* metacestode factor nonspecifically inhibits cytokine production. Parasitol Res 1998; 84:117–122.

38. Rolfs A, Muhschlegel F, Jansen-Rosseck R, et al. Clinical and immunologic follow-up study of patients with neurocysticercosis after treatment with praziquantel. Neurology 1995; 45:532–538.

39. Del Brutto OH, Sotelo J, Aguirre R, Diaz-Calderon E, Alarcon TA. Albendazole therapy for giant subarachnoid cysticerci. Arch Neurol 1992; 49:535–538.

40. Estanol B, Juarez H, Irigoyen MDC, Gonzalez-Barranco D, Corona T. Humoral immune response in patients with cerebral parenchymal cysticercosis treated with praziquantel. Neurol Neurosurg Psychiatry 1989; 52:254–257.

41. Robinson P, Atmar RL, Lewis DE, White AC Jr. Granuloma cytokines in murine cysticercosis. Infect Immunol 1997; 65:2925–2931.

42. Rejshekhar V. Rate of spontaneous resolution of a solitary cysticercus granuloma in patients with seizures. Neurology 2001; 57:2315–2317.

43. Earnest MP, Reller LB, Filley CM, Grek AJ. Neurocysticercosis in the United States: 35 cases and a review. Rev Infect Dis 1987; 9:961–979.

44. Shandera WX, White AC, Chen JC, Diaz P, Armstrong R. Neurocysticercosis in Houston, Texas. A report of 112 cases. Medicine 1994; 73:37–52.

45. White AC Jr. Neurocysticercosis: a major cause of neurological disease worldwide. Clin Infect Dis 1997; 24:101–115.

46. Del Brutto OH, Santibanez R, Noboa CA, Aguirre R, Diaz E, Alarcon TA. Epilepsy due to neurocysticercosis: analysis of 203 patients. Neurology 1992; 42:389–392.

47. Castillo M, Quencer RM, Post JD. MR of intramedullary spinal cysticercosis. AJNR Am J Neuroradiol 1988; 9:393–395.

48. Akiguchi I, Fujiwara T, Matsuyama H. Intramedullary spinal cysticercosis. Neurology 1979; 29:1531–1534.

49. McDonald JB, Turner PT, Miller AH. Cysticercosis and spinal cord compression. Ann Neurol 1979; 6:367–368.

50. Garcia HH, Evans CAW, Nash TE, et al. Current consensus guidelines for treatment of neurocysticercosis. Clin Microbiol Rev 2002; 15:747–756.

51. Zee C-S, Segall HD, Boswell W, Ahmadi J, Nelson M, Colletti P. MR imaging of neurocysticercosis. J Comput Assist Tomogr 1988; 12:927–934.
52. Suss RA, Maravilla KRT, Thompson J. MR imaging of intracranial cysticercosis: comparison with CT and anatomopathologic features. AJNR Am J Neuroradiol 1986; 7:234–242.
53. Vazquez V, Sotello J. The course of seizures after treatment for cerebral cysticercosis. N Eng J Med 1992; 327:696–701.
54. Garcia HH, Pretell EJ, Gilman RH, et al. A trial of antiparasitic treatment to reduce the rate of seizures due to cerebral cysticercosis. N Engl J Med 2004; 350:249–58.
55. Bickerstaff ER, Cloake PCP, Hughes B, Smith WT. The racemose form of cerebral cysticercosis. Brain 1952; 75:1–18.
56. Valkounova J, Zdarska Z, Slais J. Histochemistry of the racemose form of *Cysticercus cellulosae*. Folia Parasitol (Praha) 1992; 39:207–226.
57. Sotelo J, Marin C. Hydrocephalus secondary to cysticercotic arachnoiditis. A long-term follow-up review of 92 cases. J Neurosurg 1987; 66:686–689.
58. Esberg G, Reske-Nielsen R. Sudden death from cerebral cysticercosis. Scand J Infect Dis 1988; 20:679–884.
59. Del Brutto OH. Cysticercosis and cerebrovascular disease: a review. J Neurol Neurosurg Psychiatr 1992; 55:252–254.
60. Alarcon F, Hidalgo F, Moncayo J, Vinan I, Duenas G. Cerebral cysticercosis and stroke. Stroke 1992; 23:224–228.
61. Rodacki MA, Detoni XA, Teixeira WR, Boer VH, Oliveira GG. CT features of cellulosae and racemosus neurocysticercosis. J Comput Assist Tomogr 1989; 13:1013–1016.
62. Kelley R, Duong DH, Locke GE. Characteristics of ventricular shunt malfunctions among patients with neurocysticercosis. Neurosurgery 2002; 50:757–762.
63. Ginier BL, Poirier VC. MR imaging of intraventricular cysticercosis. AJNR Am J Neuroradiol 1992; 13:1247–1248.
64. Apuzzo MLJ, Dobkin WR, Zee C-S, Chan JC, Giannotta SL, Weiss MH. Surgical considerations in treatment of intraventricular cysticercosis. An analysis of 45 cases. J Neurosurg 1984; 60:400–407.
65. Madrazo I, Garcia-Renteria JA, Sandoval M, Lopez Vega F. Intraventricular cysticercosis. Neurosurgery 1983; 12:148–152.
66. Cuetter AC, Garcia-Bobadilla J, Guerra LG, Martinez FM, Kaim B. Neurocysticercosis: focus on intraventricular disease. Clin Infect Dis 1997; 24:157–164.
67. Kramer J, Carrazana EJ, Cosgrove GR, Kleefield J, Edelman RR. Transaqueductal migration of a neurocysticercus cyst. J Neurosurg 1992; 77:956–958.
68. Pushker N, Bajaj MS, Chandra M. Ocular and orbital cysticercosis. Acta Ophthalmol Scand 2001; 79:408–413.
69. Cardenas F, Quiroz H, Plancarte A, Meza A, Dalma A, Flisser A. *Taenia solium* ocular cysticercosis: findings in 30 cases. Ann Ophthalmol 1992; 24:25–28.
70. Sihota R, Honavar SG. Oral albendazole in the management of extraocular cysticercosis. Br J Ophthalmol 1994; 78:621–623.
71. Sekhar GC, Lemke BN. Orbital cysticercosis. Ophthalmology 1997; 104:1599–1604.
72. Rajshekhar V. Etiology and management of single small CT lesions in patients with seizures: understanding a controversy. Acta Neurol Scand 1991; 84:465–470.

73. Scharf D. Neurocysticercosis. Arch Neurol 1988; 45:777–780.

74. Greenlee JE, Carroll KC. Cerebrospinal fluid in CNS infections. In: Scheld WM, Whitley RJ, Durack DT, eds. Infections of the Central Nervous System. 2nd ed. Philadelphia: Lippincott-Raven, 1997:899–922.

75. Gekeler F, Eichenlaub S, Mendoza EG, Sotelo J, Hoelscher M, Loscher T. Sensitivity and specificity of ELISA and immunoblot for diagnosing neurocysticercosis. Eur J Clin Microbiol Infect Dis 2002; 21:227–229.

76. Wilson M, Bryan RT, Fried JA, Ware DA, Schantz PM, Pilcher JB, Tsang VCW. Clinical evaluation of the cysticercosis enzyme-linked immunoelectrotransfer blot in patients with neurocysticercosis. J Infect Dis 1991; 164:1007–1009.

77. Garcia HH, Herrera G, Gilman RH, Tsang VC, Pilcher JB, Diaz JF, et al. Discrepancies between cerebral computed tomography and western blot in the diagnosis of neurocysticercosis. Am J Trop Med Hyg 1994; 50:152–157.

78. Ramos-Kuri M, Montoya RS, Padilla A, et al. Immunodiagnosis of neurocysticercosis: disappointing performance of serology (ELISA) in an unbiased sample of neurologic patients. Arch Neurol 1992; 49:633–636.

79. Garcia HH, Harrison LJ, Parkhouse RM, et al. A specific antigen-detection ELISA for the diagnosis of human neurocysticercosis. The cysticercosis Working Group in Peru. Trans R Soc Trop Med Hyg 1998; 92:411–414.

80. Garcia HH, Parkhouse RM, Gilman RH et al. Serum antigen detection in the diagnosis, treatment and follow-up of neurocysticercosis patients. Trans R Soc Trop Med Hyg 2002; 94:673–676.

81. Garcia HH, Gonzalez AE, Gilman RH, et al. Circulating parasite antigen in patients with hydrocephalus secondary to neurocysticercosis. Am J Trop Med Hyg 2002; 66:427–430.

82. Sotelo J, Jung H. Pharmacokinetic optimization of the treatment of neurocysticercosis. Clin Pharmacokinet 1998; 34:503–515.

83. Jung H. Hurtado M, Medina MT, Sanchez M, Sotello J. Dexamethasone increases plasma levels of albendazole. J Neurol 1990; 237:279–280.

84. Overbosch D, van de Nes JCM, Groll E, Diekmann HW, Polderman AM, Mattie H. Penetration of praziquantel into cerebrospinal fluid and cysticerci in human cysticercosis. Eur J Clin Pharmacol 1987; 33:287–292.

85. King CH, Mahmoud AAF. Drugs five years later: praziquantel. Ann Intern Med 1989; 110:290–296.

86. Vasquez ML, Jung H, Sotelo J. Plasma levels of praziquantel decrease when dexamethasone is given simultaneously. Neurology 1987; 37:1561–1562.

87. Sotelo J, Escobedo F, Rodriguez-Carbajal J, Torres B, Rubio-Donnadieu F. Therapy of parenchymal brain cysticercosis with praziquantel. N Engl J Med 1984; 310:1001–1007.

88. Bittencourt PRM, Carcia CM, Martins R, Fernandes AG, Diekman HW, Jung W. Phenytoin and carbamazepine decrease oral bioavailability of praziquantel. Neurology 1992; 42:492–496.

89. Castro N, Medina R, Sotelo J, Jung H. Bioavailability of praziquantel increases with concomitant administration of food. Antimicrob Agents Chemother 2000; 44:2903–2904.

90. Proano JV, Madrazo I, Avelar F, Lopez-Felix B, Diaz G, Grijalva I. Medical treatment for neurocysticercosis characterized by giant subarachnoid cysts. N Engl J Med 1001; 345:879–885.

91. Davis LE. Neurocysticercosis and seizures: avoiding the cost of antihelminthic treatment. Neurology 2002; 59:1669.
92. Del Brutto OH, Sotelo J, Roman GC. Therapy for neurocysticercosis: a reappraisal. Clin Infect Dis 1993; 17:730–735.
93. Singhi P, Ray M, Singhi S, Khandelwal N. Clinical spectrum of 500 children with neurocysticercosis and response to albendazole therapy. J Child Neurol 2000; 15:207–213.
94. Padma MV, Behari M, Misra NK, Ahuja GK. Albendazole in single CT ring lesions in epilepsy. Neurology 1994; 44:1344–1346.
95. Baranwal AK, Singhi PD, Khandelwal N, Singhi SC. Albendazole therapy in children with focal seizures and single small enhancing computerized tomographic lesions: a randomized, placebo-controlled, double blind trial. Pediatr Infect Dis 1998; 7:696–700.
96. Carpio A, Santillan F, Leon P, Flores C, Hauser WA. Is the course of neurocysticercosis modified by treatment with antihelminthic agents? Arch Intern Med 1995; 155:1982–1988.
97. Salinas R, Prasad K. Drugs for treating neurocysticercosis (tapeworm infection of the brain) [Cochrane Review]. Cochrane Database Syst Rev 2000; 2:CD00215.
98. Sotelo J, Marin C. Hydrocephalus secondary to cysticercotic arachnoiditis. A long-term follow-up review of 92 cases. J Neurosurg 1987; 66:686–689.
99. Keane JR. Death from cysticercosis: seven patients with unrecognized obstructive hydrocephalus. West J Med 1984; 140:787–789.
100. Del Brutto OH, Sotelo J. Albendazole therapy for subarachnoid and ventricular cysticercosis: case report. J Neurosurg 1990; 72:816–817.
101. Bergsneider M, Holly LT, Lee JH, King WA, Frazee FG. Endoscopic management of cysticercal cysts within the lateral and third ventricles. J Neurosurg 2000; 92:14–23.
102. Roman S, Soto-Hernandez JL, Sotelo J. Effects of prednisone on ventriculoperitoneal shunt function in hydrocephalus secondary to cysticercosis. A preliminary study. J Neurosurg 1996; 84:629–633.
103. Biagi F, Velez G, Gutierrrez ML. Destruccion de los cisticercos en la carne de cerdo prensa. Med Mex 1963; 28:253–257.
104. Sotelo J, Rosas N, Palencia G. Freezing of infested pork muscle kills cysticerci. JAMA 1986; 256:893–894.
105. Lightowlers MW, Gauci CG. Vaccines against cysticercosis and hydatidosis. Vet Parasitol 2001; 101:337–352.
106. Lightowlers MW. Eradication of *Taenia solium* cysticercosis: a role for vaccination of pigs. Int J Parasitol 1999; 29:811–817.
107. Garcia-Noval J, Allan JC, Fletes C, et al. Epidemiology of *Taenia solium* taeniasis and cysticercosis in two rural Guatemalan communities. Am J Trop Med Hyg 1996; 55:282–289.

11

The Problem of Human African Trypanosomiasis

Peter G. E. Kennedy

*Division of Clinical Neurosciences, Department of Neurology,
Institute of Neurological Sciences, University of Glasgow,
Southern General Hospital, Glasgow, U.K.*

1. THE NATURE AND SCALE OF THE PROBLEM

Human African trypanosomiasis (HAT), which is also known as sleeping sickness, has for several decades been one of the most important parasitic infections affecting man in the African continent. The disease is caused by protozoan parasites of the Trypanosoma species, with the East African form of the disease caused by Trypanosoma brucei rhodesiense and the West African form caused by Trypanosoma brucei gambiense. The disease is fatal if left untreated. The parasites in both cases are transmitted by the tsetse fly of the genus Glossina so that the control of this insect vector is a major challenge in the fight against HAT. A landmark World Health Organization (WHO) report published in 1986 (1) estimated that 50 million people worldwide are at risk of developing HAT, and it is likely that the current figure is closer to 60 million. The disease is a major health problem in Africa and occurs in no less than 36 countries in sub-Saharan Africa between latitudes 14(N and 29(S reflecting the distribution of the tsetse fly (2) (Fig. 1). The area of land which is effectively "held captive" by the tsetse fly is massive and in the region of 10 million square km (3). Precise figures for the incidence of HAT are very difficult to define in large part because only a small percentage (about 5–15%) of the susceptible population is usually under active surveillance and the disease is often inadequately reported (2). In an insightful analysis of the problem, Kuzoe (2) reported in 1993 that

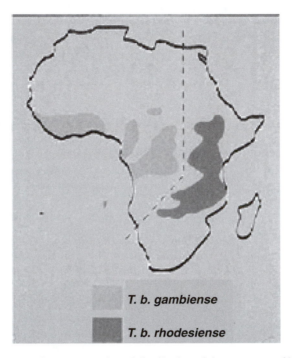

Figure 1 Diagrammatic representation of distribution of the two types of human African trypanosomiasis in Africa. (From Ref. 5.)

about 25,000 new cases are reported annually. However, it is likely that the true incidence of the disease is in the region of 300,000 cases per year (4).

If human-to-human transmission of the disease occurs, then it must be a rare event (M. Murray, personal communication). Animal trypanosomiasis is a major socioeconomic problem in Africa not only because of the severe disruption to domestic livestock breeding programs that it causes, but also because animals themselves may act as reservoirs of the human Trypanosoma parasites which can be transmitted to man by the tsetse fly (5). Thus massive regions of Africa are unable to sustain the breeding of domestic animals such as cattle, goats, horses, and camels (5). It should be noted that only a few of over 20 species of tsetse fly actually transmit HAT, 2–10% of the latter are usually infected in an endemic area, and a tsetse fly remains infective for the duration of its entire life (5,6). A description of the parasite and tsetse fly biology and ecology in relation to the West and East African forms of the disease is outside the scope of this chapter and has been given in detail elsewhere (5).

As Kuzoe has pointed out (2), HAT was virtually brought under control during the early 1950s, but then a series of factors led to its emergence as such a major threat to the health of African populations. These factors have been identified as including, for example, failure of national governments to allocate adequate financial resources to the disease, in part due to competing health priorities, political unrest and the deteriorating economic health of the countries where the disease is endemic (2). At the present time the problem in several regions of sub-Saharan Africa continues to deteriorate with continued evidence of the characteristic waves of epidemics, resurgences and outbreaks (2,5). For example, very significant focal resurgences of the disease have been reported in recent years in Angola, the Congo, and Uganda (5). Additional factors which have led to this increase in the scale of the problem include increases in man-fly contact as a result of significant population movements of both humans and infected animal reservoirs, the emergence and/or introduction of new virulent parasite strains, climatic and vegetation changes, and disruption of existing medical surveillance programs (2). Of course these various factors are not mutually exclusive and several of these may be present simultaneously further increasing the risks of focal epidemics. Another relevant factor is likely to be changes in the disease susceptibility of the human population itself. A particular and topical aspect of the latter is the recent occurrence of HAT in several European tourists returning from Africa. With increasing tourism to the African game parks and easier and more frequent air travel between sub-Saharan Africa and both North America and Europe, there is a real possibility that HAT could emerge as an increasing threat to susceptible individuals in several Western populations.

2. NEUROLOGICAL FEATURES

A variety of neurological symptoms and signs occur in HAT. Central nervous system (CNS) involvement in East African Rhodesian disease is generally an acute disease lasting a few months, in contrast to than that seen in West African Gambian sleeping sickness which is characterized by a protracted and progressive course lasting months to years (5,7). In both cases the disease is ultimately fatal. During the early (hemolymphatic) stage of HAT CNS involvement is minimal, but during the late stage of the disease CNS features predominate. However, the transition from early to late stages is not always distinct. The neurological features are summarized in Table 1.

2.1. Early Stage Features

The CNS involvement at this stage is not prominent and will occur against a background of a constellation of possible systemic features including constitutional such as fever and headache, cutaneous, cardiovascular, gastrointestinal, endocrine, lymphatic gland and eye symptoms and signs which are described in detail elsewhere (5,7,8). Patients may show some of the mental disturbances listed in Table 1, in particular somnolence, alteration of personality and irritability (5,8). Such features, which are non-specific and non-diagnostic, have been reported as being

Table 1   Central nervous system involvement in late-stage human trypanosomiasis

Mental Disturbances	Motor System Disturbances	Sensory System Involvement	Abnormal Reflexes
Indifference	Tremors of tongue and fingers	Hyperaesthesia	Pout
Lassitude	Muscular fasciculation	Generalized pruritus	Palmo-mental
Irritability	Choreiform or oscillatory movements	Paraesthesia	Babinski
Anxiety	Increased muscular tonicity	Anaesthesia	
Sleep disturbances	Increased muscular rigidity		
Agitation/mania episodes	Slurred speech		
Uncontrolled sexual impulses	Cerebellar ataxia		
Violet mood	Paralysis of one or more muscular groups		
Delirium and hallucinations	Neuritis/polyneuritis		
Increased suicidal tendencies			

Reprinted with permission (Butterworth-Heinemann) from Ref 5.

more typical of disease in European patients (8). This should clearly be borne in mind when considering a possible diagnosis of HAT in Europeans returning from endemic regions of Africa. Another feature which may occur early and especially in Europeans is spontaneous or pressure-induced skeletal pain (Kerandel's sign).

2.2.   Late-Stage Features

The timing of onset of CNS disease depends on the type of HAT; invasion of the CNS by the parasite occurs weeks to a few months after the disease has started in Rhodesian disease but many months or years in Gambian disease (5,7). The CNS disease develops insidiously and may show a varied phenotype, although some features such as severe and continuous headache, sleep and motor dysfunction are usually present (5). The CNS abnormalities will now be considered briefly in turn.

2.2.1.   Neuropsychiatric Disturbances

Mental disturbances may be prominent with frank psychosis occurring in some patients, particularly in Europeans (8), and at the later stages the irritability and personality change mentioned above may also occur. The personality change may also manifest itself as excessive familiarity and indecency with uncontrolled sexual impulses and suicidal behavior (9). Other features that may be seen include anxiety and agitation, manic episodes, depression, apathy, confusion, delirium, and hallucinations (10,11).

2.2.2. Motor and Sensory Disturbances

Numerous motor and sensory signs may occur, summarized in Table 1. For instance, focal weakness may occur in different limbs and most patients show limb, or more rarely, postural hypertonia (11). Muscle fasciculation may be seen, and tremors of the tongue and fingers are also common. Extrapyramidal features which are also well recognized include akinesia, gait disturbances, a semi-flexed posture, and choreiform movements of the head, limbs, and trunk (5,11), and athetoid movements of the upper limbs (11). Cerebellar involvement is also characteristic with slurred speech and cerebellar ataxia. A variety of abnormal, but not diagnostic, reflexes may be elicited including positive palmo-mental, pout, and Babinski reflexes, the last clearing implicating pyramidal system involvement. As well as the limb pain mentioned above, patients may complain of unpleasant hyperesthesia as well as anesthesia and paresthesia, and generalized pruritus.

2.2.3. Disturbances of Sleep Patterns

These are probably the most well-known of the features and indeed gave rise to the term "sleeping sickness." A variety of striking alterations of the normal sleep–wake cycle may occur. Typically, the patient at this stage of the illness has an uncontrollable desire to sleep, with the usual picture being excessive somnolence during the day with nocturnal insomnia (9,11). Episodes known as "narcoleptic crises" may occur in which the patient may exhibit an uncontrollable urge to sleep at any time or place (5,8). Because of the variability of the disordered sleep pattern, however, it can seldom be used as a diagnostic criterion (11).

In the final stage of the meningo-encephalitic illness, the sleep disturbances become more severe and virtually continuous. In the terminal phase of the CNS illness the patient develops seizures, double incontinence, excessive somnolence, sometimes florid psychiatric features such as mania, cerebral oedema, and finally coma leading to death (5,9,12). These features may well be exacerbated by the concomitant systemic features which will also contribute to the overall picture. Patients surviving late-stage HAT may still be left with a number of possible sequelae. These include a variety of neuropsychiatric syndromes such as cognitive impairment, depression, psychosis, and personality changes, and also neurological sequelae, which are particularly common in children, such as ataxia, hemiplegia, seizures, and movement disorders (5,13,14). While some of these improve or recover by 1 year after the illness, others may be permanent (5).

2.2.4. Post-treatment Reactive Encephalopathy

This is an extremely important drug-induced complication of HAT which may occur usually after the first course of melarsoprol treatment (see later under therapy). Once the CNS is invaded by the parasite the only available drug that can cross the blood–brain barrier is the arsenical melarsoprol, and its administration is followed by the post-treatment reactive encephalopathy (PTRE) in up to about 10% of cases, with a mortality rate of up to 10–50% (5,15). The onset of the PTRE may be gradual or sudden, with many of the features similar to untreated CNS HAT, including fever, seizures, confusion, agitation, cerebral oedema, and coma. The neuropathogenesis of this condition is discussed below.

2.3. Clinical Diagnosis and Differential Diagnosis

The diagnosis of HAT is based on a number of clinical and investigative criteria. Clearly, a critical factor is the geographical location, something which needs to be particularly noted in the case of Europeans becoming ill following a recent visit to a region of Africa where HAT is known to be endemic. Thus an obvious and important factor is to actually think of the possible diagnosis of HAT with a high index of suspicion. In African regions the presence of an existing HAT outbreak will also immediately point toward the likely diagnosis. Since the initial symptoms typical of early stage disease are non-specific, the diagnosis at this stage is often difficult to make. Even at the later stage when the CNS is involved, the diagnosis may not be easy. Most of the individual systemic and CNS features of HAT have their own wide differential diagnosis (5), so it is important to note the presence of the various systemic features which are present together with the CNS signs. When a constellation of typical signs are present together with excessive somnolence, the diagnosis becomes clearer.

One of the most important conditions that may be confused with HAT is malaria, and this is confounded by the frequent coexistence of these two diseases (5,8). Moreover, inappropriate treatment of HAT alone with anti-malarial drugs may actually reduce the patient's fever which will then produce a false sense of security and can lead to a cycle of confusion, and delay in correct diagnosis (5). Other conditions which may need to be considered in the differential diagnosis of HAT include TB meningitis, viral encephalitis, HIV infection of the CNS, fungal infections such as cryptococcal meningitis, toxoplasmosis, neurosyphilis, hookworm infection, cerebral lymphoma, typhoid and paratyphoid fever, tick typhus, brucellosis, relapsing fever, visceral leishmaniasis, and infectious mononucleosis (5). There is, at present, no particular disease which is known to be associated with HAT.

2.4. General Investigations

The general and specific non-neurological investigations in suspected HAT have been described elsewhere (5), and will not be detailed here. In brief, routine hematology and biochemistry is carried out to detect such factors as anemia, raised ESR, abnormal liver function, evidence of raised plasma kinins, evidence of DIC, immune complexes, and raised IgM levels, all of which may be seen in HAT.

There are also a variety of specific laboratory tests to diagnose HAT that have also been described in considerable detail elsewhere (5). They include different methods to directly demonstrate the parasite in the peripheral blood and bone marrow, tests to detect antibody to the trypanosome, e.g., by ELISA, methods of parasite antigen detection, e.g., ELISA, immunoassay, and more recently methods of trypanosome DNA detection (5). There is a need to develop a simple and reliable diagnostic test that could be used in field conditions.

2.5. Neurological Investigations

There are three types of neurological investigation that are used in the diagnosis of HAT, namely neuroradiology, electroencephalography (EEG), and cerebrospinal fluid (CSF) examination. While each will now be mentioned briefly, it should be appreciated that in many situations in the field, only CSF examination is likely to be available for diagnosis in field conditions.

2.5.1. Neuroradiology

To date there have not been any pathognonomic computerized tomographic (CT) or magnetic resonance imaging (MRI) features described in HAT. However, there are a few reports of radiological abnormalities in HAT (5,16), and clearly, neuroimaging should be carried out where it is available. Radiological abnormalities are more likely to be detectable at the later stages of the disease and include lesions in different regions of the brain such as white matter areas, basal nuclei and brainstem, cerebral edema, demyelination and ventricular enlargement following multiple treatment regimes (5). Serial CT or MRI also have a potential value in monitoring patients during and after therapy.

2.5.2. EEG Monitoring

While EEG abnormalities are not usually evident during the early hemolymphatic stage of HAT, during the meningo-encephalitic stage the EEG shows abnormalities which are not specific, but correlated with the severity of the CNS disease (5). The sleep–wake patterns characteristic of the disease are accompanied by various

EEG abnormalities, described in detail elsewhere (5,11,17). There are three main types of abnormal EEG patterns which may indicate the type of cerebral involvement which has occurred (5,18). Abnormalities described include, for example, the absence of transition changes during the initial phase of sleep, various types of high- and low-voltage delta wave activity, bursts of theta and alpha bursts, relative preservation of REM sleep, paroxysmal waves and sustained low voltage activity (5,11,17,18). Clinical improvement is accompanied by EEG normalization, and EEG is another way of monitoring the response to treatment.

2.5.3.   CSF Analysis

It is essential to perform a lumbar puncture to examine the CSF for the presence of trypanosomes during the meningo-encephalitic phase. If the parasites are detected then this is definite evidence of CNS involvement requiring treatment. At this stage there is typically a CSF lymphocytic pleocytosis of 10–1000/L with a moderately raised protein level of 40–200 mg/100 mL and a markedly elevated IgM level (5). The WHO criteria for diagnosing CNS involvement are the presence of trypanosomes in the CSF or a CSF WBC of >5/L. However, not all authorities would accept these criteria and the precise definition of CNS involvement in HAT remains controversial and is an active area of investigation. This is a crucial issue in view of the potentially severe side effects of drug treatment for CNS HAT (see below).

3.   CNS PATHOLOGY AND NEUROPATHOGENESIS OF HAT

3.1.   CNS Pathology of HAT

Several studies over many years have defined the most characteristic and consistent features of HAT and will be summarized briefly here. While, based on experimental studies, there is early trypanosome invasion of brain regions which lack the blood–brain or blood–nerve barrier (19), the parasites are not found in the brain parenchyma in patients who have died from the disease, although they may be found in systemic organs (20). At the macroscopic level, cerebral oedema, leptomeningitis, ependymitis, and occasionally brain herniation, and hydrocephalus can occur (20). The microscopic changes are those of a meningoencephalitis and are characterized by a diffuse perivascular and leptomeningeal inflammatory cell infiltration which occurs mainly in the white matter (20,21), and the pia and the arachnoid show marked cellular proliferation (5,21,22). The inflammatory infiltrates consist of lymphocytes, plasma cells, and macrophages. Two highly associated, but not pathognomonic, features of HAT are lymphophagocytosis and the presence in the white matter of morular or Mott cells which are probably modified plasma cells, containing large eosinophilic inclusions consisting of IgM (5,21). Both the perivascular cuffs and the surrounding brain parenchyma contain markedly activated astrocytes and microglial cells (20,23), and the inflammatory changes extend to the white matter of the cerebral hemispheres, periventricular regions, choroid plexus, cerebellum, brain stem and also the basal ganglia (20). There may also be evidence of tissue necrosis in periventricular regions (20). Despite the extensive involvement of white matter by the disease process, the degree of demyelination is minimal (21), although occasionally a diffuse white matter degeneration may develop (20). The pathological changes seen in the PTRE are mainly an exacerbation of the changes seen in CNS HAT described above, in particular the perivascular cuffs, cellular proliferation and infiltration of the brain parenchyma and astrocyte activation (5,24). There may, however, be additional features which are typical of an acute hemorrhagic leukocncephalopathy (24).

3.2. Neuropathogenesis of CNS HAT

Our knowledge of this subject has accrued from both human studies and experimental animal models of HAT. Specific findings have been correlated with particular features of the disease. For example, prostaglandin D_2 levels have been found to be elevated in the CSF in patients during the meningoencephalitic stage of HAT and may be related to both immunosuppression and somnolence (23). Tissue damage may be in part a consequence of polyclonal B-cell proliferation (25). The role of elevated endotoxin levels has also been described and may be of pathogenetic importance (26). Trypanosomes may also generate a variety of other toxins or biologically active substances in the CNS which could alter neuronal function. For example, products of trypanosome tryptophan metabolism may influence sleep patterns (20), and dead trypanosomes may release proteases, phospholipases, and free fatty acids which could produce deleterious effects on brain function (20). Regarding disordered immune function, in a rat model of HAT it was shown that various chemokines such as MIP-2, RANTES and MIP-1(are produced early during the CNS infection by astrocytes, microglia and T cells, and may be of immunopathological importance (27). It is likely that the astrocyte plays an important role in the generation of the CNS immune response in HAT as well as the PTRE, especially in view of the known astrocyte activation which occurs in the disease, and the ability of the astrocyte to present antigens and produce several cytokines (28,29) (see also below). It has also been shown in rat and mouse models of HAT that trypanosomes produce a molecule, known as trypanosome-derived lymphocyte triggering factor (TLTF), which triggers the $CD8^+$ T-cell to produce interferon (IFN)-(which has a growth-enhancing effect on trypanosomes (30,31). Moreover, increased levels of antibodies to IFN-(have been detected both in humans and in trypanosome-infected rats (32). Following trypanosome infection in rats, major histocompatability complex (MHC) class 1 antigens are induced in the neurons of the supraoptic nuclei and hypothalamic paraventricular nuclei (33) which may be of functional relevance.

The abnormalities of sleep–wake cycles seen in HAT have been modeled by Bentivoglio et al. in rats which have been shown to have disruption of the normal circadian rhythm with sleep dysregulation following experimental infection with trypanosomes (33). Melatonin and its agonist S-20,098 can restore the normal sleep rhythm in such trypanosome-infected animals (34). The suprachiasmatic nuclei (SCN) of the hypothalamus contain the circadian pacemaker for endogenous rhythms in mammals, and have therefore investigated in models of HAT. When rats were infected with Trypanosoma brucei (T. brucei), there was a selective decrease in glutamate receptor expression in the SCN of the animals, and the spontaneous neuronal activity of the SCN neurons was disrupted (35). Thus this experimental trypanosome infection provides a valuable model of the sleep disturbance in HAT. This dysregulation of the biological clock observed in these infected rats is associated with changes in gene expression in SCN neurons. Thus, c-fos expression was dramatically reduced in the SCN of trypanosome-infected rats after photic stimulation (36).

Considerable work has been carried out to establish the cause of the PTRE, mainly in animal models. This issue is of great importance in view of the very high mortality of this treatment complication. Mechanisms for the PTRE which have been proposed include immune complex deposition, autoimmunity, subcurative chemotherapy, immune responses against glial antigens released from dead parasites following chemotherapy, and direct arsenical toxicity (5,15,28). One or more or none of these possibilities may be important. We have investigated this question for over a decade in a reproducible mouse model of the PTRE which closely mirrors many of the neuropathological features of the human late-stage CNS disease (15). Intraperitoneal injection of T. brucei into mice leads to a chronic infection in which the parasites can be detected in the CNS at 21 days, and characteristic CNS histopathology is evident at a late stage of infection. The critical procedure in this model is the administration of the drug diminazene aceturate (berenil) 21–28 days after infection. Berenil cannot cross the blood–brain barrier and therefore clears the parasites from the extravascular compartments but not the CNS. The result of this treatment is the production of a post-treatment meningoencephalitis which persists after the disappearance of the parasitemia and mirrors the clinical and histopathological features of the PTRE in humans. If a second dose of berenil is given then the meningoencephalitis is even more severe.

A number of key observations have been made in this model, in particular regarding the modulation of the inflammatory reaction. It is established that the astrocyte plays a central role in the generation of the inflammatory response (15,29). Astrocytes become activated 14–21 days post-infection prior to the development of the CNS inflammatory response (29). Correlating with this onset of astrocyte activation is the appearance of several cytokines within the CNS including tumor necrosis factor (TNF)-(, IL-1, 1L-4, MIP-1 and occasionally IFN and IL-6 (37). It is likely that other cytokines will also be detected as new ones are identified and as molecular technology becomes more sensitive, but it is highly likely that astrocytes are the source of some of these cytokines. Other observations in this model include increased levels of acute phase proteins at the time of the PTRE (38), and the appearance of several autoantibodies against, e.g., myelin basic protein, galactocerebrosides, and gangliosides (39).

A number of drugs have been shown to modulate the PTRE in this mouse model. For example, the immunosuppressant drug azathiaprine can prevent the onset of the PTRE if given prior to the berenil treatment, but it is not effective in either altering the degree of astrocyte activation or treating an established PTRE (40). The drug eflornithine (DFMO) is of particular interest as it has been shown to be effective in the treatment of HAT in humans and may lead to a remarkable clinical improvement in seriously ill patients with HAT (41). It is very expensive and has only recently become widely available as a result of a public campaigns (42). DFMO is an ornithine decarboxylase inhibitor, is trypanostatic rather than trypanocidal, and its efficacy is dependent on an intact immune response (43). DFMO is able to prevent the establishment of the PTRE in this model, reduces the level of astrocyte activation, and also effectively ameliorates an established PTRE (43). More recently, we have shown that the non-peptide substance P (SP) antagonist, RP-67,580, can both significantly ameliorate the histopathological features of an established PTRE and reduce the level of astrocyte activation, thereby showing that SP plays a key role in the generation of the PTRE (44).

4. CONTROL AND TREATMENT OF HAT

The WHO report of 1986 (1) identified the two key principles of control of HAT which are first, the control of the parasite reservoir which includes both the active case detection and treatment of the disease in man, and secondly, the control of the vector, i.e., tsetse fly. Both these aspects will now be outlined.

4.1. Case Detection

Several aspects of case detection in humans using clinical and investigative methods have already been covered above in the discussion of the diagnosis of HAT and will not be reiterated here. A very detailed account of the principal techniques of parasite, parasitic antigen, and parasite DNA detection has also been given elsewhere (5). Nevertheless, it is clear from the previous discussion that for various reasons, case detection in HAT is currently suboptimal and improvements in early and reliable diagnosis of HAT, especially in field conditions, is a prerequisite for better control of the disease. In particular it is critical to have in place an integrated strategy of continuous surveillance of the susceptible human population (1,2). In recent times a major factor in significantly decreasing the level of case ascertainment and population surveillance has been political instability including war since this inevitably undermines the infrastructure required to achieve these aims. In order for surveillance to be effective it requires a massive increase in financial input and manpower in the affected countries. The result of successful active case detection and treatment of the disease will be to maintain HAT at low levels in the endemic areas and to control epidemics (1,2). The use of more sensitive and advanced techniques for detection than are currently available of parasites will be essential to realize this goal. Ideally, a diagnostic test for HAT should be inexpensive, rapid, robust, easy to carry out and allow effective decision support which will be based in large part on the high sensitivity of the test. Vaccination for HAT to prevent the disease is currently unlikely not only because of the major problem of antigenic variation seen in the disease, but also because of the very high cost of development and field testing of a vaccine (M. Murray, personal communication).

4.2. Specific Treatment of HAT

The main drugs for treatment of HAT and some general principles for future drug development will now be outlined briefly. The pharmacology and dose regimes of the main drugs used have recently been given in considerable detail elsewhere (5). It should be appreciated that the emphasis is on treatment of affected humans. Treatment of wild animal reservoirs with trypanocidal drugs as a control measure is not practical (1). However, treatment of domestic animals such as cattle is feasible (1) and indeed there is much current interest in this aspect of control of the disease.

Current available treatment for HAT is essentially based on the use of just a few drugs, namely suramin, pentamidine, berenil, melarsoprol , eflornithine and the nitrofurans such as nifurtimox (5). The side effects of some of these drugs are so severe that they would probably not be acceptable to current drug safety committees (45). All of these drugs, apart from Nifurtimox, have to be administered parenterally which is a longstanding and major problem, and even Nifurtimox, which is given orally, is poorly tolerated with a very high incidence of systemic and CNS side effects (5). To summarize typical treatment approaches, in early stage Trypanosoma rhodiense infection suramin is usually given for with berenil as an alternative, although the toxicity of the latter drug can be very severe and has not been fully evaluated in man (5). The fact that berenil is used in the mouse model to induce the PTRE adds to the concerns about using this drug in humans. Suramin is contraindicated in patients with renal disease and about one person in 20,000 develops a hypersensitivity to the drug (1). In early stage *Trypanosoma gambiense* infection, pentamidine is the drug of first choice although it also has an array of side effects (5). In late-stage disease when the CNS is involved melarsoprol is currently the first-line drug of choice and it is able to cross the blood–brain barrier. It can only be given intravenously and, as has been described above, it has the considerable drawback of producing the PTRE in up to 10% of cases. Various treatment regimes have been described. For example, in the Alupe treatment center of the Kenya Trypanosomiasis Research Institute (KETRI), four courses of three injections per week are given, and following the final course the CSF is examined to check for parasite clearance from the CNS. After discharge the patient is followed up at 3 monthly intervals with repeat CSF examinations on each occasion if practical. If the patient is well and the CSF is clear of parasites at 2 years after the disease then the patient is considered cured (46). Relapses may nevertheless occur which will require further courses of melarsoprol. However, other units will use different melarsoprol regimes such as that described by Burri et al. (47). If the PTRE develops during treatment then the melarsoprol injections are temporarily discontinued, seizures are treated with anti-convulsants, the patient given general medical support, and steroids for cerebral edema have been used by some physicians (5) although there is no current consensus on the use of steroids either prophylactically to prevent the PTRE or therapeutically during the episode (5). In the author's opinion steroids should be given during the acute PTRE.

Eflornithine has been used as a second choice drug for patients with late stage, i.e., CNS disease who relapse after melarsoprol treatments (5), and it has been shown to be particularly effective in the treatment of melarsoprol-refractory *Trypanosoma gambiense* disease (41). The history of this drug is remarkable. After it was shown in the 1980s to be effective in treating West African HAT it subsequently became an "orphan drug" in 1990 as a result of economic, pharmaceutical, and political factors (41). The drug, though effective, was both expensive and non-profitable. However, the organization Medecins Sans Frontieres and WHO, working together with the drug companies Aventis Pharma and Bristol-Myers, spearheaded a new interest in the drug (42). Currently, because of these admirable efforts, several million doses of DFMO have been made available for treatment of patients with HAT. It will be recalled that eflornithine was also highly effective in preventing and treating experimental PTRE in the mouse model. While the nitrofurans have also been used to treat melarsoprol relapses, as has been mentioned they have severe side effects and the standard and most effective treatment protocols with this drug have not been extensively evaluated (5).

There are several potential future directions for drug development in HAT, which are not necessarily mutually exclusive. For example, there is a pressing need to develop new and more effective drugs, in particular a drug which can be given orally early in the disease analogous to the situation which pertains in malaria. Affected individuals in remote rural areas could thereby start a course of oral treatment early on to prevent disease progression. New drug regimens for existing drugs may also be valuable as has recently been described with melarsoprol (47). The use of new drug combinations has particular promise, e.g., the combined use of eflornithine and melarsoprol (48), and there are various other potentially efficacious combinations (49). Indeed, it is possible that a more effective and imaginative use of the existing drugs for HAT may be in the short term almost as important as the development of new drugs for the disease, in part because of the massive cost of developing and testing new drugs. The development of new drug formulations is also a potential avenue for advance in this field such as has been shown with a topical melarsoprol gel in experimental mouse HAT (50). While it is very difficult to conceive of the latter as first-line therapy in humans, nevertheless it might have some role as adjunct therapy in the future. Finally, a new approach would be to combine melarsoprol with a drug or drugs which can target specific inflammatory responses in CNS. An example might be the use of humanized antagonists to the neuropeptide SP which has been noted above to play a role in the generation of the inflammatory CNS response in the mouse model of the PTRE.

4.3. Vector Control

The key element of control of the parasite vector (i.e., the testse fly) is to significantly reduce the level of man-fly contact (1,2,51). In brief, the methods used to achieve this aim have included: (a) ground application of insecticides, e.g., with DDT to kill the flies in their resting sites (1); (b) aerial spraying of tsetse-infested vegetation and drainage sites from fixed-wing aircraft and helicopters which generally has only a limited efficacy in control (1). While this expensive method can under some circumstances be effective in controlling tsetse fly populations in specific areas of land, it is seldom used at present because of its perceived environmental side effects (M. Murray. personal communication); (c) insecticide-impregnated fly traps baited with synthetic host odors with many different configurations have been used in several African countries (1). For example, in the Nguruman Field Station of KETRI located on a Maasai ranch in Kenya a distribution of four fly traps per square km has been found to be effective in reducing the local tsetse population (J. Ndung'u , personal communication), and increasingly sophisticated traps should lead to improved tsetse control; and (d) incorporating infrastructural changes, which may be quite simple, to villages in rural areas. For example, the installation of a well in the center of a village may obviate the need for the local population to walk through heavily tsetse-infected areas, e.g., bushes, near their homes in order to gain access to a nearby river to obtain water. Such a simple measure could reduce the incidence of HAT in a village population. There is a clear and pressing need for massive investment in both personnel, including training, and infrastructure to achieve a significant reduction in man-fly contact throughout Africa, and this will also require large scale and adequately funded programs which will need to be well coordinated, long term and integrated with the existing infrastructure and government Institutions. An ultimate goal would be the total eradication of the tsetse fly in Africa, but this is perceived as unrealistic by many experts.

ACKNOWLEDGMENTS

I wish to thank Professor Max Murray for critical reading of the manuscript and for very helpful discussions. Personal research work refereed to here was carried out with the financial support of the Jules Thorn Charitable Trust and the Wellcome Trust.

REFERENCES

1. World Health Organization. Epidemiology and control of African trypanosomiasis. Rep WHO Expert Committee Tech Rep Ser 1986; 739:1–125.
2. Kuzoe FA. Current situation of African trypanosomiasis. Acta Tropica 1993; 54(3/4):153–162.
3. Williams BI. African Trypanosomiasis. In: Cox FEAG, ed. The Wellcome Trust Illustrated History of Tropical Diseases. London: The Wellcome Trust, 1996:178–191.
4. Schieppati A, Remuzzi S, Garattini S. Modulating the profit motive to meet needs of the less-developed world. Lancet 2001; 358:1638–1641.
5. Atouguia JLM, Kennedy PGE. Neurological aspects of human African trypanosomiasis. In: Davis LE, Kennedy PGE, eds. Infectious Diseases of the Nervous System. Oxford: Butterworth-Heinemann, 2000; 11:321–372.
6. Cruz Ferreira, F. Tripanossomíase africana. In: Epidemiologia e profilaxia das doenças infecciosas e parasitárias. Lisboa: Junta de Investigação do Ultramar, 1973:361–380.
7. Apted FIC. Clinical manifestations and diagnosis of sleeping sickness. In: Mulligan HW, ed. The African Trypanosomiases. London: George Allen & Unwin, 1970:661–683.
8. Duggan AJ, Hutchington MP. Sleeping sickness in Europeans: a review of 109 cases. J Trop Med Hyg 1966; 69:124–131.
9. Antoine Ph. Étude neurologique et psychologique de malades trypanosomés et leur evolution. Annales de la Société Belge de Médicine Tropicale 1977; 57(4/5):227–247.
10. Dutertre J. La trypanosomiase humaine africaine. I. Generalités—Historique. Médicine d'Afrique Noire 1968; 4:147–157.
11. Kristensson K, Grassi-Zucconi G, Bentivoglio M. Nervous system dysfunctions in African trypanosomiasis. In: Clifford Rose F, ed. Recent Advances in Tropical Neurology. Amsterdam: Elsevier Science BV, 1995:165–174.
12. Giordano C. Les signes neurologiques et électro-encephalographiques de la trypanosomiase humaine africaine. Médicine d'Afrique Noire 1973; 20(4):317–324.
13. Kazumba M., Kazadi K, Mulumba MP. Caracteristiques de la trypanosomiase de l'enfant. A propos de 19 observations effectuées au CNPP, Cliniques Universitaires de Kinshasa, Zaire. Annales de la Société Belge de Médicine Tropicale 1993; 73:253–259.
14. Collomb H, Miletto G. Les séquelles de la trypanosomiase humaine africaine. Bulletin de la Société de Pathologie Exotique 1957; 50:573–585.
15. Kennedy PGE. The pathogenesis and modulation of the post-treatment reactive encephalopathy in a mouse model of human African trypanosomiasis. J Neuroimmunol 1999; 100:36–41.
16. Sabbah P, Brosset C, Imbert P. et al. Human African trypanosomiasis: MRI. Neuroradiology 1997; 39(10):708–710.
17. Tapie P, Buguet A, Tabaraud F. et al. Electroencephalographic and polygraphic features of 24-hour recordings in sleeping sickness and healthy African subjects. J Clin Neurophysiol 1996; 13(4):339–344.
18. Hamon JF, Camara P, Gauthier P. et al. Waking electroencephalograms in the blood-lymph and encephalitic stages of Gambian trypanosomiasis. Ann Trop Med Parasitol 1993; 87(2):149–155.

19. Schultzberg M, Ambatsis M, Samuelsson E-B, Kristensson K, van Meirvenne N. Spread of the Trypanosoma brucei to the nervous system: early attack on circumventricular organs and sensory ganglia. J Neurosci Res 1988; 21:56–61.

20. Kristensson K, Bentivoglio M. Pathology of African trypanosomiasis. In: Dumas M, Bouteille B, Buguet A, eds. Progress in Human African Trypanosomiasis, Sleeping Sickness. Springer, 157–181.

21. Cook GC. Protozoan and helminthic infections. In: Lambert HP, ed. Infections of the Central Nervous System. Philadelphia: BC Decker Inc., 1991:264–282.

22. Van Bogaert L, Janssen P. Contribuition à létude de la neurologie et neuropathologie de la trypanosomiase humaine. Annales de la Société Belge de Médicine Tropicale 1957; 37:379–412.

23. Pentreath VW. Neurobiology of sleeping sickness. Parasitol Today 1989; 5(7):215–218.

24. Adams JH, Haller L, Boa FY et al. Human African trypanosomiasis (T. b. gambiense): a study of 16 fatal cases of sleeping sickness with some observations on acute reactive arsenical encephalopathy. Neuropathol Appl Neurobiol 1986; 12:81–94.

25. Greenwood BM, Whittle HC. The pathogenesis of sleeping sickness. Trans R Soc Trop Med Hyg 1980; 74:716–725.

26. Pentreath VW, Alafiatayo RA, Crawley B, et al. (1996) Endotoxins in the blood and cerebrospinal fluid of patients with African sleeping sickness. Parasitology 1996; 112:67–73.

27. Sharafeldin A, Eltayeb R, Pashendov M, Bakhiet M. Chemokines are produced in the brain early during the course of experimental African trypanosomiasis. J Neuroimmunol 2000; 103:165–170.

28. Hunter CA, Kennedy PGE. Immunopathology in central nervous system human African trypanosomiasis. Neuroimmunology 1992; 36:91–95.

29. Hunter CA, Jennings FW, Kennedy PGE, Murray M. Astrocyte activation correlates with cytokine production in central nervous system of Trypanosoma brucei brucei-infected mice. Lab Invest 1992; 67:635–642.

30. Olsson T, Bakhiet M, Hojeberg B, Ljungdahl A, Edlund C, Andersson G, Ekre H-P, Fung-Leung W-P, Mak T, Wigzell H, Fiszer U, Kristensson K. VD8 is critically involved in lymphocyte activation by a T. brucei brucei-released molecule. Cell 1993; 72:715–727.

31. Vaidya T, Bakhiet M, Hill KL, Olsson T, Kristennson K, Donelson JE. The gene for a T lymphocyte triggering factor from African trypanosomes. J Exp Med 1997; 186:433–438.

32. Bonfanti C, Caruso A, Bakhiet M, Olsson T, Turano A, Kristensson K. Increased levels of antibodies to IFN-y in human and experimental African trypanosomiasis. Scand J Immunol 1995; 41:49–52.

33. Bentivoglio M, Grassi-Zucconi G, Olsson T, Kristennson K. Trypanosoma brucei and the nervous system. TINS 1994; 17:325–329.

34. Grassi-Zucconi G, Semprevivo M, Mocaer E, Kristensson K, Bentivoglio M. Melatonin and its new agonist S-20098 restore synchronized sleep fragmented by experimental trypanosome infection in the rat. Brain Res Bull 1996; 39:63–68.

35. Lundkvist GB, Christenson J, Eltayeb RAK, Peng Z-C, Grillner P, Mhlanga J, Bentivoglio M, Kristensson K. Altered neuronal activity rhythm and glutamate receptor expression in the suprachiasmatic nuclei of Trypanosoma brucei-infected rats. J Neuropathol Exp Neurol 1998; 57:21–29.

36. Peng Z-C, Kristensson K, Bentivoglio M. Dysregulation of photic induction of Fos-related protein in the biological clock during experimental trypanosomiasis. Neurosci Lett 1994; 182:104–106.
37. Hunter CA, Gow JW, Kennedy PGE, Jennings FW, Murray M. Immunopathology of experimental African sleeping sickness: detection of cytokine mRNA in the brains of Trypanosoma brucei brucei-infected mice. Infect Immun 1991; 59:4636–4640.
38. Eckersall PD, Gow JW, McComb C, Bradley B, Rodgers J, Murray M, Kennedy PGE. Cytokines and the acute phase response in post-treatment reactive encephalopathy of Trypanosoma brucei brucei-infected mice. Parasitol Int 2001; 50:15–26.
39. Hunter CA, Jennings FW, Tierney JF, Murray M, Kennedy PGE. Correlation of autoantibody titres with central nervous system pathology in experimental African trypanosomiasis. J Neuroimmunol 1992; 41:143–148.
40. Hunter CA, Jennings FW, Kennedy PGE, Murray M. The use of azathioprine to ameliorate post-treatment encephalopathy associated with African trypanosomiasis. Neuropathol Appl Neurobiol 1992; 18:619–625.
41. Sjoerdsma A, Schechter PJ. Eflornithine for African sleeping sickness. Lancet 1999; 354:254.
42. Kennedy PGE, Murray M, Jennings F, Rodgers J. Sleeping sickness: new drugs for old? Lancet 2002; 359:1695–1696.
43. Jennings FW, Gichuki CW, Kennedy PGE, Rodgers J, Hunter CA, Murray M, Burke JM. The role of polyamine inhibitor eflornithine in the neuropathogenesis of experimental murine African trypanosomiasis. Neuropathol Appl Neurobiol 1997; 23:225–234.
44. Kennedy PGE, Rodgers J, Jennings FW, Murray M, Leeman SE, Burke JM. A substance P antagonist, RP-67,580, ameliorates a mouse meningoencephalitic response to Trypanosoma brucei brucei. Proc Natl Acad Sci U S A 1997; 94:4167–4170.
45. Fairlamb AH. Future prospects for the chemotherapy of human trypanosomiasis. 1. Novel approaches to the chemotherapy of trypanosomiasis. Trans R Soc Trop Med Hyg 1990; 84:613–617.
46. Kennedy PGE. Human African trypanosomiasis (sleeping sickness). A neurologist's perspective. Bull R Coll Phys Surgs Glas 1999; 28:21–25.
47. Burri C, Nkunku S, Merolle A, Smith T, Blum J, Brun R. Efficacy of a new, concise schedule for melarsoprol in treatment of sleeping sickness caused by Trypanosoma brucei gambiense: a randomised trial. Lancet 2000; 355:1419–1425.
48. Simarro PP, Asumu PN. Gambian trypanosomiasis and synergism between melarsoprol and eflornithine: first case report. Trans R Trop Med Hyg Soc 1996; 90:315.
49. Jennings FW, Rodgers J, Bradley B, Gettinby G, Kennedy PGE, Murray M. Human African trypanosomiasis: potential therapeutic benefits of an alternative suramin and melarsoprol regimen. Parasitol Int 2002; 51:381–388.
50. Atouguia JM, Jennings FW, Murray M. Successful treatment of experimental murine Trypanosoma brucei infection with topical melarsoprol gel. Trans R Soc Trop Med Hyg 1995; 89:531–533.
51. Willett KC. Some principles of the epidemiology of human trypanosomiasis in Africa. Bull World Health Organ 1963; 28:645–652.

12

Enterovirus 71 Encephalitis

Chao-Ching Huang

Department of Pediatrics, National Cheng Kung University Hospital, Tainan City, Taiwan

Ying-Chao Chang

Department of Pediatrics, Chang Gung Children's Hospital, Kaohsiung, Taiwan

Cheng-Yu Chen

Department of Radiology, Tri-Service General Hospital and National Defense Medical Center, Taipei, Taiwan

1. INTRODUCTION

The enteroviruses include coxsackievirus group A and B, poliovirus, echovirus, and enteroviruses 68–71. Spread by the fecal–oral or oral–oral transmission, the non-polio enteroviruses, coxsackieviruses, and echoviruses produce several distinct syndromes, including pharyngitis, herpangina, hand-foot-and-mouth disease (HFMD), neonatal sepsis, myocarditis, pericarditis, chronic infections among persons with compromised immune systems, and a variety of neurologic disorders (1,2). The spectrum of neurologic complications caused by enteroviruses includes aseptic meningitis, acute ataxia, opso-clonus–myoclonus, encephalitis, polio-like syndrome, and Guillain–Barré syndrome (2). Enteroviral meningoencephalitis generally has a good prognosis, except when the cause is enterovirus 71 (EV71), in which case there is a substantial mortality rate (1,2).

2. EPIDEMIOLOGY

Since its first identification in 1969, EV71 infection has been found in several parts of the world, either sporadically or in epidemics (1,3–14). EV71, like coxsackievirus A16, is one of the two common causes of epidemic HFMD, and young children are most commonly affected. The HFMD is characterized by several days of fever and vomiting, and ulcerative lesions of the buccal mucosa, tongue and palate, and vesicular lesions on the surfaces of the palms and soles (1). The epidemic seasons of EV71 are in the summer and fall. Although the initial viral illness is self-limited, it is sometimes followed by aseptic meningitis, meningoencephalitis, or even acute flaccid paralysis (AFP) similar to that caused by poliovirus (1,10).

Aseptic meningitis was the commonest manifestation in early EV71 outbreaks before 1975, and serious central nervous system (CNS) complications were uncommon in the outbreak in New York, Sweden, Japan, and Australia (9,11–14). However, since 1975 there are at least four major EV71 outbreaks resulting in rapid clinical deterioration and death among young children. In the 1975 Bulgarian epidemic, 77% of patients had aseptic meningitis, 7.4% had a poliomyelitis-like syndrome, and 9.6% had bulbar meningoencephalitis, but none had HFMD (5). In the Hungarian epidemic in 1978, fever, HFMD and acute neurologic complications including aseptic meningitis, encephalitis and poliomyelitis-like paralysis were reported, and 47 patients had died (6). The 1997 outbreak in Peninsular Malaysia affected thousands of young children. This outbreak involved children who had febrile illness and HFMD followed by rapid clinical deterioration (7). Malaysian autopsy report showed that the extensive destruction of the important vital centers located in the lower brainstem was responsible for the rapid cardiopulmonary collapse in the affected young children. In 1998, the largest and most severe EV71 and HFMD epidemic to date occurred in Taiwan, which affected 129,106 cases. Among the 405 children hospitalized with acute neurologic diseases, 78 (19%) died of rapid clinical deterioration (1,10). The Taiwan EV71 fatal outbreak even continues through 2003 although at a smaller scale. The Taiwan epidemic is unique in its potential fatality. Most of those who died were young children, and the majority died of brainstem encephalitis and acute cardiopulmonary collapse within hours after admission. The outbreaks of EV71-associated neurologic diseases or fatality also occurred in Western Australia in 1999, in Japan and Singapore in 2000 (15–17).

Studies using neutralization tests for antibody against EV71 in all the age groups had shown that the incidence of EV71 infection during the Taiwan 1998 epidemic was 13–22%, with higher rates in younger children (18,19). The EV71 seroprevalence rate in children aged 6 months to 2 years was <10%, which is in contrast to that in other older children (22% in children aged 2–3 years, 36% in aged 3–6 years, 63% in aged 6–12 years, and 66% in aged 12–19 years). The age-specific pre-epidemic EV71 seroprevalence rates inversely correlated with age-specific EV71-related mortality rates. Higher post-epidemic EV71 seropositive rates among children who were younger than 3 years positively correlated with their higher mortality rates. The case-fatality rate was highest (96.96 per 100,000) in infants aged 6–11 months. Seroepidemiological studies suggest that children aged from 0.5 to 4 years old are most susceptible while the rest of the population are over 50% immune. The lack of protective antibody in younger children may account for the high incidence and high case-fatality rate in this age group (18,19).

3. NEUROLOGIC COMPLICATIONS AND MR IMAGING CORRELATES

The clinical spectrum of complications during acute EV71 infection is summarized in Table 1. Most patients with EV71-related HFMD/herpangina in this Taiwan epidemic have experienced various degrees of myoclonic jerks, especially at sleep. However, most recover without progression into neurological complications, and they usually have normal findings in cerebrospinal fluid (CSF).

3.1. Prodrome

EV71 infection usually has a biphasic course in those who develop neurologic complications: a prodrome of HFMD or herpangina, vomiting, poor feeding and fever lasted an average of 3 days, followed by neurologic manifestations. The mean age at the disease onset of EV71-related neurologic complication is 2.5 years. The highest incidence is among children who are aged 1–2 years, and 90% are 5 years of age or younger. During acute infection, EV71 is most commonly isolated from throat swab (60%), and less often from rectal swabs or vesicular fluids (40%). EV71 virus can rarely (0–2%) be isolated from CSF (1).

3.2. Neurologic Syndromes

Neurologic disorders begin 2 to 5 days after the onset of skin or mucosal lesions or fever. Three major neurologic syndromes are recognized based on the extent of neurologic involvement during the Taiwan EV71 epidemic: (1) aseptic meningitis (7%), (2) AFP (10%), and (3) brainstem encephalitis (90%). The mean ($\pm$SD) white-cell counts in CSF were $33 \pm 15/mm^3$ among patients with aseptic meningitis, $151 \pm 174/mm^3$ among those with AFP, and $194 \pm 185/mm^3$ among those with brainstem encephalitis. There was no significant difference in white-cell counts or levels of glucose, protein, and lactate in CSF among the three groups (1).

Table 1   The Clinical Spectrum of Complications During Enterovirus 71 Infection

Clinical manifestations	Involvement	Sequelae
HFMD/herpangina only	Skin, mucosan	None
HFMD/herpangina with myoclonus only	Skin, mucosa	None
HFMD/herpangina, aseptic meningitis	Skin, mucosa, meninges	None
HFMD/herpangina, acute flaccid paralysis of the upper or lower extremities	Skin, mucosa, anterior horns of spinal cord	Most have complete recovery, some are left with limb paresis
HFMD/herpangina, grade I brainstem encephalitis: mycoclonic jerks with tremor, ataxia, or both	Skin, mucosa, dorsal tegmentum of brain stem	None
HFMD/herpangina, grade II$_A$ brainstem encephalitis: myoclonus with ocular conjugation disturbance	Skin, mucosa, dorsal tegmentum of brain stem	None
HFMD/herpangina, grade III$_B$ brainstem encephalitis: myoclonus with ocular conjugation disturbance, bulbar palsy, and facial weakness	Skin, mucosa, dorsal stegmentum of brain stem extending to medulla oblongata	Many have bulbar palsy, and ataxic gait
HFMD/herpangina, grade III brainstem encephalitis: transient myoclonus, gaze abnormalities followed by rapid onset of pulmonary edema, cardiovascular dysfunction, cyanosis, shock, coma, loss of doll's eye sign, and apnea	Skin, mucosa, extensive brain stem involvement triggering systematic neurogenic inflammatory response	Most have acute fatality or neurologic disability such as long-term bulbar palsy, ventilator-dependent apnea, and spastic paresis
HFMD: hand-foot-and-mouth disease; brainstem encephalitis may also be complicated with acute flaccid paralysis		

3.2.1. Aseptic Meningitis

In contrast to the high incidence of aseptic meningitis in the 1975 Bulgaria epidemic, only a smaller percentage (<10%) of patients in this Taiwan epidemic have signs of aseptic meningitis, such as headache, vomiting, fever, and neck stiffness. All recovered within 5 days of admission. None had neurologic sequelae at follow up.

3.2.2. Acute Flaccid Paralysis

EV71 infection has become the important causes of poliomyelitis-like paralysis in several outbreaks worldwide since 1975, and EV71 is now considered one of the leading causes of AFP after the worldwide eradication of poliomyelitis (1). Cases of AFP with encephalomyelitis have been mentioned in several EV71 epidemics, with varying rates of incidence reported: 2% in Japan (1973), 21% in Bulgaria (1975), 17% in New York (1977), 4% in Hungary (1978), 9% in the United States (1985–1989), 58% in Brazil (1988–1990), 10% in Taiwan (1998), and 14% in Western Australia (1999) (1,4–6,8,9,12–15,20). Both EV71 and poliovirus infections affect mainly young children and clinically are very similar in the presentations of AFP or brainstem involvement (1,2). However, in contrast to the poliovirus infection, most patients with AFP in this Taiwan EV71 epidemic have HFMD or herpangina.

The MR studies in seven young children with EV71-related AFP of extremities showed unilateral or bilateral hyperintense lesions in the anterior horn regions of the spinal cord on T2-weighted images in six patients (Fig. 1A,B) (21). Two of three patients who received intravenous injections of contrast material had ventral root enhancement on T1-weighted images. One of them also had enhancement of the unilateral anterior horn cells. At follow-up, both patients with bilateral anterior horn abnormalities had residual motor weakness, whereas only one of the five patients with unilateral involvement had residual weakness. The MR study demonstrated that EV71-related radiculomyelitis tends to be unilateral and to specifically involve both the anterior horn of the cord and the ventral roots. The AFP is most likely reversible if it is unilateral, however, patients with bilateral flaccid paralysis and documented bilateral anterior horn lesions may have a less favorable outcome. MR imaging can allow early detection of spinal cord and root lesions in patients with EV71-related AFP (21).

Clinical manifestations of transverse myelitis of rapid onset of flaccid quadriparesis has been reported in two of the 14 patients with EV71-related neurological diseases from the 1999 epidemic in Western Australia (15). MR studies revealed a diffuse flame-shaped signal abnormality localized in the dorsal columns of the cervical cord in one patient, and a diffusely swelling lesion extending from lower medulla to the thoracic cord in the other patient. At 1 year of follow up, both patients had spastic quadriparesis, and one was ventilator-dependent.

3.2.3. Brainstem Encephalitis

Brainstem encephalitis (rhombencephalitis) is the main cause of EV71 epidemics with acute fatality in four countries: 1975 Bulgaria, 1978 Hungary, 1997 Malaysia, and 1998 Taiwan. The fatality rate of EV71-related brainstem encephalitis is 14% in the 1998 Taiwan epidemic.

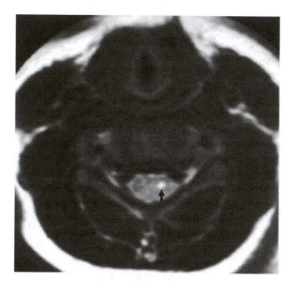

Figure 1A Acute flaccid monoplegia during EV71 infection in two patients who were completely recovered from the paresis at follow up. An axial fast short tau inversion recovery (STIR) MR image shows a high signal lesion (arrow) in the left anterior horn region of the cervical cord in a 1-year-old girl with left upper arm paresis.

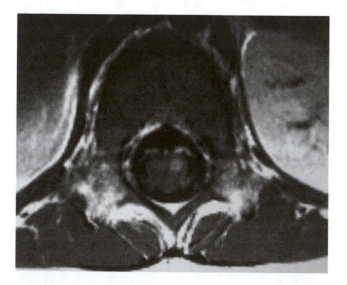

Figure 1B Acute flaccid monoplegia during EV71 infection in two patients who were completely recovered from the paresis at follow up. Contrast-enhanced axial T1-weighted image shows enhancement in the left anterior horn area and left ventral root of the lumbar cord in a 2-year-old boy who had left lower limb paresis.

In the study on 37 patients with brainstem encephalitis in southern Taiwan, 86% had myoclonus with a severity ranging from mild sleep myoclonic jerks to frequent sleeping and waking hours myoclonus, and 62% had tremor, ataxia, or both (1). The severity of brainstem encephalitis also varied. Twenty patients (54%) had grade I brainstem encephalitis, defined as generalized myoclonic jerks with tremor, ataxia, or both. Ten patients (27%) had grade II brainstem encephalitis, defined as myoclonus with cranial-nerve involvement, including ocular disturbances in nine patients (nystagmus, strabismus, or gaze paresis), and bulbar palsy in one (dysphagia, dysarthria, dysphonia, and facial weakness). Seven patients (19%) had grade III brainstem encephalitis, defined as transient myoclonus followed by the rapid onset of respiratory distress, cyanosis, poor peripheral perfusion, shock, coma, loss of the doll's eye reflex, and apnea. All seven patients with grade III brainstem encephalitis required mechanical ventilation and cardiopulmonary support immediately after admission because of fulminant neurogenic pulmonary edema or hemorrhage, and five died within 12 hr after admission. Many of the patients in grade III disease had copious pink frothy secretions noted at endotracheal intubation. Hyporeflexia or areflexia was found in 12 patients, transient visual hallucination or panic expression was noted in four, and acute transient urinary retention found in three. The frequency of hyperventilation or Cheyne–Stokes respiration, increased with the severity of brainstem encephalitis: 30% in grade II, and 86% in grade III brainstem encephalitis. A chest x-ray film revealed no lung abnormalities in patients with grade I or grade II brainstem encephalitis, whereas all except one patient with grade III brainstem encephalitis had diffuse bilateral pulmonary edema. The mean CSF lactate level was significantly higher in patients with grade III disease (12.2 ± 12.6 mmol/L) than in those with grade I disease (2.1 ± 0.8 mmol/L) or grade II disease (2.2 ± 0.6 mmol/L) (all $P < 0.001$).

Seventy percent of the patients with EV71 brainstem encephalitis who underwent MR examinations showed lesions of high signal intensity in the brainstem on T2-weighted images (Fig. 2A–C). T2-weighted hyperintense lesions extending from the midbrain to the medulla oblongata, and sometimes abnormal enhancement in the dorsal tegmentum of the brainstem on T1-weighted images after contrast medium administration can be demonstrated in patients with grade III brainstem encephalitis with pulmonary edema (Fig. 3A,B). The most common brainstem lesions are in the pontine tegmentum (72%), followed by the medulla oblongata (55%), midbrain (44%), and dentate nuclei (22%) (1). The frequency of brainstem abnormalities on MR images increase with increasing severity of brainstem encephalitis: 46% among patients with grade I disease vs. 100% among those with grade II or grade III disease (1). Except for the patient who had bulbar palsy and grade II brainstem encephalitis, no obvious difference was found in the extent of MR brainstem lesions between patients with grade I and those with grade II brainstem encephalitis. Patients with grade III disease tend to have brainstem lesions extending to the basis pontis and the whole medulla oblongata. The high sig-

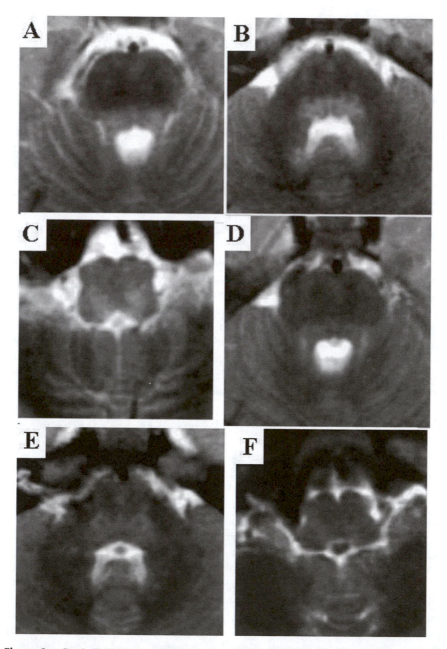

Figure 2 Grade II EV71 brainstem encephalitis in a 3-year-old girl. (A–C) T2-weighted MRI obtained at acute stage showed increased signal intensity of the tegmentum of the isthmus pontis, pons, and medulla oblongata. (D–F) A follow-up MRI 6 months later when the girl was recovered from the illness revealed complete disappearance of the high signal abnormalities in the brainstem.

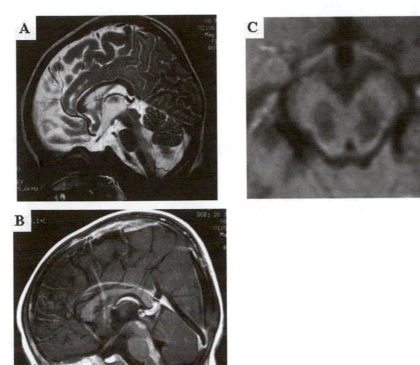

Figure 3   Grade III EV71 brainstem encephalitis and pulmonary edema in a 2-year-old boy with ventilator-dependent apnea. At acute stage: (A) The brainstem lesions are of hyperintense extending from the midbrain to the medulla oblongata best demonstrated on this sagittal T2-weighted image. (B) The high signal abnormalities in the tegmentum of the brainstem are enhanced with intravenous injection of gadolinium on this sagittal T1-weighted image. At chronic stage: (C) Axial T1-weighted image at the level of midbrain obtained 2 months after acute brainstem encephalitis shows hypointense cavitary lesions.

nals T2-weighted lesions as demonstrated on MR images in patients with grade I disease or grade II disease without bulbar palsy are reversible, as complete normal findings can be found on follow-up imaging performed months after disease onset (Fig. 2D,F). However, patients with chronic grade III brainstem encephalitis had brainstem atrophy and cavitation that extended from the tegmentum of the midbrain (Fig. 3C) to the lower medulla oblongata and upper cervical cord (1,22). These MR studies strongly suggest that the characteristic features of brainstem and spinal cord involvement during EV71 infection can be diagnostic of enteroviral encephalomyelitis (23).

3.2.4.   Other Neurologic Syndromes

Few patients were reported to develop Guillain–Barré syndrome or opso-
clonus–myoclonus syndrome without CSF pleocytosis 3–4 weeks after onset of
EV71 (15). These findings suggest the potential immune-mediated mechanisms
in the pathogenesis of some EV71-associated neurologic diseases.

4.   ASSOCIATED COMPLICATIONS: ACUTE CARDIOPULMONARY
DYSFUNCTION

4.1.   Pulmonary Edema

A distinctive, severe phenotype of EV71 infection affects young children, and is
characterized by a prodrome of HFMD, followed by acute pulmonary edema,
brainstem encephalitis, and AFP. Of the 78 patients who died in the Taiwan epidemic, 65 cases (83%) had pulmonary edema. Most of these patients died of a
fulminant course within 1–2 days after admission (1). There was a significant association between severe brainstem involvement and pulmonary edema. In a study
including 154 children with EV71 infection 11 patients was found to have pulmonary edema (24). All the 11 patients with pulmonary edema had sudden appear-
ances of tachypnea, tachycardia (135–250 beats/min), and cyanosis 1–3 days after
disease onset. Their arterial blood gas all showed hypoxia with metabolic acidosis. The risk factors for developing pulmonary edema included hyperglycemia,
leukocytosis, and upper limb weakness, with hyperglycemia the most significant
prognostic factor. Chest radiographs after endotracheal intubation all showed diffuse and bilateral alveolar density without cardiomegaly (Fig. 4), and became
completely whiteout within 12 hr in eight of the 11 patients. After intubation, all
had copious and pink frothy fluid secreted from the airway. Progressive shock and
hypoxia, oliguria or anuria, tachycardia and decreased consciousness developed in
all the 11 patients, and all of them died. Postmortem MR imaging showed hyperintensity of brainstem and spinal cord, with most severe involvement extending
from the midbrain to upper cervical spinal cord on T2-weighted images.

4.2.   Cardiovascular Dysfunction

Left ventricular dysfunction with ejection fraction of 27–56% is a frequent finding
during acute stage in young children with EV71 infection and pulmonary edema. Of
the 24 fatal cases reported in Sarawak, Malaysia, all had left ventricular dysfunction,
and 17 had pulmonary edema. Cardiac tissue from 10 patients showed normal
myocardium, but CNS tissue from five patients had inflammatory changes (25).
    Detailed hemodynamic study determined by implanted pulmonary arterial
and central venous catheters was reported in one study from five patients during

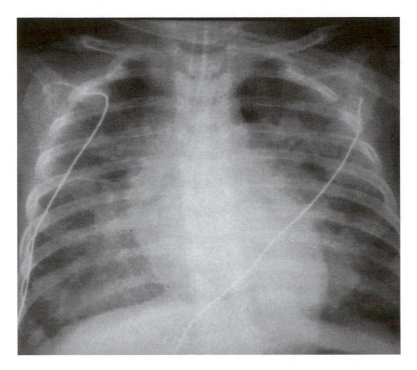

Figure 4 Chest radiographs in a young boy with grade III brainstem encephalitis shows bilateral alveolar pulmonary edema without cardiomegaly.

acute stage of EV71 brainstem encephalitis and pulmonary edema (26). Transient systolic hypertension was noted only in one patient, and hypotension presented in another. Their serum CK-MB/CK ratios were within normal range. All five patients had normal or mildly elevated pulmonary artery pressure and pulmonary artery occlusion pressure, and their central venous pressure ranged from 10 to 22 mmHg. Systemic and pulmonary vascular resistances were transiently increased in only one patient. The stroke volume index decreased to 15.3–35.7 mL/M² (normal: 30–60 mL/M²), but because of the elevated heart rate, the cardiac index did not decrease. All hemodynamic and cardiopulmonary function became normalized within days, but the neurologic sequelae was severe and usually permanent in three patients who presented with pulmonary edema, pulmonary hemorrhage, and extensive brainstem lesions. Pulmonary edema secondary to myocarditis is very unlikely since no evidence of cardiomegaly was found, no arrhythmia by electrocardiography, and no obvious myocardium inflammation in the necropsy sample. In addition, only a small proportion of patients with brainstem encephalitis and pulmonary edema had systemic arterial hypertension or increased systemic vascular resistance (24–26), suggesting pulmonary edema during the acute stage of fulminant EV71 infection may not be directly due to excessive sympathetic activation (26). In contrast, the mechanism of pulmonary edema may be related to increased pulmonary vascular permeability caused by systemic inflammatory responses triggered by extensive brainstem lesions (1,26).

5.   CYTOKINE LEVELS AND THE CLINICAL SEVERITY OF EV71 BRAINSTEM ENCEPHALITIS

Cytokine reactions during EV71 infection were examined and compared in patients with different categories complications of EV71 infection. The CSF interleukin-6 (IL-6) levels during acute stage were not significantly different among patients with brainstem encephalitis and pulmonary edema, brainstem encephalitis without pulmonary edema, or those with aseptic meningitis. The CSF IL-6 levels in patients who died or in neurologically impaired survivors did not differ significantly from the levels in patients who recovered completely. The CSF levels of IL-1$_\beta$ also had little bearing on the clinical outcome (27). This study suggests that although brain produces high levels of proinflammatory cytokines during acute stage of EV71 CNS infection, not all of them develop fulminant pulmonary edema.

In contrast, patients with EV71 brainstem encephalitis and pulmonary edema were found to have significantly higher blood levels of IL-6, tumor necrosis factor-alpha TNF-α, IL-1β, white blood cell count, and blood glucose than patients with EV71 brainstem encephalitis alone (27,28). The C-reactive protein levels did not differ significantly. The blood cytokine levels in patients with brainstem encephalitis only or in those without complications were not significantly different from that in normal children. The sensitivity, specificity, positive and negative predictive values of serum IL-6 >70 pg/mL for EV71 encephalitis with pulmonary edema were all 100% (28). Another study also found a marked elevation of plasma levels of interferon-γ (IFN-γ), IL-10, and IL-13 in patients with EV71 brainstem encephalitis and pulmonary edema compared to those without pulmonary edema (29). The significance and mechanism of elevated plasma levels of anti-inflammatory cytokines, IL-10, and IL-13, in patients with pulmonary edema during EV71 brainstem encephalitis remain to be elucidated. IFN-γ can enhance microvascular leakage through reduced endothelial barrier and tight junction (29). These studies suggest that systemic inflammatory responses, instead of local CNS cytokine reactions, during acute brainstem inflammation is related to cardiopulmonary collapse in patients with fulminant EV71 infection.

6.   AUTOPSY FINDINGS

6.1.   Brain

Postmortem studies reveal extensive inflammation in the meninges and CNS. The brainstem and spinal cord are most severely involved (7,25,30–32). The most prominent inflammatory lesions are seen in the dentate nuclei of the cerebellum, posterior two-thirds of the medulla oblongata and pons, and the anterior two-thirds of the spinal cord (30–32). The involved areas include inferior olivary nuclei, cranial nerve nuclei, nucleus tractus solitarius, and reticular formation of the medulla and pons, basis pontis, substantia nigra, and red nuclei of midbrain, and gray matter of the cervical, thoracic, and lumbar spinal cords. The histopathological findings in the spinal cord mimic those in poliomyelitis. The basal ganglia, thalamus, hypothalamus, and midbrain also shows acute inflammation, but to a lesser degree. The inflammatory infiltrates consist largely of neutrophils involving primarily the gray matter with perivascular lymphocytic cuffing, and neuronophagia. EV71 is isolated from the fresh brain tissues and also identified by immunofluorescence method with type-specific EV71 monoclonal antibody (7,25,30–32).

6.2.   Other Organs

The heart shows mild hypertrophy with a small focus of mononuclear cell infiltration in the myocardium of right ventricle. However, no accompanying myocyte damage or viral inclusion is seen. The lungs reveals primarily marked pulmonary edema with multifocal hemorrhage, but without notable inflammatory reaction (25,30–32). Although no diffuse alveolar damage is present, the beginning of the hyaline membrane formation is noted in several areas. Mild inflammatory reaction accompanied by destruction of ducts and acini is also found in the pancreas. The liver shows mild microvesicular fatty change. The rest of the visceral organs are unremarkable. The heart, lung and pancreas are all negative for EV71 immunostaining. These autopsy findings provide evidence that the brainstem and spinal cord are the main targets of EV71 infection in the patients with a rapidly fatal outcome (7,25,30–32).

7.   PATHOGENESIS OF ACUTE FATALITY WITH EV71 BRAINSTEM ENCEPHALITIS AND PULMONARY EDEMA

The EV71 outbreak is unique in its manifestations of pulmonary edema in the potentially fatal cases in young children (1,7,19). The underlying mechanisms for the acute pulmonary edema during fulminant EV71 infection is not completely understood. Neurogenic pulmonary edema can develop very rapidly after CNS insult and death may occur within minutes. Baker described 15 patients with bulbar poliomyelitis who had preceding limb weakness or dysphagia and subsequent sudden pulmonary edema, which resisted all forms of treatment and led to the death of all 15 patients (33). Extensive damage to the crucial vasomotor center located in the dorsal vagus nuclei and medial reticular formation in the medulla may be responsible for pulmonary edema (34). Animal models suggests that injury to this region may induce neurogenic pulmonary edema via massive adrenergic discharge, generalized vasoconstriction, high systemic vascular resistance, and redistribution of blood to the more distensible pulmonary bed, which can be prevented by adrenergic blockade (35). The clinical observations and pathological findings in poliomyelitis were similar to the damage caused by EV71 infection (7,30–32,33).

Almost all the fatal cases in the Taiwan EV71 epidemic had symptoms of autonomic nervous system dysfunction, such as increased heart rates and central fever, suggesting the involvement of reticular formation (24). The autonomic nervous system can continuously control heart rate and blood pressure, respiratory rate, gastrointestinal motility, body temperature, and other essential life functions. In addition, this system can also interact with the limbic system, brainstem, and hypothalamus to control systemic inflammatory responses (35). Inflammatory products produced in damaged tissues activate afferent signals that are relayed to the nucleus tractus solitarius, and subsequent activation of vagus efferent activity inhibits inflammatory cytokine synthesis through the cholinergic anti-inflammatory pathway (35). This anti-inflammatory pathway may be impaired during severe EV71 brainstem infection because of the specific destruction in the nucleus tractus solitarius and reticular formation of the medulla oblongata and pons, resulting in unchecked neurogenic inflammatory responses in the peripheral tissue.

Furthermore, injured or irritated sensory nerves can initiate inflammation or amplify the inflammatory responses initiated by noxious stimuli. Neurokinins are thought to be stored primarily in unmyelinated nerve fibers and released antidromically as part of the nociceptive response. Neurokinin-1 receptor (NK-1R) has the highest affinity for substance P, and overactivation of NK-1R in smooth muscle cells, endothelial cells, and leukocytes decreases vascular tone, and increases endothelial permeability, thereby enhancing the inflammation induced by the original stimulus (36).

In addition, excess activation of N-methyl-D-aspartate (NMDA) glutamate receptors, a major mechanism of neuronal cell death in several neurologic diseases, can also cause damage in peripheral organ (37), such as neurogenic pulmonary edema in the lung during fulminant EV71 infection. Further studies are needed to examine whether extensive brainstem involvement by EV71 during grade III brainstem encephalitis can trigger systemic neurogenic inflammations, by dysregulation of cytokine, neuropeptides or neurokinins production, or by overactivation of NMDA receptors, and results in catastrophic pulmonary edema or hemorrhage (35–37).

8. NEUROVIRULENT STRAINS VS. HOST SUSCEPTIBILITY

EV71 possesses 60 copies of four capsid proteins, VP1, VP2, VP3, and VP4 in the virion. The amino acid sequences of the VP4 region are highly conserved among EV71 isolates. The conserved 5′-untranslated region (UTR), approximately 740 nucleotides, has a crucial role in the viral life cycle. In contrast to the highly conserved 5'-UTR, the capsid protein VP1 is more variable and confers distinct antigenic properties to the virus. Molecular analysis of the VP4 and VP1 genes of recent EV71 strains indicates that several genotypes of the virus have been circulating in the Asia-Pacific region since 1997. The first of these recent outbreaks, in Sarawak, Malaysia in 1997, was caused by genotype B3. This outbreak was followed by large outbreaks by genotype C2 in Taiwan in 1998, and by genotypes B3 and C2 co-circulated in Western Australia in 1999. Singapore, Taiwan, and Sarawak had EV71 epidemics in 2000, caused predominantly by viruses belonging to genotype B4; however, large numbers of fatalities were only observed in Taiwan (38). Genetic analyses of the 5'-untranslated and VP1 regions of EV71 isolates in Taiwan epidemics from 1998 to 2000 by reverse transcription-PCR and sequencing again showed that most EV71 isolates from the 1998 epidemic belonged to genotype C, while only one-tenth of the isolates were genotype B. In contrast, all EV71 isolates from 1999 to 2000 in Taiwan belonged to genotype B (39). This study indicated that two genotypes of EV71 capable of inducing severe brainstem encephalitis have been circulating in Taiwan from 1998 to 2000.

Attempts have been made to determine the neurovirulence of EV71 among patients with differing severity of disease. Shih et al. further analyzed complete sequences of two EV71 strains isolated from the spinal cord of a fatal patient and from vesicles in a patient with mild HFMD (40). A high degree of identification (97–100%) in nucleotide sequence was confirmed throughout the entire genome, except in the focal regions of 3C-encoding viral proteinase and the 3'-NCR, where the nucleotide homology was 90–91%. In Singapore, the genomes of two representative EV71 strains isolated from a fatal case and a surviving patient were completely sequenced. Comparative sequence analysis of the two strains revealed 99% nucleotide similarity, while their deduced amino acid sequences were almost identical except for residue 1506 in the 3A non-structural region (41). No definitive marker of neurovirulence has been identified yet.

Since the EV71 outbreaks involve closely related genetic variants of EV71, the broad spectrum of disease severity may be attributed to different host immune responses following infection, but is less likely to be due to the emergence of EV71 strains with heightened virulence (41).

Patients with CD40-ligand deficiency who show hypo-IgG and elevated IgM levels are also susceptible to enterovirus meningoencephalitis (42). T-lymphocyte antigen-4 (CLTA-4) polymorphism is an important negative regulator of T-cell cytotoxicity and its polymorphism at position 49 with A or G genotype of exon 1 is linked to some autoimmune diseases. This specific polymorphism is much more common among Chinese, Japanese patients than among white patients (43). Yang et al. found that the CD40-ligand expression on CD4 T cells was significantly decreased during acute stage in children with than in those without brainstem encephalitis (43). Children with EV71 brainstem encephalitis had a significantly higher frequency of position 49 polymorphism with G/G allele in the CTLA-4 gene (58.1%) than did those without brainstem encephalitis (29.8%) and control subjects (26.9%) (43). In the

Australia EV71 epidemic, a relatively high proportion of Asian children was noted among the severely affected patients (44). These studies suggests that the pathogenesis of EV71 brainstem encephalitis may involve the dose of virus load, genetic susceptibility, such as CTLA-4 polymorphism, and younger age with altered cellular immunity (43,44).

9. POTENTIAL TREATMENT AND PREVENTION

At present, there is no known efficacious treatment for EV71 brainstem encephalitis. Before the endemic seasons of EV71, habit of hand washing should be promoted for the teachers, parents, and children. In addition, health educational pamphlets on EV71 infection which lists the symptoms and signs of HFMD, and especially the potential manifestations of brainstem encephalitis, such as high fever, persistent vomiting, and myoclonic jerks, should be widely distributed.

All patients should be treated according to the extent of the disease involvement. In patients who present with HFMD/herpangina only require symptomatic treatment, but close follow-up for manifestations of potential deterioration is recommended.

Young children with HFMD/herpangina who presents with persistently high fever, myoclonus, poor activity, vomiting, or ataxia, should be identified and admitted to hospitals for close observation of disease progression. At hospital, arterial blood pressure, heart rate, respiratory rate, oximeter readings, brainstem function examination (especially oculomotor function, bulbar function, and doll eye's sign), Glasgow Coma Scale score, and blood sugar levels should be closely and regularly monitored.

Early recognition of risk factors and intensive care are crucial to successful treatment of the fulminant infection. Patients who develop tachypnea, hypertension or hypotension, hypoxemia, hyperglycemia, or abnormal brainstem function should be admitted to the intensive care unit. The management of pulmonary edema and pulmonary hemorrhage in patients with EV71 infection is important but difficult. At the onset of respiratory distress, early endotracheal intubation is needed to allow positive-pressure mechanical ventilation with increased positive end-expiratory pressure for the treatment of pulmonary edema. High-frequency oscillatory ventilation is recommended if pulmonary edema or hemorrhage persists or if severe hypoxemia develops. Pediatric cardiologist consultation for continuous monitoring of cardiovascular hemodynamics is important and necessary for patients who develop pulmonary edema. The use of phosphodiesterase inhibitor-milrinone is recommended, even if the patient's arterial blood pressure is within normal limits, when echocardiographic examination shows signs of left ventricular dysfunction or patients have signs of decreased perfusion (26,45). Milrinone can be used to improve cardiac contractility and decrease the afterload. Use of vasodilators, especially nitroprusside, for severe hypertension should be cautious, because arterial blood pressure sometimes could drop very quickly (45).

In patients who develop hypotension, inotropic agents, such as dopamine and epinephrine become necessary to maintain sufficient perfusion pressure. The use of extracorporeal membrane oxygenation or a left ventricular assisted device is still controversial. Because most studies suggest that cardiopulmonary failure has a central origin, indications for these therapies remain undefined (26,44,45).

Despite the widespread use of intravenous immunoglobulin in patients with EV71 brainstem encephalitis in the Taiwan epidemic, there are no case–control study data available to support the effectiveness of this treatment. The use of intravenous corticosteroids was reported to ameliorate long-term neurologic deficits in a small number of patients with pulmonary edema, but convincing data are lacking (44). Rapid clinical improvement after early treatment of IFN-γ was observed in two patients who presented with poliovirus brainstem encephalitis and bulbar paralysis (46). The therapeutic effect of IFN-γ on EV71 CNS infection remains unknown.

After recovery from brainstem encephalitis and cardiopulmonary dysfunction, most survivors of fulminant EV71 infection have moderate to severe neurologic sequelae, such as spastic quadriparesis, ventilator-dependent apnea, or bulbar palsy. Coordinated programs for their long-term medical care, sufficient mechanical ventilator support and chest care, and neuro-rehabilitation are necessary and important for the functional improvement (44,45).

10. FUTURE PRESPECTIVES

Since EV71 is not susceptible to newly developed antiviral agents, and a vaccine is not currently available, control of EV71 epidemics through high-level surveillance and public health intervention are critical to maintain and extend throughout the Asia-Pacific region (47). Future research should focus on (1) understanding the molecular genetics of EV71 neurovirulence and of host susceptibility, (2) development of rapid and accurate methods for early diagnosis of EV71 infection, such as testing for IgM antibody by ELISA and PCR microchips, (3) establishment of a sensitive monitor system useful for early detection of autonomic nervous dysfunction in patients at risk for pulmonary edema, (4) development of antiviral agents to ameliorate the severity of neurologic disease, (5) development of an effective EV71 vaccine for children under age 5 years.

ACKNOWLEDGMENT

This work was supported by grants from Taiwan National Science Counsel (NSC 91-2314-B006-041).

REFERENCES

1. Huang CC, Liu CC, Chang YC, Chen CY, Yeh TF. Neurologic complications in children with enterovirus 71 infection. New Engl J Med 1999; 341:936–942.
2. Cherry JD. Enteroviruses: coxsackievirus, echoviruses, and polioviruses. In: Feigin RD, Cherry JD, eds. Textbook of Pediatric Infectious Diseases. 4th ed. Philadelphia: W.B. Saunders, 1998:1787–1839.
3. Schmidt NJ, Lennette EH, Ho HH. An apparently new enterovirus isolated from patients with disease of the central nervous system. J Infect Dis 1974; 129:304–309.
4. Chumakov M, Voroshilova M, Shindarov L, et al. Enterovirus 71 isolated from cases of epidemic poliomyelitis-like disease in Bulgaria. Arch Virol 1979; 60:329–340.
5. Shindarov LM, Chumakov MP, Voroshilova MK, et al. Epidemiological, clinical and pathomorphological characteristics of epidemic poliomyelitis-like disease caused by enterovirus 71. J Hyg Epidemiol Microbiol Immunol 1979; 23:284–295.
6. Nagy G, Takatsy S, Kukan E, Mihaly I, Domok I. Virological diagnosis of enterovirus type 71 infections: experiences grained during an epidemic of acute CNS diseases in Hungary in 1978. Arch Virol 1982; 71:217–227.
7. Lum LCS, Wong KT, Lam SK, et al. Fatal enterovirus 71 encephalomyelitis. J Pediatr 1998; 133:795–798.
8. Ishimaru H, Nakano S, Yamaoka K, Takami S. Outbreaks of hand, foot and mouth disease by enterovirus 71: high incidence of complication disorders of central nervous system. Arch Dis Child 1980; 55:583–588.
9. Alexander JP Jr, Baden L, Pallansch MA, Anderson LJ. Enterovirus 71 infections and neurogenic disease—United States, 1977–1991. J Infect Dis 1994; 169:905–908.
10. Ho M, Chen ER, Hsu KH, et al. The enterovirus type 71 epidemic of Taiwan, 1998. N Engl J Med 1999; 341:929–935.
11. Blomberg J, Lycke E, Ahlfors K, et al. New enterovirus type associated with epidemic of aseptic meningitis and/or hand, foot, and mouth disease. Lancet 1974; 2:112.
12. Chonmaitree T, Menegus MA, Schervish-Swierkosz EM, Schwalenstocker E. Enterovirus 71 infection: report of an outbreak with two cases of paralysis and a review of the literature. Pediatrics 1981; 67:489–493.
13. Melnick JL. Enterovirus type 71 infections: a varied clinical pattern sometimes mimicking paralytic poliomyelitis. Rev Infect Dis 1984; 6(suppl 2):S387–S390.
14. Gilbert GL, Dickson KE, Waters MJ, Kennett ML, Land SA, Sneddon M. Outbreak of enterovirus 71 infection in Victoria, Australia, with a high incidence of neurologic involvement. Pediatr Infect Dis J 1988; 7:484–488.
15. McMinn P, Stratov I, Nagarajan L, Davis S. Neurological manifestations of enterovirus 71 infection in children during an outbreak of hand, foot, and mouth disease in Western Australia. Clin Infect Dis 2001; 32:236–242.
16. Fujimoto T, Chikahira M, Yoshida S, et al. Outbreak of central nervous system disease associated with hand, foot, and mouth disease in Japan during the summer of 2000: detection and molecular epidemiology of enterovirus 71. Microbiol Immunol 2002; 46:621–627.
17. Chan KP, Goh KT, Chong CY, et al. Epidemic hand, foot and mouth disease caused by human enterovirus 71, Singapore. Emerg Infect Dis 2003; 9:78–85.
18. Lu CY, Lee CY, Kao CL, et al. Incidence and case-fatality rates resulting from the 1998 enterovirus 71 outbreak in Taiwan. J Med Virol 2002; 67:217–223.

19. Chang LY, King CC, Hsu KH, et al. Risk factors of enterovirus 71 infection and associated hand, foot, and mouth disease/herpangina in children during an epidemic in Taiwan. Pediatrics 2002; 109:e88.

20. Takimoto S, Waldman EA, Moreira RC, et al. Enterovirus 71 infection and acute neurological disease among children in Brazil (1988–1990). Trans R Soc Trop Med Hyg 1998; 92:25–28.

21. Chen CY, Chang YC, Huang CC, et al. Acute flaccid paralysis in infants and young children with enterovirus 71 infection: MR imaging findings and clinical correlates. Am J Neuroradiol 2001; 22:200–205.

22. Shen WC, Chiu HH, Chow KC, Tsai CH. MR imaging findings of enteroviral encephalomyelitis: an outbreak in Taiwan. Am J Neuroradiol 1999; 20:1889–1895.

23. Zimmerman RD. MR imaging findings of enteroviral encephalomyelitis: an outbreak in Taiwan. Am J Neuroradiol 1999; 20:1775–1776.

24. Chang LY, Lin TY, Hsu KH, et al. Clinical features and risk factors of pulmonary oedema after enterovirus-71-related hand, foot, and mouth disease. Lancet 1999; 354:1682–1686.

25. Chan LG, Parashar UD, Lye MS, et al. Deaths of children during an outbreak of hand, foot, and mouth disease in Sarawak, Malaysia: clinical and pathological characteristics of the disease. For the Outbreak Study Group. Clin Infect Dis 2000; 31:678–683.

26. Wu JM, Wang JN, Tsai YC, et al. Cardiopulmonary manifestations of fulminant enterovirus 71 infection. Pediatrics 2002; 109:e26.

27. Lin TY, Hsia SH, Huang YC, Wu CT, Chang LY. Proinflammatory cytokine reactions in enterovirus 71 infections of the central nervous system. Clin Infect Dis 2003; 36:269–274.

28. Lin TY, Chang LY, Huang YC, et al. Different proinflammatory reactions in fatal and non-fatal enterovirus 71 infections: implications for early recognition and therapy. Acta Paediatr 2002; 91:632–635.

29. Wang SM, Lei HY, Huang KJ, et al. Pathogenesis of enterovirus 71 brainstem encephalitis in pediatric patients: the roles of cytokines and cellular immune activation in patients with pulmonary edema. J Infect Dis 2003; 188:564–570.

30. Shieh WJ, Jung SM, Hsueh C, et al. Pathologic studies of fatal cases in outbreak of hand, foot, and mouth disease, Taiwan. Emerg Infect Dis 2001; 7(1):146–148.

31. Yan JJ, Wang JR, Liu CC, Yang HB, Su IJ. An outbreak of enterovirus 71 infection in Taiwan 1998: a comprehensive pathological, virological, and molecular study on a case of fulminant encephalitis. J Clin Virol 2000; 17:13–22.

32. Hsueh C, Jung SM, Shih SR, et al. Acute encephalomyelitis during an outbreak of enterovirus type 71 infection in Taiwan: report of an autopsy case with pathologic, immunofluorescence, and molecular studies. Mod Pathol 2000; 13:1200–1205.

33. Baker AB. Poliomyelitis: a study of pulmonary edema. Neurology 1957; 7:743–751.

34. Theodore J, Rubin E. Speculations on neurogenic pulmonary edema (NPE). Am Rev Respir Dis 1976; 119:637–641.

35. Tracey KJ. Inflammatory reflex. Nature 2002; 420:853–859.

36. Carter, MS, Krause, JE. Structure, expression, and some regulatory mechanisms of the rat preprotachykinin gene encoding substance P, neurokinin A, neuropeptide K, and neuropeptide-γ J Neurosci 1990; 10:2203–2214.

37. Said SI, Berisha HI, Pakbaz H. Excitotoxicity in the lung: *N*-Methyl-D-aspartate-induced, nitric oxide-dependent, pulmonary edema is attenuated by vasoactive

intestinal peptide and by inhibitors of poly(ADP-ribose) polymerase. Proc Natl Acad Sci U S A 1996; 93:4688–4692.

38.   Cardosa MJ, Perera D, Brown BA, et al. Molecular epidemiology of human enterovirus 71 strains and recent outbreaks in the Asia-Pacific region: comparative analysis of the VP1 and VP4 genes. Emerg Infect Dis 2003; 9:461–468.

39.   Wang JR, Tuan YC, Tsai HP, et al. Change of major genotype of enterovirus 71 in outbreaks of hand-foot-and-mouth disease in Taiwan between 1998 and 2000. J Clin Microbiol 2002; 40:10–15.

40.   Shih SR, Ho MS, Lin KH, et al. Genetic analysis of enterovirus 71 isolated from fatal and non-fatal cases of hand, foot and mouth disease during an epidemic in Taiwan, 1998. Virus Res 2000; 68:127–136.

41.   Singh S, Poh CL, Chow VT. Complete sequence analyses of enterovirus 71 strains from fatal and non-fatal cases of the hand, foot and mouth disease outbreak in Singapore (2000). Microbiol Immunol 2002; 46:801–808.

42.   Cunningham CK, Bonville CA, Ochs HD, et al. Enteroviral meningoencephalitis as a complication of X-linked hyper IgM syndrome. J Pediatr 1999; 134:584–588.

43.   Yang KD, Yang MY, Li CC, et al. Altered cellular but not humoral reactions in children with complicated enterovirus 71 infections in Taiwan. J Infect Dis 2001; 183:850–856.

44.   Nolan MA, Craig ME, Lahra MM, et al. Survival after pulmonary edema due to enterovirus 71 encephalitis. Neurology 2003; 60:1651–1656.

45.   Lin TY, Chang LY, Hsia SH, et al. The 1998 enterovirus 71 outbreak in Taiwan: pathogenesis and management. Clin Infect Dis 2002; 34(suppl 2):S52–S57.

46.   Arya S. Antiviral therapy for neurological manifestations of enterovirus 71 infection. Clin Infect Dis 2000; 30:988.

47.   McMinn PC. An overview of the evolution of enterovirus 71 and its clinical and public health significance. FEMS Microbiol Rev 2002; 26:91–107.

13

Guillain–Barré Syndrome and *Campylobacter* Infection

Kazim A. Sheikh

Department of Neurology, School of Medicine, Johns Hopkins University, Baltimore, Maryland, U.S.A.

Irving Nachamkin

Department of Pathology and Laboratory Medicine, School of Medicine, University of Pennsylvania, Philadelphia, Pennsylvania, U.S.A.

1. INTRODUCTION

Guillain–Barré syndrome (GBS) comprises a group of clinically and pathophysiologically related acute monophasic neuropathic disorders, likely of autoimmune origin, with an incidence of 1–1.5 per 100,000 population per year (1–3). After the near eradication of polio, GBS has become the commonest cause of acute flaccid paralysis throughout the world. It is now widely accepted that GBS encompasses demyelinating and axonal forms, as well as the Fisher syndrome (FS) and other minor variants. Advances made over the last 15 years indicate that (a) GBS is pathophysiologically heterogeneous, and (b) post-infectious autoimmunity is probably the predominant pathophysiologic mechanism in some forms of GBS. Post-infectious molecular mimicry in the peripheral nervous system (PNS) implies shared antigenic determinants between the infectious agents and nerve fibers of the PNS. This results in an immune response to the organism that initiates immune-mediated damage to nerve fibers. The support for this concept derives largely from both clinical and experimental studies on the acute motor axonal neuropathy (AMAN) and Fisher variants of GBS. In this context the most commonly recognized antecedent infection is *Campylobacter jejuni* enteritis. Specific anti-ganglioside antibodies are associated with different variants of

GBS. The lipooligosaccharides (LOSs) of *C. jejuni* isolates from patients with GBS carry relevant ganglioside-like moieties and gangliosides, the purported target antigens, are enriched in the nerve fibers. Pathological studies in the AMAN variant of GBS show antibody-mediated, complement-dependent injury of nerve fibers, supporting the important pathogenetic role of antibodies in the axonal variants of GBS.

Molecular mimicry has been invoked as a mechanism in a variety of autoimmune diseases. Evidence supporting the role of molecular mimicry is increasing in disorders such as post-infectious arthropathies, but critical review suggests that, as applied to post-infectious disorders, this mechanism remains an attractive but an unproved hypothesis. Nevertheless, GBS variants like AMAN and FS provide the best available evidence to support the hypothesis of molecular mimicry as a pathogenetic mechanism underlying post-infectious autoimmune disorders. This chapter highlights the hypothesis of molecular mimicry in the context of post-*Campylobacter* cases of GBS.

2. CLINICAL FEATURES OF GBS AND ITS VARIANTS

Motor symptoms predominate in GBS: the most common initial symptom is weakness, usually beginning in the lower limbs and characteristically ascending and involving both proximal and distal muscles. Areflexia or hyporeflexia is seen in almost all patients. Cranial nerve involvement is common and can be seen in up to two-thirds of the cases most often affecting facial or oculomotor nerves. Two-thirds of cases may present with sensory symptoms at the onset of the disease; however, abnormalities on sensory examination are often minimal. Pain, particularly low back, buttock, or thigh, is an early symptom in approximately 50% of patients. Autonomic dysfunction is present in one-third of patients and can manifest as reduced sinus arrthymias, sinus tachycardia, arrthymias, labile blood pressure, orthostatic hypotension, abnormal sweating, and pupillary abnormalities (4,5). Autonomic instability and bulbar weakness are major causes of morbidity and mortality in GBS.

In recent years it has become increasingly clear that clinically and pathophysiologically GBS is not a single entity, and the terms GBS and acute inflammatory demyelinating polyradiculoneuropathy (AIDP) can no longer be used synonymously as in the past. AIDP remains the most common form of GBS in Europe, North America, and the rest of the developed world, probably accounting for over 95% of patients. However, an axonal form is now widely recognized (6–8). A pure motor axonal subtype (AMAN), which is more common in developing countries, has been extensively characterized by our group in northern China (8), and it also occurs frequently in Mexico (Nachamkin I, McKhann G, unpublished data). AMAN is strongly associated with preceding *Campylobacter* infection (9,10). Other significant epidemiologic features of GBS in northern

China are a clear seasonal pattern, with peak incidence in the summer months, and an apparent predilection for rural areas and children.

The motor-sensory axonal type (AMSAN) is a more severe form with less complete recovery (6). The Fisher variant (FS) represents approximately 5% of cases of GBS. In the pure form of FS, patients present with ataxia, ophthalmoplegia and areflexia without significant weakness, although overlapping forms, with bulbar, facial and/or generalized weakness are also seen. Other rarer forms without significant motor weakness that may be classified under the term GBS include a predominantly sensory variant, brachio-pharyngeal variant, and acute idiopathic autonomic neuropathy or acute pandysautonomia.

2.1. Investigations

Electrophysiology provides the most critical diagnostic evaluation, supporting clinical diagnosis and useful prognostic information; however nerve conduction studies may be normal early in the disease particularly within the first week. Lumbar puncture is extremely useful. Cerebrospinal fluid (CSF) protein is increased in 80–90% of cases, characteristically without a significant increase in white cells (the so-called albumino-cytologic dissociation). An elevated CSF protein supports the diagnosis but, more importantly, CSF examination excludes other differential diagnoses; for example, a marked pleocytosis should raise doubt about a diagnosis of idiopathic GBS. Of note, the absence of elevated CSF protein, particularly early on, does not refute the diagnosis of GBS. There is now a large body of literature on the association of anti-ganglioside antibodies with various clinical and electrophysiological features and prognosis in GBS (also see below). Anti-ganglioside serology can provide useful support for the diagnosis in incomplete forms and unusual variants of GBS, particularly when electrodiagnostic testing and CSF are normal. In cases with typical clinical and electrodiagnostic features we do not routinely check anti-ganglioside serology for diagnosis or clinical decision-making.

2.2. Clinical Course and Prognosis

Antecedent infection is common and approximately two-thirds of patients give a history of a respiratory or diarrheal illness within the 3–4 weeks prior to onset of clinical disease (3,11,12). Neurologic symptoms usually progress over days to weeks, with a nadir within 2 weeks in the majority of patients and within 4 weeks in virtually all. The disease is monophasic and recovery begins within 2–4 weeks of this nadir in a vast majority of patients. Approximately 20% of patients remain ambulant throughout, but up to half become chair- or bed-bound, one-third require intensive care admission, and one-quarter require mechanical ventilation

(1,13–15). The severity of disease increases with increasing age (14) and antecedent infection with either *Campylobacter* (13,16) or Cytomegalovirus (CMV) (17) is also associated with more severe disease.

Most patients make a complete functional recovery over 6–12 months, but one-quarter are left with significant disability and approximately 10% are unable to walk unaided. Despite the availability of modern intensive care facilities, the mortality rate remains 3–8% in recent series (1,18). Mortality is due to cardiac arrest attributed to dysautonomia, respiratory failure or infection, or pulmonary embolism.

Poor prognostic factors include a short interval from onset to maximal deficit, the need for ventilator assistance, age >40 years, preceding *Campylobacter* infection, and small or absent CMAPs on distal stimulation (1,19,20). The most important determinant of rate and efficiency of recovery is the degree of axonal degeneration. Axonal degeneration usually indicates slow or incomplete recovery, except in cases with very distal axonal degeneration where regeneration is needed over only a short distance. The outcome is better in children (21,22) and the presence of decreased CMAP amplitudes and denervation potentials may not predict poor outcome in this age group, although a prolonged interval to the start of clinical recovery does (23).

3. PATHOLOGY

The pathology of AIDP and AMAN is well characterized, whereas the pathology of minor variants including FS is not well documented. Demyelination is a characteristic feature of AIDP and typically is concentrated in the mixed spinal roots and plexuses. Distal or terminal nerve demyelination is another site commonly involved in some patients (24–26). Leukocyte infiltration is considered a diagnostic hallmark for AIDP; however, the extent of lymphocytic infiltration varies markedly. Immunopathological studies indicate breakdown of blood–nerve barrier and deposition of activated complement components can be seen in some but not all cases of AIDP (27). These observations raise the possibility that T-cell- or antibody-mediated immune injury can predominate in an individual case.

In contrast to AIDP, axonal cases show evidence of primary axonal injury, but minimal T-cell inflammation and demyelination. Axonal degeneration selectively involves ventral roots or motor axons in AMAN and both motor and sensory axons in AMSAN. In AMAN, immunopathological studies indicate the deposition of IgG and complement activation products on nodal and internodal axolemma (28). In axonal cases, a prominent feature is the presence of macrophages within the periaxonal space, surrounding or displacing the axon, and surrounded by an intact myelin sheath (29,30). These observations suggest that the antigen of interest is present on the axon and that antibody binding to motor axolemma leads to complement activation, macrophage recruitment, and axonal degeneration.

4. PATHOGENESIS

Post-*Campylobacter* cases of AMAN and FS provide one of the best disease models for the possibility of molecular mimicry. This section discusses the role of *C. jejuni* infection (trigger), anti-ganglioside antibodies (immune response to *C. jejuni*), distribution of gangliosides in PNS (target antigens), and evidence demonstrating the role of anti-ganglioside antibodies in the pathogenesis of AMAN and FS.

4.1. *Campylobacter jejuni*

4.1.1. General Characteristics

Campylobacter jejuni infection is the most frequently recognized event preceding AMAN and other variants of GBS [reviewed in Ref. (31)]. *Campylobacter jejuni* is one of the most common causes of bacterial gastroenteritis worldwide, especially in children (32,33). This organism is a spiral-shaped, gram-negative non-spore-forming rod that is highly motile, with a single polar flagellum at one or both poles of the bacterium. Unlike other common enteric pathogens, *C. jejuni* has unique growth requirements and optimal growth is achieved in a microaerophilic environment consisting of 5% O_2, 10% CO_2, and 85% N_2.

Most *Campylobacter* infections in the United States are sporadic and occur in the summer and early fall. Sporadic infections are usually associated with ingestion of improperly handled or cooked food, and poultry products are a major source for human infections. There is a bimodal age distribution of patients with *Campylobacter* infection with peaks in infants and young children, followed by a second peak in young adults 20–40 years old. Outbreaks of *Campylobacter* infection are relatively uncommon and usually occur in the spring and winter. Food and water are major sources for reported outbreaks and prior to the early 1990s milk-borne outbreaks were common. A recently reported outbreak (34) prompted concern over a possible resurgence in milk-borne infections. Although sporadic *Campylobacter* infections show seasonal distributions in the United States, there is no evidence for seasonality of GBS cases. In contrast, the AMAN form of GBS as studied in China shows a strong seasonal pattern (9). Infection with *C. jejuni* typically results in an acute, self-limited gastroenteritis characterized by watery or bloody diarrhea usually accompanied by fever and abdominal cramps, although infection can be asymptomatic. Bacteremia is uncommon and is most likely to occur in children, the elderly, and immunocompromised individuals (35). The incidence of transient bacteremia in immunocompetent hosts is not known. In the context of GBS, both stool culture and serologic methods are needed to diagnose *Campylobacter* infection, because by the time neurological symptoms are present the yield of *C. jejuni* from stool culture is relatively low (36).

4.1.2. *Campylobacter* and GBS

The first case of GBS following *C. jejuni* gastroenteritis was described in 1982 by Rhodes and Tattersfied (37). Since then a large number of reports have documented this association, ranging from 4% in North America to 74% in northern China (31,38), with an overall prevalence estimated around 30% [(reviewed in Ref. (39)]. Some of the variations reported by different studies reflect the different assays used to define the occurrence of *C. jejuni* infection. Based on the known incidences of GBS and *C. jejuni* enteritis it is estimated that one in 1000 cases of *Campylobacter* infection is complicated by GBS and the risk may be greater for certain *Campylobacter* serotypes (Penner) such as HS:19 (40). The association of *C. jejuni* infection and GBS is considered relatively specific because GBS is rarely reported after other bacterial intestinal infections. The observation that GBS follows very rarely after *C. jejuni* infection has focused attention on the "organism" and "host" properties that may lead to this complication. The issue of organism-related factors has been examined mainly by two different but complementary approaches, namely, serotyping and characterizing the ganglioside-like mimicry in the LOS of the GBS and enteritis isolates. The host properties that could confer susceptibility to GBS after *C. jejuni* infection are not well established. Although some reports have indicated an association of both MHC class I and II alleles with post-*Campylobacter* GBS (41,42), these findings have not been confirmed. Recent studies from our group, however, show a strong association of MHC class II alleles with AIDP in Northern China (43).

Campylobacter jejuni is genetically heterogeneous and a large number of serotypes are recognized. Several classification schemes are used based on the nature of antigens, either heat-stable (Penner serotyping) or heat-labile (Lior serotyping), or molecular typing (44). Penner serotyping is most commonly used for the classification of clinical isolates including those from GBS patients. Although it was originally thought that LOS structures provide the basis of Penner serotyping, recent studies indicate that the Penner system determinants are mainly associated with capsular polysaccharide (45).

Numerous *C. jejuni* serotypes have been associated with GBS and of particular interest is the observation that some GBS-associated strains are uncommon in patients with uncomplicated gastroenteritis. Penner serotype HS:19 is overrepresented in Japanese GBS patients (up to 81%) compared to diarrhea isolates (~2%) (46–48). HS:19 is also a common isolate among northern Chinese and Mexican patients with GBS (49,50). This serostrain has also been isolated from GBS patients in Ireland and the United States (39,51) but HS:19 may not be overrepresented in all populations (52–54). Another striking example of the association of uncommon serostrains with GBS is provided by studies from South Africa. Goddard et al. (55) isolated *C. jejuni* serostrain HS:41 from nine of 17 children with GBS admitted to a hospital in Capetown. These GBS-associated organisms were collected over a 20-month period and belonged to the same genotype, as determined by DNA analysis (56). This serotype was rarely isolated from patients with uncomplicated gastroenteritis [12 of 7119 (0.16%)] over the same time period. The striking overrepresentation of serostrains HS:19 and HS:41 in patients with GBS has given support to the notion that as yet undefined properties related to the organism are critical in determining whether or not GBS follows *C. jejuni* infection. GBS-associated isolates are not restricted to these two uncommon serotypes and other *C. jejuni* serotypes isolated from GBS include HS:1, HS:2, HS:2/44, HS:4, HS:4/59, HS:5, HS:10, HS:13, HS:15, HS:16, HS:18, HS:21, HS:23/36, HS:24, HS:30, HS:37, HS:44, and HS:64 [reviewed in Ref. (57)].

4.1.3. *Campylobacter* and Molecular Mimicry

Multiple studies have characterized the core regions of lipopolysaccharide (LPS)/LOS of GBS- and diarrhea-associated *C. jejuni* strains. Biochemical, mass spectroscopy, and solid-phase immune assays with anti-ganglioside antibodies and bacterial toxins and lectins are the techniques most commonly used for this purpose. Moran and co-workers initially described the presence of sialic acid in *C. jejuni* strains in 1991 (58). Yuki et al. first described the presence of a GM1-like structure in *C. jejuni* LPS isolated from a GBS patient (59) and subsequent studies have shown the presence of GM1-, GD1a-, GalNAc-GD1a-, GM1b-, GT1a-, GD2-, GD3-, and GM2-like structures (49,60–67). Figure 1 shows the ganglioside-like structures in *C. jejuni* LOS implicated in AMAN and FS.

It is clear that both GBS- and diarrhea-associated isolates carry ganglioside-like moieties but GBS-related organisms are more likely to do so (66,67). Further, different *C. jejuni* isolates within the same serotype can have different

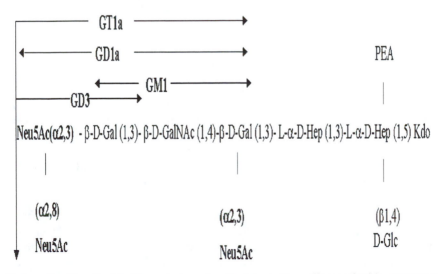

Figure 1 Ganglioside-like mimicry in *C. jejuni* core oligosaccharide structures described in various serotypes as determined by structural mass spectroscopy studies.

ganglioside-like moieties and a single isolate can have multiple ganglioside-like moieties in its LPS (49,62,63). This issue is complicated by the fact that the LPS/LOS structures, including ganglioside-like moieties, in the same isolate undergo phase variation and, not uncommonly, genomic mutational events that alter the expression of different glycosyltransferases and thus core oligosaccharide/LPS structure (68,69). Whether host factors can influence the genomic mutational events or transcription of glycosyltransferases of the infecting organism still remains to be addressed. On the whole it appears that expression of ganglioside-structures in LPS by itself is not sufficient to impart the GBS inducing properties to the infecting organism, but this is an area for further research.

The two critical findings that support the hypothesis of molecular mimicry are (a) studies that demonstrate that either human GBS sera or purified human anti-ganglioside antibodies bind to ganglioside-like moieties contained in the core oligosaccharide region of the LPS/LOS (49,70–72), and (b) immunization with *C. jejuni* LPSs/LOSs can successfully induce anti-ganglioside antibodies (73–76). These immune responses in experimental animals have generally induced low-affinity non-T-cell-dependent antibodies of IgM and IgG3 type, despite the use of adjuvants to recruit T-cell help (73,74) reflecting a high level of tolerance to self-gangliosides restricting antibody responses to *C. jejuni* LPSs (76). This high level of tolerance to self-gangliosides can be reproducibly overcome, likely with successful recruitment of T-cell help and production of T-cell-dependent IgG subclasses, by immunization with gangliosides or *C. jejuni* LPSs in transgenic animals lacking complex gangliosides (76,77). The density of ganglioside-like moieties in LPS used for immunization and manipulation of CD40 on B cells can also enhance anti-ganglioside antibody responses (40). Such observations support the notion that under some conditions the high level of tolerance to self-gangliosides can be overcome after *C. jejuni* infection, leading to induction of T-cell-dependent IgG anti-ganglioside responses similar to those seen in human GBS cases. These experimental findings raise the possibility that breakdown of tolerance to self-gangliosides is critical in the pathogenesis of post-*Campylobacter* GBS. Further, this ganglioside mimicry may not be restricted to *C. jejuni,* as recent studies indicate that *Haemophilus influenzae* also contains GM1-like structures (78,79). This observation provides support to the hypothesis that non-*Campylobacter* organisms can trigger induction of anti-ganglioside antibodies in GBS patients with no history of enteritis or serological evidence of *C. jejuni* infection (52,80).

Similar to other GBS variants, infections are the most common triggering event preceding FS, with upper respiratory viral infections and *C. jejuni* enteritis the two most frequently recognized. Post-*Campylobacter* cases provide strong support for the concept of molecular mimicry. Mass spectroscopy studies have demonstrated GD3- and GT1a-like oligosaccharides in LPS/LOSs of *C. jejuni* isolates from both GBS and FS patients (81,82) (63), but a GQ1b-like structure has not been established by this technique. Antibody binding assays with human or murine monoclonal antibodies have shown the presence of GT1a and GQ1b cross-reactive moieties in *C. jejuni* LPS/LOSs (53,83,84).

In an important study, Goodyear et al. (74) demonstrated that mice immunized with *C. jejuni* LPS containing GT1a-like moieties produce antibodies that recognize GQ1b and other cross-reactive disialylated gangliosides, thus supporting the notion that immune responses to *C. jejuni* LPS can elicit anti-ganglioside antibodies. It is not yet clear whether a similar mechanism is operative in human cases. Anti-ganglioside antibodies generated in this experimental paradigm were mostly of IgM type, typical of T-cell-independent responses to carbohydrate or glycolipid antigens. In contrast, serological studies in FS indicate class switching to IgG and subclass restriction to IgG1 and IgG3, both usually features of T-cell help and atypical of the human anti-carbohydrate antibody responses. Further experimental work in this area may clarify the mechanisms involved in the generation of human anti-ganglioside antibodies after *C. jejuni* infection. The immune mechanisms involved in the generation of anti-GQ1b antibodies in FS cases preceded by other inciting events, particularly cases with upper respiratory viral infections, are likely to be different from those in *C. jejuni* cases and are not known.

4.2. Anti-ganglioside Antibodies in Patients with GBS

Anti-glycolipid serological studies have generally attempted to correlate the specificity of antibody responses with: (a) specific clinical and pathological features such as motor vs. sensory fiber involvement or axonal vs. demyelinating injury; (b) preceding events such as *C. jejuni* infection; and (c) prognosis and recovery. These correlations are generally imperfect but, despite the limitations inherent to such large population-based serological studies, certain patterns/associations are emerging. Anti-ganglioside antibodies with multiple specificities, including those against GM1, have been reported in AIDP. The antibody correlations for this variant are both less well defined and accepted. In contrast, two major—GM1 and GD1a, and two minor—GalNAc-GD1a and GM1b gangliosides, are implicated as target antigens in AMAN. Anti-GQ1b antibodies are common in patients with FS and this correlation provides the strongest association between antibodies to a specific ganglioside and clinical phenotype. The antibodies directed against these ganglioside antigens in AMAN and FS are predominantly of IgG isotype, generally complement-fixing subtypes IgG1 and IgG3 (38,85,86). These anti-ganglioside antibody responses in GBS are almost always polyclonal and can have a broad range of cross-reactivity with related gangliosides (85–87). It has been proposed that differences in geography and or genetic background may affect the specificity and isotype distribution of anti-ganglioside responses in different populations (88,89).

4.2.1. Acute Motor Axonal Neuropathy

Yuki et al. first described the presence of high titer IgG anti-GM1 antibodies in two Japanese patients who developed AMAN with preceding *Campylobacter* infection (7). Walsh et al. (90) reported IgG anti-GM1antibodies in 14 of 95 (15%) of GBS cases and noted a correlation between the presence of these antibodies and poor recovery. Rees et al. also noted the presence of anti-GM1 antibodies in 24 of 96 (25%) of their English GBS patients, these antibodies were seen both in AIDP and axonal variants but were significantly associated with axonal subtypes (80). Jacobs et al. reported on anti-GM1antibodies in 22 of 154 (14%) of their Dutch cohort; the antibody-positive cases were classified as demyelinating and had predominant distal motor involvement, sensory sparing, and an association with preceding *C. jejuni* infection (91). In a recent analysis of more than 300 GBS patients enrolled in a multicenter trial comparing plasma exchange and IVIg, 22% of patients had anti-GM1 antibodies. This subgroup of patients was more likely to have a motor-predominant syndrome, preceding diarrhea, and axonal neurophysiology or inexcitable nerves (92). A recent Japanese report examining the relationship between anti-ganglioside antibodies and the axonal form of GBS classified 86 GBS patients as AIDP (36%), AMAN (38%), or inexcitable/unclassifiable (26%) on the basis of electrophysiological studies (88). Anti-ganglioside antibodies were almost exclusively present in the axonal group and more than 50% of patients with AMAN had anti-GM1 antibodies. The presence of anti-ganglioside antibodies was frequently associated with preceding *C. jejuni* infection.

Notably, not all studies confirm these associations. For example, Enders et al. (93) and Vriesendorp et al. (94) found no correlation between anti-GM1 antibodies and GBS subtypes or prognosis, whereas Ho et al. detected the presence of anti-GM1 antibodies equally frequently in both AMAN and AIDP patients in a northern Chinese cohort (9,38). In short, the bulk of the evidence supports the association of IgG anti-GM1 antibodies with motor-predominant and axonal forms of GBS and preceding *C. jejuni* infection. This association is not confirmed in all patient populations, however, and the frequency of this correlation varies between different populations. Whether the presence of anti-GM1 antibodies is correlated with rate of recovery remains unresolved. A recent study classified patients with AMAN and IgG anti-GM1 antibodies into two subgroups, one with rapid recovery and the other with slower recovery compared to a group of patients with AIDP (95). These authors propose that AMAN patients with IgG anti-GM1 antibodies and rapid recovery have a reversible axonal conduction failure (95), whereas those with poor recovery and anti-GM1 antibodies have axonal degeneration.

Yuki et al. (96) initially described IgG anti-GD1a antibodies in two Japanese patients with severe motor axonal injury and subsequently extended this observation in a case series of 37 patients, showing an association of these antibodies with the severity of clinical disease and axonal injury (97). In a large prospective series including Chinese 138 GBS patients, Ho et al. reported that 60% of AMAN and 4% of AIDP patients had IgG anti-GD1a antibodies, confirming the association with motor axonal injury, whereas IgG anti-GM1 antibodies were frequently detected in both variants (38). In this series serological evidence of recent *C. jejuni* infection was present in 80% of AMAN and 50% of AIDP cases. Subsequently, two large serological studies of Japanese GBS cases have confirmed the association between anti-GD1a antibodies and AMAN (88,98). Both studies show, however, that anti-GM1antibodies are more common than GD1a antibodies in Japanese patient populations. A recent European study found IgG anti-GD1a antibodies in six patients with post-*Campylobacter* severe motor axonal GBS (99). It seems that antibodies to GD1a are found in a proportion of patients with the motor axonal variant but that the frequency of these antibodies varies in different patient populations.

Kusunoki et al. initially described antibodies against the minor gangliosides GM1b and GalNAc-GD1a in Japanese patients with GBS (100,101). Other investigators have confirmed this finding in Dutch and Chinese populations (102–104). These studies indicate that 12–20% of patients with GBS have antibodies against these minor gangliosides. Patients with these antibodies are more likely to have distal motor weakness, lack sensory and cranial nerve involvement, and more frequently have preceding *C. jejuni* infection (103,105). Immunogenetic repertoire of a population may influence anti-ganglioside antibody responses is supported by a recent comparative study of Japanese and Dutch patients with GBS, Ang et al. found that Dutch patients had a stronger IgM response against GM1b and GalNAc-GD1a, whereas Japanese patients were more likely to mount an IgG response against these antigens (89).

The anti-ganglioside antibodies associated with the motor-predominant syndrome are relatively specific and sensory predominant syndromes have different antibody associations. For example, GBS cases with serological evidence of preceding CMV infection are more likely to have severe acute disease and sensory symptoms compared with those preceded by *C. jejuni* infection (17,106). Cumulatively, several studies indicate that antibodies to GM2 are present in about half the patients with CMV-associated GBS (54,107,108); nevertheless, antibodies to GM2 are also frequently present after uncomplicated CMV and EBV infection (108,109), suggesting that antibodies to GM2 are not sufficient to produce neuropathy and other factors are necessary for manifestation of disease. Moreover, a recent study examining serum anti-glycolipid antibodies in more than 400 GBS patients found a subgroup of nine patients with sensory disturbance, no electrophysiologic evidence of axonal injury, and monospecific IgG GD1b antibodies. Notably, eight of these nine patients had a preceding respiratory infection and one had gastroenteritis (110). These findings lend some support to the notion that motor dominant syndromes are more likely to be preceded by *C. jejuni* infection, whereas patients with prominent sensory features are more likely to have preceding viral respiratory infections.

4.2.2. Fisher Syndrome

The first report by Chiba et al. described the presence of antibodies against the complex ganglioside GQ1b in FS (111). Subsequent studies by other investigators have confirmed this initial observation (112–114). The fine specificity of anti-GQ1b antibodies in FS has been further defined and correlated with specific clinical features. Antibodies to GQ1b in FS almost always cross-react with a closely related minor ganglioside GT1a (115,116). Serum reactivity to gangliosides such as GD3, GD1b, and occasionally GT1b is seen in about half the patients with FS, giving rise to the suggestion that these sera recognize a disialosyl moiety shared by these gangliosides and GQ1b (117). More recent work has attempted to correlate the fine specificity of FS sera with clinical features and there is a suggestion that oropharyngeal weakness is preferentially associated with GT1a and ophthalmoplegia is associated with GQ1b reactivity (118–121). The presence of ophthalmoplegia in patients with generalized GBS has also been correlated with the presence of anti-GQ1b reactivity (122,123). Moreover, anti-GQ1b antibodies have been reported in patients with Bickerstaff's brainstem encephalitis that manifests as ophthalmoplegia, coma, pyramidal tract dysfunction, and in some cases responsiveness to plasma exchange (124,125). Because of these findings, some investigators now consider Bickerstaff's encephalitis and FS as related conditions. The basis of ataxia seen in FS remains controversial; both cerebellar and proprioceptive loss have been implicated. Areflexia in FS is likely due to afferent defects. The reversibility of both the areflexia and ataxia suggests that the sensory lesion(s) is peripheral to the dorsal root ganglion. It is possible that in some cases the cerebellum can be targeted directly (126). The anti-ganglioside antibody specificity for ataxia and areflexia is not clear, but indirect reasoning indicates that among disialylated gangliosides reactivity against GD1b may be most relevant, as some patients with acute sensory ataxic neuropathy have antibodies that cross-react with GD1b and/or GD3 but not with GQ1b/GT1a (117,127). It is now generally accepted that more than 85% of cases with FS have anti-GQ1b antibodies that reach a peak at the clinical presentation and decline with recovery (128). FS sera contain IgM, IgA, and IgG anti-GQ1b reactivity, but the IgG response is the most robust and persistent (129) and IgG anti-GQ1b antibodies are of complement-fixing isotypes (130).

4.3.   Distribution of Gangliosides in PNS

A major reason for defining the associations between anti-ganglioside antibody specificity and clinical variants of GBS is the simple hypothesis that differences in clinical manifestations are related to differences in the distribution of target antigens (gangliosides) in different regions of the nervous system. A substantial literature now exists on the distribution of gangliosides in the PNS and this clearly indicates that the absolute presence or absence of gangliosides is insufficient to explain the clinicopathologic findings seen in different variants of GBS. This issue is much more complex, however, as discussed below.

Gangliosides are sialic acid-containing glycosphingolipids that are widely distributed in mammalian tissues but are particularly enriched in the nervous system. Gangliosides are classified on the basis of the number and linkages of the sugar backbone and attached sialic acids. All complex gangliosides have a tetraose (four sugars) backbone/core, consisting of galactose, *N*-acetylgalactosamine, galactose, and glucose, to which variable numbers of sialic acids are attached; the ceramide or lipid portion of the molecule is attached to the internal glucose. For example, the four most abundant complex gangliosides in the nervous system are GM1, GD1b, GD1a, and GT1b. Simpler gangliosides have a shorter core structure instead of the tetraose backbone. The structures of gangliosides implicated as target antigens in AMAN and Fisher variants of GBS are depicted in Fig. 2. Anti-ganglioside antibody binding to these carbohydrate moieties determines their specificities. Although the antibody specificity is determined by the sequence of sugars contained in the carbohydrate core of gangliosides, some studies suggest that the length of fatty acid contained in the ceramide/lipid portion of gangliosides can affect the affinity of antibody binding to gangliosides in solid-phase immunoassays (131,132).

Biochemical extraction and tissue immunohistochemistry are the two analytical techniques used most widely to study the distribution of gangliosides in the PNS. The data obtained by these two approaches have generally been consistent and complementary. Biochemical studies indicate that there are no consistent differences in the ganglioside content of motor and sensory nerves (133–137), except that the fatty acid chains in the ceramide portion of gangliosides from sensory nerves has a larger proportion of long chain C20–26 fatty acids than do those from motor nerves (136). Our own work confirms these earlier findings that there are no quantitative differences in the major nervous system gangliosides, including GM1 and GD1a, between human motor and sensory roots. Nevertheless, qualitative differences in motor and sensory GD1a mobility on thin-layer chromatography (TLC) was observed and this likely indicates the differences in fatty acid length in the ceramide portion of sensory and motor GD1a (137). The implication of this finding is that anti-GD1a antibodies can have different affinities for sensory vs. motor GD1a. Expression of GalNAc-GD1a and GM1b in peripheral nerves has been reported (138) and one report suggests that GalNAc-GD1a may only be expressed by motor neurons and axons (139). A large number of immunolocalization studies have been done in the context of GM1. These studies, including our own (140), are limited by the use of either very-high-affinity toxins/lectins or low-affinity IgM antibodies (140–145). They demonstrate that GM1 is localized to nodes of Ranvier and paranodal myelin in both sensory and motor nerve fibers. Immunoelectronmicroscopic studies show that ganglioside GM1 is localized to nodal and internodal axolemma (140). Available data suggest that GM1 ligands bind to the Schwann cell surface but do not significantly stain compact myelin (140). We have recently generated several IgG anti-ganglioside

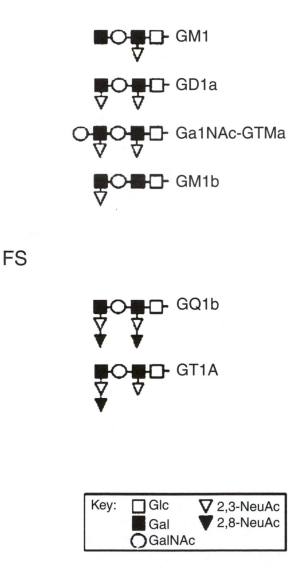

Figure 2   Ganglioside structures invoked as target antigens in AMAN and FS.

monoclonal antibodies (77,146) and used them for immunolocalization studies. Notably, anti-GD1a monoclonal antibody preferentially stained the motor nerve axons and only a subpopulation of small sensory fibers (Fig. 3). In contrast, no preferential motor axon binding with anti-GM1 antibodies was clearly recognized (137). Our results are consistent with a recent report of preferential motor nerve

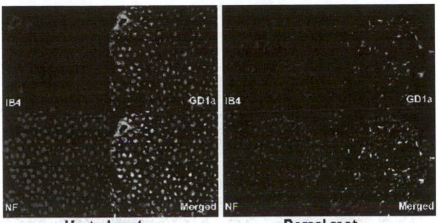

Figure 3 Fresh frozen cross-sections of rat ventral and dorsal root triple labeled with anti-ganglioside antibody GD1a-2a (green), neurofilament (red), and IB-4 (blue). Co-localization of three labels is also shown (merged). Neurofilament stains all myelinated fibers, whereas IB-4 stains unmyelinated fibers in dorsal root. This figure shows that anti-GD1a-2a antibody preferentially binds to myelinated motor axons in the ventral root and unmyelinated C fibers in the dorsal roots.

staining by serum from an AMAN patient with IgG reactivity to GD1a and GalNAc-GD1a (147,148). The localization of the minor target gangliosides GalNAc-GD1a and GM1b is not well characterized due in part to lack of mono-specific antibodies. There are no published reports on GM1b localization.

The distribution of GQ1b and related cross-reactive gangliosides in peripheral and cranial nerves has also been studied by biochemical and immunohisto-chemical techniques. The possible reasons for imprecise correlation of pathology and clinical features with the tissue distribution of target gangliosides have been alluded to above and are also relevant to the current discussion. Chiba et al. showed binding of anti-GQ1b antibodies to paranodal myelin and nodes of Ranvier and subsequently showed that the extraocular cranial nerves contain about twice as much of GQ1b as do other cranial and peripheral nerves (115,149). That GQ1b is not restricted to cranial nerves was also supported by two studies showing binding of disialosyl antibodies to the nodes of Ranvier in somatic nerves (74,150). Anti-disialosyl antibodies stain DRG neurons in several species including humans have been reported by several studies (143,144,151,152) and a recently generated GD1b-specific monoclonal antibody was shown to bind preferentially to large sensory neurons in DRG in several species including humans (137). Muscle spindles, proprioceptive transducers containing specialized muscle fibers and motor and sensory innervation, and intrafusal muscle fibers are also labeled by antibodies to disialylated antibodies (150). The distribution studies support the notion that FS-specific antibodies can target the extraocular nerves, peripheral proprioceptive sensory connections, and alter the muscle stretch reflexes. Antibodies with FS reactivity also bind to neuromuscular junctions (NMJ) in both somatic and extraocular muscles (74,150). This observation has been exploited by investigators for experimental modeling (see below) and may be relevant to FS pathogenesis, as NMJs are enriched in target gangliosides and are easily accessible to circulating antibodies.

In summary, ganglioside distribution studies do not show any quantitative differences in the distribution of gangliosides in the human sensory and motor nerves except for minor differences in the ceramide fatty acids. This difference in fatty acid length may affect ganglioside orientation and presentation in their native membranes and thus affect antibody binding. The immunolocalization studies provide convincing examples of preferential staining of myelinated motor nerve fibers by GD1a-related antibodies (see Fig. 3), but the basis of this differential antibody binding to motor fibers remains unclear (137). It is more than likely that other factors besides ganglioside density and distribution also play important roles in anti-ganglioside antibody-mediated injury. These factors include relative differences in the blood–nerve barrier in different regions of the nerve fibers and between sensory and motor spinal roots; the motor nerve terminal provides such an example. One favored explanation for the absence of CNS involvement in AMAN despite a high level of ganglioside expression in the CNS is the different permeability of blood–brain and blood–nerve barriers. The existence of such differences in barrier permeability between sensory and motor roots, however, has not been reported. Further, the conduction properties of motor fibers are significantly different from those of sensory fibers and one could speculate that these fibers are more prone to antibody-mediated conduction failure; this may be particularly relevant early in pathogenesis. Moreover, susceptibility to injury could also differ between motor and sensory fibers or different regions of the same nerve fiber based on the differences in expression of cellular protective molecules such as complement regulatory proteins. It is fair to say that the basis of preferential motor injury in AMAN remains incompletely understood and ongoing work is likely to provide further clues to this interesting pathogenetic issue. Similarly, target antigens relevant to FS syndrome are widely distributed and may be slightly more enriched in target neural elements responsible for clinical manifestations. Nevertheless, a satisfactory explanation(s) for the restriction of pathology to ocular and sensory nerves despite more widespread distribution of target antigens in the peripheral nerves is not yet established.

4.4. Evidence for Anti-ganglioside Antibody-Mediated Neural Injury

The pathogenetic significance of anti-ganglioside antibodies in GBS continues to be debated despite the development of animal models by immunization with gangliosides or *Campylobacter jejuni* (153,154). This reflects in part difficulty in reproducing these models as well as failure to induce clinical and pathological disease by the passive transfer of anti-ganglioside antibodies—a requisite for fulfillment of the Koch–Witebsky postulates for autoimmune disorders (155). Further, low affinity anti-ganglioside antibodies are part of the normal immune repertoire and are commonly found in several disease conditions. Lack of easy and reliable assays to distinguish between naturally occurring and pathogenic anti-ganglioside antibodies also contributes to the controversy surrounding this issue. Despite these caveats, the data discussed below strongly support the pathogenic role of anti-ganglioside antibodies.

Both human and experimental studies provide circumstantial evidence for the role of anti-ganglioside antibodies in the pathogenesis of axonal forms of GBS. The human data stems from the retrospective analysis of the incidence of GBS in patient populations receiving parenteral gangliosides for various neurological disorders and a clinical trial in which anti-GD2 antibodies were parenterally administered to patients with metastatic melanoma. Experimental studies can be divided into two broad categories. One group of studies has utilized various immunization strategies with gangliosides or *C. jejuni* to induce experimental neuropathy in animal models. A second group of studies examined the electrophysiological or morphological effects of either GBS-derived or experimentally induced anti-ganglioside antibodies in various in vivo or in vitro models. Notably, some of the experimental models have not always been reproducible, raising controversy about the role of anti-ganglioside antibodies.

In Europe, administration of GM1 or brain gangliosides was a not uncommon treatment for various neurological disorders and several cases of acute neuropathy following parenteral administration of gangliosides were reported in the early 1990s (156–158). However, a retrospective study in Italy failed to find a correlation between ganglioside administration and acute neuropathy (156). Subsequently, a retrospective case–control study with a much larger population sample in the Latium region of Italy reported a positive correlation between ganglioside treatment and GBS (159). This study reports that 4% of the total 4.5 million population received parenteral gangliosides over a 1-year period. A total of 42 cases of GBS were diagnosed during the same period. Six of the 42 GBS patients had received gangliosides and this was calculated to be a significantly increased incidence compared to that in patients not receiving ganglioside treatment. Serological, electrophysiological, and clinical details were not available on these cases. In an important study, Illa et al. described the clinical, electrophysiological, and serological features of seven patients with post-ganglioside GBS and compared them with eight controls who received gangliosides but did not develop GBS (160). The seven GBS patients had IgG anti-ganglioside antibodies, sera from six patients reacted with GM1 and serum from one patient reacted with GD1a and GT1b, whereas controls had no IgG anti-ganglioside reactivity. The clinical and electrophysiological features of these GBS cases were consistent with AMAN. The disease onset varied between 5 and 15 days after the initiation of ganglioside therapy, a short time course for a primary immune response for

production of IgG anti-ganglioside antibodies. The antibody titers did not correlate with severity of disease, and antibody titers remained high in two patients
after recovery. One patient had evidence of *C. jejuni* and another had evidence of
herpes zoster infection, but the remaining five cases had no serological evidence
of preceding infection. These observations support the notion that antibody
responses against gangliosides can be involved in the pathogenesis of axonal
GBS.

A phase I trial of murine monoclonal anti-GD2 antibody in metastatic
melanoma patients provides the closest approximation to a human passive transfer experiment with anti-ganglioside antibodies (161). In this trial, 12 patients
were enrolled and a monoclonal anti-GD2 antibody was administered in four
doses over an 8-day period with total doses ranging from 10 to 120 mg. All
patients receiving more than 10 mg of antibody developed acute pelvic and
abdominal pain. Five patients developed delayed neuropathic type pain after the
third and fourth infusion and four of the five patients developed neurological side
effects, including two patients with significant but reversible neuropathy. In a
subsequent study, Yuki et al. reported that this antibody binds to human peripheral nerve myelin (162). Although anti-GD2 antibodies are not frequently
reported in patients with GBS or its variants (162), these studies provide strong
support for the hypothesis that anti-ganglioside antibodies can cause peripheral
nerve injury.

Immunization with gangliosides or *C. jejuni* and passive transfer with
human GBS sera or purified anti-ganglioside antibodies, which have been used
by a number of investigators in an attempt to induce animal models of GBS produced mixed results. Immunization of rabbits with gangliosides generally does
not give rise to experimental neuritis or neuropathy except for three reports from
Japan. Nagai and colleagues reported paralytic disease after immunization with
GM1 (163), but serological studies were not done and the pathology was not
described in detail. Twenty years later Kusunoki et al. induced sensory neuropa-
thy/neuronopathy after immunization with GD1b (164) (see below). A recent
exciting report by Yuki et al. showed that rabbits immunized with mixed brain
gangliosides or GM1 developed clinical weakness, high titers of IgG anti-GM1
antibodies, and pathology consistent with axonal degeneration confined to ventral
roots (153). The induction of anti-ganglioside antibodies in various experimental
animals is not always associated with clinical symptoms and/or pathology, as suggested by several negative studies (73,74,165–167). The generation of an animal
model of *C. jejuni*-induced experimental neuropathy is complicated by the fact
that there are no animal models of *Campylobacter*-related enteritis. Nevertheless,
Li et al. used a *C. jejuni* strain isolated from a child with AMAN and induced
paralysis and pathological changes in the nerves, similar to those seen in AMAN,
in half the chickens fed with this organism (154). The LPS of the organism used
to generate this model carries ganglioside-like moieties (49), however, serological studies were not done on these animals. Subsequent attempts by other laboratories including our own (Nachamkin I, unpublished data) to reproduce this

model with the same organism were unsuccessful. Several studies indicated that *C. jejuni* LPS extracted from different GBS-related strains induce anti-ganglioside antibodies but these did not produce clinical or pathological disease (73–75). The difference in the relative affinity of experimentally induced anti-ganglioside antibodies has been proposed to relate to the dissociation of serological responses and experimental disease (167). This study provides one potential explanation for the disparate results reported by different investigators.

Electrophysiological and morphological effects of anti-ganglioside antibodies associated with AMAN have been studied in vitro. The physiologic studies have focused on the effects of antibodies on nerve fiber conduction and ion channels. Some in vitro electrophysiological studies have reported anti-GM1 antibody-mediated conduction failure at the nodes of Ranvier or motor nerve terminals (168–171) and this conduction failure could be secondary to blockade of voltage-gated sodium channels (170,172). All investigators have not been able to reproduce these findings (173–175), partly because of differences in the methodology. The studies supporting the blockade of sodium channels by anti-GM1 antibodies have given rise to a concept in evolution that conduction failure could be on an axonal basis. Although this concept originates from controversial experimental findings support for this concept is largely derived from the following clinical observations: some patients with AMAN recover rapidly (95,176), the pathological changes in some cases with AMAN are very mild despite severe clinical weakness (177), the rapid resolution of distal conduction block in some patients with AMAN and anti-GM1 antibodies (95), and the reversible conduction abnormalities myelinated fibers caused by specific sodium channel toxins like tetrodotoxin and saxitoxin (178,179).

We have recently established two in vitro models to study the morphologic consequences of anti-GD1a antibodies. First, a cell lysis assay indicates that these antibodies lyse neuronal cell lines by targeting GD1a, and complement is required for neuronal injury in this model (Zhang G, Sheikh K, unpublished observations). Second, anti-GD1a-related antibodies can cause motor nerve degeneration in an organotypic spinal cord culture model (180). One can conclude from these studies that anti-ganglioside antibodies have pathophysiologic effects, but, the exact molecular and cellular mechanisms of anti-ganglioside antibody-mediated neural injury need further elucidation.

Evidence for the pathophysiologic effects of anti-GQ1b antibodies or FS sera is largely derived from the studies done on phrenic nerve hemi-diaphragm preparations focusing on antibody-mediated effects at the NMJ (181–183). The pathology of FS is not well documented but few autopsy studies in FS have indicated that segmental demyelination is a pathological feature of this form of GBS. The focus of research in FS has shifted away from paranodal demyelination because an in vitro study on isolated, desheathed mouse sciatic nerve incubated with FS antibodies demonstrated anti-disialosyl antibody binding and complement deposition at the nodes of Ranvier without acute conduction failure (175). These data are interpreted as evidence against antibody-mediated physiological conduction block at the nodes of Ranvier and imply that paranodal demyelination may be less relevant to pathogenesis of FS-related antibodies.

Roberts et al. (181) reported that in phrenic nerve hemi-diaphragm preparations anti-GQ1b-positive FS sera and IgG caused a temporary and moderate increase in spontaneous quantal acetylcholine release at the NMJ, as assessed by a rise in miniature end plate potential frequency, and subsequent at nerve terminal failure of the conduction. In passive transfer experiments with a human IgM anti-disialosyl antibody in mice no clinical disease was induced despite deposition of IgM at motor nerve terminals, nevertheless, ex vivo hemi-diaphragm preparations from these animals showed conduction failure as described above (150). In a series of in vitro studies with mouse hemi-diaphragm preparations, Willison et al. have demonstrated that FS sera, FS IgG fractions, and a human monoclonal anti-GQ1b IgM antibody bind to NMJs, cause massive quantal release of acetycholine from nerve terminals and eventually blockade of neuromuscular transmission primarily through pre-synaptic mechanisms, resembling the effects of the paralytic neurotoxin alpha-latrotoxin (183). Further, these antibody-mediated effects on NMJs required complement, although, the conduction failure at NMJs required neither activation of classical pathway nor formation of membrane attack complex (183), as C1q- and C8-deficient sera reproduced alpha-latrotoxin-like effects. These findings were further extended to the monoclonal anti-diasialosyl antibodies generated by immunization with *C. jejuni* LPS, thus supporting a connection among the infecting organism, anti-ganglioside antibody, and nerve injury (74). Recently, the same group has shown that in this model there are morphological changes at the light and electron microscope level, consistent with degeneration of motor nerve terminals (184).

In a parallel set of studies by Buchwald et al. (182,185,186) using a perfused macropatch clamp electrode technique on the phrenic nerve hemi-diaphragm preparation, IgG fractions from both GQ1b-positive and -negative FS cases blocked evoked acetylcholine release and depressed the amplitude of post-synaptic potentials, implicating both a pre- and postsynaptic blocking effect. This effect was reversible and was independent of complement. The different findings from the two groups likely reflect both differences in methodology and more than one mechanism of NMJ blockade mediated by these antibodies.

There are no animal models of FS, either with passive transfer of antibodies or active immunization with LPS or gangliosides. Sensory ataxic neuropathy model of Kusunoki et al. (164), however, is extremely instructive for the acute and chronic sensory ataxic neuropathies (including FS) associated with anti-disialosyl antibodies. In this model repeated injection of the disialosyl ganglioside GD1b and KLH mixed with Freund's adjuvant led to sensory ataxia in a significant proportion of animals after 4 or more weeks of immunization. All animals developed anti-GD1b antibodies, but neuropathy was restricted to animals with antibody reactivity restricted to GD1b and not cross-reactive with other related gangliosides (187). The diseased animals demonstrated degeneration of

DRG neurons with secondary nerve fiber degeneration in dorsal roots and dorsal columns. Although the pathophysiology of FS is unlikely to be on the basis of degeneration of DRG neurons, this model, however, provides support for the concept that antibodies with reactivity to disialosyl gangliosides could cause sensory ataxia and areflexia. Of note a passive transfer of sera from sick rabbits to healthy animals has not produced significant clinicopathologic disease (188).

5. UNRESOLVED ISSUES

Although significant advances have been made in our understanding of the pathogenesis of AMAN and FS over the last 15 years, clearly several fundamental issues remain unresolved. These issues include: (a) Why only a small proportion of patients develop GBS after *C. jejuni* infection GBS? (b) What is the mechanism(s) underlying development of anti-ganglioside antibodies? (c) Since the ganglioside content of CNS is much higher than that in the PNS, why is CNS spared? (d) What is the basis of regional localization of pathology along the neuraxis or the course of a nerve fiber? e) Do antibodies have intrinsic properties that allow them to cross the blood–tissue barriers and is this capability tissue- or nerve-specific? (f) What are the cellular and molecular mechanisms of antibody-mediated neural injury? (g) Why it has been difficult to establish reproducible animal model(s)?

In the absence of an animal model of *C. jejuni* enteritis it is difficult to understand the basis of aberrant enteric mucosal immune responses that lead to induction of anti-ganglioside antibody and susceptibility to development of GBS after *Campylobacter* infection. The existing tools and experimental models of anti-ganglioside antibody-mediated neural injury are likely to provide further insights into the pathogenesis of this interesting group of disorders. Although AMAN and FS are rare diseases, detailed dissection of the mechanisms involved in the pathogenesis of these variants of GBS is likely to increase our understanding of post-infectious autoimmunity in general.

6. RECONSTRUCTION OF PATHOGENESIS

Despite the caveats mentioned above analysis of the clinical and experimental data suggests that post-*Campylobacter* AMAN and FS are among the best-understood acute inflammatory neuropathic disorders. A simplistic formulation of the pathogenesis would start with a primary immune antibody response to infectious organisms bearing ganglioside-like moieties. The immune response consists of specific IgG anti-ganglioside antibodies related to these variants, causing preferential motor fiber injury in AMAN and damage to oculomotor nerves, sensory ganglion neurons or fibers in FS, leading to specific clinical and physiological features associated with these variants. Clinical recovery occurs with a decline in antibody titers. The experimental models clearly show that these antibodies have pathogenic effects, thus supporting the hypothesis of post-infectious molecular mimicry in the pathogenesis of AMAN and Fisher variants of GBS.

7. COMMENT

Witebsky in 1957 proposed a set of criteria (189), consciously modeled on Koch's postulates, which should ideally be fulfilled in order to prove the role of an aberrant immune response in the pathogenesis of a human autoimmune disease. The original criteria included 1) direct demonstration or recognition of autoimmune response in the form of free circulating antibodies; 2) recognition of the corresponding specific antigen for this auto-antibody; 3) generation of antibodies against the same antigen in experimental animals; and 4) an actively immunized animal must also develop pathological features similar to those in the human disease. These original criteria were proposed in the context of auto-antibodies and chronic thyroiditis, but can be easily applied to other effectors of the immune system such as cell-mediated autoimmunity. Although not included in the original criteria, the most direct, stringent, widely accepted (190), and sat-

Witebsky criteria	AMAN	FS	Myastheni gravis
Original			
Demonstration of circulating Abs	✓	✓	✓
Recognition of Ab's target antigen	✓	✓	✓
Ab production against these target antigens in experimental animals	✓	✓	✓
Active immunization in animals causes pathology similar to that of human disease	✓	✗	✓
Extended			
Passive transfer reproduces pathology similar to that of human disease	✗	✗	✓
Triggering events	✓	✓	✗

Figure 4 Comparison of the number of original and extended Witebsky criteria fulfilled by AMAN, FS, and myasthenia gravis.

isfying evidence for the autoimmune nature of a human disease is the reproduction of clinical and pathological features by passive transfer of autoreactive antibodies or lymphocytes. We think in this context an attempt should also be made to determine the triggering event(s) that could lead to an aberrant autoimmune response and disease. The analysis of clinical and experimental evidence presented above would argue that AMAN and FS fulfill most of the original and extended Witebsky criteria for autoimmune diseases and these variants arguably can now be compared to the prototypic antibody-mediated autoimmune disorders like myasthenia gravis (see Fig. 4). In conclusion, AMAN and FS provide the best disease models that strongly support the hypothesis of molecular mimicry as a pathogenetic mechanism underlying some post-infectious autoimmune disorders.

REFERENCES

1. Rees JH, Thompson RD, Smeeton NC, Hughes RA. Epidemiological study of Guillain–Barre syndrome in southeast England. J Neurol Neurosurg Psychiatry 1998; 64(1):74–77.
2. Arnason BGW, Soliven B. Acute inflammatory demyelinating polyradiculopathy. In: Dyck PJ, Thomas PK, Griffin JW, Low PA, Poduslo JF, eds. Peripheral Neuropathy. Philadelphia: W.B. Saunders, 1993:1437–1497.
3. Emilia-Romagna Study Group on Clinical and Epidemiological Problems in Neurology. Guillain–Barre syndrome variants in Emilia-Romagna, Italy, 1992–3: incidence, clinical features, and prognosis. J Neurol Neurosurg Psychiatry 1998; 65(2):218–224.
4. Tuck RR, McLeod JG. Autonomic dysfunction in Guillain–Barre syndrome. J Neurol Neurosurg Psychiatry 1981; 44(11):983–990.
5. Fuller GN, Jacobs JM, Lewis PD, Lane RJM. Pseudoaxonal Guillain–Barre syndrome: severe demyelination mimicking axonopathy. A case with pupillary involvement. J Neurol Neurosurg Psychiatry 1992; 55:1079–1083.
6. Feasby TE, Gilbert JJ, Brown WF, et al. An acute axonal form of Guillain–Barre polyneuropathy. Brain 1986; 109:1115–1126.
7. Yuki N, Yoshino H, Sato S, Miyatake T. Acute axonal polyneuropathy associated with anti-GM1 antibodies following *Campylobacter* enteritis. Neurology 1990; 40:1900–1902.
8. McKhann GM, Cornblath DR, Griffin JW, Ho TW, Li CY, Jiang Z, et al. Acute motor axonal neuropathy: A frequent cause of acute flaccid paralysis in China. Ann Neurol 1993; 33:333–342.
9. Ho TW, Mishu B, Li CY, Gao CY, Cornblath DR, Griffin JW, et al. Guillain–Barre syndrome in northern China: Relationship to *Campylobacter jejuni* infection and anti-glycolipid antibodies. Brain 1995; 118:597–605.
10. Visser LH, van der Meché FG, Van Doorn PA, Meulstee J, Jacobs BC, Oomes PG, et al. Guillain–Barré syndrome without sensory loss (acute motor neuropathy). A subgroup with specific clinical, electrodiagnostic and laboratory features. Dutch Guillain–Barré study group. Brain 1995; 118:841–847.

11. Winer JB, Hughes RAC, Osmond C. A prospective study of acute idiopathic neu-
    ropathy. 2. Antecedent events. J Neurol Neurosurg Psychiatry 1988; 51:613–618.
12. Jacobs BC, Rothbarth PH, van der Meche FG, Herbrink P, Schmitz PI, De Klerk
    MA, et al. The spectrum of antecedent infections in Guillain–Barre syndrome: a
    case–control study. Neurology 1998; 51(4):1110–1115.
13. Winer JB, Hughes RAC, Osmond C. A prospective study of acute idiopathic neu-
    ropathy. 1. Clinical features and their prognostic value. J Neurol Neurosurg
    Psychiatry 1988; 51:605–612.
14. Sheth RD, Riggs JE, Hobbs GR, Gutmann L. Age and Guillain–Barre syndrome
    severity. Muscle Nerve 1996; 19(3):375–377.
15. Haass A, Trabert W, Grebnich N, Schimrigk. High-dose steroid therapy in
    Guillain–Barre syndrome. J Neuroimmunol 1988; 20:305–309.
16. Kaldor J, Speed BR. Guillain–Barre syndrome and *Campylobacter jejuni*: a sero-
    logical study. Br Med J 1984; 288:1867–1870.
17. Visser LH, van der Meché FGA, Meulstee J, Rothbarth PPh, Jacobs BC, Schmitz
    PIM, et al. Cytomegalovirus infection and Guillain–Barré syndrome: the clinical,
    electrophysiologic, and prognostic features. Neurology 1996; 47:668–673.
18. Guillain–Barre Study Group. Plasmapheresis and acute Guillain–Barre syndrome.
    Neurology 1985; 35:1096–1104.
19. McKhann GM, Griffin JW, Cornblath DR, Mellits D, Fisher RS, Quaskey SA, et al.
    Plasmapheresis and Guillain–Barre syndrome: analysis of prognostic factors and
    the effect of plasmapheresis. Ann Neurol 1988; 23:347–353.
20. Ropper AH. Severe acute Guillain–Barre syndrome. Neurology 1986; 36:429–432.
21. Delanoe C, Sebire G, Landrieu P, Huault G, Metral S. Acute inflammatory demyeli-
    nating polyradiculopathy in children: clinical and electrodiagnostic studies. Ann
    Neurol 1998; 44(3):350–356.
22. Bradshaw DY, Jones HR Jr. Guillain–Barre syndrome in children: clinical course,
    electrodiagnosis, and prognosis. Muscle Nerve 1992; 15:500–506.
23. Eberle E, Brink J, Azen S, White D. Early predictors of incomplete recovery in chil-
    dren with Guillain–Barré polyneuritis. J Pediatr 1975; 86(3):356–359.
24. Massaro ME, Rodriguez EC, Pociecha J, Arroyo HA, Sacolitti M, Taratuto AL, et
    al. Nerve biopsy in children with severe Guillain–Barre syndrome and inexcitable
    motor nerves. Neurology 1998; 51(2):394–398.
25. Reisin RC, Cersosimo R, Garcia AM, Massaro M, Fejerman N. Acute "axonal"
    Guillain–Barre syndrome in childhood. Muscle Nerve 1993; 16(12):1310–1316.
26. Hall SM, Hughes RA, Atkinson PF, McColl I, Gale A. Motor nerve biopsy in severe
    Guillain–Barre syndrome. Ann Neurol 1992; 31:441–444.
27. Hafer-Macko C, Sheikh KA, Li CY, Ho TW, Cornblath DR, McKhann GM, et al.
    Immune attack on the Schwann cell surface in acute inflammatory demyelinating
    polyneuropathy. Ann Neurol 1996; 39:625–635.
28. Hafer-Macko C, Hsieh S-T, Li CY, Ho TW, Sheikh K, Cornblath DR, et al. Acute
    motor axonal neuropathy: an antibody-mediated attack on axolemma. Ann Neurol
    1996; 40:635–644.
29. Griffin JW, Li CY, Ho TW, Xue P, Macko C, Cornblath DR, et al. Guillain–Barre
    syndrome in northern China: the spectrum of neuropathologic changes in clinically
    defined cases. Brain 1995; 118:577–595.
30. Griffin JW, Li CY, Ho TW, Tian M, Gao CY, Xue P et al. Pathology of the motor-
    sensory axonal Guillain–Barre Syndrome. Am Neurol Assoc 1996; 39:17–28.

31. Hughes RA, Rees JH. Clinical and epidemiologic features of Guillain–Barre syndrome. J Infect Dis 1997; 176(suppl 2):S92–S98.

32. Friedman CR, Neimann J, Wegener HC, Tauxe RV. Epidemiology of *Campylobacter jejuni* infections in the United States and other industrialized nations. In: Nachamkin I, Blaser MJ, eds. *Campylobacter*. Washington, DC: American Society for Microbiology, 2000:121–138.

33. Oberhelman RA, Taylor DN. Campylobacter infections in developing countries. In: Nachamkin I, Blaser MJ, eds. *Campylobacter*. Washington, DC: American Society for Microbiology, 2000:139–153.

34. Harrington P, Archer J, Davis JP, Croft DR, Varma JK. Outbreak of *Campylobacter jejuni* infections associated with drinking unpasteurized milk procured through a cow-leasing program, Wisconsin, 2001. MMWR Morb Mort Wkly Rep 2002; 51:548–549.

35. Skirrow MB, Jones DM, Sutcliffe E, Benjamin J. *Campylobacter bacteraemia* in England and Wales, 1981–91. Epidemiol Infect 1993; 110(3):567–573.

36. Nachamkin I. Microbiologic approaches for studying *Campylobacter* species in patients with Guillain–Barre syndrome. J Infect Dis 1997; 176(suppl 2):S106–S114.

37. Rhodes KM, Tattersfield AE. Guillainv–Barre syndrome associated with *Campylobacter* infection. Br Med J (Clin Res Ed) 1982; 285(6336):173–174.

38. Ho TW, Willison HJ, Nachamkin I, Li CY, Veitch J, Ung H, et al. Anti-GD1a antibody is associated with axonal but not demyelinating forms of Guillain–Barre syndrome. Ann Neurol 1999; 45(2):168–173.

39. Moran AP, Prendergast MM, Hogan EL. Sialosyl-galactose: a common denominator of Guillain–Barre and related disorders? 2002.

40. Allos BM. Association between *Campylobacter* infection and Guillain–Barre syndrome. J Infect Dis 1997; 176(suppl 2):S125–S128.

41. Yuki N, Sato S, Itoh T, Miyatake T. HLA-B35 and acute axonal polyneuropathy following *Campylobacter jejuni* infection. Neurology 1991; 41:1561–1563.

42. Rees JH, Vaughan RW, Kondeatis E, Hughes RAC. HLA-class II alleles in Guillain–Barre syndrome and Miller Fisher syndrome and their association with preceding *Campylobacter jejuni* infection. J Neuroimmunol 1995; 62:53–57.

43. Magira EE, Papaioakim M, Nachamkin I, Asbury AK, Li CY, Ho TW, et al. Differential distribution of HLA-DQ beta/DR beta epitopes in the two forms of Guillain–Barre syndrome, acute motor axonal neuropathy and acute inflammatory demyelinating polyneuropathy (AIDP): identification of DQ beta epitopes associated with susceptibility to and protection from AIDP. J Immunol 2003; 170(6):3074–3080.

44. Patton CM, Wachsmuth IK, Evins GM, Kiehlbauch JA, Plikaytis BD, Troup N, et al. Evaluation of 10 methods to distinguish epidemic-associated *Campylobacter* strains. J Clin Microbiol 1991; 29(4):680–688.

45. Karlyshev AV, Linton D, Gregson NA, Lastovica AJ, Wren BW. Genetic and biochemical evidence of a *Campylobacter jejuni* capsular polysaccharide that accounts for Penner serotype specificity. Mol Microbiol 2000; 35(3):529–541.

46. Yuki N, Sato S, Fujimoto S, Yamada Y, Kinoshita A, Itoh T. Serotype of *Campylobacter jejuni*, HLA, and the Guillain–Barre syndrome. Muscle Nerve 1992; 16:968–969.

47. Fujimoto S, Yuki N, Itoh T, Amako K. Specific serotype of *Campylobacter jejuni* associated with Guillain–Barre syndrome. J Infect Dis 1992; 165:183 (Letter).

48. Kuroki S, Saida T, Nukina M, Haruta T, Yoshioka M, Kobayashi Y, et al. *Campylobacter jejuni* strains from patients with Guillain–Barre syndrome belong mostly to Penner serogroup 19 and contain beta-*N*-acetylglucosamine residues. Ann Neurol 1993; 33:243–247.

49. Sheikh KA, Nachamkin I, Ho TW, Willison HJ, Veitch J, Ung H, et al. *Campylobacter jejuni* lipopolysaccharides in Guillain–Barre syndrome: molecular mimicry and host susceptibility. Neurology 1998; 51(2):371–378.

50. Arzate BP, Garcia GR, Ponce NE, Nachamkin I. Comparison of two selective media for the isolation of *Campylobacter* species from a pediatric population in Mexico. Diagn Microbiol Infect Dis 1999; 34(4):329–332.

51. Mishu B, Ilyas AA, Koski CL, Vriesendorp F, Cook SA, Mithen F, et al. Serologic evidence of previous *Campylobacter jejuni* infection in patients with the Guillain–Barre syndrome. Ann Intern Med 1993; 118:947–953.

52. Rees JH, Soudain SE, Gregson NA, Hughes RA. *Campylobacter jejuni* infection and Guillain–Barré syndrome. N Engl J Med 1995; 333:1374–1379.

53. Jacobs BC, Hazenberg MP, Van Doorn PA, Endtz HPh, van der Meché FGA. Cross-reactive antibodies against gangliosides and *Campylobacter jejuni* lipopolysaccharides in patients with Guillain–Barré or Miller Fisher syndrome. J Infect Dis 1997; 175:729–733.

54. Jacobs BC, Van Doorn PA, Groeneveld JH, Tio-Gillen AP, van der Meche FG. Cytomegalovirus infections and anti-GM2 antibodies in Guillain–Barre syndrome. J Neurol Neurosurg Psychiatry 1997; 62(6):641–643.

55. Goddard EA, Lastovica AJ, Argent AC. Campylobacter 0:41 isolation in Guillain–Barre syndrome. Arch Dis Child 1997; 76(6):526–528.

56. Lastovica AJ, Goddard EA, Argent AC. Guillain–Barre syndrome in South Africa associated with *Campylobacter jejuni* O:41 strains. J Infect Dis 1997; 176(suppl 2):S139–S143.

57. Prendergast MM, Moran AP. Lipopolysaccharides in the development of the Guillain–Barre syndrome and Miller Fisher syndrome forms of acute inflammatory peripheral neuropathies. J Endotoxin Res 2000; 6(5):341–359.

58. Moran AP, Rietschel ET, Kosunen TU, Zahringer U. Chemical characterization of *Campylobacter jejuni* lipopolysaccharides containing N-acetylneuraminic acid and 2,3-diamino-2,3-dideoxy-D-glucose. J Bacteriol 1991; 173(2):618–626.

59. Yuki N, Handa S, Taki T, Kasama T, Takahashi M, Saito K. Cross-reactive antigen between nervous tissue and a bacterium elicits Guillain–Barre syndrome: molecular mimicry between gangliocide GM1 and lipopolysaccharide from Penner's serotype 19 of *Campylobacter jejuni*. Biomed Res 1992; 13:451–453.

60. Yuki N, Taki T, Inagaki F, et al. A bacterium lipopolysaccharide that elicits Guillain–Barre syndrome has a GM1 ganglioside-like structure. J Exp Med 1993; 178:1771–1775.

61. Yuki N, Taki T, Takahashi M, et al. Penner's serotype 4 of *Campylobacter jejuni* has a lipopolysaccharide that bears a GM1 ganglioside epitope as well as one that bears a GD1a epitope. Infect Immun 1994; 62:2101–2103.

62. Aspinall GO, McDonald AG, Raju TS, Pang H, Moran AP. Chemical structures of the core regions of *Campylobacter jejuni* serotypes O:1, O:4, O:23, and O:36 lipopolysaccharides. Eur J Biochem 1993; 213:1017–1027.

63. Aspinall GO, McDonald AG, Pang H, Kurjanczyk LA, Penner JL. Lipopolysaccharides of *Campylobacter jejuni* serotype O:19: structures of core

oligosaccharide regions from the serostrain and two bacterial isolates from patients with the Guillain–Barré syndrome. Biochemistry 1994; 33:241–249.

64. Aspinall GO, Fujimoto S, McDonald AG, et al. Lipopolysaccharides from *Campylobacter jejuni* associated with Guillain–Barre syndrome patients mimic human gangliosides in structure. Infect Immun 1994; 62:2122–2125.

65. Yuki N, Taki T, Handa S. Antibody to GalNAc-GD1a and GalNAc-GM1b in Guillain–Barre syndrome subsequent to *Campylobacter jejuni* enteritis. J Neuroimmunol 1996; 71:155–161.

66. Nachamkin I, Ung H, Moran AP, Yoo D, Prendergast MM, Nicholson MA, et al. Ganglioside GM1 mimicry in *Campylobacter* strains from sporadic infections in the United States [published erratum appears in J Infect Dis 1999 Jun;179(6):1593]. J Infect Dis 1999; 179(5):1183–1189.

67. Nachamkin I, Liu J, Li M, Ung H, Moran AP, Prendergast MM, et al. *Campylobacter jejuni* from patients with Guillain–Barre syndrome preferentially expresses a GD(1a)-like epitope. Infect Immun 2002; 70(9):5299–5303.

68. Gilbert M, Karwaski MF, Bernatchez S, Young NM, Taboada E, Michniewicz J, et al. The genetic bases for the variation in the lipo-oligosaccharide of the mucosal pathogen, *Campylobacter jejuni*. Biosynthesis of sialylated ganglioside mimics in the core oligosaccharide. J Biol Chem 2002; 277(1):327–337.

69. Guerry P, Szymanski CM, Prendergast MM, Hickey TE, Ewing CP, Pattarini DL, et al. Phase variation of *Campylobacter jejuni* 81–176 lipooligosaccharide affects ganglioside mimicry and invasiveness in vitro. Infect Immun 2002; 70(2):787–793.

70. Wirguin I, Suturkova-Milosevic Lj, Della-Latta P, Fisher T, Brown RH Jr, Latov N. Monoclonal IgM antibodies to GM1 and asialo-GM1 in chronic neuropathies cross-react with *Campylobacter jejuni* lipopolysaccharides. Ann Neurol 1994; 35:698–703.

71. Yuki N, Handa S, Tai T, Takahashi M, Saito K, Tsujino Y, et al. Ganglioside-like epitopes of lipopolysaccharides from *Campylobacter jejuni* (PEN 19) in three isolates from patients with Guillain–Barre syndrome. J Neurol Sci 1995; 130(1):112–116.

72. Oomes PG, Jacobs BC, Hazenberg MPH, Banffer JRJ, van der Meché FGA. Anti-GM1 IgG antibodies and *Campylobacter jejuni* bacteria in Guillain–Barre syndrome: evidence of molecular mimicry. Ann Neurol 1995; 38:170–175.

73. Wirguin I, Briani C, Suturkova-Milosevic L, Fisher T, Della-Latta P, Chalif P, et al. Induction of anti-GM1 ganglioside antibodies by *Campylobacter jejuni* lipopolysaccharides. J Neuroimmunol 1997; 78(1/2):138–142.

74. Goodyear CS, O'Hanlon GM, Plomp JJ, Wagner ER, Morrison I, Veitch J, et al. Monoclonal antibodies raised against Guillain–Barre syndrome- associated *Campylobacter jejuni* lipopolysaccharides react with neuronal gangliosides and paralyze muscle-nerve preparations [published erratum appears in J Clin Invest 1999 Dec;104(12):1771]. J Clin Invest 1999; 104(6):697–708.

75. Ang CW, De Klerk MA, Endtz HP, Jacobs BC, Laman JD, van der Meche FG, et al. Guillain–Barre syndrome- and Miller Fisher syndrome-associated *Campylobacter jejuni* lipopolysaccharides induce anti-GM1 and anti-GQ1b antibodies in rabbits. Infect Immun 2001; 69(4):2462–2469.

76. Bowes T, Wagner ER, Boffey J, Nicholl D, Cochrane L, Benboubetra M, et al. Tolerance to self gangliosides is the major factor restricting the antibody response to lipopolysaccharide core oligosaccharides in *Campylobacter jejuni* strains associated with Guillain–Barre syndrome. Infect Immun 2002; 70(9):5008–5018.

77. Lunn MP, Johnson LA, Fromholt SE, Itonori S, Huang J, Vyas AA, et al. High-affinity anti-ganglioside IgG antibodies raised in complex ganglioside knockout mice: reexamination of GD1a immunolocalization. J Neurochem 2000; 75(1):404–412.

78. Mori M, Kuwabara S, Miyake M, Noda M, Kuroki H, Kanno H, et al. Haemophilus influenzae infection and Guillain–Barre syndrome. Brain 2000; 123(Pt 10):2171–2178; 2001; 123(Pt 10):2171–2178.

79. Mori M, Kuwabara S, Miyake M, Dezawa M, Adachi-Usami E, Kuroki H, et al. Haemophilus influenzae has a GM1 ganglioside-like structure and elicits Guillain–Barre syndrome. Neurology 1999; 52(6):1282–1284.

80. Rees JH, Gregson NA, Hughes RAC. Anti-ganglioside GM1 antibodies in Guillain–Barre syndrome and their relationship to *Campylobacter jejuni* infection. Ann Neurol 1995; 38:809–816.

81. Salloway S, Mermel LA, Seamans M, Aspinall GO, Nam Shin JE, Kurjanczyk LA, et al. Miller-Fisher syndrome associated with *Campylobacter jejuni* bearing lipopolysaccharide molecules that mimic human ganglioside GD3. Infect Immun 1996; 64(8):2945–2949.

82. Shin JE, Ackloo S, Mainkar AS, Monteiro MA, Pang H, Penner JL, et al. Lipo-oligosaccharides of *Campylobacter jejuni* serotype O:10. Structures of core oligosaccharide regions from a bacterial isolate from a patient with the Miller-Fisher syndrome and from the serotype reference strain. Carbohydr Res 1997; 305(2):223–232.

83. Jacobs BC, Endtz H, van der Meché FGA, Hazenberg MP, Achtereekte HA, Van Doorn PA. Serum anti-GQ1b IgG antibodies recognize surface epitopes on *Campylobacter jejuni* from patients with Miller Fisher syndrome. Ann Neurol 1995; 37:260–264.

84. Yuki N, Taki T, Takahashi M, Saito K, Yoshino H, Tai T, et al. Molecular mimicry between GQ1b ganglioside and lipopolysaccharides of *Campylobacter jejuni* isolated from patients with Fisher's syndrome. Ann Neurol 1994; 36:791–793.

85. Ogino M, Orazio N, Latov N. IgG anti-GM1 antibodies from patients with acute motor neuropathy are predominantly of the IgG1 and IgG3 subclasses. J Neuroimmunol 1995; 58(1):77–80.

86. Yuki N, Ichihashi Y, Taki T. Subclass of IgG antibody to GM1 epitope-bearing lipopolysaccharide of *Campylobacter jejuni* in patients with Guillain–Barre syndrome. J Neuroimmunol 1995; 60(1/2):161–164.

87. Koga M, Tatsumoto M, Yuki N, Hirata K. Range of cross reactivity of anti-GM1 IgG antibody in Guillain–Barre syndrome. J Neurol Neurosurg Psychiatry 2001; 71(1):123–124.

88. Ogawara K, Kuwabara S, Mori M, Hattori T, Koga M, Yuki N. Axonal Guillain–Barre syndrome: relation to anti-ganglioside antibodies and *Campylobacter jejuni* infection in Japan. Ann Neurol 2000; 48(4):624–631.

89. Ang CW, Koga M, Jacobs BC, Yuki N, van der Meche FG, Van Doorn PA. Differential immune response to gangliosides in Guillain–Barre syndrome patients from Japan and The Netherlands. J Neuroimmunol 2001; 121(1/2):83–87.

90. Walsh FS, Cronin M, Koblar S, Doherty P, Winer J, Leon A, et al. Association between glycoconjugate antibodies and Campylobacter infection in patients with Guillain–Barre syndrome. J Neuroimmunol 1991; 34:43–51.

91. Jacobs BC, Van Doorn PA, Schmitz PI, et al. *Campylobacter jejuni* infections and anti-GM1 antibodies in Guillain–Barré syndrome. Ann Neurol 1996; 40:181–187.

92. Hadden RD, Cornblath DR, Hughes RA, Zielasek J, Hartung HP, Toyka KV, et al. Electrophysiological classification of Guillain–Barre syndrome: clinical associations and outcome. Plasma Exchange/Sandoglobulin Guillain–Barre Syndrome Trial Group. Ann Neurol 1998; 44(5):780–788.

93. Enders U, Karch H, Toyka KV, Michels M, Zielasek J, Pette M, et al. The spectrum of immune responses to *Campylobacter jejuni* and glycoconjugates in Guillain–Barre syndrome and in other neuroimmunological disorders. Ann Neurol 1993; 34:136–144.

94. Vriesendorp FJ, Mishu B, Blaser M, Koski CL. Serum antibodies to GM1, peripheral nerve myelin, and *Campylobacter jejuni* in patients with Guillain–Barre syndrome and controls: correlation and prognosis. Ann Neurol 1993; 34:130–135.

95. Kuwabara S, Asahina M, Koga M, Mori M, Yuki N, Hattori T. Two patterns of clinical recovery in Guillain–Barre syndrome with IgG anti-GM1 antibody. Neurology 1998; 51(6):1656–1660.

96. Yuki N, Yoshino H, Sato S, Shinozawa K, Miyatake T. Severe acute axonal form of Guillain–Barre syndrome associated with IgG anti-GD1a antibodies. Muscle Nerve 1992; 15:899–903.

97. Yuki N, Yamada M, Sato S, Ohama E, Kawase Y, Ikuta F, et al. Association of IgG anti-GD1a antibody with severe Guillain–Barre syndrome. Muscle Nerve 1993; 16:642–647.

98. Tagawa Y, Yuki N, Hirata K. High anti-GM1 and anti-GD1a IgG antibody titers are detected in Guillain–Barre syndrome but not in chronic inflammatory demyelinating polyneuropathy. Eur Neurol 2002; 48(2):118–119.

99. Caudie C, Vial C, Bancel J, Petiot P, Antoine JC, Gonnaud PM. Antiganglioside antibody profiles in 249 cases of Guillain–Barre syndrome. Ann Biol Clin (Paris) 2002; 60(5):589–597.

100. Kusunoki S, Chiba A, Kon K, Ando S, Arisawa K, Tate A, et al. N-acetylgalactosaminyl GD1a is a target molecule for serum antibody in Guillain–Barre syndrome. Ann Neurol 1994; 35:570–576.

101. Kusunoki S, Iwamori M, Chiba A, et al. GM1b is a new member of antigen for serum antibody in Guillain–Barré syndrome. Neurology 1996; 47:237–242.

102. Ang CW, Yuki N, Jacobs BC, Koga M, Van Doorn PA, Schmitz PI, et al. Rapidly progressive, predominantly motor Guillain–Barre syndrome with anti-GalNAc-GD1a antibodies. Neurology 1999; 53(9):2122–2127.

103. Yuki N, Ang CW, Koga M, Jacobs BC, Van Doorn PA, Hirata K, et al. Clinical features and response to treatment in Guillain–Barre syndrome associated with antibodies to GM1b ganglioside [In Process Citation]. Ann Neurol 2000; 47(3):314–321; 2000; 47(3):314–321.

104. Yuki N, Ho TW, Tagawa Y, Koga M, Li CY, Hirata K, et al. Autoantibodies to GM1b and GalNAc-GD1a: relationship to *Campylobacter jejuni* infection and acute motor axonal neuropathy in China. J Neurol Sci 1999; 164(2):134–138.

105. Hao Q, Saida T, Yoshino H, Kuroki S, Nukina M, Saida K. Anti-GalNAc-GD1a antibody-associated Guillain–Barre syndrome with a predominantly distal weakness without cranial nerve impairment and sensory disturbance. Ann Neurol 1999; 45(6):758–768.

106. Hughes RA, Hadden RD, Gregson NA, Smith KJ. Pathogenesis of Guillain–Barre syndrome. J Neuroimmunol 1999; 100(1/2):74–97.

107. Irie S, Saito T, Nakamura K, Kanazawa N, Ogino M, Nukazawa T, et al. Association of anti-GM2 antibodies in Guillain–Barre syndrome with acute cytomegalovirus infection. J Neuroimmunol 1996; 68(1/2):19–26.

108. Khalili-Shirazi A, Gregson N, Gray I, Rees J, Winer J, Hughes R. Antiganglioside antibodies in Guillain–Barre syndrome after a recent cytomegalovirus infection. J Neurol Neurosurg Psychiatry 1999; 66(3):376–379.

109. Yuki N, Tagawa Y. Acute cytomegalovirus infection and IgM anti-GM2 antibody. J Neurol Sci 1998; 154(1):14–17.

110. Miyazaki T, Kusunoki S, Kaida K, Shiina M, Kanazawa I. Guillain–Barre syndrome associated with IgG monospecific to ganglioside GD1b. Neurology 2001; 56(9):1227–1229.

111. Chiba A, Kusunoki S, Shimizu T, Kanazawa I. Serum IgG antibody to ganglioside GQ1b is a possible marker of Miller Fisher syndrome. Ann Neurol 1992; 31:677–679.

112. Willison HJ, Veitch J, Patterson G, Kennedy PGE. Miller Fisher syndrome is associated with serum antibodies to GQ1b ganglioside. J Neurol Neurosurg Psychiatry 1993; 56:204–206.

113. Yuki N, Sato S, Tsuji S, Ohsawa T, Miyatake T. Frequent presence of anti-GQ1b antibody in Fisher's syndrome. Neurology 1993; 43:414–417.

114. Carpo M, Pedotti R, Lolli F, Pitrola A, Allaria S, Scarlato G, et al. Clinical correlate and fine specificity of anti-GQ1b antibodies in peripheral neuropathy. J Neurol Sci 1998; 155(2):186–191.

115. Chiba A, Kusunoki S, Obata H, Machinami R, Kanazawa I. Serum anti-GQ1b IgG antibody is associated with ophthalmoplegia in Miller Fisher syndrome and Guillain–Barre syndrome: clinical and immunohistochemical studies. Neurology 1993; 43:1911–1917.

116. Ilyas AA, Cook SD, Mithen FA, Taki T, Kasama T, Handa S, et al. Antibodies to GT1a ganglioside in patients with Guillain–Barre syndrome. J Neuroimmunol 1998; 82(2):160–167.

117. Willison HJ, Almemar A, Veitch J, Thrush D. Acute ataxic neuropathy with cross-reactive antibodies to GD1b and GD3 gangliosides. Neurology 1994; 44(12):2395–2397.

118. Mizoguchi K, Hase A, Obi T, Matsuoka H, Takatsu M, Nishimura Y, et al. Two species of antiganglioside antibodies in a patient with a pharyngeal-cervical-brachial variant of Guillain–Barre syndrome. J Neurol Neurosurg Psychiatry 1994; 57(9):1121–1123.

119. O'Leary CP, Veitch J, Durward WF, Thomas AM, Rees JH, Willison HJ. Acute oropharyngeal palsy is associated with antibodies to GQ1b and GT1a gangliosides. J Neurol Neurosurg Psychiatry 1996; 61(6):649–651.

120. Koga M, Yuki N, Ariga T, Morimatsu M, Hirata K. Is IgG anti-GT1a antibody associated with pharyngeal-cervical-brachial weakness or oropharyngeal palsy in Guillain–Barre syndrome? J Neuroimmunol 1998; 86(1):74–79.

121. Kashihara K, Shiro Y, Koga M, Yuki N. IgG anti-GT1a antibodies which do not cross react with GQ1b ganglioside in a pharyngeal-cervical-brachial variant of Guillain–Barre syndrome. J Neurol Neurosurg Psychiatry 1998; 65(5):799.

122. Ter Bruggen JP, van der Meche FG, de Jager AE, Polman CH. Ophthalmoplegic and lower cranial nerve variants merge into each other and into classical Guillain–Barre syndrome. Muscle Nerve 1998; 21(2):239–242.

123. Odaka M, Yuki N, Hirata K. Anti-GQ1b IgG antibody syndrome: clinical and immunological range. J Neurol Neurosurg Psychiatry 2001; 70(1):50–55.

124. Yuki N. Successful plasmapheresis in Bickerstaff's brain stem encephalitis associated with anti-GQ1b antibody. J Neurol Sci 1995; 131(1):108–110.

125. Kikuchi M, Tagawa Y, Iwamoto H, Hoshino H, Yuki N. Bickerstaff's brainstem encephalitis associated with IgG anti-GQ1b antibody subsequent to *Mycoplasma pneumoniae* infection: favorable response to immunoadsorption therapy. J Child Neurol 1997; 12(6):403–405.

126. Kornberg AJ, Pestronk A, Blume GM, Lopate G, Yue J, Hahn A. Selective staining of the cerebellar molecular layer by serum IgG in Miller-Fisher and related syndromes. Neurology 1996; 47(5):1317–1320.

127. O'Leary CP, Willison HJ. Autoimmune ataxic neuropathies (sensory ganglionopathies). Curr Opin Neurol 1997; 10(5):366–370.

128. Mizoguchi K. Anti-GQ1b IgG antibody activities related to the severity of Miller Fisher syndrome. Neurol Res 1998; 20(7):617–624.

129. Koga M, Yuki N, Takahashi M, Saito K, Hirata K. Close association of IgA antiganglioside antibodies with antecedent *Campylobacter jejuni* infection in Guillain–Barré and Fisher's syndromes. J Neuroimmunol 1998; 81(1/2):138–143.

130. Willison HJ, Veitch J. Immunoglobulin subclass distribution and binding characteristics of anti-GQ1b antibodies in Miller Fisher syndrome. J Neuroimmunol 1994; 50:159–165.

131. Itonori S, Hidari K, Sanai Y, Taniguchi M, Nagai Y. Involvement of the acyl chain of ceramide in carbohydrate recognition by an anti-glycolipid monoclonal antibody: the case of an anti-melanoma antibody, M2590, to GM3-ganglioside. Glycoconj J 1989; 6(4):551–560.

132. Tagawa Y, Laroy W, Nimrichter L, Fromholt SE, Moser AB, Moser HW, et al. Antiganglioside antibodies bind with enhanced affinity to gangliosides containing very long chain fatty acids. Neurochem Res 2002; 27(7/8):847–855.

133. Svennerholm L, Boström K, Fredman P, Jungbjer B, Lekman A, Månsson J-E, et al. Gangliosides and allied glycosphingolipids in human peripheral nerve and spinal cord. Biochim Biophys Acta 1994; 1214:115–123.

134. Svennerholm L, Bostrom K, Fredman P, Jungbjer B, Mansson JE, Rynmark BM. Membrane lipids of human peripheral nerve and spinal cord. Biochim Biophys Acta 1992; 1128(1):1–7.

135. Ogawa-Goto K, Abe T. Gangliosides and glycosphingolipids of peripheral nervous system myelins—a minireview. Neurochem Res 1998; 23(3):305–310.

136. Ogawa-Goto K, Funamoto N, Abe T, Nagashima K. Different ceramide compositions of gangliosides between human motor and sensory nerves. J Neurochem 1990; 55:1486–1493.

137. Gong Y, Tagawa Y, Lunn MP, Laroy W, Heffer-Lauc M, Li CY, et al. Localization of major gangliosides in the PNS: implications for immune neuropathies. Brain 2002; 125:2491–2506.

138. Ilyas AA, Li SC, Chou DK, Li YT, Jungalwala FB, Dalakas MC, et al. Gangliosides GM2, IV4GalNAcGM1b, and IV4GalNAcGC1a as antigens for monoclonal

immunoglobulin M in neuropathy associated with gammopathy. J Biol Chem 1988; 263(9):4369–4373.

139. Yoshino H. Distribution of gangliosides in the nervous tissues recognized by axonal form of Guillain–Barre syndrome (in Japanese). Neuroimmunology 1997; 5:174–175.

140. Sheikh KA, Deerinck TJ, Ellisman MH, Griffin JW. The distribution of ganglioside-like moieties in peripheral nerves. Brain 1999; 122(Pt 3):449–460.

141. Ganser AL, Kirschner DA, Willinger M. Ganglioside localization on myelinated nerve fibres by cholera toxin binding. J Neurocytol 1983; 12:921–938.

142. Corbo M, Quattrini A, Latov N, Hays AP. Localization of GM1 and Gal(beta1–3)GalNAc antigenic determinants in peripheral nerve. Neurology 1993; 43:809–814.

143. Kusunoki S, Chiba A, Tai T, Kanazawa I. Localization of GM1 and GD1b antigens in the human peripheral nervous system. Muscle Nerve 1993; 16:752–756.

144. O'Hanlon GM, Paterson GJ, Wilson G, Doyle D, McHardie P, Willison HJ. Anti-GM1 ganglioside antibodies cloned from autoimmune neuropathy patients show diverse binding patterns in the rodent nervous system. J Neuropath Exp Neurol 1996; 55:184–195.

145. Molander M, Berthold C-H, Persson H, Andersson K, Fredman P. Monosialoganglioside (GM1) immunofluoresence in rat spinal roots studied with a monoclonal antibody. J Neurocytol 1997; 26:101–111.

146. Schnaar RL, Fromholt SE, Gong Y, Vyas AA, Laroy W, Wayman DM, et al. IgG-class mouse monoclonal antibodies to major brain gangliosides. Anal Biochem 2002; 302:276–284.

147. Lugaresi A, Ragno M, Torrieri F, Di Guglielmo G, Fermani P, Uncini A. Acute motor axonal neuropathy with high titer IgG and IgA anti-GD1a antibodies following Campylobacter enteritis. J Neurol Sci 1997; 147(2):193–200.

148. De Angelis MV, Di Muzio A, Lupo S, Gambi D, Uncini A, Lugaresi A. Anti-GD1a antibodies from an acute motor axonal neuropathy patient selectively bind to motor nerve fiber nodes of Ranvier. J Neuroimmunol 2001; 121(1/2):79–82; 2002; 121(1/2):79–82.

149. Chiba A, Kusunoki S, Obata H, Machinami R, Kanazawa I. Ganglioside composition of the human cranial nerves, with special reference to pathophysiology of Miller Fisher syndrome. Brain Res 1997; 745(1/2):32–36.

150. Willison HJ, O'Hanlon GM, Paterson G, Veitch J, Wilson G, Roberts M, et al. A somatically mutated human antiganglioside IgM antibody that induces experimental neuropathy in mice is encoded by the variable region heavy chain gene, V1–18. J Clin Invest 1996; 97(5):1155–1164.

151. Kusunoki S, Mashiko H, Mochizuki N, Chiba A, Arita M, Hitoshi S, et al. Binding of antibodies against GM1 and GD1b in human peripheral nerve. Muscle Nerve 1997; 20:840–845.

152. Maehara T, Ono K, Tsutsui K, Watarai S, Yasuda T, Inoue H, et al. A monoclonal antibody that recognizes ganglioside GD1b in the rat central nervous system. Neurosci Res 1997; 29(1):9–16.

153. Yuki N, Yamada M, Koga M, Odaka M, Susuki K, Tagawa Y, et al. Animal model of axonal Guillain–Barre syndrome induced by sensitization with GM1 ganglioside. Ann Neurol. In press.

154. Li CY, Xue P, Gao CY, Tian WQ, Liu RC, Yang C. Experimental *Campylobacter jejuni* infection in the chicken: an animal model of axonal Guillain–Barré syndrome. J Neurol Neurosurg Psychiatry 1996; 61:279–284.

155. Sheikh KA, Griffin JW. Variants of the Guillain–Barre syndrome: progress toward fulfilling "Koch's postulates". Ann Neurol 2001; 49(6):694–696.

156. Granieri E, Casetta I, Govoni V, Tola MR, Paolino E, Rocca WA. Ganglioside therapy and Guillain–Barre syndrome. A historical cohort study in Ferrara, Italy, fails to demonstrate an association. Neuroepidemiology 1991; 10(4):161–169.

157. Schonhofer PS. Guillain–Barre syndrome and parenteral gangliosides. Lancet 1991; 338(8769):757.

158. Figueras A, Morales-Olivas FJ, Capella D, Palop V, Laporte JR. Bovine gangliosides and acute motor polyneuropathy. BMJ 1992; 305(6865):1330–1331.

159. Raschetti R, Maggini M, Popoli P, Caffari B, Da Cas R, Menniti-Ippolito F, et al. Gangliosides and Guillain–Barre syndrome. J Clin Epidemiol 1995; 48(11):1399–1405.

160. Illa I, Ortiz N, Gallard E, Juarez C, Grau JM, Dalakas MC. Acute axonal Guillain–Barre syndrome with IgG antibodies against motor axons following parenteral gangliosides. Ann Neurol 1995; 38:218–224.

161. Saleh MN, Khazaeli MB, Wheeler RH, Dropcho E, Liu T, Urist M, et al. Phase I trial of the murine monoclonal anti-GD2 antibody 14G2a in metastatic melanoma. Cancer Res 1992; 52(16):4342–4347.

162. Yuki N, Yamada M, Tagawa Y, Takahashi H, Handa S. Pathogenesis of the neurotoxicity caused by anti-GD2 antibody therapy. J Neurol Sci 1997; 149:127–130.

163. Nagai Y, Momoi T, Saito M, Mitsuzawa E, Ohtani S. Ganglioside syndrome, a new autoimmune neurologic disorder, experimentally induced with brain gangliosides. Neurosci Lett 1976; 2:107–111.

164. Kusunoki S, Shimizu J, Chiba A, Ugawa Y, Hitoshi S, Kanazawa I. Experimental sensory neuropathy induced by sensitization with ganglioside GD1b. Ann Neurol 1996; 39(4):424–431.

165. Gregson NA, Hammer CT. Some immunological properties of antisera raised against the trisialoganglioside GT1B. Mol Immunol 1982; 19(4):543–550.

166. Saez-Torres I, Diaz-Villoslada P, Martinez-Caceres E, Ferrer I, Montalban X. Gangliosides do not elicit experimental autoimmune encephalomyelitis in Lewis rats and SJL mice. J Neuroimmunol 1998; 84(1):24–29.

167. Lopez PH, Villa AM, Sica RE, Nores GA. High affinity as a disease determinant factor in anti-GM(1) antibodies: comparative characterization of experimentally induced vs. disease-associated antibodies. J Neuroimmunol 2002; 128(1/2):69–76.

168. Arasaki K, Kusunoki S, Kudo N, Kanazawa I. Acute conduction block in vitro following exposure to antiganglioside sera. Muscle Nerve 1993; 16:587–593.

169. Roberts M, Willison HJ, Vincent A, Newsom-Davis J. Multifocal motor neuropathy human sera block distal motor nerve conduction in mice. Ann Neurol 1995; 38:111–118.

170. Takigawa T, Yasuda H, Kikkawa R, Shigeta Y, Saida T, Kitasato H. Antibodies against GM1 ganglioside affect K+ and Na+ currents in isolated rat myelinated nerve fibers. Ann Neurol 1995; 37:436–442.

171. Arasaki K, Kusunoki S, Kudo N, Tamaki M. The pattern of antiganglioside antibody reactivities producing myelinated nerve conduction block in vitro. J Neurol Sci 1998; 161(2):163–168.

172. Weber F, Rudel R, Aulkemeyer P, Brinkmeier H. Anti-GM1 antibodies can block neuronal voltage-gated sodium channels. Muscle Nerve 2000; 23(9):1414–1420.
173. Harvey GK, Toyka KV, Zielasek J, Kiefer R, Simonis C, Hartung H-P. Failure of anti-GM1 IgG or IgM to induce conduction block following intraneural transfer. Muscle Nerve 1995; 18:388–394.
174. Hirota N, Kaji R, Bostock H, Shindo K, Kawasaki T, Mizutani K, et al. The physiological effect of anti-GM1 antibodies on saltatory conduction and transmembrane currents in single motor axons. Brain 1997; 120:2159–2169.
175. Paparounas K, O'Hanlon GM, O'Leary CP, Rowan EG, Willison HJ. Anti-ganglioside antibodies can bind peripheral nerve nodes of Ranvier and activate the complement cascade without inducing acute conduction block in vitro [see comments]. Brain 1999; 122(Pt 5):807–816.
176. Ho TW, Li CY, Cornblath DR, Gao CY, Asbury AK, Griffin JW, et al. Patterns of recovery in the Guillain–Barré syndromes. Neurology 1997; 48:717–724.
177. Griffin JW, Li CY, Macko C, Ho TW, Hsieh S-T, Xue P, et al. Early nodal changes in the acute motor axonal neuropathy pattern of the Guillain–Barre syndrome. J Neurocytol 1996; 25:33–51.
178. Oda K, Araki K, Totoki T, Shibasaki H. Nerve conduction study of human tetrodotoxication. Neurology 1989; 39(5):743–745.
179. Long RR, Sargent JC, Hammer K. Paralytic shellfish poisoning: a case report and serial electrophysiologic observations. Neurology 1990; 40(8):1310–1312.
180. Umapathi T, Li Y, Lunn MP, Ho TW, Schnaar RL, Griffin JW, et al. A high affinity monoclonal anti-ganglioside antibody causes degeneration of motor nerves in organotypic spinal cord cultures. Neurology 2001; 56:290–291 (Abstract).
181. Roberts M, Willison H, Vincent A, Newsom-Davis J. Serum factor in Miller-Fisher variant of Guillain–Barre syndrome and neurotransmitter release. Lancet 1994; 343:454–455.
182. Buchwald B, Weishaupt A, Toyka KV, Dudel J. Immunoglobulin G from a patient with Miller-Fisher syndrome rapidly and reversibly depresses evoked quantal release at the neuromuscular junction of mice. Neurosci Lett 1995; 201:163–166.
183. Plomp JJ, Molenaar PC, O'Hanlon GM, Jacobs BC, Veitch J, Daha MR, et al. Miller Fisher anti-GQ1b antibodies: alpha-latrotoxin-like effects on motor end plates [published erratum appears in Ann Neurol 1999 Jun;45(6):823]. Ann Neurol 1999; 45(2):189–199.
184. O'Hanlon GM, Plomp JJ, Chakrabarti M, Morrison I, Wagner ER, Goodyear CS, et al. Anti-GQ1b ganglioside antibodies mediate complement-dependent destruction of the motor nerve terminal. Brain 2001; 124(Pt 5):893–906.
185. Buchwald B, Weishaupt A, Toyka KV, Dudel J. Pre- and postsynaptic blockade of neuromuscular transmission by Miller-Fisher syndrome IgG at mouse motor nerve terminals. Eur J Neurosci 1998; 10(1):281–290.
186. Buchwald B, Toyka KV, Zielasek J, Weishaupt A, Schweiger S, Dudel J. Neuromuscular blockade by IgG antibodies from patients with Guillain–Barre syndrome: a macro-patch-clamp study. Ann Neurol 1998; 44(6):913–922.
187. Kusunoki S, Hitoshi S, Kaida K, Arita M, Kanazawa I. Monospecific anti-GD1b IgG is required to induce rabbit ataxic neuropathy. Ann Neurol 1999; 45(3):400–403.

188. Kusunoki S, Hitoshi S, Kaida K, Murayama S, Kanazawa I. Degeneration of rabbit sensory neurons induced by passive transfer of anti-GD1b antiserum. Neurosci Lett 1999; 273(1):33–36.

189. Witebsky E, Rose NR, Terplan P, Paine JR, Egan RW. Chronic thyroiditis and autoimmunization. J A M A 1957; 164:1439–1447.

190. Rose NR, Bona C. Defining criteria for autoimmune diseases (Witebsky's postulates revisited). Immunol Today 1993; 14(9):426–430.

14

Latent and Activated Brain Flora: Human Herpesviruses, Endogenous Retroviruses, Coronaviruses, and *Chlamydia* and Their Role in Neurological Disease

Michael Mayne

Department of Pharmacology and Therapeutics, University of Manitoba, Winnipeg, Manitoba, Canada

J. B. Johnston

Robarts Research Institute, London, Ontario, Canada

1. INTRODUCTION

Several latent infectious agents have been associated recently with human neurological disease. However, the appearance of infectious agents within the central nervous system (CNS) does not always induce pathogenesis. Here, we will discuss the putative association of specific human herpesvirus family members, endogenous retroviruses, coronaviruses and *Chlamydia pneumoniae* in the pathogenesis of the demyelinating disease, multiple sclerosis (MS) as well as other diseases of the CNS. Because human herpesvirus type 6 (HHV-6) has received extensive attention in recent years, we will discuss in detail the pros and cons for involvement of this virus in the pathogenesis of MS. Other research has implicated a role for the reactivation of endogenous retroviruses or coronaviruses in MS. Further, a non-viral entity *C. pneumoniae* also is implicated as a causative agent. How can so many different agents cause a selective pathological response? Current thinking suggests that a two-step process is involved in the autoimmunity of MS which individuals who are genetically predisposed are exposed to an infectious trigger that removes tolerance of T cells. Removal of T-cell tolerance by infectious agents activating the Toll receptor family for example, would enable autoimmune cells to attack self-antigens. If true, this hypothesis would help to explain why so many infectious agents have been associated with MS.

2. OVERVIEW OF LATENT INFECTIOUS AGENTS ASSOCIATED WITH NEUROLOGICAL DISEASE

Although many latent viruses have been associated with multiple forms of neurological disease, this review will focus on the checkered and long-standing argument that various latent viruses are associated with the pathogenesis of MS. At least 10 viral families and one non-viral entity have been associated with this human demyelinating disease (Table 1). Viral etiology is not limited to MS as an etiology has also been established for other human demyelinating diseases including progressive multifocal leukoencephalopathy that has been linked to papovavirus, and postinfectious encephalitis and subacute sclerosing panencephalitis that have been linked to measles infections (1). In addition, myelopathy/tropical spastic paraparasis has been linked to human T-cell lymphotropic lentivirus type 1 (2,3) and human immunodeficiency virus type 1 (HIV-1) dementia and encephalopathy has been linked to HIV-1 infection (4,5). Clearly, there appears to be a strong link between various latent viruses and demyelination. Here, we will summarize arguments for and against an association between latent viral infections and MS with emphasis on HHV-6, coronaviruses, endogenous retroviruses, and the non-viral entity, *C. pneumoniae*. In addition, we propose a theory to explain how so many different infectious agents can trigger a common pathological event.

3. HHV-6 EPIDEMIOLOGY, ROSEOLA, AND ASSOCIATION WITH IMMUNOCOMPROMISED PATIENTS

3.1. Epidemiology

Most adults in North America and Europe are seropositive for HHV-6 and the virus appears to be prevalent in all populations throughout the world (6). HHV-6 is often shed in the saliva of asymptomatic seropositive children and adults and this is the most likely mode of transmission (7). The peak age of acquisition in North America is 6–12 months of age (median 9 months), and the mother and baby usually have the same strain of virus. Perinatal or congenital infection has not been detected (8). HHV-6 infection accounts for the majority of roseola infections in the United States (97%) (9). The closely related beta herpesvirus, human herpesvirus type 7 (HHV-7) has a median age of acquisition of 26 months and acquisition of this virus is associated with different risk factors compared to HHV-6 (10).

3.2. Roseola

Over 50 years ago, a possible viral etiology for roseola was proposed however, it was not until the late 1980s when Yamanishi showed that HHV-6 caused roseola (11). Variant B (there are two main variants of HHV-6; A and B) is responsible for almost all roseola-associated HHV-6 infection (9,12) and at least 50% of primary episodes of infant fever are due to HHV-6 infection (13). Primary HHV-6 infections are associated with a rash in greater than 60% of infants in Japan whereas in the United States only one in four infants appears to develop a rash (14). In rare cases (approximately one in 50) a child with roseola may develop seizures and require hospitalization (11).

3.3. HHV-6 Reactivation in Immunocompromised Patients

Primary HHV-6 infection or reactivation in healthy adults is rare. However, reactivation or primary infection, when it occurs, can be associated with significant consequences. In immunocompromised individuals, specifically organ or stem cell transplant recipients or in cancer patients, HHV-6 often reactivates or new infection occurs as indicated by increased antibody titers or increased frequency of detection of HHV-6 DNA using polymerase chain reaction (PCR). In organ transplant recipients, HHV-6 reactivation occurs usually 1 month following transplant and can be associated frequently with CMV (15) and HHV-6 reactivation has been associated with organ rejection. In severe cases of HHV-6 reactivation in transplant recipients, encephalitis can occur and in some events be fatal. However, in prospective studies, HHV-6 reactivation in transplant recipients is often limited and may cause a mild fever or rash (16,17) and may have serious implications among recipients of major organ or stem cell transplants during which HHV-6 viremia can lead to organ rejection, or failure and can in some cases, be fatal (18–20).

4. HHV-6 ASSOCIATION WITH NEUROLOGICAL DISEASE

4.1. HHV-6 Associated Encephalitis

In children, CNS manifestations were recognized long before HHV-6 was clearly implicated as the etiological agent of roseola. Infants may show symptoms including bulging fontanels, irritability, febrile seizures, meningoencephalitis and, residual encephalopathy [for review see Ref. (14)]. However, because the prognosis for HHV-6 infection in young children is excellent, only rarely does significant neurological disease occur. In a prospective examination of 2716 children with primary HHV-6 infection, the HHV-6A variant was identified more frequently in CSF samples from children with acute febrile illness than in PBMC isolates from children with primary infection (21) suggesting a greater neurotropism of HHV-6A than HHV-6B.

There have been several recent reports that have implicated HHV-6 as a pathogenic agent following solid organ or bone marrow transplantation (16,17,22–24) and in rare cases, patients have developed acute encephalitis or other neurological disease (24–27). Clearly, reactivation and infection from donor organs can occur and although HHV-6A and B have been detected post-transplantation, B is the predominant variant that is detected suggesting that reactivation of HHV-6 may occur in the host. Prospective studies show that there is little clinical impact on the success of organ transplantations (22,28). However, subgroup analysis has linked HHV-6 reactivation with delayed engraftment, graft vs. host disease, and rash (29).

4.2. HHV-6 and HIV

The role of HHV-6 as a co-factor in HIV disease and acquired immune deficiency syndrome (AIDS) has received considerable attention. HHV-6 has been suggested to directly enhance HIV replication (30) and may also act as a pathogenic factor in HIV replication through several mechanisms (7,29–32). There have been multiple reports of direct interactions between HIV and HHV-6. HHV-6 infection increases CD4 expression (32) possibly rendering cells vulnerable to further HIV infection. Recently HHV-6 has also been shown to act as a co-factor during AIDS development (33). At autopsy, HIV victims often have higher HHV-6 viral load throughout the body compared to non-HIV-infected controls (29). However, HHV-6 is lower in peripheral blood of HIV patients with lower CD4 cell counts suggesting that HHV-6 levels in blood may not play an important role in HIV replication (34,35). HHV-6 cannot induce immune deficiency per se, and thus, it is likely that HHV-6 may only act as an opportunistic agent in immunocompromised HIV/AIDS patients similar to organ transplant patients. It is not clear whether HHV-6 reactivation in HIV-infected patients directs the progression of dementia. The human herpesvirus type 8 (HHV-8) however, is believed to be the causative agent of Kaposi's sarcoma in AIDS patients (36). Recent data shows a negative association between Kaposi's sarcoma and AIDS dementia complex suggesting that active HHV-8 may actually protect AIDS patients from the development of cognitive disorders (37). Although HHV-8 is detected at similar frequency in the normal and diseased brain (38), it does not appear to have any correlation with other neurological diseases including AIDS dementia (39) or subacute sclerosing panencephalitis (40).

4.3. HHV-6 Association with Multiple Sclerosis

There is accumulating evidence that links HHV-6 with MS pathogenesis. Etiologically, genetic factors including race, sex, ethnicity, family history and HLA haplotype and non-genetic factors such as age, weather, diet, and socioeconomic status are all linked with development of MS (41). Perhaps the strongest epidemiological data is that the rate of concordance is eight times greater in monozygotic than dizygotic twins (42) however, the concordance rate among monozygotic twins remains only 25%. Experimentally, oligoclonal bands specific for viral or bacterial epitopes can be found in high frequencies in cerebrospinal fluid (CSF) of MS patients suggesting the presence of an infectious agent. Elevation in CSF immunoglobulins, which demonstrate an oligoclonal pattern when separated by electrophoretic methods, are found in >90% MS patients and several other chronic neurological diseases (43). Thus oligoclonal bands are a useful predictor of MS that may aide in the identification of agent(s) that cause MS.

One of the first reports that HHV-6 may be associated with MS was from Challoner et al. who detected HHV-6 DNA in MS plaques (44) by means of non-biased search using representational difference analysis (RDA) that allowed the selection and amplification of previously unknown DNA sequences present by means of successive cycles of subtractive hybridization and subsequent PCR amplification. When applied to material from MS brains, RDA amplified a DNA fragment that was determined to be similar to a specific gene from the Z29 isolate of HHV-6B. Consistent with data demonstrating CNS as a site of HHV-6 latency (45), the percentage of HHV-6 DNA positive MS brains was not significantly different from that of control brains (78% vs. 74%, respectively). However, monoclonal antibodies against the HHV-6 virion proteins 101K and p41 were able to detect HHV-6 antigen expression in MS plaques and not in control brains.

A recent study by Blumberg et al. demonstrated the presence of HHV-6 DNA in chronic MS white matter plaques using a two-step in situ PCR (ISPCR) technique (46). Two additional studies have also shown that HHV-6 can be detected with high frequency in autopsy or fresh biopsy specimens from MS patients (46a,46b).

Of these studies, we noted that HHV-6 DNA can be detected approximately 60% of the time in MS lesions whereas approximately 25% of the case studies of normal appearing white matter from patients with other neurological disease or healthy controls were positive for HHV-6 DNA (Fig. 1). Although these studies detected viral DNA at lesion sites, much more work needs to be completed. Specifically, it will be critical to determine if live HHV-6 virus is present and active during lesion development, progression and repair. Further, if virus is present and active during the chronological event of lesion development, what role does it play in mediating oligodendrocyte viability and/or differentiation.

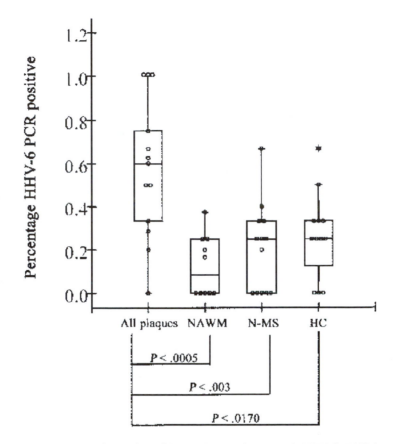

Figure 1 Frequency of detection of human herpesvirus type 6 (HHV-6) DNA in multiple sclerosis (MS) plaques, non-MS neurologic disease (N-MS) brains, and healthy control (HC) brains. HHV-6 DNA was significantly increased in MS plaque samples [37/64 (57.8%)], compared with samples from N-MS [10/46 (21.7%)] and HC brains [11/41 (26.8%)]. There was no difference in the frequency of HHV-6 DNA in normal-appearing white matter [NAWM; 7/44 (15.9%)], compared with N-MS or HC brains. Each box shows the median, interquartile range, and extreme values (*) of the proportion of HHV-6-positive samples for each subject within the sample classification. Pairwise comparisons were done by Scheffe post hoc test on a generalized linear model analysis of variance. (From the Journal of Infectious Diseases, University of Chicago Press.)

A conclusion from these studies is that HHV-6 appears to localize in oligodendrocytes and microglial cells. HHV-6 DNA was also unexpectedly detected in white matter lesions from PML brains at higher amounts than JC virus, the etiologic agent of PML. These findings have added to the debate of whether HHV-6 can be considered a commensal agent in brain or a potentially pathogenic virus in MS.

Another study performed on brain tissues from patients having either secondary progressive or relapsing/remitting MS demonstrated the presence of HHV-6 DNA in 17 of 19 diseased tissue sections and in three of 23 uninvolved regions (47). The presence of viral DNA was statistically significant in brain tissues from MS patients (eight of 11) with respect to control CNS tissues (two of 28). Furthermore, 54% of total blood samples from MS patients were positive for active HHV-6 infection, as demonstrated by a highly difficult rapid culture assay (47). This latter observation is controversial as several groups have reported a lack of clinical correlation between the detection of HHV-6 in blood samples and the development of MS (48–50).

The presence of different HHV-6 variants may also account for contrasting results. HHV-6B variant has been detected in cell-associated compartments such as saliva and PBMC at comparable frequencies from normal donors and MS patients. In contrast, the HHV-6A variant has been demonstrated in serum and urine of MS patients but not controls (51). Ablashi et al. have demonstrated that PBMC from MS patients were mostly variant B (87%), similar to isolates from healthy donors (67%) (52). These data are in agreement with the higher frequency of HHB-6B variant infection in the normal population. Because HHV-6A has been suggested to be a more neurotropic (21) it is possible that the association of HHV-6 and MS is variant-specific (51,53,54).

In summary, it appears that the presence of HHV-6 in brain rather than blood may be more closely associated with the pathogenesis of MS. However, what is lacking from all studies to date is actual detection of live HHV-6 virus in brain tissue. Unless this can be shown in biopsy samples from MS patients or it can be demonstrated that HHV-6 can cause demyelination (e.g., in an animal model) researchers should remain cautious about closely associating HHV-6 with the development and/or progression of MS.

4.4. Association of Other Herpesvirus Family Members and Neurological Disease

In addition to HHV-6, other herpesvirus family members notably Epstein–Barr virus (EBV; HHV-4) and herpes simplex virus type 1also known as oral herpes (HSV-1; HHV-1) have been implicated in the pathogenesis of MS. A recent longitudinal study found that in 19 patients, EBV early antigens (p54 + p138) and positive serum DNA was seen in 72.7% of patients with exacerbations and in none of the patients with clinically stable disease (55). Although others have shown that there are no primary EBV infections in MS patients (56), the results of the longitudinal study suggest that EBV may reactivate in MS patients. A recent systematic review of case–control studies comparing EBV serology in MS patients and controls found that the summary odds ratio of MS comparing EBV seropositive individuals with EBV seronegative individuals was 13.5 (95% CI: 6.3–31.4) indicating that EBV may have a role in the pathogenesis of MS (57).

Of all the other human herpesviruses (there have been eight members identified in the family) HSV-1 is the leading etiological candidate for MS. HSV-1 is a common neurotropic virus that is capable of long latencies and can cause focal demyelination in animals. A study conducted by Tourtelotte's group in 1996 found that HSV-1 was present in more MS cases than in controls and in more active than inactive plaques (58,59). Although they found HSV-1 DNA in white and gray matter in MS patients, which lessens the clinical correlation of HSV-1 with MS, cellular localization of HSV to oligodendrocytes suggested that HSV-1 may remain latent and reactivate during relapse and damage oligodendrocytes (58). Others have also observed that HSV-1 reactivates in peripheral blood of acute relapsing MS patients (60). An interesting yet unproved suggestion is that HSV-1 induces MS (or other autoimmune disorders) via molecular mimicry in which a protein encoded by HSV-1 induces a host immunologic response to attack self-antigens. In support of this argument, Cortese et al. found that IgG antibodies raised against phage-displayed peptide mimics (mimotopes) recognized by oligoclonal immunoglobulins were found to cross-react with an epitope shared by a brain-specific factor conserved from rodents to humans, and the surface glycoprotein gB of HSV-1 (61). Thus, in addition to HHV-6, other members of the HHV family have been implicated in the pathogenesis of MS. In summary, it is safe to conclude that different human herpesviruses are associated with the pathogenesis of MS. However, the conclusion that herpesviruses cause MS remains unfounded. It will be critical for researchers to determine if any (or all) herpesvirus family members are essential, necessary or involved in the development of MS.

5. CHLAMYDIA PNEUMONIAE

The genus *Chlamydia* is composed of four species of obligate intracellular parasites, *C. psittacci*, *C. pecorum*, *C. trachomatis* and *C. pneumoniae*, three of which have been shown to be pathogenic to humans [reviewed in Refs. (62–64)]. By virtue of the presence of trilaminar membranes *Chlamydiae* are considered to be gram-negative bacteria. However, they are among the smallest known prokaryotes and have no close relationship to other known organisms. Therefore, they likely represent a novel eubacterial phylogenetic branch. The *Chlamydiae* are also distinguished by an unusual development cycle that involves two distinct morphological forms. The small, highly infective elementary body is capable of survival outside the host cell and represents the transmissible form of the pathogen. Within infected cells, the elementary body reorganizes to form a reticulate body that undergoes multiple division cycles over a 24-hr period. Progeny elementary bodies are released by lysis approximately 48 hr after the initial infection.

Chlamydiae normally infect mucosal surfaces and establish chronic and persistent infections in which tissue damage is believed to be immune-mediated

(64,65). *Chlamydia trachomatis* is responsible for diverse infections of the urogenital tract, eyes and respiratory system, while *C. pneumoniae* was first identified as a respiratory pathogen that causes community-acquired pneumonia, pharyngitis, and bronchitis. Because an animal reservoir has yet to be identified for either of these species, they are considered to be strictly human pathogens. Although humans are not its natural host species, inhalation of airborne *C. psittacci* from avian droppings can cause the respiratory tract infection, psittacosis. *Chlamydia pecorum* infection of humans has not been reported. Infection by all four species has also been shown to involve invasion of the CNS with the attendant development of neurological complications in their host organism (66). For example, *C. pecorum* causes sporadic bovine encephalomyelitis in cattle, while meningoencephalitis has been reported following infection by *C. psittacci* and *C. trachomatis. Chlamydia pneumoniae* has also been implicated in cases of undiagnosed encephalitis (67,68), including a report that attributed a case of acute disseminated encephalomyelitis that responded to treatment with antibiotics and corticosteroids (69). Recent studies linking *C. pneumoniae* to chronic brain diseases such as MS (70–72) and Alzheimer's disease (AD) (73) have generated even greater interest in the bacteria as a potential CNS pathogen.

Chlamydia pneumoniae is normally encountered before 15 years of age and it exhibits high adult seroprevalence rates, approaching 70%. *Chlamydia pneumoniae* preferentially targets the oral and nasal mucosa of the respiratory tract, infecting vascular endothelium, macrophages/monocytes and smooth muscle cells. In addition to respiratory aliments, *C. pneumoniae* has also been associated with a diverse array of human diseases, including chronic syndromes with autoimmune components. These include asthma, sarcoidosis, coronary artery disease, erythema nodosum, stroke, endocarditis, thyroiditis, arthritis, Reiter's syndrome, artherosclerosis, and temporal giant cell arteritis (74–80). The sheer volume of diseases in which *C. pneumoniae* has been implicated has led to the speculation that it represents an opportunistic infection rather than the etiological agent in these conditions. In this section, we will concentrate on the potential role of the bacterium in MS and AD.

A link between *C. pneumoniae* infection and the development of MS was first suggested in 1998 following the detection of the bacterium in the CSF of an MS patient with high EDSS who improved neurologically following antibiotic therapy (70). Further support for this association was provided by larger follow-up studies from the same group showing that *C. pneumoniae* was detectable by PCR amplification of the major outer membrane protein gene (ompA) in approximately two-thirds of clinically defined MS patients and up to 50% of monosymptomatic MS patients (71,72). In contrast, the protein was evident in less than 20% of control patients with other neurological diseases (OND) (71,72). Moreover, the bacterium could be cultured from CSF obtained from the majority of MS patients, but it was infrequently detected in control samples (71). Several independent laboratories have failed to confirm these results, however. In these studies, attempts to detect *C. pneumoniae* in the CSF of MS patients by culture or PCR have yielded variable results that range from very low rates of positive MS patients (<10%) to no positive patients to higher prevalence of the pathogen in control groups than in MS patients (81–87). Further obscuring a putative role for this bacterium in MS is the fact that different results are obtained by different investigators when the same samples are analyzed (72,88), emphasizing the need for more accurate and reproducible means of analyzing these results.

Increased production of immunoglobulins and the formation within the CSF of oligoclonal bands with alkaline isoelectric points is a hallmark of chronic CNS diseases with infectious origins (89). These properties, which are thought to represent an intrathecal immune response to a pathogen, are also evident in more than 90% of MS patients, supporting a role for infection in the development of the disease (89). ELISA analyses have detected elevated titers of anti-chlamydia antibodies in CSF from MS patients compared to controls (71) Moreover, antigens derived from the *C. pneumoniae* elementary body have been reported to partially or completely adsorb oligoclonal bands from the CSF of the majority of MS patients studied (90). As with the prevalence studies discussed above, however, other studies dispute these findings. Although higher intrathecal Ig responses to *C. pneumoniae* antigens were detected in MS patients compared to controls, a recent study has reported that the oligoclonal bands present in the CSF of MS patients do not recognize these antigens (91), suggesting that the observed immune responses to *C. pneumoniae* were simply part of a polyspecific antibody response to CNS pathogens. The reported failure of anti-chlamydia antibody titers to correlate with disease progression, clinical markers or oligoclonal banding patterns further weakens arguments favoring *C. pneumoniae* as the etiological agent in MS (92,93).

Magnetic resonance imaging (MRI) has provided some evidence to support an association between *C. pneumoniae* and enhanced spinal, but not brain, lesions in MS patients (94). However, animal studies using the experimental allergic encephalitis (EAE) model of MS in rodents may support a potential role for the bacterium in initiating or enhancing an adverse immune response that contributes to MS pathology. In these experiments, the severity of EAE induced in rodents by immunization with neural antigens was reported to be increased following intraperitoneal injection with live infectious *C. pneumoniae* (95,96). This response was specific to *C. pneumoniae*, involved colonization of the CNS by the pathogen and could be attenuated with therapeutic agents aimed at reducing the infection (95). *Chlamydia pneumoniae* has also been shown to encode a 20 amino acid peptide that shares a seven residue domain with myelin basic protein (MBP), the primary antigen targeted by the host autoimmune response in MS (96). This peptide was found to induce EAE by activating a different population of autoreactive T cells than MBP, supporting a potential role for *C. pneumoniae* in the amplification of autoreactive lymphocytes. Furthermore, infection with *C. pneumoniae* has been shown to induce expression of proinflammatory cytokines, such as tumor necrosis factor (TNF) (97), and to promote breakdown of the blood–brain barrier (BBB) by contributing to endothelial damage and changes in junctional complex proteins of microvascular endothelial cells (98).

Alzheimer's disease is a chronic neurodegenerative CNS disease in which deposition of β-amyloid within the brain is thought to promote the development of an adverse host inflammatory response that contributes to neuronal damage and death. However, recent evidence suggests that the inflammation associated with AD may also involve an infectious component, most likely acting as a triggering stimulus (99). As with MS, some researchers believe that *C. pneumoniae* may contribute to this process. To that end, PCR amplification of bacterial DNA and mRNA revealed that *C. pneumoniae* was 16-fold more prevalent in postmortem brain tissue from late onset AD patients than in brain samples from OND controls (73). This finding was confirmed by the ability to both culture the pathogen from these samples and to detect chlamydial bodies by electron microscopy in AD, but not control, brain tissue (73). In addition, *C. pneumoniae* was shown by immunohistochemistry to be present primarily in pericytes and glial cells within areas of active AD neuropathology (73). Thus, *C. pneumoniae* was present, viable and transcriptionally active within the CNS of AD patients. As with MS, however, these results have proven difficult to confirm. Other studies have found that Chlamydia serum antibody titers do not correlate the incidence or progression of AD (97,100) while the ability to detect *C. pneumoniae* in the CNS of AD patients has been sporadic (101,102). As with MS, the link between *C. pneumoniae* infection and development of AD remains unclear.

Of interest to the study of both MS and AD is the potential link between the possession of the ε4 allele type at the apolipoprotein E (APOE) locus and the pathobiology of *C. pneumoniae*. The presence of this allele, which is considered by many to represent a high risk factor for the earlier onset and rapid progression of sporadic AD (103), has also been suggested to contribute to the susceptibility to *C. pneumoniae* infection and influence disease profile (104). Although studies have failed to show increased prevalence the ε4 allele in MS patients, indicating that it is not a risk factor for the disease, MS patients who possess the allele do present with earlier onset and more rapid progression of the disease when compared to MS patients lacking the allele (105,106). However, this association has yet to be confirmed and remains highly speculative.

6. HUMAN CORONAVIRUSES

The *Coronaviridae* are a ubiquitous family of RNA viruses of the order *Nidovirales* that are associated with respiratory and gastrointestinal infections in diverse vertebrates, including humans, rodents and birds [reviewed in Refs. (107–110)]. The coronavirus genome is the largest among RNA viruses at 27–30 kb in size, consisting of a single strand of positive-sense RNA that possesses both a 5′ methyl cap and a 3′ polyadenylated tail.

Human coronaviruses (HCoV) were first isolated in 1965 and all known strains fall into either the OC43 or 229E mammalian serological groups (110). Generally, HCoV infections are seasonal, being most common in winter and early spring, and exhibit a periodicity with an interval of 2–3 years in which infections in a particular period are caused primarily by a single serotype. Seroprevalence is high in the adult population and most individuals are exposed to the virus by 5 years of age (110). HCoV preferentially target epithelial cells of the upper respiratory tract and infection by either serotype can be asymptomatic or present as a common cold lacking lower respiratory tract complications. In fact, HCoV are now thought to be responsible for 10–30% of all common colds in humans. Although active primary infections are resolved within a week, chronic persistent infections can develop in susceptible hosts and reinfection with the same serotype often occurs within 4 months of first infection. In addition to the common cold, pathologies such as pneumonia, diarrhea, meningitis, MS and Parkinson's disease have also been attributed to the virus.

Although HCoV are recognized primarily as respiratory pathogens, growing evidence supports their neurotropic, neuroinvasive, and neurovirulent potential. Like many members of the nidoviruses, HCoV exhibit the potential to invade the CNS and infect neural cells (111). In addition to macrophages/monocytes (112,113), HCoV have been shown to infect astrocytes and microglia in primary culture and acutely and to persistently infect immortalized human glial cells in a viral strain-dependent fashion (114,115). Infection of brain endothelial cells has also been reported. The receptor that mediates HCoV neurotropism has been identified as CD13, an aminopeptidase found on oligodendrocytes, neurons and astrocytes that determines the susceptibility of these cells to infection (116). Thus, HCoV has the potential to invade the CNS through either a hematogenous route via infected monocytes or infection of endothelial cells or an intranasal routes via the olfactory nerve.

A potential link between HCoV infection and the development of human neurological diseases has been suggested for several decades. Most notable is the body of evidence supporting a role for these viruses in MS, a theory based largely on the finding that some coronaviruses are neurovirulent and cause a demyelinating syndrome with clinical manifestations that closely resemble MS. MHV (strain JHM) is a naturally occurring murine coronavirus that induces a acute and chronic demyelinating disease in mice (117–120). Moreover, MHV has also been shown to infect cells within the primate CNS, leading to subacute panencephalitis and demyelination (121,122). Like MS, the disease course following MHV infection is influenced by diverse factors, such as host genetics, age and immune status (118) and the virus serves as an animal model for MS. Within the CNS, MHV targets neurons, astrocytes and oligodendrocytes (118) and early studies suggested that demyelination was the product of virus-induced damage or destruction of these cells (123,124). In fact, the demyelination properties of MHV have recently been shown to map to the viral spike gly-coprotein (125).

More recent reports have suggested that this process is far more complex and likely includes an immunopathological component involving T-cell targeting of viral antigens expressed in infected tissues (126–129). In support of this concept, infection of mice lacking B and T cells does not result in demyelination, although demyelination mediated by $\gamma\delta$ T cells rather than the conventional CD4 and CD8 $\alpha\beta$ T cells has been reported in these mice (130,131). Virus-activated CD8 T cells have also been shown to have the potential to contribute to MHV-mediated demyelination through a bystander effect, even after antigen has been cleared from the CNS (132). This finding is supported by evidence that MHV infection of the CNS promotes upregulation of normally low expression MHC I on oligodendrocytes, neurons, microglia and endothelia and class II MHC on microglia providing the potential to present antigen to T-cell and facilitate auto-damage (133).

The association between HCoV infection and MS in humans is less clear. As early as 1976, particles resembling coronaviruses were observed the in cister-nae of autopsied brains from MS patients (134) and coronaviruses that were molecularly similarly to MHV were isolated from MS brain tissue (135). In addition, expression of coronavirus RNA and antigen was detected in MS brains and CSF (136–138), concurrent with the presence of intrathecal antibodies against the virus (139,140). Anti-coronavirus antibodies were detected in 25–50% of MS patients depending on viral strain, but not in control patients (139,140). More recent studies have confirmed that HCoV RNA is present in brain samples from many MS patients and that the prevalence of the virus varies with viral strain (44% positive for 229E and 23% positive for OC43) (111). Viral RNA was local-ized primarily outside of blood vessels, within both plaques and normal tissue in the brain parenchyma (111). In addition, OC43 viral RNA was preferentially detected in MS brains compared to controls (36% vs. 14%) and mutations were evident in the viral nucleocapsid gene with greater frequency in MS patients (111). As with other pathogens implicated in MS, independent studies dispute these findings and have either found no comparable increase in viral levels or failed to detect the virus at all (141–143). Similarly, no differences in anti-coron-avirus serum and CSF antibody titers were observed by some groups (144,145).

Mechanistically, evidence exists in support of a potential role for HCoV as a contributor to the pathology of MS. Recent studies have identified long-term, cross-reactive T cells in the blood of MS patients who recognize both MBP and antigens of the 229E serotype of HCoV (146,147), supporting a potential role for the virus as a contributor to molecular mimicry. Similarly, in vitro infection stud-ies with OC43 have shown that the virus activates glial cells leading to increased production of proinflammatory cytokines and MMPs that may contribute to neu-ral cell death and damage (148). Finally, coronavirus infection of macrophages has been shown to induce apoptosis in viral strain-specific manner (229E but not OC43) (149).

7. HUMAN ENDOGENOUS RETROVIRUSES

Retroviral elements, such as human endogenous retroviruses (HERV), comprise approximately 8% of the human genome (150,151). HERV are structurally similar to other retroviruses and, presumably, were derived from exogenous retroviruses that became integrated into the germ-line and inherited in a classic Mendelian fashion (150,151). Although thousands of distinct HERV are present in the human genome, most HERV are replication incompetent and do not produce viral particles. However, specific subsets of HERV are transcriptionally active and can encode protein with enzymatic activity or viral particles with unknown infectious potential (150,151). Consequently, some HERV are posited to influence cellular gene expression and contribute to normal physiological processes important to growth and development, such as cellular differentiation and morphogenesis (152).

It has also been suggested that HERV play important roles in pathological processes, including several autoimmune conditions, possibly through their ability to alter immune function or encode gene products that promote disease development or progression (153–156). For example, several reports have implicated multiple HERV families in diseases with a presumed autoimmune etiology such as MS (157–161), rheumatoid arthritis (RA) (162,163), type I diabetes (164) and Sjogren's syndrome (165), as well such diverse conditions as schizophrenia (166–168) and Addison's disease (169). Similarly, HERV have been implicated in cell transformation and tumor development in diverse cancers, including breast cancer (170), melanoma (171), leukemia (172,173) and seminoma (174). However, a causative role for HERV in a specific disease or syndrome has yet to be shown.

A potential role for HERV in MS was suggested following the discovery that extracellular particles with associated RT activity could be isolated from leptomeningeal cells (LM7) (175) and monocytes (159) isolated from patients with the disease. Antibodies that cross-reacted with the reverse transcriptase gene of the exogenous retroviruses, HIV and HTLV, were subsequently detected in serum and CSF from MS patients (176). These findings culminated in the identification of a novel retrovirus detected preferentially in CSF, serum and conditioned media from MS patients (177). RNA corresponding to this virus, termed MS-associated retrovirus (MSRV), was detected in both healthy and MS brain tissue (178) and shown to share significant identity (82–88%) with HERV-W/ERV-9 family of endogenous retroviruses (160,179,180). In addition, antibodies that recognized two different regions of the MSRV envelope (*env*) gene were detected with greater frequency in CSF from MS patients (181), suggesting that MSRV/HERV-W may represent an extracellular variant of an activated and viable HERV.

HERV-W is thought to have first entered the primate genome following divergence of old and new world monkeys approximately 25 million years ago

(182). In humans it is present at a frequency of 30–100 proviral copies per haploid genome, with notable insertions at chromosome 7q21-22 (HERV-7q) and within the TCR gene on chromosome 14q11.2 (HERV-TcR) (183). HERV-W is expressed in normal placenta as a 7.6-kb retroviral element and encodes a fusogenic membrane glycoprotein (syncytin) that may play a role in placental development (184). Syncytin is expressed specifically in placental syncytiatrophoblasts, but the protein has also been shown to induce syncytia in human, simian and porcine cells (185). This property likely stems from its ability to interact with the hASCT-1 and -2 amino acid transporters on target cells (186). Of interest, HIV pseudotyping experiments have shown that the HERV-W *env* gene encodes a functional envelope protein that can confer infectivity on *env*-deleted HIV particles (187). These findings suggest that HERVs may exhibit the potential for vertical or horizontal transmission via transcomplementation of virion proteins from other HERV species.

A putative role for HERVs in MS etiology was strengthened by independent studies that identified a second genetically distinct family of HERV, the RGH/HERV-H family, in retroviral particles produced from cell cultures obtained from MS patients (157,158). Moreover, low-level transmission of these particles was observed in cell culture (188). Both viruses have been shown to have proviral insertions in close proximity to each other on chromosome 7q21-22, a genetic locus previously associated with the multigenic susceptibility to MS (183). These findings suggested that coactivation of multiple HERVs may form part of a pathogenic chain reaction in autoimmune diseases that is induced by diverse infectious agents. For example, herpesviruses, such as HHV-6 and EBV discussed above, may play an etiological role in MS by triggering HERV reactivation in predisposed individuals. In support of this theory, the HSV-1 ICP0 protein has been shown to transactivate the HERV-K long-terminal repeats (LTR) (189). In addition, co-infection with EBV and retroviruses has been proposed to contribute to the development and progression of MS (190,191), a concept supported by the finding that concurrent EBV infection leads to transactivation of a superantigen encoded by the HERV-K18 *env* gene (192).

In terms of CNS pathology, HERVs may also play more direct roles in autoimmune diseases. For example, the HERV-W syncytin protein has been shown to function as a superantigen in lymphocyte cultures, possibly contributing to the generation of autoreactive T cells (193). In related experiments, HERV peptides were also found to preferentially stimulate proliferation of and cytokine production by peripheral blood mononuclear cells (PBMC) from acute, but not stable, MS patients (194). This process was CD4 cell-mediated and independent of HLA type II molecules (194). Similarly, MS patients have been found to exhibit a more frequent and potent type 2 immune response to HERV sequences (195). Conditioned media from cell cultures of monocyte/macrophages obtained from MS patients and expressing HERV-W have also been shown to contain a 17-kDa glycosylated protein with cytotoxic activity, termed gliotoxin (196). As the name implies, this cytotoxin exhibits a narrow specificity for neuroglial cells (oligodendrocytes, astrocytes), a finding of some significance to degenerative CNS diseases. To that end, gliotoxin has also been detected in the CSF of patients with active MS, concurrent with the presence of retroviral particles containing HERV-W sequences (196).

In addition to MS, considerable interest has been expressed in a putative role for HERV in other neurological disorders, such as schizophrenia. The potential for retroviruses to contribute to the pathogenesis of schizophrenia is not novel and was initially proposed several decades ago with the theory that retroviral infection during pregnancy may lead to impairment in fetal brain development that culminates in the disease (197–199). However, this theory remained unproven and was largely dismissed. However, more recent experiments have shown that retroviral sequences were detectable in the CSF of 30% of individuals with rapid onset schizophrenia, but not detectable in any of the OND controls (168). In addition, representational difference analyses of twins discordant for schizophrenia detected the presence of sequences homologous to HERV-W in individuals with schizophrenia (166,167), a finding supported by subsequent experiments that found that transcription of members of the HERV-W family was increased in the frontal cortex of patients of schizophrenia compared to controls (168). These studies provided the first evidence in support of an association between activation of retroviral elements in the CNS and the development of the schizophrenia and led to the classification of a family of schizophrenia-associated retroviruses (SZRV). These retroviral elements have been shown to contain an intact polymerase (*pol*) gene, which has been used to identify three subtypes (SZRV-1, -3, and -4) on the basis of sequence homology (167).

It should be noted that macrophage activation and increased expression of proinflammatory cytokines are features common to the pathogenesis of many of the autoimmune diseases in which HERVs have been implicated (200). Moreover, both of these events have been shown to profoundly influence the expression and release of endogenous retroviruses and their gene products (201–204). Thus, it is conceivable that the increased HERV expression observed in inflammatory conditions is a consequence of heightened macrophage activity. In support of this hypothesis, activation and differentiation of monocytoid cells in vitro was recently shown to increase the expression of several HERV families (HERV-E, HERV-H, HERV-K, HERV-W) implicated in inflammatory diseases (205). This induction was virus- and stimulus-dependent and mimicked by treatment with proinflammatory cytokines commonly elevated in conditions associated with enhanced HERV expression, such as TNF-α ((205). Moreover, monocyte differentiation was accompanied by evidence of the release of particles containing HERV sequences and possessing reverse transcriptase activity. A link between elevated levels of proinflammatory molecules and altered expression of several HERV families was also observed in autopsied brain tissue from patients diagnosed with CNS diseases characterized by altered macrophage and microglia activity, including MS, and AD (205). These findings are consistent with other reports demonstrating that HERV expression in non-monocytic cells is influenced by cellular differentiation and cytokine-stimulation (201,203). Furthermore, they suggest that increased HERV expression may be a consequence of immune activation rather than indicative of a causative role for these agents in autoimmune diseases.

Although it is difficult to assign a role for HERV as causative agents in inflammatory diseases, their contribution to disease progression cannot be precluded. Thus, it is conceivable that the increased expression of HERV-specific transcripts and proteins detected in autoimmune diseases initiates a response that exacerbates the inflammation associated with a particular disease and promotes tissue damage. Subsequent analysis of the actions of individual HERV-encoded proteins may elucidate potential relationships and mechanisms by which HERV are involved in the pathogenesis of inflammatory CNS diseases.

8. CONCLUSION: HOW CAN DIFFERENT LATENT INFECTIOUS AGENTS CAUSE A COMMON NEUROLOGICAL OUTCOME? A POTENTIAL ROLE FOR TOLL-LIKE RECEPTORS

While there has been considerable basic and clinical study in the field of MS research, the cause of MS has yet to be identified. Importantly, it was determined recently that MS may not be a single disease but rather a syndrome with multiple differentiating neuropathologies (206). This concept may help to advance research as MS populations (post-mortem) can be stratified based on their neuropathological profiles. Different neuropathologies suggest that perhaps different disease-induced triggers exist although this assumption is puzzling because it is difficult to envision how so many separate "triggers" could induce a common pathological outcome. We have summarized here how multiple stimuli could engage and activate the human immune system and damage myelin sheaths and impair neuronal activity (Fig. 2).

Others have suggested that viruses may represent one of many putative environmental triggers (207). In fact, it was suggested over 100 years ago that various infectious agents could trigger MS (207). How can so many different viruses induce a similar response that could lead to autoimmunity? This question may have been partially answered recently by Ichikawa et al. (208). Because myelin-reactive $CD4^+$ cells are effectors of EAE and are presumed to the primary effector of MS, they hypothesized that tolerance of these cells must be removed prior to the induction of auto-immunity. They showed that myelin specific T cells from tolerized donor mice (SJL mice injected with proteolipid-protein) are converted into pathogenic effector cells that proliferate, secrete cytokines and transfer EAE following the activation of CD40R or the Toll-like receptor type 9 (TLR-9). Reactivation of the MBP-specific cells and induction of autoimmunity

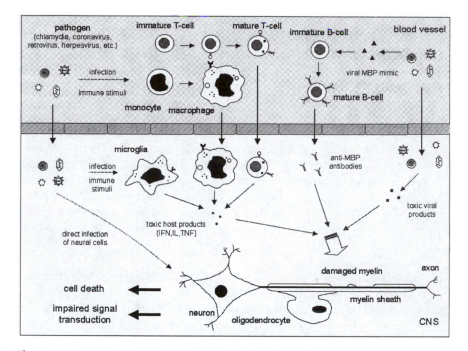

Figure 2   Proposed direct and indirect mechanisms by which a pathogen may contribute to the development and progression of multiple sclerosis. In the indirect model, an exogenous infection or re-activation of a latent or endogenous pathogen may stimulate the activation and proliferation of immune cells. These cells include macrophages and T and B lymphocytes within the peripheral circulation (blood vessel), which can migrate into the central nervous system (CNS) upon activation, and resident CNS cells such as microglia. Within the CNS, a toxic cascade is initiated that manifests as impaired neuronal signaling due to myelin sheath damage and neural and neuronal cell death. Components of this cascade include proinflammatory cytokines, including interferons (IFN), interleukins (IL) and tumor necrosis factor-α (TNF-α), and antibodies against viral peptides that mimic breakdown products of myelin, such as myelin basic protein (MBP). In the direct model, infection of neurons or the myelin-producing oligodendrocytes by a pathogen may lead to cell death or loss of neural function. Similarly, proteins encoded by the pathogen may be inherently toxic and promote myelin damage or cell death.

was dependent on IL-12; a protein known to be important for the pathogenesis of MS (209,210). Thus, activation of systems that remove tolerance of auto-reactive T cells may induce autoimmunity. TLR receptors are important cellular sensors of pathogenic invasion and are critical players in the host innate immune response [for reviews see Refs. (211–213)]. In the case of MS, it can be envisioned that many different infectious agents could potentially activate the TLR system (there are many TLR receptors that respond to bacterial or viral infections), remove tolerance and induce autoimmunity. Experimentally, it will be important to determine if the latent viruses outlined above alter TLR expression and function. In addition, it will be critical to confirm the involvement of TLR receptors in the removal of T cells tolerance by conducting experiments in which TLR-receptor systems are removed/knockout. However, there is likely much more to this story, as it is clear that although viral or bacterial infections in the general population are frequent, the prevalence of MS is not. Therefore, removal of T-cell tolerance would most likely occur after the initial expansion of myelin (or other peptide) specific autoimmune cells, placing the involvement of TLR receptors downstream of the initial disease-inducing event. Nevertheless, the above observations may help to understand how many different latent infectious agents are associated with a common pathological event.

REFERENCES

1. Johnson RT. The virology of demyelinating diseases. Ann Neurol 1994; 36:S54–S60.
2. Osame M, Izumo S, Igata A, Matsumoto M, Matsumoto T, Sonoda S, Tara M, Shibata Y. Blood transfusion and HTLV-I associated myelopathy. Lancet 1986; 2:104–105.
3. Osame M, Usuku K, Izumo S, Ijichi N, Amitani H, Igata A, Matsumoto M, Tara M. HTLV-I associated myelopathy, a new clinical entity. Lancet 1986; 1:1031–1032.
4. Brew BJ. AIDS dementia complex. Neurol Clin 1999; 17:861–881.
5. Tardieu M. HIV-1-related central nervous system diseases. Curr Opin Neurol 1999; 12:377–381.
6. Ranger S, Patillaud S, Denis F, Himmich A, Sangare A, M'Boup S, Itoua-N'Gaporo A, Prince-David M, Chout R, Cevallos R. Seroepidemiology of human herpesvirus-6 in pregnant women from different parts of the world. J Med Virol 1991; 34:194–198.
7. Levy JA, Ferro F, Greenspan D, Lennette ET. Frequent isolation of HHV-6 from saliva and high seroprevalence of the virus in the population. Lancet 1990; 335:1047–1050.
8. Stoeckle MY. The spectrum of human herpesvirus 6 infection: from roseola infantum to adult disease. Annu Rev Med 2000; 51:423–430.
9. Dewhurst S, McIntyre K, Schnabel K, Hall CB. Human herpesvirus 6 (HHV-6) variant B accounts for the majority of symptomatic primary HHV-6 infections in a population of U.S. infants. J Clin Microbiol 1993; 31:416–418.
10. Caserta MT, Hall CB, Schnabel K, Long CE, D'Heron N. Primary human herpesvirus 7 infection: a comparison of human herpesvirus 7 and human herpesvirus 6 infections in children. J Pediatr 1998; 133:386–389.
11. Yamanishi K, Okuno T, Shiraki K, Takahashi M, Kondo T, Asano Y, Kurata T. Identification of human herpesvirus-6 as a causal agent for exanthem subitum. Lancet 1988; 1:1065–1067.
12. Dewhurst S, Chandran B, McIntyre K, Schnabel K, Hall CB. Phenotypic and genetic polymorphisms among human herpesvirus-6 isolates from North American infants. Virology 1992; 190:490–493.

13. Asano Y, Yoshikawa T, Suga S, Kobayashi I, Nakashima T, Yazaki T, Kajita Y, Ozaki T. Clinical features of infants with primary human herpesvirus 6 infection (exanthem subitum, roseola infantum). Pediatrics 1994; 93:104–108.

14. Kimberlin DW, Whitley RJ. Human herpesvirus-6: neurologic implications of a newly-described viral pathogen. J Neurovirol 1998; 4:474–485.

15. DesJardin JA, Gibbons L, Cho E, Supran SE, Falagas ME, Werner BG, Snydman DR. Human herpesvirus 6 reactivation is associated with cytomegalovirus infection and syndromes in kidney transplant recipients at risk for primary cytomegalovirus infection. J Infect Dis 1998; 178:1783–1786.

16. Cone RW, Huang ML, Corey L, Zeh J, Ashley R, Bowden R. Human herpesvirus 6 infections after bone marrow transplantation: clinical and virologic manifestations. J Infect Dis 1999; 179:311–318.

17. Lau YL, Peiris M, Chan GC, Chan AC, Chiu D, Ha SY. Primary human herpes virus 6 infection transmitted from donor to recipient through bone marrow infusion. Bone Marrow Transplant 1998; 21:1063–1066.

18. Buchbinder S, Elmaagacli AH, Schaefer UW, Roggendorf M. Human herpesvirus 6 is an important pathogen in infectious lung disease after allogeneic bone marrow transplantation. Bone Marrow Transplant 2000; 26:639–644.

19. Desachy A, Ranger-Rogez S, Francois B, Venot C, Traccard I, Gastinne H, Denis F, Vignon P. Reactivation of human herpesvirus type 6 in multiple organ failure syndrome. Clin Infect Dis 2001; 32:197–203.

20. Yoshikawa T, Asano Y. Central nervous system complications in human herpesvirus-6 infection. Brain Dev 2000; 22:307–314.

21. Hall CB, Caserta MT, Schnabel KC, Long C, Epstein LG, Insel RA, Dewhurst S. Persistence of human herpesvirus 6 according to site and variant: possible greater neurotropism of variant A. Clin Infect Dis 1998; 26:132–137.

22. Imbert-Marcille BM, Tang XW, Lepelletier D, Besse B, Moreau P, Billaudel S, Milpied N. Human herpesvirus 6 infection after autologous or allogeneic stem cell transplantation: a single-center prospective longitudinal study of 92 patients. Clin Infect Dis 2000; 31:881–886.

23. Kadakia MP. Human herpesvirus 6 infection and associated pathogenesis following bone marrow transplantation. Leuk Lymphoma 1998; 31:251–266.

24. Rogers J, Rohal S, Carrigan DR, Kusne S, Knox KK, Gayowski T, Wagener MM, Fung JJ, Singh N. Human herpesvirus-6 in liver transplant recipients: role in pathogenesis of fungal infections, neurologic complications, and outcome. Transplantation 2000; 69:2566–2573.

25. Bosi A, Zazzi M, Amantini A, Cellerini M, Vannucchi AM, De Milito A, Guidi S, Saccardi R, Lombardini L, Laszlo D, Rossi Ferrini P. Fatal herpesvirus 6 encephalitis after unrelated bone marrow transplant. Bone Marrow Transplant 1998; 22:285–288.

26. Paterson DL, Singh N, Gayowski T, Carrigan DR, Marino IR. Encephalopathy associated with human herpesvirus 6 in a liver transplant recipient. Liver Transpl Surg 1999; 5:454–455.

27. Singh N, Paterson DL. Encephalitis caused by human herpesvirus-6 in transplant recipients: relevance of a novel neurotropic virus. Transplantation 2000; 69:2474–2479.

28. Schmidt CA, Wilbron F, Weiss K, Brinkmann V, Oettle H, Lohmann R, Langrehr JM, Neuhaus P, Siegert W. A prospective study of human herpesvirus type 6 detected by polymerase chain reaction after liver transplantation. Transplantation 1996; 61:662–664.

29. Clark DA. Human herpesvirus 6. Rev Med Virol 2000; 10:155–173.

30. Knox KK, Carrigan DR. Active HHV-6 infection in the lymph nodes of HIV-infected patients: in vitro evidence that HHV-6 can break HIV latency. J Acquir Immune Defic Syndr Hum Retrovirol 1996; 11:370–378.

31. Lusso P, Ensoli B, Markham PD, Ablashi DV, Salahuddin SZ, Tschachler E, Wong-Staal F, Gallo RC. Productive dual infection of human CD4+ T lymphocytes by HIV-1 and HHV- 6. Nature 1989; 337:370–373.

32. Lusso P, De Maria A, Malnati M, Lori F, DeRocco SE, Baseler M, Gallo RC. Induction of CD4 and susceptibility to HIV-1 infection in human CD8+ T lymphocytes by human herpesvirus 6. Nature 1991; 349:533–535.

33. Grivel JC, Ito Y, Faga G, Santoro F, Shaheen F, Malnati MS, Fitzgerald W, Lusso P, Margolis L. Suppression of CCR5—but not CXCR4-tropic HIV-1 in lymphoid tissue by human herpesvirus 6. Nat Med 2001; 7:1232–1235.

34. Dolcetti R, Di Luca D, Carbone A, Mirandola P, De Vita S, Vaccher E, Sighinolfi L, Gloghini A, Tirelli U, Cassai E, Boiocchi M. Human herpesvirus 6 in human immunodeficiency virus-infected individuals: association with early histologic phases of lymphadenopathy syndrome but not with malignant lymphoproliferative disorders. J Med Virol 1996; 48:344–353.

35. Fabio G, Knight SN, Kidd IM, Noibi SM, Johnson MA, Emery VC, Griffiths PD, Clark DA. Prospective study of human herpesvirus 6, human herpesvirus 7, and cytomegalovirus infections in human immunodeficiency virus-positive patients. J Clin Microbiol 1997; 35:2657–2659.

36. Geraminejad P, Memar O, Aronson I, Rady PL, Hengge U, Tyring SK. Kaposi's sarcoma and other manifestations of human herpesvirus 8. J Am Acad Dermatol 2002; 47:641–655.

37. Grulich AE, Dore GJ, Brew BJ. Human herpesvirus 8 and protection from AIDS dementia complex. Herpes 2000; 7:38–40.

38. Chan PK, Ng HK, Cheung JL, Cheng AF. Survey for the presence and distribution of human herpesvirus 8 in healthy brain. J Clin Microbiol 2000; 38:2772–2773.

39. Polk S, Munoz A, Sacktor NC, Jenkins FJ, Cohen B, Miller EN, Jacobson LP. A case–control study of HIV-1-related dementia and co-infection with HHV-8. Neurology 2002; 59:950–953.

40. Anlar B, Pinar A, Yasar Anlar F, Engin D, Ustacelebi S, Kocagoz T, Us D, Akduman D, Yalaz K. Viral studies in the cerebrospinal fluid in subacute sclerosing panencephalitis. J Infect 2002; 44:176–180.

41. Ebers GC, Kukay K, Bulman DE, Sadovnick AD, Rice G, Anderson C, Armstrong H, Cousin K, Bell RB, Hader W, Paty DW, Hashimoto S, Oger J, Duquette P, Warren S, Gray T, P OC, Nath A, Auty A, Metz L, et al. A full genome search in multiple sclerosis. Nat Genet 1996; 13:472–476.

42. Ebers GC, Sadovnick AD. The role of genetic factors in multiple sclerosis susceptibility. J Neuroimmunol 1994; 54:1–17.

43. Paty DW, Noseworthy JH, Ebers GC. Diagnosis of multiple sclerosis. In: Paty DW, Ebers GC, eds. Multiple Sclerosis. Philadelphia: FA Davis Company, 1998:93–97.

44. Challoner PB, Smith KT, Parker JD, MacLeod DL, Coulter SN, Rose TM, Schultz ER, Bennett JL, Garber RL, Chang M, et al. Plaque-associated expression of human herpesvirus 6 in multiple sclerosis. Proc Natl Acad Sci U S A 1995; 92:7440–7444.

45. Caserta MT, Hall CB, Schnabel K, McIntyre K, Long C, Costanzo M, Dewhurst S, Insel R, Epstein LG. Neuroinvasion and persistence of human herpesvirus 6 in children. J Infect Dis 1994; 170:1586–1589.

46. Blumberg BM, Mock DJ, Powers JM, Ito M, Assouline JG, Baker JV, Chen B, Goodman AD. The HHV6 paradox: ubiquitous commensal or insidious pathogen? A two-step in situ PCR approach. J Clin Virol 2000; 16:159–178.

46a. Goodman AD, Mock DJ, Powers JM, Baker JV, Blumberg BM. Human herpesvirus 6 genome and antigen in acute multiple sclerosis lesions. J Infect Dis 2003; 187(9):1365–1376.

46b. Cermelli C, Berti R, Soldan SS, Mayne M, D'ambrosia JM, Ludwin SK, Jacobson S. High frequency of human herpesvirus 6 DNA in multiple sclerosis plaques isolated by laser microdissection. J Infect Dis 2003; 187(9):1377–1387.

47. Knox KK, Brewer JH, Henry JM, Harrington DJ, Carrigan DR. Human herpesvirus 6 and multiple sclerosis: systemic active infections in patients with early disease. Clin Infect Dis 2000; 31:894–903.

48. Alvarez-Lafuente R, Martin-Estefania C, de Las Heras V, Castrillo C, Picazo JJ, Varela de Seijas E, Gonzalez RA. Active human herpesvirus 6 infection in patients with multiple sclerosis. Arch Neurol 2002; 59:929–933.

49. Mayne M, Krishnan J, Metz L, Nath A, Auty A, Sahai BM, Power C. Infrequent detection of human herpesvirus 6 DNA in peripheral blood mononuclear cells from multiple sclerosis patients. Ann Neurol 1998; 44:391–394.

50. Rotola A, Cassai E, Tola MR, Granieri E, Di Luca D. Human herpesvirus 6 is latent in peripheral blood of patients with relapsing–remitting multiple sclerosis. J Neurol Neurosurg Psychiatry 1999; 67:529–531.

51. Akhyani N, Berti R, Brennan MB, Soldan SS, Eaton JM, McFarland HF, Jacobson S. Tissue distribution and variant characterization of human herpesvirus (HHV)-6: increased prevalence of HHV-6A in patients with multiple sclerosis. J Infect Dis 2000; 182:1321–1325.

52. Ablashi DV, Eastman HB, Owen CB, Roman MM, Friedman J, Zabriskie JB, Peterson DL, Pearson GR, Whitman JE. Frequent HHV-6 reactivation in multiple sclerosis (MS) and chronic fatigue syndrome (CFS) patients. J Clin Virol 2000; 16:179–191.

53. Kim JS, Lee KS, Park JH, Kim MY, Shin WS. Detection of human herpesvirus 6 variant A in peripheral blood mononuclear cells from multiple sclerosis patients. Eur Neurol 2000; 43:170–173.

54. Soldan SS, Leist TP, Juhng KN, McFarland HF, Jacobson S. Increased lymphoproliferative response to human herpesvirus type 6A variant in multiple sclerosis patients. Ann Neurol 2000; 47:306–313.

55. Wandinger K, Jabs W, Siekhaus A, Bubel S, Trillenberg P, Wagner H, Wessel K, Kirchner H, Hennig H. Association between clinical disease activity and Epstein–Barr virus reactivation in MS. Neurology 2000; 55:178–184.

56. Wagner HJ, Hennig H, Jabs WJ, Siekhaus A, Wessel K, Wandinger KP. Altered prevalence and reactivity of anti-Epstein–Barr virus antibodies in patients with multiple sclerosis. Viral Immunol 2000; 13:497–502.

57. Ascherio A, Munch M. Epstein–Barr virus and multiple sclerosis. Epidemiology 2000; 11:220–224.

58. Sanders VJ, Waddell AE, Felisan SL, Li X, Conrad AJ, Tourtellotte WW. Herpes simplex virus in postmortem multiple sclerosis brain tissue. Arch Neurol 1996; 53:125–133.

59. Sanders VJ, Felisan S, Waddell A, Tourtellotte WW. Detection of herpesviridae in postmortem multiple sclerosis brain tissue and controls by polymerase chain reaction. J Neurovirol 1996; 2:249–258.

60. Ferrante P, Mancuso R, Pagani E, Guerini FR, Calvo MG, Saresella M, Speciale L, Caputo D. Molecular evidences for a role of HSV-1 in multiple sclerosis clinical acute attack. J Neurovirol 2000; 6(suppl 2):S109–S114.

61. Cortese I, Capone S, Luchetti S, Cortese R, Nicosia A. Cross-reactive phage-displayed mimotopes lead to the discovery of mimicry between HSV-1 and a brain-specific protein. J Neuroimmunol 2001; 113:119–128.

62. Beatty WL, Morrison RP, Byrne GI. Persistent chlamydiae: from cell culture to a paradigm for chlamydial pathogenesis. Microbiol Rev 1994; 58:686–699.

63. Peeling RW, Brunham RC. Chlamydiae as pathogens: new species and new issues. Emerg Infect Dis 1996; 2:307–319.

64. Ward ME. The immunobiology and immunopathology of chlamydial infections. Apmis 1995; 103:769–796.

65. Beatty WL, Byrne GI, Morrison RP. Repeated and persistent infection with Chlamydia and the development of chronic inflammation and disease. Trends Microbiol 1994; 2:94–98.

66. Korman TM, Turnidge JD, Grayson ML. Neurological complications of chlamydial infections: case report and review. Clin Infect Dis 1997; 25:847–851.

67. Koskiniemi M, Gencay M, Salonen O, Puolakkainen M, Farkkila M, Saikku P, Vaheri A. *Chlamydia pneumoniae* associated with central nervous system infections. Eur Neurol 1996; 36:160–163.

68. Yucesan C, Sriram S. *Chlamydia pneumoniae* infection of the central nervous system. Curr Opin Neurol 2001; 14:355–359.

69. Heick A, Skriver E. *Chlamydia pneumoniae*-associated ADEM. Eur J Neurol 2000; 7:435–438.

70. Sriram S, Mitchell W, Stratton C. Multiple sclerosis associated with *Chlamydia pneumoniae* infection of the CNS. Neurology 1998; 50:571–572.

71. Sriram S, Stratton CW, Yao S, Tharp A, Ding L, Bannan JD, Mitchell WM. *Chlamydia pneumoniae* infection of the central nervous system in multiple sclerosis. Ann Neurol 1999; 46:6–14.

72. Sriram S, Yao SY, Stratton C, Calabresi P, Mitchell W, Ikejima H, Yamamoto Y. Comparative study of the presence of *Chlamydia pneumoniae* in cerebrospinal fluid of patients with clinically definite and monosymptomatic multiple sclerosis. Clin Diagn Lab Immunol 2002; 9:1332–1337.

73. Balin BJ, Gerard HC, Arking EJ, Appelt DM, Branigan PJ, Abrams JT, Whittum-Hudson JA, Hudson AP. Identification and localization of *Chlamydia pneumoniae* in the Alzheimer's brain. Med Microbiol Immunol (Berl) 1998; 187:23–42.

74. Braun J, Laitko S, Treharne J, Eggens U, Wu P, Distler A, Sieper J. *Chlamydia pneumoniae*—a new causative agent of reactive arthritis and undifferentiated oligoarthritis. Ann Rheum Dis 1994; 53:100–105.

75. Elkind MS, Lin IF, Grayston JT, Sacco RL. *Chlamydia pneumoniae* and the risk of first ischemic stroke : The Northern Manhattan Stroke Study. Stroke 2000; 31:1521–1525.

76. Gran JT, Hjetland R, Andreassen AH. Pneumonia, myocarditis and reactive arthritis due to *Chlamydia pneumoniae*. Scand J Rheumatol 1993; 22:43–44.

77. Heuschmann PU, Neureiter D, Gesslein M, Craiovan B, Maass M, Faller G, Beck G, Neundoerfer B, Kolominsky-Rabas PL. Association between infection with *Helicobacter pylori* and *Chlamydia pneumoniae* and risk of ischemic stroke subtypes: results from a population-based case–control study. Stroke 2001; 32:2253–2258.

78. Madre JG, Garcia JL, Gonzalez RC, Montero JM, Paniagua EB, Escribano JR, Martinez JD, Cenjor RF. Association between seropositivity to *Chlamydia pneumoniae* and acute ischaemic stroke. Eur J Neurol 2002; 9:303–306.

79. Moling O, Pegoretti S, Rielli M, Rimenti G, Vedovelli C, Pristera R, Mian P. *Chlamydia pneumoniae*—reactive arthritis and persistent infection. Br J Rheumatol 1996; 35:1189–1190.

80. Saario R, Toivanen A. *Chlamydia pneumoniae* as a cause of reactive arthritis. Br J Rheumatol 1993; 32:1112.

81. Gieffers J, Pohl D, Treib J, Dittmann R, Stephan C, Klotz K, Hanefeld F, Solbach W, Haass A, Maass M. Presence of *Chlamydia pneumoniae* DNA in the cerebral spinal fluid is a common phenomenon in a variety of neurological diseases and not restricted to multiple sclerosis. Ann Neurol 2001; 49:585–589.

82. Hammerschlag MR, Ke Z, Lu F, Roblin P, Boman J, Kalman B. Is *Chlamydia pneumoniae* present in brain lesions of patients with multiple sclerosis? J Clin Microbiol 2000; 38:4274–4276.

83. Ke Z, Lu F, Roblin P, Boman J, Hammerschlag MR, Kalman B. Lack of detectable *Chlamydia pneumoniae* in brain lesions of patients with multiple sclerosis. Ann Neurol 2000; 48:400.

84. Layh-Schmitt G, Bendl C, Hildt U, Dong-Si T, Juttler E, Schnitzler P, Grond-Ginsbach C, Grau AJ. Evidence for infection with *Chlamydia pneumoniae* in a subgroup of patients with multiple sclerosis. Ann Neurol 2000; 47:652–655.

85. Sotgiu S, Piana A, Pugliatti M, Sotgiu A, Deiana GA, Sgaramella E, Muresu E, Rosati G. *Chlamydia pneumoniae* in the cerebrospinal fluid of patients with multiple sclerosis and neurological controls. Mult Scler 2001; 7:371–374.

86. Sriram S. Failure to detect *Chlamydia pneumoniae* in the central nervous system of patients with MS. Neurology 2000; 55:1423–1424.

87. Tsai JC, Gilden DH. *Chlamydia pneumoniae* and multiple sclerosis: no significant association. Trends Microbiol 2001; 9:152–154.

88. Kaufman M, Gaydos CA, Sriram S, Boman J, Tondella ML, Norton HJ. Is *Chlamydia pneumoniae* found in spinal fluid samples from multiple sclerosis patients? Conflicting results. Mult Scler 2002; 8:289–294.

89. Correale J, de los Milagros Bassani Molinas M. Oligoclonal bands and antibody responses in multiple sclerosis. J Neurol 2002; 249:375–389.

90. Yao SY, Stratton CW, Mitchell WM, Sriram S. CSF oligoclonal bands in MS include antibodies against Chlamydophila antigens. Neurology 2001; 56:1168–1176.

91. Derfuss T, Gurkov R, Then Bergh F, Goebels N, Hartmann M, Barz C, Wilske B, Autenrieth I, Wick M, Hohlfeld R, Meinl E. Intrathecal antibody production against *Chlamydia pneumoniae* in multiple sclerosis is part of a polyspecific immune response. Brain 2001; 124:1325–1235.
92. Krametter D, Niederwieser G, Berghold A, Birnbaum G, Strasser-Fuchs S, Hartung HP, Archelos JJ. *Chlamydia pneumoniae* in multiple sclerosis: humoral immune responses in serum and cerebrospinal fluid and correlation with disease activity marker. Mult Scler 2001; 7:13–18.
93. Krametter D, Niederwieser G, Berghold A, Birnbaum G, Strasser-Fuchs S, Hartung HP, Archelos JJ. *Chlamydia pneumoniae*-specific humoral immune responses and clinical disease parameters in multiple sclerosis. Ann Neurol 2001; 49:135.
94. Hao Q, Miyashita N, Matsui M, Wang HY, Matsushima T, Saida T. *Chlamydia pneumoniae* infection associated with enhanced MRI spinal lesions in multiple sclerosis. Mult Scler 2002; 8:436–440.
95. Du C, Yao SY, Ljunggren-Rose A, Sriram S. *Chlamydia pneumoniae* infection of the central nervous system worsens experimental allergic encephalitis. J Exp Med 2002; 196:1639–1644.
96. Lenz DC, Lu L, Conant SB, Wolf NA, Gerard HC, Whittum-Hudson JA, Hudson AP, Swanborg RH. A *Chlamydia pneumoniae*-specific peptide induces experimental autoimmune encephalomyelitis in rats. J Immunol 2001; 167:1803–1808.
97. Bruunsgaard H, Ostergaard L, Andersen-Ranberg K, Jeune B, Pedersen BK. Proinflammatory cytokines, antibodies to *Chlamydia pneumoniae* and age-associated diseases in Danish centenarians: is there a link? Scand J Infect Dis 2002; 34:493–499.
98. MacIntyre A, Hammond CJ, Little CS, Appelt DM, Balin BJ. *Chlamydia pneumoniae* infection alters the junctional complex proteins of human brain microvascular endothelial cells. FEMS Microbiol Lett 2002; 217:167–172.
99. Balin BJ, Appelt DM. Role of infection in Alzheimer's disease. J Am Osteopath Assoc 2001; 101:S1–S6.
100. Renvoize EB, Awad IO, Hambling MH. A sero-epidemiological study of conventional infectious agents in Alzheimer's disease. Age Ageing 1987; 16:311–314.
101. Gieffers J, Reusche E, Solbach W, Maass M. Failure to detect *Chlamydia pneumoniae* in brain sections of Alzheimer's disease patients. J Clin Microbiol 2000; 38:881–882.
102. Ring RH, Lyons JM. Failure to detect *Chlamydia pneumoniae* in the late-onset Alzheimer's brain. J Clin Microbiol 2000; 38:2591–2594.
103. Mahley RW, Rall SC Jr. Apolipoprotein E: far more than a lipid transport protein. Annu Rev Genomics Hum Genet 2000; 1:507–537.
104. Gerard HC, Wang GF, Balin BJ, Schumacher HR, Hudson AP. Frequency of apolipoprotein E (APOE) allele types in patients with Chlamydia-associated arthritis and other arthritides. Microb Pathog 1999; 26:35–43.
105. Chapman J, Vinokurov S, Achiron A, Karussis DM, Mitosek-Szewczyk K, Birnbaum M, Michaelson DM, Korczyn AD. APOE genotype is a major predictor of long-term progression of disability in MS. Neurology 2001; 56:312–316.
106. Fazekas F, Strasser-Fuchs S, Kollegger H, Berger T, Kristoferitsch W, Schmidt H, Enzinger C, Schiefermeier M, Schwarz C, Kornek B, Reindl M, Huber K, Grass R, Wimmer G, Vass K, Pfeiffer KH, Hartung HP, Schmidt R. Apolipoprotein E epsilon

4 is associated with rapid progression of multiple sclerosis. Neurology 2001; 57:853–857.

107. Compton SR, Barthold SW, Smith AL. The cellular and molecular pathogenesis of coronaviruses. Lab Anim Sci 1993; 43:15–28.

108. Lai MM. Coronavirus: organization, replication and expression of genome. Annu Rev Microbiol 1990; 44:303–333.

109. Lai MM, Cavanagh D. The molecular biology of coronaviruses. Adv Virus Res 1997; 48:1–100.

110. Myint SH. Human coronaviruses—a brief review. Rev Med Virol 1994; 4:35–46.

111. Arbour N, Day R, Newcombe J, Talbot PJ. Neuroinvasion by human respiratory coronaviruses. J Virol 2000; 74:8913–8921.

112. Collins AR. Human macrophages are susceptible to coronavirus OC43. Adv Exp Med Biol 1998; 440:635–639.

113. Patterson S, Macnaughton MR. Replication of human respiratory coronavirus strain 229E in human macrophages. J Gen Virol 1982; 60:307–314.

114. Arbour N, Cote G, Lachance C, Tardieu M, Cashman NR, Talbot PJ. Acute and persistent infection of human neural cell lines by human coronavirus OC43. J Virol 1999; 73:3338–3350.

115. Arbour N, Ekande S, Cote G, Lachance C, Chagnon F, Tardieu M, Cashman NR, Talbot PJ. Persistent infection of human oligodendrocytic and neuroglial cell lines by human coronavirus 229E. J Virol 1999; 73:3326–3337.

116. Lachance C, Arbour N, Cashman NR, Talbot PJ. Involvement of aminopeptidase N (CD13) in infection of human neural cells by human coronavirus 229E. J Virol 1998; 72:6511–6519.

117. Lane TE, Buchmeier MJ. Murine coronavirus infection: a paradigm for virus-induced demyelinating disease. Trends Microbiol 1997; 5:9–14.

118. Houtman JJ, Fleming JO. Pathogenesis of mouse hepatitis virus-induced demyelination. J Neurovirol 1996; 2:361–376.

119. Matthews AE, Weiss SR, Paterson Y. Murine hepatitis virus—a model for virus-induced CNS demyelination. J Neurovirol 2002; 8:76–85.

120. Stohlman SA, Hinton DR. Viral induced demyelination. Brain Pathol 2001; 11:92–106.

121. Murray RS, Cai GY, Hoel K, Zhang JY, Soike KF, Cabirac GF. Coronavirus infects and causes demyelination in primate central nervous system. Virology 1992; 188:274–284.

122. Murray RS, Cai GY, Soike KF, Cabirac GF. Further observations on coronavirus infection of primate CNS. J Neurovirol 1997; 3:71–75.

123. Haspel MV, Lampert PW, Oldstone MB. Temperature-sensitive mutants of mouse hepatitis virus produce a high incidence of demyelination. Proc Natl Acad Sci U S A 1978; 75:4033–4036.

124. Weiner LP. Pathogenesis of demyelination induced by a mouse hepatitis. Arch Neurol 1973; 28:298–303.

125. Das Sarma J, Fu L, Tsai JC, Weiss SR, Lavi E. Demyelination determinants map to the spike glycoprotein gene of coronavirus mouse hepatitis virus. J Virol 2000; 74:9206–9213.

126. Dandekar AA, Wu GF, Pewe L, Perlman S. Axonal damage is T cell mediated and occurs concomitantly with demyelination in mice infected with a neurotropic coronavirus. J Virol 2001; 75:6115–6120.

127. Fleming JO, Wang FI, Trousdale MD, Hinton DR, Stohlman SA. Interaction of immune and central nervous systems: contribution of anti-viral Thy-1+ cells to demyelination induced by coronavirus JHM. Reg Immunol 1993; 5:37–43.

128. Lane TE, Liu MT, Chen BP, Asensio VC, Samawi RM, Paoletti AD, Campbell IL, Kunkel SL, Fox HS, Buchmeier MJ. A central role for CD4(+) T cells and RANTES in virus-induced central nervous system inflammation and demyelination. J Virol 2000; 74:1415–1424.

129. Wang FI, Stohlman SA, Fleming JO. Demyelination induced by murine hepatitis virus JHM strain (MHV-4) is immunologically mediated. J Neuroimmunol 1990; 30:31–41.

130. Dandekar AA, Perlman S. Virus-induced demyelination in nude mice is mediated by gamma delta T cells. Am J Pathol 2002; 161:1255–1263.

131. Matthews AE, Lavi E, Weiss SR, Paterson Y. Neither B cells nor T cells are required for CNS demyelination in mice persistently infected with MHV-A59. J Neurovirol 2002; 8:257–264.

132. Haring JS, Pewe LL, Perlman S. Bystander CD8 T cell-mediated demyelination after viral infection of the central nervous system. J Immunol 2002; 169:1550–1555.

133. Redwine JM, Buchmeier MJ, Evans CF. In vivo expression of major histocompatibility complex molecules on oligodendrocytes and neurons during viral infection. Am J Pathol 2001; 159:1219–1224.

134. Tanaka R, Iwasaki Y, Koprowski H. Intracisternal virus-like particles in brain of a multiple sclerosis patient. J Neurol Sci 1976; 28:121–126.

135. Burks JS, DeVald BL, Jankovsky LD, Gerdes JC. Two coronaviruses isolated from central nervous system tissue of two multiple sclerosis patients. Science 1980; 209:933–934.

136. Cristallo A, Gambaro F, Biamonti G, Ferrante P, Battaglia M, Cereda PM. Human coronavirus polyadenylated RNA sequences in cerebrospinal fluid from multiple sclerosis patients. New Microbiol 1997; 20:105–114.

137. Murray RS, Brown B, Brian D, Cabirac GF. Detection of coronavirus RNA and antigen in multiple sclerosis brain. Ann Neurol 1992; 31:525–533.

138. Stewart JN, Mounir S, Talbot PJ. Human coronavirus gene expression in the brains of multiple sclerosis patients. Virology 1992; 191:502–505.

139. Salmi A, Ziola B, Hovi T, Reunanen M. Antibodies to coronaviruses OC43 and 229E in multiple sclerosis patients. Neurology 1982; 32:292–295.

140. Salmi A, Ziola B, Reunanen M, Julkunen I, Wager O. Immune complexes in serum and cerebrospinal fluid of multiple sclerosis patients and patients with other neurological diseases. Acta Neurol Scand 1982; 66:1–15.

141. Dessau RB, Lisby G, Frederiksen JL. Coronaviruses in brain tissue from patients with multiple sclerosis. Acta Neuropathol (Berl) 2001; 101:601–604.

142. Dessau RB, Lisby G, Frederiksen JL. Coronaviruses in spinal fluid of patients with acute monosymptomatic optic neuritis. Acta Neurol Scand 1999; 100:88–91.

143. Sorensen O, Collins A, Flintoff W, Ebers G, Dales S. Probing for the human coronavirus OC43 in multiple sclerosis. Neurology 1986; 36:1604–1606.

144. Fleming JO, el Zaatari FA, Gilmore W, Berne JD, Burks JS, Stohlman SA, Tourtellotte WW, Weiner LP. Antigenic assessment of coronaviruses isolated from patients with multiple sclerosis. Arch Neurol 1988; 45:629–633.

145. Madden DL, Wallen WC, Houff SA, Leinikki PA, Sever JL, Holmes KA, Castellano GA, Shekarchi IC. Coronavirus antibodies in sera from patients with multiple sclerosis and matched controls. Arch Neurol 1981; 38:209–210.

146. Boucher A, Denis F, Duquette P, Talbot PJ. Generation from multiple sclerosis patients of long-term T-cell clones that are activated by both human coronavirus and myelin antigens. Adv Exp Med Biol 2001; 494:355–362.

147. Talbot PJ, Paquette JS, Ciurli C, Antel JP, Ouellet F. Myelin basic protein and human coronavirus 229E cross-reactive T cells in multiple sclerosis. Ann Neurol 1996; 39:233–240.

148. Edwards JA, Denis F, Talbot PJ. Activation of glial cells by human coronavirus OC43 infection. J Neuroimmunol 2000; 108:73–81.

149. Collins AR. In vitro detection of apoptosis in monocytes/macrophages infected with human coronavirus. Clin Diagn Lab Immunol 2002; 9:1392–1395.

150. Lower R, Lower J, Kurth R. The viruses in all of us: characteristics and biological significance of human endogenous retrovirus sequences. Proc Natl Acad Sci U S A 1996; 93:5177–5184.

151. Wilkinson DA, Mager DL, Leong JC. Endogenous human retroviruses. In: Levy JA, ed. The Retroviridae. New York, NY: Plenum Press, 1994:465–535.

152. Larsson E, Andersson G. Beneficial role of human endogenous retroviruses: facts and hypotheses. Scand J Immunol 1998; 48:329–338.

153. Krieg AM, Gourley MF, Perl A. Endogenous retroviruses: potential etiologic agents in autoimmunity. FASEB J 1992; 6:2537–2544.

154. Lower R. The pathogenic potential of endogenous retroviruses: facts and fantasies. Trends Microbiol 1999; 7:350–356.

155. Nakagawa K, Harrison LC. The potential roles of endogenous retroviruses in autoimmunity. Immunol Rev 1996; 152:193–236.

156. Rasmussen HB, Clausen J. Possible involvement of endogenous retroviruses in the development of autoimmune disorders, especially multiple sclerosis. Acta Neurol Scand Suppl 1997; 169:32–37.

157. Christensen T, Dissing Sorensen P, Riemann H, Hansen HJ, Moller-Larsen A. Expression of sequence variants of endogenous retrovirus RGH in particle form in multiple sclerosis. Lancet 1998; 352:1033.

158. Christensen T, Dissing Sorensen P, Riemann H, Hansen HJ, Munch M, Haahr S, Moller-Larsen A. Molecular characterization of HERV-H variants associated with multiple sclerosis. Acta Neurol Scand 2000; 101:229–238.

159. Perron H, Lalande B, Gratacap B, Laurent A, Genoulaz O, Geny C, Mallaret M, Schuller E, Stoebner P, Seigneurin JM. Isolation of retrovirus from patients with multiple sclerosis. Lancet 1991; 337:862–863.

160. Perron H, Garson JA, Bedin F, Beseme F, Paranhos-Baccala G, Komurian-Pradel F, Mallet F, Tuke PW, Voisset C, Blond JL, Lalande B, Seigneurin JM, Mandrand B. Molecular identification of a novel retrovirus repeatedly isolated from patients with multiple sclerosis. The Collaborative Research Group on Multiple Sclerosis. Proc Natl Acad Sci U S A 1997; 94:7583–7588.

161. Rasmussen HB, Geny C, Deforges L, Perron H, Tourtelotte W, Heltberg A, Clausen J. Expression of endogenous retroviruses in blood mononuclear cells and brain tissue from multiple sclerosis patients. Mult Scler 1995; 1:82–87.

162. Nakagawa K, Brusic V, McColl G, Harrison LC. Direct evidence for the expression of multiple endogenous retroviruses in the synovial compartment in rheumatoid arthritis. Arthritis Rheum 1997; 40:627–638.

163. Nelson PN, Lever AM, Smith S, Pitman R, Murray P, Perera SA, Westwood OM, Hay FC, Ejtehadi HD, Booth JC. Molecular investigations implicate human endogenous retroviruses as mediators of anti-retroviral antibodies in autoimmune rheumatic disease. Immunol Invest 1999; 28:277–289.

164. Conrad B, Weissmahr RN, Boni J, Arcari R, Schupbach J, Mach B. A human endogenous retroviral superantigen as candidate autoimmune gene in type I diabetes. Cell 1997; 90:303–313.

165. Konttinen YT, Kasna-Ronkainen L. Sjogren's syndrome: viewpoint on pathogenesis. One of the reasons I was never asked to write a textbook chapter on it. Scand J Rheumatol Suppl 2002:15–22.

166. Deb-Rinker P, Klempan TA, O'Reilly RL, Torrey EF, Singh SM. Molecular characterization of a MSRV-like sequence identified by RDA from monozygotic twin pairs discordant for schizophrenia. Genomics 1999; 61:133–144.

167. Deb-Rinker P, O'Reilly RL, Torrey EF, Singh SM. Molecular characterization of a 2.7-kb, 12q13-specific, retroviral-related sequence isolated by RDA from monozygotic twin pairs discordant for schizophrenia. Genome 2002; 45:381–390.

168. Karlsson H, Bachmann S, Schroder J, McArthur J, Torrey EF, Yolken RH. Retroviral RNA identified in the cerebrospinal fluids and brains of individuals with schizophrenia. Proc Natl Acad Sci U S A 2001; 98:4634–4639.

169. Pani MA, Seidl C, Bieda K, Seissler J, Krause M, Seifried E, Usadel KH, Badenhoop K. Preliminary evidence that an endogenous retroviral long-terminal repeat (LTR13) at the HLA-DQB1 gene locus confers susceptibility to Addison's disease. Clin Endocrinol (Oxf) 2002; 56:773–777.

170. Wang-Johanning F, Frost AR, Johanning GL, Khazaeli MB, LoBuglio AF, Shaw DR, Strong TV. Expression of human endogenous retrovirus k envelope transcripts in human breast cancer. Clin Cancer Res 2001; 7:1553–1560.

171. Schiavetti F, Thonnard J, Colau D, Boon T, Coulie PG. A human endogenous retroviral sequence encoding an antigen recognized on melanoma by cytolytic T lymphocytes. Cancer Res 2002; 62:5510–5516.

172. Depil S, Roche C, Dussart P, Prin L. Expression of a human endogenous retrovirus, HERV-K, in the blood cells of leukemia patients. Leukemia 2002; 16:254–259.

173. Patzke S, Lindeskog M, Munthe E, Aasheim HC. Characterization of a novel human endogenous retrovirus, HERV-H/F, expressed in human leukemia cell lines. Virology 2002; 303:164–173.

174. Sauter M, Schommer S, Kremmer E, Remberger K, Dolken G, Lemm I, Buck M, Best B, Neumann-Haefelin D, Mueller-Lantzsch N. Human endogenous retrovirus K10: expression of Gag protein and detection of antibodies in patients with seminomas. J Virol 1995; 69:414–421.

175. Perron H, Geny C, Laurent A, Mouriquand C, Pellat J, Perret J, Seigneurin JM. Leptomeningeal cell line from multiple sclerosis with reverse transcriptase activity and viral particles. Res Virol 1989; 140:551–561.

176. Perron H, Geny C, Genoulaz O, Pellat J, Perret J, Seigneurin JM. Antibody to reverse transcriptase of human retroviruses in multiple sclerosis. Acta Neurol Scand 1991; 84:507–513.

177. Perron H, Firouzi R, Tuke P, Garson JA, Michel M, Beseme F, Bedin F, Mallet F, Marcel E, Seigneurin JM, Mandrand B. Cell cultures and associated retroviruses in multiple sclerosis. Collaborative Research Group on MS. Acta Neurol Scand Suppl 1997; 169:22–31.

178. Lefebvre S, Hubert B, Tekaia F, Brahic M, Bureau JF. Isolation from human brain of six previously unreported cDNAs related to the reverse transcriptase of human endogenous retroviruses. AIDS Res Hum Retroviruses 1995; 11:231–237.

179. Blond JL, Beseme F, Duret L, O. Bouton O, F. Bedin F, H. Perron H, B. Mandrand B, Mallet F. Molecular characterization and placental expression of HERV-W, a new human endogenous retrovirus family. J Virol 1999; 73:1175–1185.

180. La Mantia G, Maglione D, Pengue G, Di Cristofano A, Simeone A, Lanfrancone L, Lania L. Identification and characterization of novel human endogenous retroviral sequences preferentially expressed in undifferentiated embryonal carcinoma cells. Nucleic Acids Res 1991; 19:1513–1520.

181. Jolivet-Reynaud C, Perron H, Ferrante P, Becquart L, Dalbon P, Mandrand B. Specificities of multiple sclerosis cerebrospinal fluid and serum antibodies against mimotopes. Clin Immunol 1999; 93:283–293.

182. Voisset C, Blancher A, Perron H, Mandrand B, Mallet F, Paranhos-Baccala G. Phylogeny of a novel family of human endogenous retrovirus sequences, HERV-W, in humans and other primates. AIDS Res Hum Retroviruses 1999; 15:1529–1533.

183. Perron H, Perin JP, Rieger F, Alliel PM. Particle-associated retroviral RNA and tandem RGH/HERV-W copies on human chromosome 7q: possible components of a 'chain-reaction' triggered by infectious agents in multiple sclerosis? J Neurovirol 2000; 6(suppl 2):S67–S75.

184. Mi S, Lee X, Li X, Veldman GM, Finnerty H, Racie L, LaVallie E, Tang XY, Edouard P, Howes S, Keith JC, McCoy JM. Syncytin is a captive retroviral envelope protein involved in human placental morphogenesis. Nature 2000; 403:785–789.

185. Blond JL, Lavillette D, Cheynet V, Bouton O, Oriol G, Chapel-Fernandes S, Mandrand B, Mallet F, Cosset FL. An envelope glycoprotein of the human endogenous retrovirus HERV-W is expressed in the human placenta and fuses cells expressing the type D mammalian retrovirus receptor. J Virol 2000; 74:3321–3329.

186. Lavillette D, Marin M, Ruggieri A, Mallet F, Cosset FL, Kabat D. The envelope glycoprotein of human endogenous retrovirus type W uses a divergent family of amino acid transporters/cell surface receptors. J Virol 2002; 76:6442–6452.

187. An DS, Xie Y, Chen IS. Envelope gene of the human endogenous retrovirus HERV-W encodes a functional retrovirus envelope. J Virol 2001; 75:3488–3489.

188. Christensen T, Pedersen L, Sorensen PD, Moller-Larsen A. A transmissible human endogenous retrovirus. AIDS Res Hum Retroviruses 2002; 18:861–866.

189. Kwun HJ, Han HJ, Lee WJ, Kim HS, Jang KL. Transactivation of the human endogenous retrovirus K long terminal repeat by herpes simplex virus type 1 immediate early protein 0. Virus Res 2002; 86:93–100.

190. Haahr S, Sommerlund M, Christensen T, Jensen AW, Hansen HJ, Moller-Larsen A. A putative new retrovirus associated with multiple sclerosis and the possible involvement of Epstein–Barr virus in this disease. Ann N Y Acad Sci 1994; 724:148–156.

191. Haahr S, Munch M. The association between multiple sclerosis and infection with Epstein–Barr virus and retrovirus. J Neurovirol 2000; 6(suppl 2):S76–S79.

192. Sutkowski N, Conrad B, Thorley-Lawson DA, Huber BT. Epstein–Barr virus transactivates the human endogenous retrovirus HERV-K18 that encodes a superantigen. Immunity 2001; 15:579–589.

193. Perron H, Jouvin-Marche E, Michel M, Ounanian-Paraz A, Camelo S, Dumon A, Jolivet-Reynaud C, Marcel F, Souillet Y, Borel E, Gebuhrer L, Santoro L, Marcel S, Seigneurin JM, Marche PN, Lafon M. Multiple sclerosis retrovirus particles and

recombinant envelope trigger an abnormal immune response in vitro, by inducing polyclonal Vbeta16 T-lymphocyte activation. Virology 2001; 287:321–332.

194. Clerici M, Fusi ML, Caputo D, Guerini FR, Trabattoni D, Salvaggio A, Cazzullo CL, Arienti D, Villa ML, Urnovitz HB, Ferrante P. Immune responses to antigens of human endogenous retroviruses in patients with acute or stable multiple sclerosis. J Neuroimmunol 1999; 99:173–182.

195. Trabattoni D, Ferrante P, Fusi ML, Saresella M, Caputo D, Urnovitz H, Cazzullo CL, Clerici M. Augmented type 1 cytokines and human endogenous retroviruses specific immune responses in patients with acute multiple sclerosis. J Neurovirol 2000; 6(suppl 2):S38–S41.

196. Menard A, Paranhos-Baccala G, Pelletier J, Mandrand B, Seigneurin JM, Perron H, Reiger F. A cytotoxic factor for glial cells: a new avenue of research for multiple sclerosis? Cell Mol Biol (Noisy-le-grand) 1997; 43:889–901.

197. Crow TJ. A re-evaluation of the viral hypothesis: is psychosis the result of retroviral integration at a site close to the cerebral dominance gene? Br J Psychiatry 1984; 145:243–253.

198. O'Reilly RL, Singh SM. Retroviruses and schizophrenia revisited. Am J Med Genet 1996; 67:19–24.

199. Yolken RH, Karlsson H, Yee F, Johnston-Wilson NL, Torrey EF. Endogenous retroviruses and schizophrenia. Brain Res Brain Res Rev 2000; 31:193–199.

200. Gonzalez-Scarano F, Baltuch G. Microglia as mediators of inflammatory and degenerative diseases. Annu Rev Neurosci 1999; 22:219–240.

201. Katsumata K, Ikeda H, Sato M, Ishizu A, Kawarada Y, Kato H, Wakisaka A, Koike T, Yoshiki T. Cytokine regulation of env gene expression of human endogenous retrovirus-R in human vascular endothelial cells. Clin Immunol 1999; 93:75–80.

202. Larsson E, Venables P, Andersson AC, et al. Tissue and differentiation specific expression on the endogenous retrovirus ERV3 (HERV-R) in normal human tissues and during induced monocytic differentiation in the U-937 cell line. Leukemia 1997; 11(suppl 3):142–144.

203. Larsson E, Venables PJ, Andersson AC, et al. Expression of the endogenous retrovirus ERV3 (HERV-R) during induced monocytic differentiation in the U-937 cell line. Int J Cancer 1996; 67:451–456.

204. Sibata M, Ikeda H, Katumata K, Takeuchi K, Wakisaka A, Yoshoki T. Human endogenous retroviruses: expression in various organs in vivo and its regulation in vitro. Leukemia 1997; 11(suppl 3):145–146.

205. Johnston JB, Silva C, Holden J, Warren KG, Clark AW, Power C. Monocyte activation and differentiation augment human endogenous retrovirus expression: implications for inflammatory brain diseases. Ann Neurol 2001; 50:434–442.

206. Lassmann H. The pathology of multiple sclerosis and its evolution. Philos Trans R Soc Lond B Biol Sci 1999; 354:1635–1640.

207. Cermelli C, Jacobson S. Viruses and multiple sclerosis. Viral Immunol 2000; 13:255–267.

208. Ichikawa HT, Williams LP, Segal BM. Activation of APCs through CD40 or Toll-like receptor 9 overcomes tolerance and precipitates autoimmune disease. J Immunol 2002; 169:2781–2787.

209. Karp CL. Interleukin-12: amiss in MS. Ann Neurol 1999; 45:689–692.

210. Karp CL, van Boxel-Dezaire AH, Byrnes AA, Nagelkerken L. Interferon-beta in multiple sclerosis: altering the balance of interleukin-12 and interleukin-10? Curr Opin Neurol 2001; 14:361–368.

211. Lien E, Ingalls RR. Toll-like receptors. Crit Care Med 2002; 30:S1–S11.

212. Zuany-Amorim C, Hastewell J, Walker C. Toll-like receptors as potential therapeutic targets for multiple diseases. Nat Rev Drug Discov 2002; 1:797–807.

213. Modlin RL. Mammalian toll-like receptors. Ann Allergy Asthma Immunol 2002; 88:543–547.

214. Simmons A. Herpesvirus and multiple sclerosis. Herpes 2001; 8:60–63.

215. Swanborg RH, Whittum-Hudson JA, Hudson AP. Human herpesvirus 6 and *Chlamydia pneumoniae* as etiologic agents in multiple sclerosis—a critical review. Microbes Infect 2002; 4:1327–1333.

216. Tomsone V, Logina I, Millers A, Chapenko S, Kozireva S, Murovska M. Association of human herpesvirus 6 and human herpesvirus 7 with demyelinating diseases of the nervous system. J Neurovirol 2001; 7:564–569.

217. Marrie RA, Wolfson C. Multiple sclerosis and varicella zoster virus infection: a review. Epidemiol Infect 2001; 127:315–325.

218. Wroblewska Z, Gilden D, Devlin M, et al. Cytomegalovirus isolation from a chimpanzee with acute demyelinating disease after inoculation of multiple sclerosis brain cells. Infect Immun 1979; 25:1008–1015.

219. McHatters GR, Scham RG. Bird viruses in multiple sclerosis: combination of viruses or Marek's alone? Neurosci Lett 1995; 188:75–76.

220. Melnick JL, Seidel E, Inoue YK, Nishibe Y. Isolation of virus from the spinal fluid of three patients with multiple sclerosis and one with amyotrophic lateral sclerosis. Lancet 1982; 1:830–833.

221. Ohara Y. Multiple sclerosis and measles virus. Jpn J Infect Dis 1999; 52:198–200.

222. Pille ER, Mzokova VM, Andreeva AP, Andzhaparidze OG. Possible role of measles, rubella and mumps viruses in multiple sclerosis. Acta Virol 1977; 21:139–145.

223. Hodge MJ, Wolfson C. Canine distemper virus and multiple sclerosis. Neurology 1997; 49:S62–S69.

224. Koprowski H, ter Meulen V. Multiple sclerosis and parainfluenza 1 virus. History of the isolation of the virus and expression of phenotypic differences between the isolated virus and Sendai virus. J Neurol 1975; 208:175–190.

225. Goswami KK, Randall RE, Lange LS, Russell WC. Antibodies against the paramyxovirus SV5 in the cerebrospinal fluids of some multiple sclerosis patients. Nature 1987; 327:244–247.

226. Stoner GL. Polyomavirus models of brain infection and the pathogenesis of multiple sclerosis. Brain Pathol 1993; 3:213–227.

227. Koprowski H, DeFreitas EC, Harper ME, et al. Multiple sclerosis and human T-cell lymphotropic retroviruses. Nature 1985; 318:154–160.

228. Graber P, Rosenmund A, Probst A, Zimmerli W. Multiple sclerosis-like illness in early HIV infection. Aids 2000; 14:2411–2413.

229. Meiering CD, Linial ML. Historical perspective of foamy virus epidemiology and infection. Clin Microbiol Rev 2001; 14:165–176.

230. Murray RS, Cai GY, Hoel K, Johnson S, Cabirac GF. Coronaviruses and multiple sclerosis. Adv Exp Med Biol 1993; 342:353–357.

231. Compston DA, Vakarelis BN, Paul E, McDonald WI, Batchelor JR, Mims CA. Viral infection in patients with multiple sclerosis and HLA-DR matched controls. Brain 1986; 109 (Pt 2):325–344.

232. Britton DE, Houff SA, Eiben RM. Possible interactions between rabies vaccination and a progressive degenerative CNS disease. Arch Neurol 1978; 35:693.

233. Nakashima I, Fujihara K, Itoyama Y. Human parvovirus B19 infection in multiple sclerosis. Eur Neurol 1999; 42:36–40.

234. Woyciechowska JL, Dambrozia J, Leinikki P, et al. Viral antibodies in twins with multiple sclerosis. Neurology 1985; 35:1176–1180.

235. Haase CG, Viazov S, Fiedler M, Koenig N, Faustmann PM, Roggendorf M. Borna disease virus RNA is absent in chronic multiple sclerosis. Ann Neurol 2001; 50:423–424.

15

Herpes Simplex Virus Drug Resistance—HSV Thymidine Kinase Mutants

Richard B. Tenser

Departments of Neurology, and Microbiology and Immunology, Penn State University College of Medicine, Hershey, Pennsylvania, U.S.A.

1. INTRODUCTION

The widespread use of nucleoside analog antivirals to treat patients infected with herpes simplex virus (HSV) is indicted by the statement in a recent publication that, "More than 2.3 million kg of these drugs have been prescribed...in >30 countries" (1). Many clinical trials have demonstrated the effectiveness of these antivirals. However, clinical studies have also reported the detection of drug-resistant viral mutants, particularly important in the care of immunosuppressed patients. Laboratory studies have indicated the mechanisms of viral resistance. The development of drug-resistant mutants of HSV has raised the issue of the potential pathogenicity of these mutants, and also mechanisms of HSV infection whereby such mutants may arise.

A biological characteristic of herpesvirus infections is the frequent establishment of a latent infection after initial acute infection. The initial acute infection may be symptomatic or asymptomatic. After latency is established, there is the potential for the virus to reactivate from latency. Reactivation may cause recurrent disease or may be asymptomatic. Herpesvirus latency may occur in various cell types and is not simply a low-level persistent infection but rather an infection in which novel viral RNAs and proteins may be expressed. Latency seems to be a biological niche to which herpesviruses such as HSV have adapted. Mechanisms of latency and reactivation have received much study, because

Table 1   Human Herpesviruses

Herpesvirus	Classification	Illness associated
Herpes simplex virus type 1 (HSV-1)	Alpha	Mucocutaneous infection, encephalitis
HSV-2	Alpha	Mucocutaneous infection, encephalitis
Varicella zoster virus	Alpha	Chicken pox, zoster (shingles)
Epstein–Barr virus	Gamma	Mononucleosis, lymphoma
Human cytomegalovirus	Beta	Renal infection, encephalitis, retinitis
Human herpesvirus 6 (HHV 6)	Beta	Exanthum subitum, multiple sclerosis? (2,3)
HHV 7	Beta	Exanthum subitum
HHV 8	Gamma	Kaposi sarcoma

although several nucleoside analog antivirals have been developed which are effective against acute infection of at least some of the human herpesviruses, these are not effective against the viruses in the latent state. HSV is probably the best studied human herpesvirus, of the eight human herpesviruses that have been identified at the present time (Table 1).

Multiple animal herpesviruses also exist, at least one of which [e.g., B virus of monkeys (cercopithecine herpesvirus)] may cause serious infection of humans (4). In considering the development of antivirals, treatment of some human herpesvirus infections has been a modest success story of modern medicine. The alpha herpesviruses particularly are effectively treated with several antivirals. The first antiviral of real value for systemic administration was acyclovir (Zostrix), followed more recently by its prodrug valacyclovir (Valtrex), and also famciclovir (Famvir), the prodrug of penciclovir. The mechanism of action of these medications is similar and is predicated on the biology of the alpha herpesviruses (HSV-1, HSV-2, varicella zoster virus). Emphasis in the discussion below will be on HSV-1 and HSV-2.

Antivirals such as acyclovir (Acv) are inactive until they are phosphorylated, initially to the monophosphate (Acv P) and then to the triphosphate (Acv PPP). Phosphorylation to Acv P is mediated by a viral encoded enzyme, the HSV encoded thymidine kinase (TK). Further phosphorylation to Acv PPP is via cellular enzymes (5–7). Acv PPP inhibits the viral DNA polymerase and acts a DNA chain terminator, both of which mechanisms inhibit HSV replication. The key to the sequence of events following administration of acyclovir is phosphorylation to Acv P by the viral TK. Without this occurrence; acyclovir and this class of antivirals are inactive, since these antivirals are poorly phosphorylated to the monophosphate by cellular enzymes. It can be thought that by expressing a viral encoded TK which phosphorylates Acv, HSV carries the seeds of its own destruction.

HSV encoded TK and the two known cellular TKs (TK 1 and TK 2, often considered as cytosolic and mitochondrial TK) have similarities but considerable differences as well. The major difference in terms of biology and medicine is the spectrum of nucleosides and nucleoside analogues that these enzymes phosphorylate to the monophosphate. Figure 1 presents phosphorylation in brief outline form. Generally, the cellular TKs are more fastidious than is the HSV TK, in terms of substrates that are phosphorylated.

HSV TK has often been considered to be a promiscuous enzyme, which phosphorylates many substrates (6,8,9), and also has thymidylate kinase activity (10). Cellular TKs are much more selective. It is the promiscuous nature of HSV TK, which allows for the selectivity and great value of the antivirals in the inhibition of these viruses. Phosphorylation to the active antiviral state is dependent on HSV infection being present. Parenthetically, it can be noted that in the treatment of human immunodeficiency virus (HIV) infection, phosphorylation of zidovudine (AZT) is necessary, in this case by cellular TK, for this to be active as an antiviral in the inhibition of HIV (10,11). Although HIV does not express an enzyme which activates AZT, some issues of HIV resistance to AZT may be similar to HSV resistance to antivirals. In summary, phosphorylation of the antiviral Acv to the active antiviral state is efficiently achieved by HSV TK and poorly so by cellular TKs. Phosphorylation of Acv to the active antiviral state by HSV TK is outlined in Fig. 2.

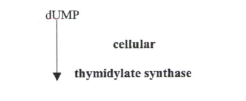

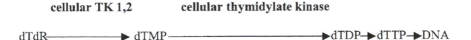

Figure 1 Schematic outline of the synthesis of thymidine nucleotides by human enzymes and by HSV TK. Thymidine (dTdR) phosphorylation by cellular and HSV TKs to the nucleotides dTMP, dTDP and dTTP is followed by incorporation of dTTP into cellular or viral DNA. In addition to being synthesized by TK-mediated phosphorylation of dTdR (ATP is the phosphate donor), dTMP is synthesized by thymidylate synthase-mediated methylation (tetrahydrofolate is the methyl donor).

HSV TK   cellular enzymes

AcV ──────►Acv P──────────► Acv PP ──►Acv PPP──

──► inhibition of viral DNA synthesis

Figure 2   Schematic outline of AcV phosphorylation by HSV TK. Acv is readily phosphorylated by the promiscuous HSV TK but not by cellular TKs. The triphosphate form (Acv PPP) inhibits viral DNA synthesis.

Related to the point of enzyme selectivity and whether substrate is or is not phosphorylated by TK is the concept of competition. For example, AZT phosphorylation by cellular TK is competed by dTdR, since the same cellular TK enzyme is required for AZT and for dTdR phosphorylation (11,12). Therefore, dTdR administration, which competes with and decreases phosphorylation of AZT, decreases the effectiveness of AZT in inhibiting HIV infection. In addition, medication, which decreases cellular TK expression, decreases the effectiveness of AZT (13), probably by decreasing AZT phosphorylation.

A last factor related to substrate competition is the issue of nucleoside and nucleotide pool levels within cells. Transport of nucleosides into cells occurs by several mechanisms (14,15), and competition among nucleosides for transport into cells is present. In addition, some medications alter nucleoside transport (16,17), and it is probable that intracellular nucleoside pools can be altered in this fashion. Intracellular levels of specific nucleosides will alter effective levels of other nucleosides, via competition for enzymes. Once within cells, dTdR is usually rapidly phosphorylated to dTTP, and little free intracellular dTdR is present (14). Purine and pyrimidine deoxyucleotide levels vary within cells, and in lymphocytes have been reported to be dTTP≥dATP≥dCTP≥dGTP (12). After HSV infection of fibroblasts levels were dTTP>dCTP>dGTP>dATP (18). The possible role-specific nucleoside–nucleotide pools in infection by HSV TK mutants, which are resistant to Acv may have biological importance will be discussed below.

2. HSV TK MUTANTS

Although Acv and related antivirals have been effective in the control of HSV, via inhibition of HSV replication, mutant HSV, which is resistant to these drugs may arise. Resistance primarily arises in three ways. First, mutation may occur in the gene coding for the viral TK, which results in the viral TK being more restrictive and not able to phosphorylate Acv (19,20). Such virus is termed TK altered. Alternatively, mutation in the TK gene may result in the absence of viral TK enzyme (21,22). This virus is termed TK negative. In these instances the viral TK is either less promiscuous or is absent. The result with either mutant is the lack of phosphorylation of Acv, which therefore is not activated to the antiviral state. Lastly, viral mutation may occur whereby even though Acv is phosphorylated, the viral DNA polymerase is altered so that it is not inhibited by Acv PPP (21,22). HSV DNA polymerase mutants may be sensitive to other antivirals which inhibit HSV DNA polymerase, such as foscarnet (23). For these three types of HSV TK mutants, Acv does not inhibit the virus. In summary, most but not all HSV mutants resistant to Acv are TK negative. HSV DNA polymerase mutants are TK positive but are resistant to Acv. Most common of these types of HSV mutants are TK negative mutants with absent TK activity (24). TK negative mutants are easily detected in cell culture studies and may also occur in patients.

Development of TK negative HSV mutants is Darwinian. That is, mutations in the HSV TK gene occur routinely with viral replication, and TK negative HSV is present in HSV populations (25,26). Ordinarily such mutants have little biological effect because of the very large majority of wild type are TK positive HSV. However, in the presence of antivirals such as Acv, which, subsequent to the phosphorylation of Acv by the viral TK inhibits the replication of TK positive HSV, TK negative HSV increases in amount. TK negative HSV, which does not phosphorylate Acv survives and replicates in the Acv environment, an environment which inhibits wild-type TK positive HSV.

TK negative HSV mutants have been particularly recognized in immunosuppressed patients treated with antivirals such as Acv (23,27,28). Presumably in non-immunosuppressed individuals, TK negative HSV is present and possibly increases after Acv treatment since mutant HSV replication is not inhibited by Acv. However, such individuals have intact immune systems, and this results in TK negative HSV being cleared by usual control mechanisms. However, in immunosuppressed individuals immune control mechanisms are defective. This results in the inability to clear TK negative HSV, with resultant further increased TK negative HSV replication. TK negative HSV is readily detected in cultures of herpes skin lesions of immunosuppressed patients treated with Acv (23,27,28). It has been estimated that approximately 5% of immunosuppressed patients undergoing antiviral treatment develop Acv-resistant HSV disease (24). Isolates from most would likely show infection by a mixture of wild-type TK positive and mutant TK negative HSV.

Figure 3 shows cell culture isolation of a mixture of TK negative mutant and wild-type TK positive HSV isolated from an immunosuppressed patient (29). HSV was isolated on HSV-susceptible monolayer cells from a swab of the lesion. Plaque autoradiography was used to differentiate TK positive from TK negative

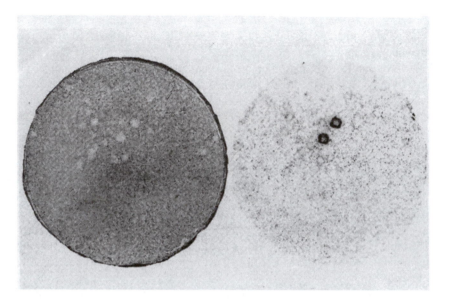

Figure 3 HSV isolated from a swab of a chronic mucocutaneous lesion in an immuno-suppressed patient treated with AcV. Rabbit kidney monolayer cells were infected with lysate from the swab. After culture for 4 days at 37°C in 5% CO_2, [14]dTDR was added (0.5 Ci/mL; 53.4 mCi/mmol), and cultures were incubated for an additional 4 hr. Monolayer cultures were then stained with neutral red and fixed with formalin. After drying, monolayers were placed in contact with x-ray film for 5 days and then the film was developed. LEFT, stained monolayer culture showing a total of 20 HSV plaques. RIGHT, radiograph of the monolayer culture showing two HSV plaques which incorporated TdR. Those two plaques (see mono-layer on the left) indicate wild-type TK positive HSV. The remaining HSV plaques in the monolayer which did not incorporate TdR are TK mutant HSV. (From Ref. 28.)

HSV. In this procedure, as HSV plaques in the monolayer cell culture developed, the cell culture was treated with radiolabeled dTdR. After this treatment the monolayer cells were fixed, stained and dried, and an autoradiograph of the monolayer was made. Total HSV plaques are seen in the fixed, stained monolayer culture (Fig. 3, left). TK positive (isotope-labeled) and TK negative (isotope-unla-beled) plaques are seen in the autoradiograph of the monolayer (Fig. 3, right). Labeled dTdR had been phosphorylated by the abundant HSV TK present in cells infected with the wild-type TK positive HSV, and infected cells in TK positive HSV plaques are seen dark in the autoradiograph. Light TK negative HSV plaques had not phosphorylated radiolabeled dTdR. In immunodeficient mice infected with mixtures of wild-type and TK mutant HSV and then treated with Acv, chronic HSV ulcers appeared with a mixture of TK negative and TK posi-tive HSV (30), as in immunosuppressed patients.

What is the effect of TK negative HSV in terms of infection of the nervous system, particularly HSV latent infection and reactivation?

3. HSV LATENCY AND REACTIVATION

Latent HSV infection of the human nervous system is the reservoir from which recurrent HSV infection of epithelial surfaces develops (31,32). Reactivation of latent HSV infection results in recurrent herpes infection of mouth and face (herpes labialis), cornea (herpes keratitis), and genitals (herpes genitalis). Reactivation may also be asymptomatic, occurring with infectious HSV shedding but without the presence of clinically apparent lesions. HSV present in latent infection has been well demonstrated to be an infection of sensory ganglion neurons in humans (33–35) and in experimental animals (36,37). Reactivation in trigeminal ganglion (TG) neurons is thought to result in clinically apparent recurrences of the face and eye. Reactivation in sacral dorsal root ganglion neurons is thought to result in genital recurrence. Latency and reactivation in autonomic ganglion neurons may also occur (35). The causes of HSV reactivation in humans are not well known, with the usual suspects including stress and UV light (38). Interestingly, a very reliable means to cause HSV reactivation in humans is the physical manipulation of the TG. Following the surgical treatment of trigeminal neuralgia, reactivation of human HSV latent infection from TG and root manipulation has been well described (39,40). It is probable that TG and trigeminal root manipulation result in altered TG neuron function, e.g., altered neuronal transcription, which results in reactivation of HSV, which is latent in TG neurons (41).

During latency, infectious HSV is not present, nor are viral proteins expressed, and only a single species of viral RNA is readily detected (36). Viral DNA is present of course, the basis for the production of infectious virus after reactivation. The HSV RNA expressed during latency, the latency-associated transcript (LAT) is detected in the nuclei of latently-infected neurons in humans (42,43) and experimental animals (36,37). As the only viral transcript readily detected during latency, understanding LAT expression has received great emphasis, including the role of the LAT promoter and other regulatory elements (44), and HSV LAT is the most commonly used molecular marker of HSV latency. In this brief discussion, LAT will be considered as being what has been termed the major LATs (1.5 and 2.0 kb) and not the low level 8.3 kb transcript (44). It has been noted in many instances that LAT expression is specific for neurons, and that LAT expression in these cells is long-term and constitutive (45,46). It has been suggested that LAT expression may decrease HSV-induced apoptosis (47,48), possibly by decrease of lytic HSV infection (37).

Experimental studies of HSV latency and reactivation have been performed by many investigators. In these studies, experimental animals, most commonly mice but sometimes guinea-pigs (often to study genital HSV infection) or rabbits (usually to study ocular HSV infection) have been used. Typically, HSV infection of the cornea is performed in order to infect TG neurons, but nasal infection does the same. Alternatively, genital or more commonly footpad infection is performed to infect dorsal root ganglion neurons. HSV is transported via retrograde axoplasmic flow to the sensory ganglion neurons from the site of primary infection (49). Presumably human TG infection occurs via similar mechanisms after initial HSV infection; acute infection of the sensory ganglion results. During the period of 3–7 days after experimental infection HSV antigens are readily detected in the ganglia. In addition, if ganglia are removed, homogenized and tested on HSV-susceptible monolayer cells, infectious virus is easily detected. However, after 7–10 days the same methods do not result in detection of HSV or HSV antigens. Latent infection is present. As noted above, at this time only HSV DNA and HSV LAT are detected. During the period of latency (operationally defined in most experimental studies as being 28 or more days after initial infection) HSV can be reactivated from latency, so that infectious virus is produced. Typically this is done by killing the animal and placing the sensory ganglia in explant culture in vitro. Within several days infectious virus is synthesized and is easily detected. It should be emphasized that during latency, removal of the sensory ganglion, homogenization of the ganglion and attempts to isolate HSV fail. Infectious virus is not present. Latency implies not simply a low-level infection of HSV but a special type of infection by HSV, a situation marked by the absence of expression of viral antigens and RNAs, other than the expression of HSV LAT in infected sensory ganglion neurons (36,50).

4.   THE ROLE OF HSV TK IN LATENCY AND REACTIVATION

As part of investigations of the pathogenesis of HSV latency and reactivation we investigated experimental HSV infection with TK negative mutants of HSV. The rationale of these studies was based on observations by others of the biology of TK negative HSV. It had been noted that TK negative HSV replicated well in monolayer cell culture and was apparently dispensable for virus replication. Specifically, it was not essential for HSV replication in most cell culture situations. However, TK negative HSV did not replicate well in cell culture under conditions in which cell culture medium contained low serum (8). Low serum medium results in minimal replication of monolayer cells in culture, cells that are used to support virus growth. Since HSV latent infection is an infection of neurons, a non-replicating cell type, and since TK negative HSV replicated poorly in nondividing cells in cell culture, we sought to determine if TK negative HSV could replicate in neurons and whether it would establish latent infection in neurons.

In initial studies we performed corneal infection of guinea-pigs (51) and mice (52) with HSV TK mutants. TK negative HSV used for these studies was developed by growth of standard TK positive HSV in the presence of drugs like Acv. Observations were threefold: first TK mutant HSV replicated well in eyes of experimental animals, almost to the level of wild-type TK positive HSV. This was determined by performing ocular swabs of experimental animals 3–5 days after infection. Second, HSV replicated poorly in TG tissue. This was determined by removal of TG 3–5 days after infection, homogenization and isolation of HSV on susceptible culture cells. Third, HSV latency was very decreased when TG were tested during the period of latency (≥28 days after infection) (51,52). Testing for latency was performed by explant culture of TG. From these studies we concluded that HSV TK expression was not important for virus replication in situations of replicating or potentially replicating cells (e.g., corneal epithelium) but was important for replication in nondividing cells (e.g., neurons). In addition, HSV TK expression seemed to be important for latent infection. Subsequent to the performance of related studies by our laboratory and those of other investigators, which supported these results, HSV LAT was discovered (53).

HSV LAT provided a molecular means to detect latency, rather than testing for HSV reactivation in explant culture. In 1989 we (54) and other groups (55,56) reported results of investigations in which experimental animals were infected with TK negative HSV, and during the period of latency, rather than explanting ganglia and assaying for infectious HSV, ganglia were removed at the time of latency (≥28 days after infection) and tested for HSV LAT. In situ hybridization studies showed HSV LAT in the nuclei of TK negative HSV-infected mice, to about the same degree as in mice infected with wild-type TK positive HSV (Fig. 4). The groups

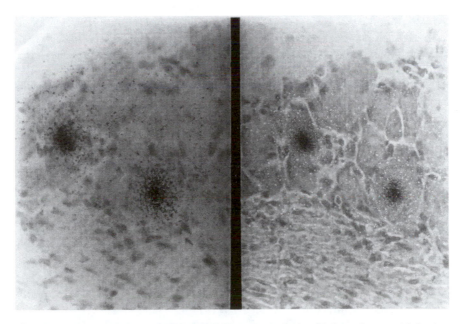

Figure 4 HSV LAT in trigeminal ganglion neurons of mice 28 days after nasal infection with TK mutant HSV (dlsactk, Ref. 57). (Left) high power photomicrograph, standard optics, (right) phase contrast, showing isotope grains over neuronal nuclei. (Infection, tissue preparation and in situ hybridization methods as in Ref. 60.)

arrived at the same conclusion: HSV TK is not important for the establishment of HSV latency (i.e., LAT is readily expressed during the period of latency) but is important for the reactivation of HSV from latency (54–56).

More recently we further investigated the role of TK expression and reactivation in studies that further demonstrates the importance of HSV TK expression for HSV reactivation, and also returns to consideration of intracellular nucleoside/nucleotide pools. We performed corneal and footpad infection of mice with TK negative HSV. During the period of latency sensory ganglia were removed and explant cultured to detect reactivation of HSV. Unlike in previous studies, while some sensory ganglia were explant cultured in standard culture medium, others were cultured in medium supplemented with dTdR. Reactivation of TK negative HSV in cell culture was markedly increased in the dTdR group (57). Addition of other nucleosides to the culture medium did not have the same effect. Second, if the explant medium containing dTdR also contained an inhibitor of nucleoside transport, the reactivation-enhancing effect of dTdR was blocked (58). These results, strongly supported the conclusion that HSV TK expression is important for reactivation from latency. Also of interest, if the nucleoside transport inhibitor was present in the explant medium used to test reactivation of wild-type TK positive HSV, reactivation was inhibited (58).

In addition to evidence that HSV TK expression is important for HSV reactivation from latency, HSV TK expression is important for acute HSV infection, at least in the nervous system. This had been suggested in early studies, which showed limited replication of TK negative HSV in TG when tested 3 days after corneal inoculation of virus (51,52). It was also indicated by the very reduced lethality of TK negative HSV after intracerebral inoculation of adult mice (59). In addition, acute infection of TG tissue in adult but not newborn mice was dependent on viral TK expression (60). Reactivation from latency may utilize similar viral replication mechanisms as acute infection. This conclusion was supported by the report that HSV TK expression was important for HSV lytic gene expression (61).

One other experimental study relates to the role of HSV TK expression and disease. In this in vivo study corneal infection of mice was performed with TK negative HSV. The goal was to investigate infection by TK negative HSV during the period of acute infection (3–5 days after infection), remembering that in previous studies acute ganglion infection by TK negative HSV was very low level (51,52,60). However in this study, similar to the in vitro study in which explant culture medium was supplemented with dTdR (58), we treated mice in vivo with dTdR. dTdR in mouse drinking water resulted in greatly increased titers of infectious TK negative HSV in TG (57). HSV isolated was shown to be TK negative by plaque autoradiography (see Fig. 3.). Therefore, in this in vivo study, TK negative HSV replication was enhanced by supplemental nucleoside.

5. THE ROLE OF HSV TK MUTANTS IN HUMAN DISEASE

Since TK mutants are usually present in large populations of HSV virus particles (26,27), it would be expected that HSV isolates from humans would contain TK negative mutants. Such mutants have been isolated, usually from immunosuppressed patients with cutaneous HSV infections who have been treated with antivirals such as Acv (23,27–29). As noted above, HSV mutants that are resistant to antivirals such as Acv usually are mutated in the viral TK gene so that TK enzyme is not expressed (TK negative mutants). Less common are mutants, which express HSV TK, which is more selective than the wild-type TK, and does not phosphorylate Acv. While there is a good correlation between resistance to Acv and defect in the viral TK gene, some HSV mutants resistant to Acv express wild-type TK. In these mutants Acv is phosphorylated by the viral TK, but resistance to Acv occurs because the HSV DNA polymerase enzyme is not inhibited by phosphorylated Acv (21,22).

In immunologically intact individuals treated for HSV infection, TK HSV mutants are likely to be present in the HSV population, but following inhibition of wild-type HSV by the antiviral, the intact immune system easily clears the relatively few TK negative virus particles present. In immunologically suppressed patients, Acv inhibits replication of wild-type HSV TK, but TK mutants resistant to Acv are not cleared, and subsequently these replicate. From experimental animal data it might be concluded that TK negative HSV would be present in humans at cutaneous sites of infection but not in the nervous system, particularly not in neurons. HSV usually enters the nervous system via neurons, secondary to axoplasmic transport to neuronal cell bodies from peripheral sites of infection (49). Therefore, one might think that TK negative HSV would be sequestered in neurons, where it would not replicate, and would not be pathogenic in the nervous system. In this scenario, the bad news might be that TK negative HSV would replicate at cutaneous sites (and possibly other non-neuronal sites), and the good news would be that it would not productively infect neurons. This scenario might be supported by the general absence of TK negative HSV encephalitis in immunosuppressed patients, including those with significant cutaneous infections. However, even wild-type TK positive HSV encephalitis is uncommon in Acv-treated immunosuppressed patients, suggesting that TK phenotype is not the sole important factor.

Several observations in experimental animals lead to caution before concluding that TK negative HSV would not infect neurons. In most situations where TK negative HSV is isolated, including from immunosuppressed patients, while TK negative HSV is isolated, wild-type TK positive HSV is also isolated (28). That is, HSV mixtures are present (30). The relative amounts of virus particles in HSV mixtures, which express each of the two TK phenotypes varies. Reversion of TK negative HSV to the TK positive phenotype occurs at different rates for different HSV mutants selected for Acv resistance (62). By plaque autoradiography it is easy to determine the relative amounts of HSV with each TK phenotype (28,30). What is the biological affect of such virus mixtures? In experimental animal studies in which mice were infected with a mixture of TK negative and TK positive HSV, it appeared that TK positive HSV complemented the TK negative virus (30,63). It appeared that TK positive HSV "assisted" the replication of TK negative HSV. Might this occur in humans where TK negative HSV is present, either by the small amount of TK positive HSV that is present, or possibly when antiviral treatment is discontinued and TK positive HSV replication increases?

In addition, TK negative HSV replication is much greater in newborn mice than adult mice (60), probably due to impaired immune responsiveness, but probably also the presence of many more replicating cells. Enhanced HSV replication in replicating cells in vivo was noted in a study of virus replication in liver of mice. In this study, partial hepatectomy was performed. Following this procedure rapid liver regeneration occurred. This produced an in vivo source of replicating cells. TK negative HSV replication was greatly increased in liver during the period of liver regeneration, supporting the concept that HSV TK expression is particularly important for replication in nondividing cells (64). Therefore, might TK negative HSV replication readily occur in humans in replicating cells?

Reports of TK negative HSV in humans have been limited to isolations from cutaneous sites (23,27–29). However, it is likely that TK negative HSV may be present at other sites including brain during HSV encephalitis. It could be argued that only wild-type TK positive HSV would be isolated (at time of post-mortem) from TG and dorsal root ganglia of normal, immunologically intact individuals, since HSV is present only in neurons during latency and since TK mutant HSV replication in neurons is restricted. In support of this speculation, it was reported that patients treated repeatedly with topical penciclovir for recurrent mucocutaneous HSV infection did not show an increase in the proportion of TK HSV mutants isolated from cutaneous sites. Although mutant HSV increased with days of treatment, showing TK mutant HSV replication, there was no increase from one course of treatment to another, suggesting that TK mutant HSV did not accumulate in sensory ganglion neurons (1). However, during acute HSV encephalitis HSV likely replicates in neuronal and glial cells, possibly providing a source within the brain of TK mutant HSV. One could speculate on whether antiviral resistant HSV is important in situations where responsiveness to antivirals appears limited. Lastly, we can speculate and return to the issue of nucleoside–nucleotide pool levels and possible enhanced TK negative HSV replication. Since dTdR treatment of mice enhanced TK negative HSV replication (57), it is reasonable to consider the same might occur in patients. Nucleoside–nucleotide pool levels, including transport into neurons are not well known, and may be of importance in patients, in terms of HSV replication in the nervous system. Increased intraneuronal dTdR might result in increased TK negative replication, as was the case in experimental animals.

In summary, it is clear that HSV TK expression is important for HSV latency, specifically for reactivation of HSV from latency. Second, HSV TK expression appears to be important for acute HSV replication in the nervous system possibly related to mechanisms important for HSV reactivation from latency.

Third, HSV TK mutants, which are resistant to antivirals such as Acv commonly develop. Such mutants can be frequently isolated from cutaneous sites of infection in immunosuppressed humans who have been treated with antivirals. Experimental animal results suggest that HSV TK mutants may be pathogenic, probably at sites of replicating cells. However, neurological disease caused by HSV TK mutants has not yet been demonstrated. Although not yet demonstrated, TK negative HSV is probably present in detectable amounts in sensory ganglion neurons of humans, at least in those who have been immunosuppressed and developed cutaneous infections with TK mutant HSV. It is likely, however, that mutant virus in that setting is no more pathological than is wild-type HSV. It would be predicted that TK negative HSV, although defective for reactivation, might reactivate in ganglion neurons when complemented by wild-type HSV that may also be present. Medications such as Acv, effective against replicating HSV, would not be expected to eliminate wild-type HSV, which is latent in ganglion neurons. In considering HSV pathogenesis, less is known of the role of TK negative, or for that matter wild-type HSV on central nervous system (CNS) disease latency and the possibility of CNS reactivation. In experimental animals HSV latent infection of the CNS can be readily demonstrated (65) (Fig. 5). Of interest,

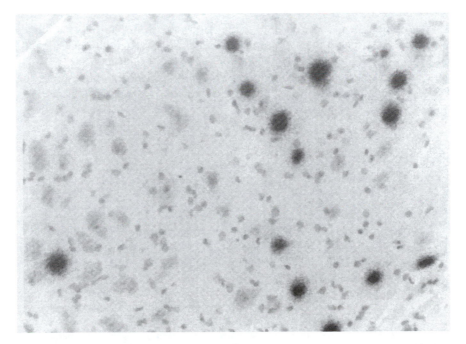

Figure 5   HSV latent infection of the CNS. HSV LAT in facial nucleus neurons 28 days after intranasal inoculation of wild-type HSV (strain KOS). Isotope grains indicate LAT in neurons. (HSV inoculation, tissue preparation and in situ hybridization was performed as in Ref. 60.)

reactivation of HSV from in vitro explants of CNS tissue occurs at much lesser rates than does reactivation from peripheral sensory ganglia (65, unpublished data).

6. HSV TK AND THE NEW BIOLOGY

Since HSV TK expression permits the phosphorylation of antivirals such as Acv with resultant inhibition of DNA synthesis, investigators have sought to use HSV TK expression in novel ways. The goal of several studies has been to incorporate the HSV TK gene into mammalian cells, which then express the viral TK enzyme. The administration of antivirals such as Acv results in drug phosphorylation by the viral TK and cell death. The HSV TK gene has generally been incorporated into mammalian cells in two ways. In some studies transgenic mice have been developed, in which the HSV TK gene is under the control of a particular cellular promotor, for example, the immunoglobulin (66) or growth hormone promotor (67). HSV TK activity was expressed in those cells, which normally express the promotor, and the administration of Acv-like medications resulted in the ablation of these cells. Immunosuppression (66) or dwarfism (67) resulted. The second approach has been to utilize a viral vector to transfer the HSV TK gene to neoplastic cells. Following treatment with Acv-like medications and drug phosphorylation by the viral TK, killing of the neoplastic cells resulted (68). In both types of studies the specificity of Acv-like medications for cells expressing the HSV TK gene is key. Development of additional methods to deliver and express the HSV TK gene in specific cell types would likely result in means to knockout those specific cell populations.

REFERENCES

1. Shin YK, Weinberg A, Spruance S, Bernard M, Bacon TH, Boon RJ, Levin MJ. Susceptibility of herpes simplex virus isolates to nucleoside analogues and the proportion of nucleoside-resistant variants after repeated topical application of penciclovir to recurrent herpes labialis. J Infect Dis 2003; 187:1241–1245.
2. Goodman AD, Mock DJ, Powers JM, Baker JV, Blumberg BM. Human herpesvirus 6 genome and antigen in acute multiple sclerosis lesions. J Infect Dis 2003; 187:1365–1376.
3. Cermelli C, Berti R, Soldan SS, Mayne M, D'ambrosia JM, Ludwin SK, Jacobson S. High frequency of human herpesvirus 6 DNA in multiple sclerosis plaques isolated by laser microdissection. J Infect Dis 2003; 187:1377–1387.
4. Benson PM, Malane SL, Banks R, Hicks CB, Hilliard JB. B virus (herpesvirus simiae) and human infection. Arch Dermatol 1989; 125:1247–1248.
5. Elion GB, Furman PA, Fyfe JA, deMiranda P, Beauchamp L, Schaeffer HJ. Proc Natl Acad Sci U S A 1977; 74:5716–5720.

6. Balzarini J, Bohman C, Walker RT, De Clerque E. Comparative cytostatic activity of different antiherpetic drugs against herpes simplex virus thymidine kinase gene-transfected tumor cells. Mol Pharmacol 1994; 45:1253–1258.
7. Saritsky RT, Quail MR, Clark PE, Nguyen TT, Halsey WS, Wittrock RJ, Bartus JD, VanHorn MM, Sathe GM, VanHorn S, Kelly MD, Bacon TH, Leary JJ. Characterization of herpes simplex viruses selected in culture for resistance to penciclovir or acyclovir. J Virol 2001; 75:1761–1769.
8. Jamieson AT, Gentry GA, Subak-Sharpe JH. Induction of both thymidine and deoxycytidine kinase activity by herpes virus. J Gen Virol 1974; 24:481–492.
9. Chen MS, Prusoff WH. Association of thymidylate kinase activity with pyrimidine deoxyribonucleoside kinase induced by herpes simplex virus. J Biochem 1979; 253:1325–1327.
10. Lowy I, Caruso M, Goff SP, Klatzmann D. Cellular thymidine kinase activity is required for the inhibition of HIV-1 replication by AZT in lymphocytes. Viriology 1994; 200:271–275.
11. Arts EJ, Wainberg MA. Mechanisms of nucleoside analog antiviral activity and resistance during human immunodeficiency virus reverse transcription. Antimicrob Agents Chemother 1996; 40:527–540.
12. Meyerhans A, Vartanian J-P, Hultgren C, Plikat U, Karlsson A, Wang L, Eriksson S, Wain-Hobson S. Restriction and enhancement of human immunodeficiency virus type 1 replication by modulation of intracellular deoxynucleoside triphosphate pools. J Virol 1994; 68:535–540.
13. Imamichi T, Murphy MA, Adelsberger JW, Yang J, Watkins CM, Berg SC, Baseler MW, Lempicki RA, Guo J, Levin JG, Lane HC. Actinomycin D induces high-level resistance to thymidine analogs in replication of human immunodeficiency virus type 1 by interfering with host cell thymidine kinase expression. J Virol 2003; 77:1011–1020.
14. Wawra E. Microinjection of deoxynuclotides into mouse cells: no evidence that precursors for DNA synthesis are channeled. J Biol Chem 1988; 263:9908–9912.
15. Plagemann PGW, Wohlhueter RM, Woffendin C. Nucleoside and nucleobase transport in animal cells. Biochim Biophys Acta 1988; 947:405–443.
16. Belt JA, Marina NM, Phelps DA, Crawford CR. Nucleoside transport in normal and neoplastic cells. Adv Enzyme Regul 1993; 33:235–252.
17. Tenser RB, Gaydos A, Hay KA. Inhibition of herpes simplex virus reactivation by dipyridamole. Antimicrob Agents Chemother 2001; 45:3657–3659.
18. Mendel DB, Barkheimer DB, Chen MS. Biochemical basis for increased susceptibility to cidofir of herpes simplex viruses with altered or deficient thymidine kinase activity. Antimicrob Agents Chemother 1995; 39:2120–2122.
19. Darby G, Field HJ, Salisbury SA. Altered substrate specificity of herpes simplex virus thymidine kinase confers acyclovir-resistance. Nature 1981; 289:81–83.
20. Ellis MN, Keller PM, Fyfe JA, Martin JL, Rooney JF, Straus SE, Lehrman SN, Barry DW. Clinical isolate of herpes simplex virus type 2 that induces a thymidine kinase with altered substrate specificity. Antimicrob Agents Chemother 1987; 31:1117–1125.
21. Coen DM, Schaffer PA. Two distinct loci confer resistance to acycloguanosine in herpes simplex virus type 1. Proc Natl Acad Sci U S A 1980; 77:2265–2269.
22. Schnipper LE, Crumpacker CS. Resistance of herpes simplex virus to acycloguanosine: role of viral thymidine kinase and DNA polymerase loci. Proc Natl Acad Sci U S A 1980; 77:2270–2273.

23. Chatis PA, Miller CH, Schrager LE, Crumpacker CS. Successful treatment with fos-carnet of an acyclovir-resistant mucocutaneous infection with herpes simplex virus in a patient with acquired immunodeficiency syndrome. N Engl J Med 1989; 320:297–300.

24. Christophers J, Clayton J, Craske J, Ward R, Collins P, Trowbridge M, Darby G. Survey of resistance of herpes simplex virus to acyclovir in northwest England. Antimicrob Agents Chemother 1998; 42:868–872.

25. Pottage JC, Kessler HA. Herpes simplex virus resistance to acyclovir: clinical relevance. Infect Agents Dis 1995; 4:115–124.

26. Parris DS, Harrington JE. Herpes simplex virus variants resistant to high concentrations of acyclovir exist in clinical isolates. Antimicrob Agents Chemother 1982; 22:71–77.

27. Sarisky RT, Nguyen TT, Duffy KE, Wittrock RJ, Leary JJ. Difference in incidence of spontaneous mutations distinct between herpes simplex virus types 1 and 2. Antimicrob Agents Chemother 2000; 44:1524–1529.

28. Erlich KS, Mills J, Chatis P, Mertz GJ, Busch DF, Follansbee SE, Grant RM, Crumpacker CS. Acyclovir-resistant herpes simplex virus infections in patients with the acquired immunodeficiency syndrome. N Engl Med 1989; 320:293–296.

29. Westheim AI, Tenser RB, Marks JG. Acyclovir resistance in a patient with chronic mucocutaneous herpes simplex virus infection. J Am Acad Dermatol 1987; 17:875–880.

30. Ellis MN, Waters R, Hill EL, Lobe DC, Sellereth DW, Barry DW. Orofacial infection of athymic mice with defined mixtures of acyclovir-susceptible and acyclovir-resistant herpes simplex virus type 1. Antimicrob Agents Chemother 1989; 33:304–310.

31. Whitley RJ, Schlitt M. Encephalitis caused by herpes viruses, including B virus. In: Scheld WM, Whitley RJ, Durack DT, eds. Infections of the Central Nervous System. New York: Raven Press, 1991:41–86.

32. Posavad CM, Koelle, Corey L. Tipping the scales of herpes simplex virus reactivation: the important responses are local. Nat Med 1998; 4:381–382.

33. Tullo AB, Shimeld C, Easty DL, Darville JM. Distribution of latent herpes simplex virus infection in human trigeminal ganglion. Lancet 1983; 1:353.

34. Baringer JR, Swoveland P. Recovery of herpes simplex virus from human trigemnial ganglions. N Engl J Med 1973; 288:648–650.

35. Warren KG, Brown SM, Wroblewska Z, Gilden D, Koprowski M, Subak-Sharpe J. Isolation of latent herpes simplex virus from the superior cervical and vagus ganglions of human beings. N Engl J Med 1978; 298:1068–1069.

36. Wagner EK, Bloom DC. Experimental investigations of herpes simplex virus latency. Clin Microbiol Rev 1997; 10:419–443.

37. Garber D, Schaffer P, Knipe D. A LAT-associated function reduces productive cycle gene expression during acute infection of murine sensory neurons with herpes simplex virus type 1. J Virol 1997; 71:5885–5893.

38. Rooney JF, Straus SE, Mannix ML, Wohlenberg CR, Banks S, Jagarrath S, Brauer JE, Notkins AL. UV light-induced reactivation of herpes simplex virus type 2 and prevention by acyclovir. J Infect Dis 1992; 166:500–506.

39. Young RF. Glycerol rhizolysis for treatment of trigeminal neuralgia. J Neurosurg 1988; 69:39–45.

40. Belber CJ, Rak RA. Balloon compression rhizolysis in the surgical management of trigeminal neuralgia. Neurosurgery 1987; 20:908–913.
41. Tenser RB. Trigeminal neuralgia-mechanisms of treatment. Neurology 1998; 51:17–19.
42. Steiner I, Spivack JG, O'Boyle DR, Lavi E, Frqser NW. Latent herpes simplex virus transcription in human trigeminal ganglia. J Virol 1988; 62:3493–3496.
43. Krause PR, Croen KD, Straus SE, Ostrove JM. Detection and preliminary characterization of herpes simplex virus type 1 transcripts in latently infected human trigeminal ganglia. J Virol 1988; 62:4819–4823.
44. Millhouse S, Wigdahl B. Molecular circuitry in regulating herpes simplex virus type 1 latency in neurons. J Neurovirol 2000; 6:6–24.
45. Batchelor AH, O'Hare P. Localization of cis-acting sequence requirements in the promotor of the latency-associated transcript of herpes simplex virus type 1 required for cell-type-specific activity. J Virol 1992; 66:3573–3582.
46. Lokensgard JR, Blom DC, Dobson AT, Feldman LT. Long-term promotor activity during herpes simplex virus latency. J Virol 1994; 68:7148–7158.
47. Ahmed M, Lock M, Miller CG, Fraser NW. Regions of the herpes simplex virus type 1 latency-associated transcript that protect cells from apoptosis in vitro and protect neuronal cells in vivo. J Virol 2002; 76:717–729.
48. Lin P, Peng W, Perng G-C, Brick DJ, Nesburn AB, Jones C, Wechsler SL. Identification of herpes simplex virus type 1 latency-associated transcript sequences that inhibit apoptosis and enhance the spontaneous reactivation phenotype. J Virol 2003; 77:6556–6561.
49. Mikloska Z, Cunningham AL. Alpha and gamma interferons inhibit herpes simplex virus type 1 infection and spread in epidermal cells after axonal transmission. J Virol 2001; 75:11,821–11,826.
50. Steiner I, Kennedy PGE. Herpes simplex virus latent infection in the nervous system. J Neurovirol 1995; 1:19–29.
51. Tenser RB, Miller RL, Rapp F. Trigeminal ganglion infection by thymidine kinase-negative mutants of herpes simplex virus. Science 1979; 205:915–917.
52. Tenser RB, Dunstan ME. Herpes simplex virus thymidine kinase expression in infection of the trigeminal ganglion. Virology 1979; 99:417–422.
53. Stevens JG, Wagner EK, Devi-Rao GB, Cook ML, Feldman L. RNA complementary to a herpesvirus alpha gene mRNA is predominant in latently infected neurons. Science 1987; 235:1056–1059.
54. Tenser RB, Hay KA, Edris WA. Latency associated transcript but not reactivatable virus is present in sensory ganglion neurons after inoculation of thymidine kinase-negative mutants of herpes simplex virus type 1. J Virol 1989; 63:2861–2865.
55. Coen DM, Kosz-Vnenchak M, Jacobson JG, Leib DA, Bogard CL, Schaffer PA, Tylker KL, Knipe DM. Thymidine kinase-negative herpes simplex virus mutants establish latency in mouse trigeminal ganglia but do not reactivate. Proc Natl Acad Sci U S A 1989; 86:4736–4740.
56. Efstathiou S, Kemp S, Darby G, Minson AC. The role of herpes simplex virus type 1 thymidine kinase in pathogenesis. J Gen Virol 1989; 70:869–879.
57. Tenser RB, Gaydos A, Hay KA. Reactivation of thymidine kinase-defective herpes simplex virus is enhanced by nucleoside. J Virol 1996; 70:1271–1276.
58. Tenser RB, Gaydos A, Hay KA. Inhibition of herpes simplex virus reactivation by dipyridamole. Antimicrob Agents Chemother 2001; 45:3657–3659.

59. Tenser RB. Intracerebral inoculation of newborn and adult mice with thymidine kinase-deficient mutants of herpes simplex virus type 1. J Infect Dis 1983; 147:956.

60. Hay KA, Gados A, Tenser RB. The role of herpes simplex thymidine kinase expression in neurovirulence and latency in newborn vs adult mice. J Neuroimmunol 1995; 61:41–52.

61. Jacobson JG, Ruffner KL, Kosz-Vnenchak K, Hwang CBC, Wobbe KK, Knipe DM, Coen DM. Herpes simplex virus thymidine kinase and specific stages of latency in murine trigeminal ganglia. J Virol 1993; 67:6903–6908.

62. Griffiths A, Coen DM. High-frequency phenotypic reversion and pathogenicity of an acyclovir-resistant herpes simplex virus mutant. J Virol 2003; 77:2282–2286.

63. Tenser RB, Edris WA. Trigeminal ganglion infection by thymidine kinase-negative mutants of herpes simplex virus after in vivo complementation. J Virol 1987; 61:2171–2174.

64. Fang Z-F, Tenser RB, Rapp F. Hepatic infection by thymidine kinase-positive and thymidine kinase-negative herpes simplex virus after partial hepatectomy. Infect Immun 1983; 42:402–408.

65. Stroop WG, Schaefer DC. Herpes simplex virus, type 1 invasion of the rabbit and mouse nervous systems reveled by in situ hybridization. Acta Neuropathol 1987; 74:124–132.

66. Heyman RA, Borrelli E, Lesley J, Anderson D, Richman DD, Baird SM, Hyman R, Evans RM. Thymidine kinase obliteration: creation of transgenic mice with controlled immune deficiency. Proc Natl Acad Sci U S A 1989; 86:2698–2702.

67. Borrelli E, Heyman RA, Arias C, Sawchenko PE, Evans RM. Transgenic mice with inducible dwarfism. Nature 1989; 339:538–541.

68. Barba D, Hardin J, Sadelin M, Gage FH. Development of anti-tumor immunity following thymidine kinase-mediated killing of experimental brain tumors. Proc Natl Acad Sci U S A 1994; 91:4348–4352.

16

Drug-Resistant Bacterial Infections: Implications for Neurosurgical and Neurological Patients

Karen L. Roos

The John and Nancy Nelson Professor of Neurology, Department of Neurology, Indiana University School of Medicine, Indianapolis, IN, U.S.A.

1. INTRODUCTION

There are three antimicrobial-resistant bacterial infections that are a threat to neurosurgical and neurological patients: penicillin and cephalosporin-resistant *Streptococcus pneumoniae*, methicillin-resistant *Staphylococcus aureus* (MRSA), and vancomycin-resistant enterococci. *Streptococcus pneumoniae* infections are typically community-acquired, whereas MRSA and vancomycin-resistant enterococci occur in patients who have undergone a neurosurgical procedure, especially those involving an intracranial device such as a ventriculostomy, have had a prolonged hospitalization, or a number of courses of antimicrobial therapy. The emergence of antimicrobial-resistant bacterial infections has changed the recommendations for the empiric therapy of community- and hospital-acquired meningitis and the management of the postoperative neurosurgical patient.

2. DEFINITIONS

The National Committee for Clinical Laboratory Standards establishes the standards for determining the susceptibility of bacteria to antibiotics based on the minimum inhibitory concentration (MIC). The MIC breakpoints are often different for central nervous system (CNS) infections compared to infections outside of the CNS. For pneumococcal meningitis, isolates with an MIC of ≤0.06 μg/mL are considered susceptible to penicillin, those with an MIC of 0.12–1 μg/mL to be intermediate and those with an MIC of ≥2 μg/mL to be resistant. A pneumococcal isolate with an MIC for cefotaxime or ceftriaxone of <0.5 μg/mL is considered susceptible, 1.0 μg/mL intermediate, and >2.0 μg/mL resistant (1). A strain of pneumococci is considered nonsusceptible to an antibiotic when the MIC is in the intermediate or resistant range (2).

The National Committee for Clinical Laboratory Standards defines staphylococci requiring concentrations of vancomycin of ≤4 μg/mL for growth inhibition as "susceptible," those requiring concentrations of 8–16 μg/mL for inhibition as "intermediate," and those requiring concentrations of ≥32 μg/mL as resistant (1,3). The term vancomycin-resistant *S. aureus* (VRSA) is reserved for isolates of *S. aureus* for which the MICs of vancomycin are ≥32 μg/mL (3).

3. EPIDEMIOLOGY

In the United States, approximately 34% of pneumococcal isolates are penicillin nonsusceptible (MICs in the intermediate and resistant ranges) and approximately 14% are resistant to ceftriaxone (2). Asymptomatic carriers play a key role in the transmission of resistant strains. Children are a reservoir for pneumococci, and after treatment for otitis media or upper respiratory tract infections may be colonized with antimicrobial-resistant pneumococci. Contact with young children is a risk factor for invasive pneumococcal disease in adults (4).

Data from the National Nosocomial Infection Surveillance System of the Centers for Disease Control and Prevention show that the rate of methicillin resistance among *S. aureus* isolates causing infection in intensive care unit (ICU) patients is a growing problem (5,6). According to recent estimates, greater than 50% of nosocomial infections in patients in the ICU are due to MRSA (5,7). This is a 37% increase in the incidence of MRSA infections from 1994 to 1998 (7). Prolonged hospitalization, care in an ICU, prolonged antimicrobial therapy, surgical procedures, and close proximity to a patient in the hospital who is infected or colonized with MRSA are the risk factors associated with nosocomial-acquired MRSA (5). The first documented case of VRSA was reported in the United States in 2002, underscoring the need to prevent the spread of antimicrobial-resistant microorganisms (8). Clinical isolates of coagulase-negative staphylococci with low-level resistance to vancomycin have been reported (3).

Even though enterococci are the second most common pathogenic causes of bloodstream infections in patients in the ICU, they are a relatively uncommon cause of CNS infections (6,9). Enterococci are part of the normal flora in the gastrointestinal tract. The most common conditions associated with enterococcal meningitis are external ventricular drains and epidural catheters, neurosurgical procedures, immunosuppressive therapy, gastrointestinal disease and *Strongyloides* species hyperinfection. Most cases of enterococcal meningitis are caused by *Enterococcus faecalis* (9). Vancomycin-resistant enterococcal infections are a major problem. Enterococci are naturally resistant to several antibiotics and have the ability to acquire resistance through the exchange of genetic material (9). Prolonged hospitalizations, prior antimicrobial therapy, severe and immunocompromising illnesses, hemodialysis, intrahospital transfer from one floor to another, and vancomycin administration for more than 7 days have all been associated with vancomycin-resistant *E. faecium* colonization or infections (10).

4. MECHANISMS OF RESISTANCE

4.1. *Streptococcus pneumoniae*

The mechanism by which *S. pneumoniae* develops resistance to beta-lactam antibiotics (penicillin and extended spectrum cephalosporins) is through alterations of one or more penicillin-binding proteins (PBPs) (11). Penicillin-binding proteins are enzymes that are important in the biosynthesis of the bacterial cell wall and are inhibited by the binding of beta-lactam antibiotics. Alterations in the PBPs lead to a decrease in their affinity for beta-lactam antibiotics and thus a decreased susceptibility to the antibiotic (2). The mechanism of resistance is acquired through a process in which a particular genome encoding the alteration is acquired from other bacteria by pneumococci and incorporated into their own DNA (11,12).

There are two major mechanisms by which *S. pneumoniae* acquires resistance to the macrolide group of antibiotics (erythromycin, clarithromycin, and azithromycin). Pneumococcal isolates with the M phenotype have developed resistance to the macrolide group of antibiotics through the acquisition of the *mefE* gene. Antimicrobial resistance is mediated through an efflux pump that removes macrolide antibiotics from the cell (2). Another form of resistance is encoded by the *ermAM* gene, and is associated with a methylase that blocks the binding of macrolides, clindamycin, and streptogramins to the bacterial 23S ribosomal RNA (2). When the antibiotic binds to the bacterial 23S ribosomal target site, it inhibits protein synthesis. When this step is blocked, the antibiotic is not able to kill the bacteria. If a pneumococcal strain is penicillin intermediate or resistant, there is a good possibility it is macrolide resistant as well.

Vancomycin-resistant strains of pneumococci have not been seen, but strains of *S. pneumoniae* tolerant to vancomycin have been reported. Tolerance is the ability of a bacteria to survive in the presence of an antibiotic, neither growing nor being eradicated by the antibiotic. Tolerance may be a precursor for the development of antimicrobial resistance because it creates survivors of antibiotic therapy (13–15). Some vancomycin-tolerant pneumococci have been reported to carry mutations in loci that normally would respond to the "death peptide" signal by secreting a protein. This protein was the effector molecule that triggered the cell death pathway (16). If this peptide is not secreted, the lysis of pneumococcal cells does not occur.

4.2. *Staphylococcus aureus*

The mechanisms of resistance of MRSA are very similar to those of *Streptococcus pneumoniae*. One particular gene, acquired from another bacteria, alters one particular PBP, resulting in absolute resistance to methicillin (17).

The enterococci are not only inherently resistant to antimicrobial agents, they are able to transfer antimicrobial resistance to other bacteria. Some isolates of VRSA contain the *vanA* vancomycin-resistant gene. This gene is acquired from vancomycin-resistant enterococci (18). Conjugative transfer of the *vanA* gene and other resistance genes from *E. faecalis* to *S. aureus* has been demonstrated in vitro, resulting in VRSA (18,19).

4.3. Vancomycin-Resistant Enterococci

Enterococci are part of the normal flora of the gastrointestinal tract. As described, they develop resistance to antibiotics through the acquisition of genes from other bacteria.

5. THERAPEUTIC IMPLICATIONS OF ANTIMICROBIAL RESISTANCE

To successfully treat an infection, an antibiotic must be selected that will provide a concentration greater than the MIC at the site of infection in the CNS for a period of time adequate to eradicate the organism (2). Central nervous system infection with an organism that is resistant to an antibiotic can often be successfully treated by either using higher doses of the antibiotic for a prolonged period of time, by using a combination of intravenous and intraventricular therapy, or by using a combination of antibiotics.

5.1. Empiric and Specific Therapy of Community-Acquired Bacterial Meningitis

Empiric therapy of community-acquired bacterial meningitis is based on the possibility that penicillin and cephalosporin-resistant pneumococci are the causative organisms of the meningitis. A combination of either ceftriaxone (pediatric dose: 100 mg/kg/day in a 12-hr dosing interval; adult dose: 2 g every 12 hr) or cefo-

Table 1 Antimicrobial Therapy of Antibiotic-Resistant CNS Bacterial Infections.

Organism	Antibiotic (adult dose)
Penicillin-resistant *Streptococcus pneumoniae*	Ceftriaxone 2 g every 12 hr (or) cefotaxime 3 g every 4 hr (or) cefepime 2 g every 12 hr
Penicillin and cephalosporin-resistant *Streptococcus pneumoniae*	Ceftriaxone (or) cefotaxime (plus) vancomycin 500 mg every 6 hr (or) 1 g every 12 hr
Methicillin-resistant *Staphylococcus aureus*	Vancomycin (or) intraventricular vancomycin 20 mg/day
Vancomycin-resistant enterococcus	Linezolid 600 mg every 12 hr

taxime (pediatric dose: 300 mg/kg/day in a 4–6-hr dosing interval; adult dose 3 g every 4 hr), or cefepime (adult dose: 2 g every 12 hr) plus vancomycin (pediatric dose: 40–60 mg/kg/day in a 6- or 12-hr dosing interval; adult dose 500 mg every 6 hr or 1 g every 12 hr) is recommended (Table 1). There are a number of clinical trials demonstrating the efficacy of the third-generation cephalosporins, ceftriaxone, and cefotaxime, in bacterial meningitis. These cephalosporins are used relatively interchangeably in the empiric therapy of bacterial meningitis for both children and adults. Cefepime is a broad spectrum fourth-generation cephalosporin with in vitro activity similar to that of cefotaxime or ceftriaxone against *Streptococcus pneumoniae* and *Neisseria meningitidis* and greater activity against *Enterobacter* species and *Pseudomonas aeruginosa* (20). Cefepime was demonstrated to be efficacious in the therapy of penicillin- and quinolone-resistant pneumococci in the rabbit meningitis model (21). Cefepime monotherapy is however not recommended. Therapy with a third- or fourth-generation cephalosporin plus vancomycin is continued until the results of antimicrobial susceptibility testing are available. Therapy can then be modified accordingly.

The results of a prospective, randomized, double-blind trial of adjunctive dexamethasone therapy for bacterial meningitis in 301 adults in five European countries over a period of 9 years demonstrated that dexamethasone improves the outcome in adults with acute bacterial meningitis. The benefits were most striking in the patients with pneumococcal meningitis (22). There has been concern that dexamethasone would decrease the penetration of vancomycin into the cerebrospinal fluid (CSF). In a prospective study of 11 adults with community-acquired pneumococcal meningitis that were treated with a combination of dexamethasone and vancomycin at a dose of 15 mg/kg every 8 hr or 7.5 mg/kg every 6 hr there were four therapeutic failures (23). The dose of vancomycin was well below the recommended dose of 60 mg/kg/day. In a prospective, randomized clinical trial of the bactericidal activity of vancomycin against cephalosporin-resistant pneumococci in CSF of children with acute bacterial meningitis, vancomycin in a dosage of 60 mg/kg/day penetrated reliably into the CSF when the children were treated concomitantly with dexamethasone (0.6 mg/kg/day, divided into four doses for 4 days) (24). The combination of dexamethasone and vancomycin is efficacious in the treatment of bacterial meningitis when the recommended dose of vancomycin is used.

Lumbar puncture should be repeated 36–38 hr after the initiation of therapy (unless contraindicated by the neurological exam) to document eradication of the pathogen. This recommendation has become increasingly important to follow with the emergence of antimicrobial-resistant organisms.

Meropenem is a carbapenem antibiotic that is structurally related to imipenem, has similar in vitro antimicrobial activity to imipenem, but reportedly less seizure proclivity (25,26). Meropenem shows good activity against penicillin-resistant pneumococci in vitro, is highly active against listeriae, and has been demonstrated to be effective in cases of meningitis caused by *Pseudomonas aeruginosa* (27). But the number of patients enrolled in clinical trials of meropenem in bacterial meningitis has not been sufficient to date to address its efficacy against penicillin-resistant pneumococci.

5.2. Empiric Therapy of Meningitis in the Postoperative Neurosurgical Patient

The majority of cases of postoperative meningitis are caused by *Staphylococcus aureus*, coagulase-negative staphylococci, aerobic gram-negative bacilli and streptococci (28). Empiric therapy for postoperative meningitis should include a combination of vancomycin, based on the possibility that MRSA is the causative organism and either cefepime, ceftazidime, or meropenum, for gram-negative coverage, including *Pseudomonas aeruginosa*. Methicillin is not recommended in empiric therapy of postoperative meningitis due to the high incidence of methicillin-resistant staphylococci in neurosurgical patients. When the results of culture and sensitivity are available, antimicrobial therapy can be modified accordingly. Staphylococci are the most common causative organisms of craniotomy bone flap infections, osteomyelitis of the skull as a complication of craniotomy wound infections, postoperative epidural abscess, and CSF shunt infections.

Either intrashunt or intraventricular vancomycin has become fairly standard therapy for the treatment of methicillin-resistant coagulase-negative staphylococci shunt infections. The toxicity of intraventricular vancomycin is fairly minimal and primarily based on anecdotal reports including rare cases of mental status changes, fever, headache, and tinnitus (29,30). Physicians who have had experience with the neurotoxicity of intrathecal penicillin or intrathecal gentamicin may be reluctant to use intraventricular vancomycin, but they should not be. This is a very effective way to deliver vancomycin to the CNS and is especially efficacious in the treatment of immunosuppressed patients with *S. aureus* meningitis due to repeated lumbar punctures for intrathecal chemotherapy. The dose is 20 mg/day in adults and 10 mg/day in children.

5.3. Vancomycin-Resistant Enterococcal Infections

Optimal therapy for vancomycin-resistant enterococcal CNS infections has not been established and recommendations are based on case reports and small series. Vancomycin-resistant *Enterococcus faecium* meningitis has been successfully treated with linezolid, a oxazolidinone antibiotic (9,31). Linezolid has good CSF penetration, and is generally well tolerated. It should not be used in patients being treated with a monoamine-oxidase inhibitor, and prolonged therapy has been associated with thrombocytopenia (31). There are unfortunately already reports of patients with linezolid-resistant *E. faecium* infections (32). Chloramphenicol may also be used to treat vancomycin-resistant enterococcal meningitis, however an increasing number of vancomycin-resistant enterococci are either intermediately susceptible or resistant to chloramphenicol in vitro (31). Quinupristin/dalfopristin are two semisynthetic streptogramin antibiotics that are combined in a 30:70 ratio, and are bacteriostatic against enterococcus (31,33). In susceptible organisms, both quinupristin and dalfopristin bind to the 50S ribosomal subunit and act synergistically to inhibit protein synthesis (33). Intravenous quinupristin/dalfopristin penetrates poorly into the subarachnoid space. The administration of quinupristin/dalfopristin by both the intravenous (7.5 mg/kg every 8 hr) and intraventricular route (2 mg daily) was successful in eradicating vancomycin-resistant *Enterococcus faecium* ventriculostomy-related meningitis (33).

6. PREVENTION

Antibiotic-resistant pneumococcal infections can be prevented by vaccinating adults at risk for community-acquired pneumonia with the 23-valent pneumococcal polysaccharide vaccine, and young children with the seven-valent protein-polysaccharide conjugate vaccine. Adults who should be vaccinated include anyone over the age of 65, those with chronic medical conditions, immunosuppressed individuals, HIV-infected individuals, and anyone who has had a splenectomy or an inherited or acquired complement deficiency. The vaccine has been demonstrated to reduce disease caused by antimicrobial-resistant pneumococci (4).

After antibiotic treatment for otitis media or respiratory tract infections, children may be colonized with antimicrobial-resistant pneumococci. A shorter course of a higher dose of an antibiotic for treatment of these infections may reduce the risk of post-treatment antibiotic-resistant pneumococcal carriage in these children and the risk of spread of these organisms to adults. This is being investigated in clinical trials (34).

To prevent the iatrogenic transmission of methicillin or VRSA, and *vancomycin-resistant enterococci*, the infected patient should be in a private room, gloves must be worn whenever there is direct contact with the patient, masks should be worn when there will be any contact with oropharyngeal secretions, gowns should be worn if any soiling of clothes is anticipated, and strict hand-washing procedures should be followed before leaving the patient's room. To examine a ventilator-dependent patient in the ICU, a mask, gloves and gown should be worn. The examiner may be splashed with respiratory secretions during the ophthalmologic exam, or while examining for brainstem reflexes.

7. KEY POINTS

- In the United States, approximately 34% of pneumococcal isolates are penicillin nonsusceptible and approximately 14% are resistant to ceftriaxone.
- Greater than 50% of nosocomial infections in patients in the ICU are due to methicillin-resistant *S. aureus*.
- The first documented case of vancomycin-resistant *S. aureus* was reported in the United States in 2002.
- Empiric therapy of community-acquired bacterial meningitis is based on the possibility that penicillin and cephalosporin-resistant pneumococci are the causative organisms of the meningitis.
- Empiric therapy of postoperative meningitis should include a combination of vancomycin and either cefepime, ceftazidime, or meropenum, based on the possibility that methicillin resistant *S. aureus* is the causative organism.
- Central nervous system infection with an organism that is resistant to an antibiotic can often be successfully treated by either using higher doses of the antibiotic for a prolonged period of time, by using a combination of intravenous and intraventricular therapy, or by using a combination of antibiotics.

8. SUMMARY

Recommendations for the empiric therapy of community- and hospital-acquired meningitis are constantly changing due to increasing antimicrobial-resistant bacterial infections. Empiric therapy of community-acquired bacterial meningitis is based on the possibility that penicillin and cephalosporin-resistant pneumococci are the causative organisms of the meningitis and includes a combination of a third- or fourth-generation cephalosporin and vancomycin. Empiric therapy of postoperative meningitis should include a combination of vancomycin, based on the possibility that MRSA is the causative organism, and either cefepime ceftazidime, or moropenum.

Inadequate empiric therapy is associated with increased mortality, but excessive antibiotic use promotes the emergence and spread of antibiotic-resistant bacterial pathogens (35). Empiric therapy should be modified when culture results are available. The need for broad-spectrum antimicrobial therapy should be re-evaluated on a daily basis. As importantly, physicians should take the necessary precautions to limit the iatrogenic spread of antimicrobial resistant organisms.

REFERENCES

1. National Committee for Clinical Laboratory Standards. Performance Standards for Antimicrobial Susceptibility Testing, Tenth Informational Supplement (Aerobic Dilution). Wayne, PA: National Committee for Clinical Laboratory Standards, 2000.
2. Kaplan SL, Mason EO. Mechanisms of pneumococcal antibiotic resistance and treatment of pneumococcal infections in 2002. Pediatr Ann 2002; 31:250–260.
3. Fridkin SK. Vancomycin-intermediate and -resistant *Staphylococcus aureus*: what the infectious disease specialist needs to know. Clin Infect Dis 2001; 32:108–115.
4. Whitney CG, Farley MM, Hadler J, Harrison LH, et al. Decline in invasive pneumococcal disease after the introduction of protein-polysaccharide conjugate vaccine. N Engl J Med 2003; 348:1737–1746.
5. Salgado CD, Farr BM, Calfee DP. Community-acquired methicillin-resistant *Staphylococcus aureus*: a meta-analysis of prevalence and risk factors. Clin Infect Dis 2003; 36:131–139.
6. National Nosocomial Infections Surveillance (NNIS). System report, data summary from January 1990–May 1999, issued June 1999. Am J Infect Control 1999; 27:520–532.
7. Cosgrove SE, Sakoulas G, Perencevich EN, Schwaber MJ, et al. Comparison of mortality associated with methicillin-resistant and methicillin-susceptible *Staphylococcus aureus* bacteremia: a meta-analysis. Clin Infect Dis 2003; 36:53–59.
8. CDC. *Staphylococcus aureus* resistant to vancomycin—United States, 2002. MMWR Morb Mortal Wkly Rep 2002; 51:565–567.
9. Zeana C, Kubin CJ, Della-Latta P, Hammer SM. Vancomycin-resistant *Enterococcus faecium* meningitis successfully managed with linezolid: case report and review of the literature. Clin Infect Dis 2001; 33:477–482.
10. Tornieporth NG, Roberts RB, John J, Hafner A, Riley LW. Risk factors associated with vancomycin-resistant *Enterococcus faecium* infection or colonization in 145 matched case patients and control patients. Clin Infect Dis 1996; 23:767–772.
11. Jacobs MR. Drug-resistant *Streptococcus pneumoniae*: rational antibiotic choices. Am J Med 1999; 106:19S–25S.
12. Bonafede M, Rice LB. Emerging antibiotic resistance. J Lab Clin Med 1997; 130:558–566.
13. McCullers JA, English BK, Novak R. Isolation and characterization of vancomycin-tolerant *Streptococcus pneumoniae* from the cerebrospinal fluid of a patient who developed recrudescent meningitis. J Infect Dis 2000; 181:369–373.

14. Novack R, Henriques B, Charpentier E, Normark S, Tuomanen E. Emergence of vancomycin tolerance in *Streptococcus pneumoniae.* Nature 1999; 399:590–593.

15. Liu HH, Tomasz A. Penicillin tolerance in multiply drug-resistant natural isolates of *Streptococcus pneumoniae.* J Infect Dis 1985; 152:365–372.

16. Robertson GT, Zhao J, Desai BV, Coleman WH, et al. Vancomycin tolerance induced by erythromycin but not by loss of vncRS, vex3, or pep27 function in *Streptococcus pneumoniae.* J Bacteriol 2002; 184(24):6987–7000.

17. Bartlett JG, Bradley SF, Herwaldt LA, Jacobs MR, Perl TM, Poole MD. A roundtable discussion of antibiotic resistance: putting the lessons to work. Am J Med 1999; 106 (5A):49S–52S.

18. Chang S, Sievert DM, Hageman JC, Boulton ML. Infection with vancomycin-resistant *Staphylococcus aureus* containing the *vanA* resistance gene. N Engl J Med 2003; 348:1342–1347.

19. Noble WC, Virani Z, Cree RG. Co-transfer of vancomycin and other resistance genes from *Enterococcus faecalis* NCTC 12201 to *Staphylococcus aureus.* FEMS Microbiol Lett 1992; 72:195–198.

20. Saez-Llorens X, Castano E, Garcia R, Baez C, et al. Prospective randomized comparison of cefepime and cefotaxime for treatment of bacterial meningitis in infants and children. Antimicrob Agents Chemother 1995; 39:937–940.

21. Cottagnoud P, Acosta F, Cottagnoud M, Tauber MG. Cefepime is efficacious against penicillin- and quinolone-resistant pneumococci in experimental meningitis. J Antimicrob Chemother 2002; 49:327–330.

22. de Gans J, van de Beek D, et al. Dexamethasone in adults with bacterial meningitis. N Engl J Med 2002; 347:1549–1556.

23. Viladrich PF, Gudiol F, Linares J, et al. Evaluation of vancomycin for therapy of pneumococcal meningitis. Antimicrob Agents Chemother 1991; 35:2467–2472.

24. Klugman KP, Friedland IR, Bradley JS. Bactericidal activity against cephalosporin-resistant *Streptococcus pneumoniae* in cerebrospinal fluid of children with acute bacterial meningitis. Antimicrob Agents Chemother 1995; 39:1988–1992.

25. Patel JB, Giles RE. Meropenem: evidence of lack of proconvulsive tendency in mice. J Antimicrob Agents Chemother 1989; 24(suppl A):307–309.

26. Fitoussi F, Doit C, Benali K, Bonacorsi S, et al. Comparative in vitro killing activities of meropenem, imipenem, ceftriaxone, and ceftriaxone plus vancomycin at clinically achievable cerebrospinal fluid concentrations against penicillin-resistant *Streptococcus pneumoniae* isolates from children with meningitis. Antimicrob Agents Chemother 1998; 42:942–944.

27. Klugman KP, Dagan R, Meropenem Meningitis Study Group. Randomized comparison of meropenem with cefotaxime for treatment of bacterial meningitis. Antimicrob Agents Chemother 1995; 39:1140–1146.

28. Neurosurgery Working Party of the British Society for Antimicrobial Chemotherapy. Antimicrobial prophylaxis in neurosurgery and after head injury. Lancet 1994; 344:1547–.

29. Wen DY, Bottini AG, Hall WA, Haines SJ. The intraventricular use of antibiotics. Neurosurg Clin North Am 1992; 3:343.

30. Golledge CL, McKenzie T. Monitoring vancomycin concentrations in CSF after intraventricular administration. J Antimicrob Chemother 1988; 21:262.

31. Steinmetz MP, Vogelbaum MA, De Georgia MA, Andrefsky JC, Isada C. Successful treatment of vancomycin-resistant enterococcus meningitis with linezoled: case report and review of the literature. Crit Care Med 2001; 29:2383–2385.

32. Zurenko GE, Todd WM, Hafkin B, et al. Development of linezolid-resistant *Enterococcus faecium* in two compassionate use program patients treated with Linezolid [abstract 848]. In: Program and Abstracts of the 38th Interscience Conference on Antimicrobial Agents and Chemotherapy (San Francisco). Washington, DC: American Society for Microbiology, 1999:117.

33. Williamson JC, Glazier SS, Peacock JE. Successful treatment of ventriculostomy-related meningitis caused by vancomycin-resistant *Enterococcus* with intravenous and intraventricular quinupristin/dalfopristin. Clin Neurol Neurolsurg 2002; 104:54–56.

34. Schrag SJ, Pena C, Fernandez J, Sanchez J, et al. Effect of short-course, high-dose amoxicillin therapy on resistant pneumococcal carriage: a randomized trial. JAMA 2001; 286(1):49–56.

35. Paterson DL, Rice LB. Empirical antibiotic choice for the seriously ill patient: are minimization of selection of resistant organisms and maximization of individual outcome mutually exclusive? CID 2003; 36:1006–1012.

17

HIV-Related Neurological Disease in the Era of HAART

C. T. Loy, S. Tomlinson, and B. J. Brew
St. Vincent's Hospital, Darlinghurst, Sydney, Australia

Highly active antiretroviral therapy (HAART) has significantly improved both the general and neurological outcome for patients with human immunodeficiency virus (HIV) infection. However, HAART has changed the nature and treatment of HIV-related neurological diseases. These complications and the HAART-induced changes will be approached by using an anatomical framework (brain, spinal cord, peripheral nerve, and muscle). Within each part of the neuraxis, the complications will be discussed according to whether they are directly related to HIV, for example, dementia, or indirectly related, for example, an opportunistic infection such as cerebral toxoplasmosis. It is essential for the reader to appreciate that this review will be highlighting the more significant complications. For a full dissertation on the neurological complications the reader is referred to the recent book by Brew (1).

There are some general principles that are important to appreciate in approaching the management of patients with neurological complications relating to HIV disease. The most important are "time locking," "parallel tracking," and "layering." Of these perhaps the most significant is that of "time locking" by which it is meant the chief factor determining the type of involvement is the degree of advancement of HIV disease as judged by the CD4 cell count. In the pre-HAART era this would be best measured by the current CD4 cell count. However, as a consequence of the immune restorative effects of HAART, the nadir count may also be important: some patients do not have full reconstitution of their immune system with HAART and remain vulnerable to certain complications that are linked to the nadir count. The second principle is that of parallel tracking: different complications affect different parts of the neuraxis within the same time frame. This may alter the manifestations of the complications. For example, a patient may have HIV spinal cord damage as well as peripheral neuropathy; each will affect the other's symptoms and signs to varying extents depending on the severity of each. The third principle is that of layering, wherein several complications are layered one upon the other within one part of the nervous system. The threshold for expression of disease may consequently be reduced: previous insults have left damage thereby reducing the amount of "reserve."

1. CONDITIONS RELATING TO THE BRAIN

As can be seen from Table 1, there is a large number of complications that may affect the brain in HIV disease. It can be clinically helpful to have a dichotomous approach and split the complications into those that have dominantly focal manifestations and those that do not. Focal manifestations usually occur in patients with CD4 cell counts below 200, while non-focal complications can occur at any stage of HIV disease.

Table 1 Complications Related to the Brain

Direct	
Early HIV (CD4 >500 cells/μL)	Seroconversion-related encephalitis and myelopathy
	Aseptic meningitis
	Mononeuropathies
Moderate HIV (CD4 200–500 cells/μL)	Aseptic meningitis
Advanced HIV (CD4 <200 cells/μL)	
	AIDS dementia complex
	Seizures
	Transient neurologic deficits
	Movement disorders
Opportunistic conditions	
	Toxoplasmosis
	Primary central nervous system lymphoma
	Progressive multifocal leukoencephalopathy
	Tuberculoma
	Cryptococcal meningitis
	VZV encephalopathy
	Tuberculous meningitis
	CMV encephalitis
	Neurosyphilis

1.1. Direct Complications

1.1.1. Early and Moderately Advanced HIV Disease [CD4 Cell Count >200 Cells/(L)]

Rarely in the context of seroconversion patients may develop a meningoencephalitis which is usually self-limiting (2). There is no specific therapy though intuitively HAART would seem to have a potential role. In early and moderately advanced disease, aseptic meningitis may also occur. Most often it is associated with only mild symptoms and again it is self-limiting in the majority (3,4). Very rarely, patients may have recurrent attacks. It is important to appreciate that some patients may have a cerebrospinal fluid (CSF) profile of aseptic meningitis but no symptoms or signs.

1.1.2. Advanced Disease [CD4 Cell Count <200 Cells/(L)]

AIDS Dementia Complex (ADC):   ADC was the first direct neurological complication that was described in the early 1980s. Initially the marked apathy that is characteristic of the disorder was mistaken for depression in patients with advanced, often pre-terminal HIV disease. It was only after careful clinical and neuropathological assessments that the true nature of the disorder was realized.

Classically, ADC is a subcortical dementing illness characterized by disorders involving cognitive, motor, and behavioral functions (5). Most commonly, patients complain of poor concentration and memory for day-to-day events, psychomotor slowing, clumsiness, and lack of interest in interpersonal relationships (6). In the pre-HAART era, it occurred at a time when HIV disease was advanced—most often when the CD4 cell count was below 200 cells/μL (5). The dominant neuropathological and neuroimaging findings were those of inflammatory mononuclear infiltrates affecting the basal ganglia and deep white matter (7). While evidence of productive HIV infection in the brain was usually found it was not always present—indeed there were some patients in whom little or no HIV was found (8). Furthermore, there was discordancy between the amount of HIV infection and the clinical deficit (8). More intensive studies revealed that the clinical deficit was best correlated with the degree of immune activation within the brain, especially in regard to microglia (9). The diagnosis was clinically based, supported by neuroimaging findings of cerebral atrophy and CSF analyses showing elevated concentrations of immune activation markers such as β_2 microglobulin and neopterin, as well as raised concentrations of HIV RNA (5). Magnetic resonance spectroscopy of the brain showed elevated peaks of choline and myoinositol indicating cell turnover and presumably inflammatory infiltrates (10). These markers correlated with the presence and severity of ADC. The disorder sometimes responded to antiviral therapy (5). However, with the advent of HAART there have been changes to ADC in its clinical manifestations as well as possibly aspects of pathogenesis and treatment.

The clinical manifestations of ADC in patients taking HAART have altered. It is no longer an illness that occurs with advanced almost pre-terminal HIV disease. The CD4 cell count at diagnosis has risen from a mean of 50–100 (5) to 160 cells/ µL (11) and, indeed, the average CD4 count of the multicenter AIDS cohort is now just over 500 (Sacktor N, personal communication). The mean survival has lengthened from 6 (6) to 44 months (12). The areas of brain involvement may also be somewhat different, with early data suggesting more "cortical" involvement neuropsychologically (13) and temporal lobe involvement on FDG PET scanning (14). These features seem to be superimposed to varying extents upon a background of the more classical basal ganglia abnormalities. However, it should be stressed that these data are preliminary and require confirmation.

Longer patient survival also allows additional factors to confound the cognitive deficit among patients with ADC. There is already some clinical evidence to implicate that co-infection with hepatitis C and testosterone deficiency may lead to more prominent cognitive deficits (15). Other interesting but more speculative confounders include accelerated amyloid beta deposition (16,17), and possible brain mitochondrial neuronal toxicity from antiretroviral drugs.

While the pathogenesis of ADC does not yet appear to be any different in HAART-treated patients it is important to discuss this possibility after a brief review of the current thinking on the topic. There are three major principles. First, HIV enters the central nervous system (CNS) early, possibly at the time of seroconversion or some time soon after. Second, as previously discussed, ADC is better correlated with the degree of microglial activation than the amount of active HIV replication in the brain. Most investigators believe that the immune activation is dependent on viral replication but that it is excessive because of lack of appropriate down-regulating signals—a pro-inflammatory environment (18). Some investigators consider, however, that such immune activation in some patients may become autonomous after it has been "kick-started" by HIV. As evidence for this, there is a TH2 shift within the brain with IL-4 and IL-10 levels being reduced (18). Additionally, there is loss of astrocytes (19). The latter is potentially important as astrocytes are necessary for maintaining microglia in a "de-activated" state. Their absence therefore may mean that the microglia in an astrocyte-deficient microenvironment become activated and autonomous. Third, most of the neuronal toxicity in the brain is mediated via activation of the N-methyl-D-aspartate (NMDA) receptor (20). The pathogenesis of the white matter changes is still unclear but most researchers consider that it is at least partly related to excess cytokine production.

How might HAART have changed these aspects of pathogenesis? In regard to the first principle of HIV brain entry, HAART paradoxically may afford HIV more opportunities to enter the brain. The long-term toxicity associated with some drugs in HAART regimens often means that patients take "drug holidays" otherwise known as treatment interruptions. These may last several weeks to months and are frequently associated with a significant rebound in plasma HIV viral load, which in some patients may facilitate entry into the CNS, if not the brain. This is predicated on the idea that "pulses" of high plasma viral load are more likely to lead to brain penetration than sustained high levels. Once in the CNS, HIV may persist because the HAART regimens have limited penetration into the brain (see below). Indeed, in the long term, subtherapeutic drug concentrations in the brain would be expected to facilitate the development of resistance. In regard to the second principle of immune activation, if it has become autonomous in some patients, further antiretroviral therapy will not alter the course of brain damage. It should be stressed, however, that at present this is only theoretical. Conversely though there appear to be some patients in whom brain damage is no longer active—there is no evidence of virological or immunological activation. Such patients appear to have a degree of irreversible damage and their disease is "inactive." This possibility was first articulated in 2001 (21) as a result of the analyses of the abacavir ADC trial. The addition of abacavir to HAART did not further improve neuropsychological function but this may in part have been related to the fact that most of the patients at entry did not have a detectable viral load or immune activation markers in the CSF raising the possibility that they had inactive ADC (22).

HAART has also altered the management of ADC. The 2002 International AIDS Society-USA Panel recommends HAART as first-line treatment for HIV infection (23). Though definitive data are still lacking, preliminary results support the effectiveness of HAART in ADC. These include substantially greater reduction in CSF viral load (24), delayed onset of AIDS-related cognitive impairment (25), improved neuropsychological measures (22,26), and partial reversal of AIDS-related cognitive impairment and its associated changes on magnetic resonance spectroscopy (27).

Despite the evidence for HAART's efficacy in ADC there are some caveats. In practice, only about 50% of patients improve (28). This may be related to some or all of the deficits being fixed or inactive as previously mentioned. Alternately, it may be a consequence of resistance to antiretroviral drugs. It is now well known that the CNS and blood compartments may have HIV quasispecies that have different patterns of resistance. Additionally, not all the currently available drugs can penetrate into the brain as discussed below. Finally, only some of the drugs used in HAART regimens are effective in non-dividing/minimally dividing cells such as microglia. The latter is critical as microglia are the only intrinsic brain cell that can support productive brain infection.

Each of the latter possibilities will now be discussed in more depth. Indeed, it is suggested that each be carefully considered in the clinical context of deciding upon an antiretroviral regimen in individual patients with ADC. Before starting treatment for ADC in a patient on HAART, the possibility that it may be inactive should be considered. The means by which this can be definitively determined in "real time" rather than retrospectively are under investigation. Nonetheless, clinical assessment by history that reveals stability over months would argue in favor of inactive disease. Other tools that would seem to be intuitively correct, such as a CSF HIV viral load below 50 cpml and a normal concentration of β_2 microglobulin, need to be rigorously evaluated. Similarly, magnetic resonance spectroscopy of the brain showing no elevation of choline or myoinositol peaks intuitively would seem to indicate inactive disease but this too remains speculative.

The next issue that should be considered before undertaking treatment for ADC is to determine whether resistance to one or more antiretroviral drugs of a proposed HAART regimen may be present. Indeed, on the basis of randomized controlled trial data, the 2002 International AIDS Society-USA Panel considers serum genotypic drug resistance testing in HIV treatment failure as standard-of-care (23). We suggest that this should be extended to include the CSF in ADC patients as resistance tends to be specific for each antiviral drug class (29), and resistance can be discordant between blood and CSF in as many as one-third of patients (30–32). This is especially true when ADC is present (33). This compartmentalization of viral behavior is accentuated by examples where CSF nucleoside reverse transcriptase inhibitor and protease inhibitor resistance mutations could not be detected in paired serum, and vice versa (31,32). Virologically, this may be explained by different selection pressures in the two compartments. In addition, it should be remembered that the resistance patterns found in the CSF may not reflect those in the brain for some patients—as shown by data suggesting the further compartmentalization of viral evolution (34), and antiretroviral resistance (35) among different regions of the brain. Nonetheless, there is no in-vivo method of assessing brain resistance patterns, and the clinical significance of regional brain variation in resistance is unknown. In this regard, early data suggest the novel approach of using peripheral blood monocyte count as a screen for CSF antiretroviral resistance (36). This is based on the rationale that low-brain monocyte/microglia turnover from the blood may encourage development of CSF antiretroviral resistance. These data still require further confirmation.

The last issue for consideration prior to ADC treatment is whether the individual drugs in the proposed HAART regimen are able to effectively penetrate and "work" in the brain. Failure of ADC to respond to HAART may be related to poor penetration of some antiretroviral drugs into the brain. However, this does remain a controversial issue as investigators have conflicting results. On the one hand, multiple CSF-penetrating antiretrovirals have been found to be more effective in lowering CSF viral load than single CSF-penetrating antiretroviral regimes (37). On the other hand, HAART with multiple CSF-penetrating antiretrovirals was not found to be more effective in improving psychomotor speed when compared to single CSF-penetrating antiretroviral regimens (38). It should be kept in mind that neither of these studies was based on randomized data, drug interactions were not assessed, and patients with ADC were not analyzed as a separate group. The last factor is potentially an important one because patients with ADC are more likely to have brain infection which is autonomous from systemic infection, thus making drug entry into the brain more crucial. Accordingly, it is recommended that "brain penetrating" drugs be used whenever possible in a HAART regimen. Antiretrovirals that penetrate the CSF, in concentrations that are efficacious as assessed by the median inhibitory concentration (IC_{50}), include zidovudine, stavudine, abacavir, lamivudine, nevirapine, efavirenz, indinavir (39) and possibly atazanavir. Ritonavir may also have a special role, as it improves indinavir CSF penetration beyond that expected from its cytochrome p450 effect (40). This phenomenon may possibly be generalizable to other antiretrovirals. This is suggested by in vitro data in which ritonivir inhibits drug efflux transporter systems, including the multidrug resistance-associated protein (MRP1) (41) and the P-glycoprotein (42). An additional aspect of the brain activity of antiretroviral drugs is their ability to inhibit replication in non-dividing cells such as microglia, where the infection is chronic and persistent. The comparative efficacy of antiretroviral drugs in such cells has not been studied. Indeed, such data in their entirety are not available even for monocytes or macrophages. Nonetheless, data derived from monocyte studies with several of the antiretroviral drugs can be used as a guide. As a general rule, nucleoside/nucleotide reverse transcriptase inhibitors do not perform well: they are effective for acute infection but are ineffective once there has been integration into the host genome. The "pecking order" for most effective to least is zidovudine, lamivudine, abacavir, stavudine, didanosine, and tenofovir (43). Efavirenz is even more potent than zidovudine but data on nevirapine are few. The protease inhibitors in general are effective in chronic persistent infection because of their post-integration mechanism of action, but comparative efficacy data are also lacking. Importantly however, the concentrations required often significantly exceed those needed for efficacy in lymphocytes (44). Thus for ADC therapy an argument can certainly be made for using maximal doses of indinavir or perhaps atazanavir boosted with ritonavir to improve penetration. At present there is a disturbing irony in ADC therapy: the very drugs that penetrate well into the brain, namely the nucleoside reverse transcriptase inhibitors, are poor at inhibiting chronic persistent infection in monocyte lineage cells, while the drugs that are effective in such cells do not penetrate into the brain very well.

HAART has also changed aspects of monitoring ADC treatment. Previously, efficacy would be able to be assessed after approximately 8 weeks and improvement beyond this time point would be very unlikely. Now, HAART efficacy in ADC may be expected by 6 weeks (22) with further improvement over the next 6 months and possibly longer (22,45). Therapeutic drug monitoring should also be considered, particularly as levels of serum protease inhibitors, and intuitively other antiretroviral medications, have been correlated with virological response (46). However, there are few data regarding the clinical value of monitoring CSF drug levels to date. While such levels probably only partly reflect brain parenchymal concentrations (47), again intuitively, they would seem to be helpful. Nonetheless, there are practical issues regarding the optimum time of sampling, not to mention the lack of properly conducted studies.

1.2.   Other Direct HIV Complications Affecting the Brain

Rarely, HIV may lead to a number of other complications: transient ischemic-like attacks (48), epilepsy (49) and movement disorders, especially chorea (5). These are often related to the presence of ADC or seem associated with an increased risk of developing ADC. Each may be caused by opportunistic conditions and so formal investigation should be performed before HIV can be determined as the cause.

1.3.   Indirect Complications Affecting the Brain:
Opportunistic Conditions

Most opportunistic CNS infections in patients with HIV occur in the context of advanced disease with low CD4 T-cell counts. Rarely, such complications occur in the context of "normal" or only mildly lowered counts. This is thought to be related to the lack of reconstitution of certain pathogen-specific clones by HAART (50). The principles of treatment for these conditions are essentially the same:

- in the short term, treat the opportunistic infection with specific therapy at induction doses followed by lower maintenance doses;
- once the condition has stabilized on specific therapy, optimize the patient's immune function by appropriate use of HAART;
- once there has been sustained (usually >3 months) improvement in CD4 cell count above the cut-off related to the risk associated with the particular opportunistic infection, maintenance therapy can be ceased (51–56).

There are some important considerations in treating such infections including:

- potential interactions between antiretroviral and antimicrobial agents which can alter the efficacy or toxicity of either, for example, rifampicin and protease inhibitors;
- emerging resistance of organisms (e.g., tuberculosis) which can be potentiated by non-adherence to treatment regimens;
- need for maintenance therapy in patients with persistently low CD4 cell counts to prevent relapse;
- potential for an immune reconstitution reaction after implementation of HAART leading to an exacerbation of the clinical features of the underlying opportunistic condition. Indeed, immune reconstitution may drive a previously subclinical opportunistic condition to clinical expression.

1.4. Cerebral Toxoplasmosis

Toxoplasmosis in the era of HAART is still probably the most common cause of a cerebral space occupying lesion in patients with advanced HIV despite the fact that HAART has led to a dramatic fall in the incidence (51). It is usually seen in patients with a CD4 count below 100 cells/µL. It is almost always a reactivation of toxoplasmosis rather than primary infection. Presentation is with headache, fever, focal deficits, and often seizures (57). Positive serum antibody and brain imaging showing ring-enhancing lesions are almost always present. Given the prevalence of cerebral toxoplasmosis, if the diagnosis is suspected on clinical grounds then a trial of therapy with monitoring for clinical response is reasonable without the need for biopsy. Improvement is most often seen within 1–2 weeks. Treatment is with sulfadiazine plus pyrimethamine for 3–6 weeks (58). Clindamycin can be used in the event of sulfur intolerance (58). Failure of therapy may indicate an alternate etiology such as lymphoma (see below) and biopsy may therefore be indicated. Prophylactic treatment with cotrimoxazole is effective in preventing toxoplasmosis in advanced HIV disease (59).

1.5. Primary Central Nervous System Lymphoma

Primary central nervous system lymphoma (PCNSL) is an intermediate or high-grade non-Hodgkin's B-cell lymphoma arising in the CNS with an incidence in the HIV population that was up to 3600 times greater than in the non-HIV population in the pre-HAART era (60). However, the incidence of PCNSL has significantly decreased with the advent of HAART regimens (61). Previously, it was the second most common cause of a cerebral space occupying lesion after toxoplasmosis and postmortem studies showed a prevalence of 9–14% (62–64). It usually occurred in patients with a low CD4 count (<50 cells/µL). Epstein–Barr virus (EBV) is strongly implicated in the pathogenesis of PCNSL. Presentation is with confusion, headache, focal deficit, and seizures. CSF PCR for EBV is positive in the majority of cases and is contributory to the diagnosis (60). Imaging shows enhancing lesions with a predilection for the deep gray matter and periventricular regions. The tumor is often multicentric. Thallium-201 SPECT scans show increased uptake and PET scans reveal increased metabolic activity; as such both can help differentiate PCNSL from cerebral toxoplasmosis. In the pre-HAART era, a diagnosis of PCNSL was associated with very poor survival. HAART leading to improvement in immune function and CD4 count can prolong survival in patients with PCNSL more than any other treatment modality (65,66). Radiotherapy can also prolong survival, but usually only in the order of months (66). Chemotherapy can also be used, but results to date have been disappointing. Steroids can help with symptom control, but their use should be minimized prior to brain biopsy because they can lead to partial tumor lysis and a false-negative biopsy result. Multicentricity and anatomic predilection render PCNSL a poor candidate for surgical resection. Despite improvement in survival with HAART, and occasional remission (67) long-term prognosis in patients with PCNSL is still poor.

1.6. Progressive Multifocal Leukoencephalopathy

Progressive multifocal leukoencephalopathy (PML) is another common cause of a focal cerebral lesion. It is caused by reactivation of latent JC virus infection. In the pre-HAART era it was the third most common cause behind toxoplasmosis and PCNSL. With the introduction of HAART, the latter conditions have become very uncommon making PML probably one of the most frequent causes. Presentation is with a focal deficit or deficits in the absence of fever or headache. Cerebral imaging shows multifocal non-enhancing lesions without mass effect often approaching but not involving the cortex (68). This appearance is virtually diagnostic but CSF PCR for JC virus DNA can be helpful; occasionally brain biopsy is necessary for definitive diagnosis. HAART has had a dramatic effect on HIV-related PML by reducing the risk of death as much as 63% (69). Unfortunately, there has been a variable effect on the degree of neurological improvement. There may be transient worsening of the clinical deficits in the first few weeks of HAART, probably as a consequence of immune reconstitution (68). However as HAART is the only effective treatment for PML, it should not be delayed. Adjunct short-term treatment with corticosteroids, though unproven, seems reasonable.

1.7. Cerebral Tuberculoma

While this is not common in the developed world, it is one of the most common causes of a cerebral mass lesion in resource poor settings. Indeed, in some areas, anecdotally at least, it appears to be more common than cerebral toxoplasmosis. HIV infection does not seem to significantly alter the natural history of the disorder but it may take longer to respond to antituberculous therapy and there is the potential for interaction between some of the medications and HAART-related drugs, especially the protease inhibitors (70).

1.8. Cryptococcal Meningitis

Cryptococcal meningitis has geographic variability in incidence but overall it occurs in approximately 7% of patients with advanced HIV disease. Presentation is with non-specific headache, and fever. Nausea, photophobia, and drowsiness are also seen. There are often few signs to elicit and only 30% or less will have neck stiffness. Features of elevated intracranial pressure correlate with poor outcome. One-third of patients will have concurrent cryptococcal infection at a distant site, for example, pulmonary or cutaneous. Serum cryptococcal antigen is almost always positive in patients with cryptococcal meningitis. CT brain scan usually does not reveal specific changes with the infrequent exception of meningeal enhancement or discrete cryptococcomas. CSF is abnormal in 75% with a mild to moderate mononuclear pleocytosis and elevated protein, sometimes with decreased CSF glucose. Occasionally, CSF can be acellular or have normal glucose. CSF cryptococcal antigen is almost always positive. India ink staining will detect the fungal infection in 70%. Ideally fungal culture for sensitivity and specificity should be performed.

Treatment with fluconazole or amphotericin B is effective against cryptococcal meningitis. A 10–12-week course is usually necessary. If repeat lumbar puncture at this stage still grows cryptococcus, treatment should be continued. Amphotericin B may lead to sterilization of CSF more quickly than fluconazole, however trials show that the 8-week outcome is similar with both treatments. The incidence of fluconazole resistance is much more common than resistance to amphotericin B, however the advantage of fluconazole is that after an i.v. induction dose, it can be given orally. Relapse after cessation of therapy is common, therefore ongoing maintenance therapy is recommended. Relapse does not necessarily indicate development of resistance. Primary prophylaxis with fluconazole is recommended in patients with CD4 counts below 100/μL (71).

1.9. Other Less Common CNS Infections in HIV-Positive Patients

Varicella zoster virus (VZV) can lead to a vasculopathy affecting large and small vessels, though in HIV disease the latter occurs more often. Clinically, patients present with focal deficits. MRI of the brain and CSF analysis for VZV DNA as well as intrathecal antibody synthesis are helpful in making the diagnosis though their sensitivity in HIV-infected patients is unknown. Treatment is with intravenous aciclovir. Poor CNS availability usually limits the use of oral agents such as famciclovir or valaciclovir (72).

Tuberculous meningitis is seen in patients with CD4 counts less than 400/μL and is more common in populations where TB is endemic, for example, developing countries, and intravenous drug users. The course of tuberculous meningitis in patients with HIV does not seem very different from the non-HIV population. It is fatal in one-third of cases. The complications seen most commonly are hydrocephalus and symptoms from focal lesions (73). Treatment for tuberculous meningitis can be problematic as the interactions with antiretroviral medications are complex, and the emergence of multidrug-resistant TB has made therapy complicated. Combination therapy with isoniazid with pyridoxine, and pyrazinamide with either rifampacin or ethambutol is often used. Adverse drug reactions appear to be more common in the HIV population, and rifampicin interacts with protease inhibitors (70,73).

CMV encephalitis occurs in patients with very advanced HIV disease (CD4 <50/μL) and high viral load (74). Patients present with fever, confusion, cognitive dysfunction, headache, brainstem features and cranial neuropathies, sometimes ataxia and rarely focal neurologic deficits. The differential diagnosis includes PML. PCR for CSF CMV DNA assists in diagnosis. Concurrent CMV retinitis or CMV at other sites is often found. Treatment usually consists of combined therapy: ganciclovir and focscarnet but response to therapy is variable.

Neurosyphilis has a broad spectrum of clinical presentations in HIV disease, including mass lesions from gummas, and focal lesions from meningovascular syphilitis. Concurrent HIV infection may predispose to earlier onset or more severe neurosyphilis (75). Serum FTA antibody and serum and CSF VDRL can aid diagnosis. Neurosyphilis requires 14 days of treatment with high-dose intravenous penicillin.

West Nile virus encephalitis is of particularly current importance. Thus far though it has only been reported in one patient with HIV (76) and it is not apparent how each disease affects the other.

2. CONDITIONS AFFECTING THE SPINAL CORD

2.1. Direct Complications

2.1.1. Early and Moderately Advanced Disease [CD4 Cell Count >200 Cells/(L)]

Rarely a myelopathy may develop in the context of seroconversion (77). Again the role of HAART for this condition has not been proved but intuitively it would seem to have a place.

2.1.2. Advanced HIV Disease (CD4 Cell Count<200 Cells/(L)

HIV Myelopathy and Myelitis: Direct involvement of the spinal cord with HIV can result in a vacuolar myelopathy or a myelitis (78,79). Vacuolar myelopathy is clinically similar to subacute combined degeneration of the cord in B12 deficiency with a spastic paraparesis, no definite sensory level, and prominent loss of vibration and proprioception. It is clinically apparent in up to 10% of patients with advanced HIV disease. Generally the condition stablilizes and although impairment in mobility may result, death does not usually ensue. The cause of the condition is unknown as HIV itself does not seem to cause the condition (79) but there is some evidence that it may be related to nef, a component of HIV (80). There is no proven therapy.

Myelitis can occur in conjunction with vacuolar myelopathy or independently. Inflammatory change in the cord, sometimes with multinucleated cells, is seen, and clinically a sensory level is more common (81). HAART may lead to very significant clinical improvement (82).

2.2. Indirect Complications Affecting the Spinal Cord

These more often occur in advanced disease and include herpes simplex, varicella zoster, and CMV. Human T-lymphotropic virus type I (HTLV-I), tuberculosis and syphilis may occur at the moderately advanced stage of HIV disease (81).

2.3. Amyotrophic Lateral Sclerosis-Like Disorder

An illness resembling amyotrophic lateral sclerosis has been described in a small number of patients with HIV. Preliminary data suggests an incidence of the disorder higher than for ALS in the general population (83–85). It appears to have a rapid course and affects both upper and lower motor neurons. The illness is associated with a high CNS viral load. Treatment with HAART has been reported to result in stabilization or remission of the condition. At present it is not apparent whether the association implies a direct causal role for HIV or other like viruses in the pathogenesis of amyotrophic lateral sclerosis or whether it is simply the co-occurrence of the two diseases with HIV simply unmasking patients who were in the pre-clinical stage of amyotrophic lateral sclerosis.

3. PERIPHERAL NERVE MANIFESTATIONS OF HIV

Peripheral neuropathies are commonly seen in patients with HIV. Indeed, with the advent of HAART, HIV-associated neuropathies have become the most common neurologic sequelae of HIV (86). The spectrum of involvement is broad. The chief factor that determines the type of peripheral nerve disorder to which a patient will be susceptible is the degree of advancement of HIV disease as judged by the CD4 cell count—probably both the nadir and the current count. Medication-related neuropathies and neuropathy secondary to concurrent infections are also seen. It is important to understand that a patient may display features of more than one peripheral nerve pathological process simultaneously, a concept known as "layering," and that a process affecting the peripheral nerves may also involve the CNS, a concept known as "parallel tracking." While these concepts are certainly applicable to all aspects of involvement of the nervous system by HIV they are particularly relevant to the peripheral nervous system. Additionally, certain non-HIV-related causes of peripheral neuropathy seem to occur more often in HIV-infected patients, for example, alcohol and diabetes-related neuropathy. This is probably a consequence of decreased "nerve reserve" as a result of peripheral nerve damage from HIV. The era of HAART has changed the face of peripheral neuropathy in patients with HIV, principally through drug side effects being seen more often as patients live longer.

Table 2 outlines the categories of neuropathy to be explored in this chapter.

3.1. Direct Complications

3.1.1. Early HIV [CD4 >500 Cells/(L)]

Peripheral nerve lesions are occasionally seen in patients with early HIV disease or as part of the seroconversion illness. Facial nerve palsy is the most common peripheral nerve manifestation of seroconversion, followed by a Guillain–Barre syndrome (GBS)-type illness (87). The key feature in HIV-related GBS is that the CSF shows a mild to moderate mononuclear pleocytosis (88) in contradistinction to its non-HIV counterpart. Other neuropathies including cranial neuropathies, brachial neuritis, and vasculitic neuropathy at seroconversion have also been described (89,90). Treatment of all of the above

Table 2   Peripheral Neuropathies Seen in Patients with HIV

Neuropathies related to HIV infection	
Early HIV (CD4 >500 cells/μL)	Seroconversion
	Guillain–Barre syndrome
	Mononeuropathies
Moderate HIV (CD4 200–500 cells/μL)	Chronic inflammatory demyelinating polyneuropathy
	Vasculitic neuropathies
	Mononeuritis multiplex
	Diffuse infiltrative lymphocytosis syndrome
Advanced HIV (CD4 <200 cells/μL)	Distal sensory polyneuropathy
	Autonomic neuropathy
Neuropathy related to concurrent infection	
	Syphilitic neuropathy
	Hepatitis C neuropathy
	CMV neuropathies
	HTLV-I neuropathy
Medication-related neuropathy in HIV patients	
	Antiretroviral agents
	Antimicrobial agents
	Chemotherapeutic agents
	Other

in general is the same as for non-HIV patients. Implementation of HAART may help but as yet is unproved.

3.1.2. Moderately Advanced HIV [CD4 200–500 Cells/(L)]

Chronic Inflammatory Demyelinating Polyneuropathy: Chronic inflammatory demyelinating polyneuropathy (CIDP) in HIV is essentially clinically identical to its non-HIV counterpart. As with HIV-related GBS, the CSF shows a mild mononuclear pleocytosis. Segmental demyelination and myelination are seen on biopsy, as well as infiltrates of macrophages and lymphocytes. The latter is probably more prominent than in non-HIV CIDP, just as there is more axonal loss (91). Patients with mild disease should not be aggressively treated, as the effects of immune suppression may outweigh the benefits. In those patients requiring treatment, intravenous gamma globulin is probably preferable to plasma exchange or steroids, to minimize immune compromise (90). The role of HAART in CIDP is not known.

Mononeuritis Multiplex and Vasculitic Neuropathies: The underlying pathogenesis of mononeuritis multiplex in HIV patients is thought to be due to a vasculitis, either as part of a systemic process or confined to the peripheral nerve. While HIV per se appears capable of leading to a vasculitis, other causes such as hepatitis B and C must be considered. When the condition is significant, treatment may consist of intravenous immunoglobulin, corticosteroids, and possibly cytotoxic agents. There is limited evidence for the role of HAART (92). In those cases where hepatitis B or C is present, specific therapy may be appropriate. For hepatitis B this would include tenofovir and lamivudine both of which are active against HIV and so could be included in a HAART regimen. Hepatitis C-related neuropathy may respond to interferon alpha and ribavirin but it should be remembered that interferon alpha may rarely cause neuropathy and complicate clinical management (93). Cytotoxic therapy is sometime required. The role for HAART is speculative but theoretically sound, given the inverse relationship between hepatitis C viral load and immunodeficiency related to HIV.

Diffuse Infiltrative Lymphocytosis Syndrome: Diffuse infiltrative lymphocytosis syndrome (DILS) results from a multivisceral infiltration of CD8 lymphocytes in association with an exaggerated peripheral CD8 hyperlymphocytosis (>1000 cells/mm^3) in HIV patients (94). The syndrome resembles Sjogren's disease by way of sicca symptoms and parotidomegaly. Lymphadenopathy and splenomegaly due to lymphocyte infiltration are sometimes seen. The neuropathy develops over days to weeks and is characterized as a painful symmetric distal sensory disturbance. Biopsy reveals CD8 infiltrates which strongly express HIV antigens (95). The lymphocytic infiltrates are angiocentric without vessel wall disruption. In contrast to angiocentric lymphoma, the infiltrates do not appear to be monoclonal (94). Response to HAART appears promising with two-thirds of patients making a full recovery.

3.2.   Advanced HIV

3.2.1.   Distal Sensory Polyneuropathy

Distal sensory polyneuropathy (DSP) is the most common disorder of peripheral nerves in patients with HIV. It occurs in approximately one-third of patients with moderate to advanced HIV disease, with still more having asymptomatic involvement (87,90). Previously DSP was seen most commonly in patients with CD4 counts below 200 cells/µL, however with the advent of HAART, DSP is now also recognized in patients with higher range CD4 counts. Risk factors for developing DSP include older age, high viral loads, and low CD4 counts (90). The incidence of DSP increases as HIV progresses, with the annual incidence in patients with advanced HIV being in the order of 7 % (87,91).

Patients describe progressive paresthesiae in the lower limbs over weeks to months beginning in the toes and moving proximally. Upper limb involvement is much less common. In at least 10% there is significant burning pain making walking difficult. Approximately two-thirds of patients have hyporeflexia or areflexia of the ankle jerks (90). However, all patients have diminished pain, temperature, and vibration sense.

It is important to exclude other causes of neuropathy especially those potentially treatable or reversible including nutritional deficiency, drug toxicity, paraproteins, thyroid dysfunction, hepatitis B and C. Nerve conduction studies show changes of an axonal sensory neuropathy but up to 20% of patients will have normal studies, because of predominant small fiber involvement. Sural nerve biopsy shows predominantly axonal degeneration of small myelinated and unmyelinated fibers, sometimes with secondary demyelination. Inflammatory infiltrates are relatively sparse, but the extent of mononuclear and macrophage infiltration appears to correlate with severity (96). Intraepidermal punch biopsy shows reduced numbers of nerve fiber density in the distal leg (97). In clinical practice, however, neither procedure is usually necessary for diagnosis.

The pathogenesis is poorly understood but there are two fundamental aspects which parallel the pathogenesis of ADC: 1) there is no HIV infection of the nerve per se (95), and 2) the best correlate of the presence and severity of DSP is the presence and degree of immune activation of the neighboring macrophages and satellite cells. The latter may be as a direct consequence of HIV infection or as a result of neurotoxic components of HIV, for example, gp120 (94).

There is no proven therapy that is significantly effective. Treatment with nerve growth factor in one trial did lead to significant improvement in the pain but not in other indices of the neuropathy (98). There is some evidence that HAART may be effective (92,99) but further studies are needed. Clearly, antiretroviral drugs that are associated with neuropathy should be avoided (see below). Consequently, treatment primarily focuses upon the identification of any other causes of neuropathy that may exacerbate DSP, such as nutritional deficiency. In addition, treatment can include measures to alleviate pain in those patients where it complicates DSP. Drugs that have been proved to be effective include lamotrigine and gabapentin. Other agents are also useful: valproic acid, tricyclic antidepressants.

3.2.2. Autonomic Neuropathy

Approximately12% of patients with advanced HIV develop autonomic neuropathy (100). Usually this is not clinically significant but on occasion postural hypotension and gastroparesis can be problematic.

3.3. Indirect Complications

3.3.1. Neuropathies Related to Intercurrent Infections

Syphilitic Polyradiculopathy: There is one case report in the literature (101) that describes lower limb polyradiculopathy in a patient with secondary syphilis. Treatment is along standard lines for meningovascular syphilis.

Hepatitis C-Related Neuropathy: Patients with hepatitis C can develop peripheral neuropathy manifesting as a mononeuritis multiplex, a distal symmetric polyneuropathy or a mononeuropathy. These almost always occur in the presence of cryoglobulins (102). Therapeutic options have been discussed in the previous section.

Cytomegalovirus-Related Neuropathies: Cytomegalovirus infection in advanced HIV disease can manifest in two different ways—via a direct insult to nerves resulting in an inflammatory polyradiculopathy or by way of a mononeuritis multiplex (95). CMV polyradiculopathy occurs in 2% of patients with a CD4 count of 50 cells/μL or below (103). It is characterized by the gradual onset of lumbosacral back pain radiating in a sciatic distribution over days followed by progression of weakness and sensory disturbance to an areflexic paraparesis, often with urinary symptoms. The presence of Babinski's sign and a thoracic sensory level are unusual and indicate spinal cord involvement. Concomitant CMV in other organs (especially CMV retinitis) is seen in one-third of patients. MRI of the cauda equina shows thickened or enhancing nerve roots in one-third of patients (104). CSF in 90% shows a significant predominantly polymorphonuclear pleocytosis with low glucose, elevated protein, and positive PCR for CMV DNA (105). Pathologically there is a lymphocytic infiltrate in the nerve roots and occasionally a mild myelitis (106). Untreated CMV polyradiculopathy can lead to death in days to weeks. Treatment options include ganciclovir or foscarnet or both (103). Ongoing maintenance therapy should be continued after induction therapy, at least for several months after CD4 count is maintained over 200 cells/μL (107). Alteration or implementation of HAART during the early stages of CMV treatment can result in an immune reconstitution reaction with worsening of symptoms. Therefore, such therapy should be delayed until several weeks after implementation of CMV treatment.

CMV mononeuritis multiplex usually occurs in patients with very low CD4 counts (108). CMV involvement in other organs is seen in one-third, and one quarter of patients will display more widespread involvement of the neuraxis such as mental slowing (108,109). CSF infrequently shows a polymorphonuclear pleocytosis but PCR for CMV DNA is positive in 90%. Most patients will improve with treatment with foscarnet or ganciclovir (108,109).

HTLV-1 Neuropathy: HIV patients with HTLV-1 co-infection have a higher incidence of peripheral neuropathy. It manifests as a distal symmetric sensory peripheral neuropathy (110).

3.3.2. Medications in HIV Patients That May Cause Neuropathy

Neurotoxic antiretroviral drugs [zalcitabine (ddC), didanosine (ddI), stavudine (d4T)]—the "d" drugs—can cause an axonal neuropathy at any stage of HIV infection though it appears to be more common as HIV disease advances (86). The incidence lies between 15% and 40% (111,112). The risk factors include dose, duration and exposure to multiple "d" drugs as well as hydroxyurea (112,113). The clinical picture is one of a DSP, often with pain, that usually develops after 4–6 months of treatment. Apart from the temporal relationship to the nucleoside analog, the clinical picture is identical to HIV-related DSP. It is important to differentiate between the two entities to avoid needless cessation of dideoxynucleosides drugs, with consequent compromise of the patient's optimal HAART regimen, when the neuropathy is in fact HIV-related DSP. At present there is no definitive laboratory test to distinguish between the two entities. However, an elevated plasma lactate is frequently seen in patients with painful nucleoside neuropathy (114). This is thought to reflect the likely pathogenesis of nucleoside neuropathy namely mitochondrial dysfunction (112–114). Pathologically, there is axonal degeneration and skin biopsy shows reduced epidermal nerve fiber density correlating with pain severity (86). The condition is reversible in most patients provided early diagnosis is made. Clinicians should be aware that some patients may continue to progress for some time after discontinuing the drug before improvement is seen (a phenomenon known as "coasting") (114). Treatment centers around removal of the drug and use of appropriate medication to control the pain as discussed in the DSP section.

Other medications are used frequently in HIV disease and may also cause a neuropathy. These include ethambutol, isoniazid, vincristine, vinblastine, paclitaxel, thalidomide, dapsone, and the statin class of lipid lowering drugs.

4. CONCLUSION

In conclusion, HAART has led to substantial changes in the clinical manifestations and treatment options for HIV involvement of the neuraxis. In the future, HIV-related neurological complications may change as patients live longer and become older. Age-related complications may "fuse" with HIV complications in novel ways further making this area of neurology challenging both clinically and scientifically. Moreover, long-term treatment-related toxicities may impact on the nervous system especially in the area of cerebrovascular diseases.

REFERENCES

1. Brew BJ. HIV Neurology. New York: Oxford University Press 2001.
2. Brew BJ, Perdices M, Cooper DA, et al. Neurological complications of HIV infection in the absence of immunodeficiency. Aust N Z J Med 1989; 19(6):700–705.
3. Hollander H, Stringari S. Human immunodeficiency virus associated meningitis: clinical course and correlations. Am J Med 1987; 83:813–816.
4. Brew BJ, Miller J. Human immunodeficiency related headache. Neurology 1993; 43:1098–1100.
5. Brew BJ (ed.). AIDS dementia complex. In: HIV Neurology. New York: Oxford University Press, 2001:53–90.
6. Navia BA, Jordan BD, Price RW. The AIDS dementia complex: I. Clinical features. Ann Neurol 1986; 19(6):517–524.
7. Navia B, Cho ES, Petito CK, et al. The AIDS dementia complex II: Neuropathology. Ann Neurol 1986; 19:525–535.
8. Brew BJ, Rosenblum M, Cronin K, et al. The AIDS dementia complex and human immunodeficiency virus type 1 brain infection: clinical–virological correlations. Ann Neurol 1995; 38:563–570.
9. Glass JD, Wesselingh SL, Selnes OA, et al. Clinical–neuropathologic correlation in HIV-associated dementia. Neurology 1993; 43:2230–2237.
10. Chang L, Ernst T, Leonido-Yee M, et al. Cerebral metabolites correlate with clinical severity of HIV-cognitive motor complex. Neurol 1999; 52:100–108.
11. Dore GJ, Correll PK, Li Y, Kaldor JM, Cooper DA, Brew BJ. Changes to AIDS dementia complex in the era of highly active antiretroviral therapy. AIDS 1999; 13(10):1249–1253.
12. Dore GJ, McDonald A, Li Y, Kaldor J, Brew BJ. Marked improvement in survival following AIDS dementia complex in the era of highly active antiretroviral therapy. AIDS 2003; 17(10):1539–1545.
13. Cysique L, Brew BJ, Maruff P. High rate of neuropsychologiocal impairment in patients with HIV infection despite long term HAART. XIV International AIDS Conference, Spain, Barcelona, 2002.

14. Brew BJ, Fulham M, Garsia R. Factors associated with AIDS dementia complex. Ninth Conference on Retroviruses and Opportunistic Infections, Seattle, 2002.

15. Brew BJ. Evidence for a change in AIDS dementia complex (ADC) in the era of highly active antiretroviral therapy and the possibility of new forms of ADC. AIDS 2003 2004; 18 (suppl.): 575–578.

16. Rempel H, Buffum D, Pulliam L. HIV-1 tat inhibits the amyloid beta degrading enzyme, neprilysin. J Neurovirol 2002; 8(suppl 1):12.

17. Nebuloni M, Pellegrinelli A, Ferri A, et al. Beta amyloid precursor protein and patterns of HIV p24 immunohistochemistry in different brain areas of AIDS patients. AIDS 2001; 15(5):571–575.

18. Wesselingh SL, Glass J, McArthur JC, Griffin JW, Griffin DE. Cytokine dysregulation in HIV-associated neurological disease. Adv Neuroimmunol 1994; 4(3):199–206.

19. Thompson KA, McArthur JC, Wesselingh SL. Correlation between neurological progression and astrocyte apoptosis in HIV-associated dementia. Ann Neurol 2001; 49(6):745–752.

20. Lipton SA, Gendelman HE. Seminars in medicine of the Beth Israel Hospital, Boston. Dementia associated with the acquired immunodeficiency syndrome. N Eng J Med 1995; 332:934–940.

21. Brew BJ. Markers of AIDS dementia complex: the role of cerebrospinal fluid assays. AIDS 2001; 15:1883–1884.

22. Brew BJ, Halman M, Catalan J, et al. Safety and efficacy of Abacavir (ABC, 1592) in AIDS dementia complex (Study CNAB 3001). 12th World AIDS Conference, Geneva, 1998.

23. Yeni PG, Hammer SM, Carpenter CC, et al. Antiretroviral treatment for adult HIV infection in 2002: updated recommendations of the International AIDS Society-USA Panel. JAMA 2002; 288(2):222–235.

24. Gisslen M, Hagberg L. Antiretroviral treatment of central nervous system HIV-1 infection: a review. HIV Med 2001; 2(2):97–104.

25. Deutsch R, Ellis RJ, McCutchan JA, et al. AIDS-associated mild neurocognitive impairment is delayed in the era of highly active antiretroviral therapy. AIDS 2001; 15(14):1898–1899.

26. Suarez S, Baril L, Stankoff B, et al. Outcome of patients with HIV-1-related cognitive impairment on highly active antiretroviral therapy. AIDS 2001; 15(2):195–200.

27. Chang L, Ernst T, et al. Highly active antiretroviral therapy reverses brain metabolite abnormalities in mild dementia. Neurology 1999; 53:782–789.

28. Dougherty RH, Skolasky RL, McArthur JC. Progression of HIV-associated dementia treated with HAART. AIDS Reader 2002; 12:69–74.

29. Menendez-Arias L. Targeting HIV: antiretroviral therapy and development of drug resistance. Trends Pharm Sci 2002; 23(8):381–388.

30. Venturi G, Catucci M, Romano L, et al. Antiretroviral resistance mutations in human immunodeficiency virus type 1 reverse transcriptase and protease from paired cerebrospinal fluid and plasma samples. J Infect Dis 2000; 181:740–745.

31. Cunningham PH, Smith DG, Satchell C, Cooper DA, Brew B. Evidence for independent development of resistance to HIV-1 reverse transcriptase inhibitors in the cerebrospinal fluid. AIDS 2000; 14(13):1949–1954.

32. Stingele K, Haas J, Zimmermann T, Stingele R, Hubsch-Muller C, Freitag M, Storch-Hagenlocher B, Hartmann M, Wildemann B. Independent HIV replication

in paired CSF and blood viral isolates during antiretroviral therapy. Neurology 2001; 56(3):355–361.

33. Ellis RJ. Clinical Implications of Divergent Evolution of HIV in the CNS. Viral and Host Genetic Factors Regulating HIV/CNS disease. Washington, DC, 2002.

34. Shapshak P, Segal DM, Crandall KA, Fujimura RK, Zhang BT, Xin KQ, Okuda K, Petito CK, Eisdorfer C, Goodkin K. Independent evolution of HIV type 1 in different brain regions. AIDS Res Hum Retroviruses 1999; 15(9):811–820.

35. Smit TK, Brew BJ, Toustellatte W, Margello S, Saksena NK. Evidence of independent evolution of HIV drug resistance in diverse areas of the brain of HIV infected patients on antiretroviral therapy. J Virol 2004; 78: 10133–10148.

36. Brew BJ, Pemberton L Ray J. Can the peripheral blood monocyte count be used as a marker of CSF resistance to antiretroviral drugs? J Neurovirol 2003 2004; 10 (suppl1): 1–60.

37. Antinori A, Giancol ML, Grisetti S, Soldani F, Alba L, Liuzzi G, Amendola A, Capobianchi M, Tozzi V, Perno CF. Factors influencing virological response to antiretroviral drugs in cerebrospinal fluid of advanced HIV-1-infected patients. AIDS 2002; 16(14):1867–1876.

38. Sacktor N, Tarwater PM, Skolasky RL, McArthur JC, Selnes OA, Becker J, Cohen B, Miller EN, Multicenter for AIDS Cohort Study. CSF antiretroviral drug penetrance and the treatment of HIV-associated psychomotor slowing. Neurology 2001; 57(3):542–544.

39. Wynn HE, Brundage RC, Fletcher CV. Clinical implications of CNS penetration of antiretroviral drugs. CNS Drugs 2002; 16(9):595–609.

40. Van Praag RME, Weverling GJ, Portegies P, Jurriaans S, Zhou X, Turner-Foisy ML, Sommadossi J, Burger DM, Lange JMA, Hoetelmans RMW, Prins JM. Enhanced penetration of indinavir in cerebrospinal fluid and semen after the addition of low-dose ritonavir. AIDS 2002; 14(9):1187–1194.

41. Olson DP, Scadden DT, D'Aquila RT, De Pasquale MP. The protease inhibitor ritonavir inhibits the functional activity of the multidrug resistance related-protein 1 (MRP-1). AIDS 2002; 16(13):1743–1747.

42. Drewe J, Gutmann H, Fricker G, Torok M, Beglinger C, Huwyler J. HIV protease inhibitor ritonavir: a more potent inhibitor of P-glycoprotein than the cyclosporine analog SDZ PSC 833. Biochem Pharmacol 1999; 57(10):1147–1152.

43. van Herrewege Y, Penne L, Vereecken C, et al. Activity of reverse transcriptase inhibitors in monocyte-derived dendritic cells: a possible in vitro model for post exposure prophylaxis of sexual HIV transmission. AIDS Res Hum Retroviruses 2002; 18:1091–1102.

44. AquaroS, Calio R, Balzarini J, et al. Macrophages and HIV infection: therapeutical approaches toward this strategic virus reservoir. Antivir Res 2002; 55:209–225.

45. Tozzi V, Balestra P, Galgani S, et al. Positive and sustained effects of highly active antiretroviral therapy on HIV-1 associated neurocognitive impairment. AIDS 1999; 13(14):1889–1897.

46. Back DJ, Khoo SH, Gibbons SE, Merry C. The role of therapeutic drug monitoring in treatment of HIV infection. Br J Clin Pharm 2001; 51(4):301–308.

47. Groothuis DR, Levy RM. The entry of antiviral and antiretroviral drugs into the central nervous system. J Neurovirol 1997; 3:387–400.

48. Brew BJ (ed.). Cerebrovascular complications and transient neurologic deficits. In: HIV Neurology. New York: Oxford University Press, 2001:146–151.

49. Brew BJ (ed.). Seizures. In: HIV Neurology. New York: Oxford University Press, 2001:142–145.

50. Gea-Banacloche JC, Lane HC. Immune reconstitution in HIV infection. AIDS 1999; 13:S25–S38.

51. Kovacs JA, Masur H. Prophylaxis against opportunistic infections in patients with human immunodeficiency virus infection. N Engl J Med 2000; 342:1416–1429.

52. Martinez E, Garcia-Viejo MA, et al. Discontinuation of secondary prophylaxis for cryptococcal meningitis in HIV-infected patients responding to highly active anti-retroviral therapy. AIDS 2000; 14(16):2615–2617.

53. Whitcup SM, Fortin E, Lindblad AS, Griffiths P, Metcalf JA, Robinson MR, Manischewitz J, Baird B, Perry C, Kidd IM, Vrabec T, Davey RT Jr, Fallon J, Walker RE, Kovacs JA, Lane HC, Nussenblatt RB, Smith J, Masur H, Polis MA. Discontinuation of anti-cytomegalovirus therapy in persons with HIV infection and cytomegalovirus retinitis. JAMA 1999; 282(17):1633–1637.

54. Macdonald JC, Torriani FJ, Morse LS, Karavellas MP, Reed JB, Freeman WR. Lack of reactivation of cytomegalovirus (CMV) retinitis after stopping CMV mainte-nance therapy in AIDS patients with sustained elevations in CD4 T cells in response to highly active antiretroviral therapy. J Infect Dis 1998, 177(5):1182–1187.

55. Miro JM, Lopez JC, Podzamczer D, et al. Discontinuation of toxoplasmic encephalitis prophylaxis is safe in HIV-1 and *T. gondii* coinfected patients after immunological recovery with HAART: preliminary results of the GESIDA 04/98B study. Proceedings of the Seventh Conference on Retroviruses and Opportunistic infections, San Francisco, January 30–February 2, 2000; abstract 230.

56. Bertschy S, Opravil M, Telenti A, et al. Discontinuation of maintenance therapy against toxoplasmosis encephalitis may not be safe despite sustained response to combination antiretroviral therapy. 9th Conference on Retroviruses and Opportunistic Infections, Seattle, 2002.

57. Luft BJ, Hafner R, Korzun AH, et al. Toxoplasmic encephalitis in patients with the acquired immune deficiency syndrome. Members of the ACTG 077p/ANRS 009 Study Team. N Engl J Med 1993; 329:995–1000.

58. Brew BJ (ed.). Toxoplasmosis. In: HIV Neurology. New York: Oxford University Press, 2001:117–123.

59. Carr A, Tindall B, Brew BJ, Marriott DJ, Harkness JL, Penny R, et al. Low dose trimethoprim-sulphamethoxazole prophylaxis for toxoplasmic encephalitis in AIDS. Ann Int Med 1992; 117:106–111.

60. Ambinder RF. Epstein–Barr associated lymphoproliferations in the AIDS setting. Eur J Can 2001; 37:1209–1216.

61. Saktor N, Lyles RH, Skolasky MA, Kleeberger C, Selnes OA, Miller EN, Becker JT, Cohen B, MacArthur J. HIV associated neurologic disease incidence changes: Multicenter AIDS Cohort Study, 1990–1998. Neurology 2001:257–260.

62. Budka H, Costanzi G, Cristina S, Lechi A, Parravicini C, Trabattoni R, Vago L. Brain pathology induced by infection with the human immunodeficiency virus (HIV). A histological, immunocytochemical and electron microscopical study of 100 autopsy cases. Acta Neuropathol 1987; 75:185–198.

63. Rosenblum ML, Levy RM, Bredesen DE, So YT, Wara W, Ziegler JL. Primary cen-tral nervous system lymphomas in patients with AIDS. Ann Neruol 1988; 23:S13–S16.

64. Rhodes RH. Histopathologic features in the central nervous system of 400 acquired immunodeficiency syndrome cases: implications of rates of occurrence. Hum Pathol 1993; 24:1189–1198.

65. Skeist DJ, Crosby C. Survival is prolonged by highly active retroviral therapy in AIDS patients with primary central nervous system lymphoma. AIDS 2003,17:1787–1793.

66. Hoffman C, Tabrizian S, Wolf E, Eggers C, Stoehr A, Plettenberg A, Buhk T, Stellbrink HJ, Horst HA, Jager H, Rosenkranz T. Survival of AIDS patients with primary central nervous system lymphoma is dramatically improved by HAART-induced immune recovery. AIDS 2001; 15:219–2127.

67. McGowan JP, Shah S. Long term remission of AIDS related primary central nervous system lymphoma associated with highly active antiretroviral therapy. AIDS 1998; 12:952–954.

68. Brew BJ (ed.). Progressive multifocal leukoencephalopathy. In: HIV Neurology. New York: Oxford University Press, 2001:1132–1141.

69. Gasnault J, Taoufik Y, Goujard C, et al. Prolonged survival without neurological improvement in patients with AIDS-related progressive multifocal leucoencephalopathy on potent combined anti-retroviral therapy. J Neurovirol 1999; 5:421–429.

70. Carpenter C, Benson C, Chaisson R. Tuberculosis and HIV infection. In: Crowe S, Hoy J, Mills J, eds. Management of the HIV Infected Patient. London: Martin Dunitz Press, 2002:385–400.

71. Brew BJ (ed.). Cryptococcal meningitis. In: HIV Neurology. New York: Oxford University Press, 2001:191–196.

72. Gilden DH, Mahalingam R, Cohrs RJ, Kleinschmidt-DeMasters BK, Forghani B. The protean manifestations of varicella-zoster virus vasculopathy. J Neurovirol 2002; 8(suppl 2):75–79.

73. Katrak SM, Shembalkar PK, Bijwe SR, Bhandarkar LD. The clinical, radiological and pathological profile of tuberculous meningitis in patients with and without human immunodeficiency virus infection. J Neurol Sci 2000; 181:118–126.

74. Erice A, Tierney C, Hirsch M, Caliendro AM, Weinberg A, Kendall MA, Polsky B. Cytomegalovirus (CMV) and human immunodeficiency virus (HIV) burden, CMV end organ disease and survival in subjects with advanced HIV infection (AIDS Clinical Trial Group Protocol 360). Clin Infect Dis 2003; 37:567–578.

75. Brew BJ (ed.). Uncommon causes of predominantly focal cerebral complications in advanced HIV disease. In: HIV Neurology. New York: Oxford University Press, 2001:158–159.

76. Szilak I, Minamoto GY. West Nile viral encephalitis in an HIV-positive woman in New York. N Engl J Med 2000; 342(1):59–60.

77. Denning DW, Anderson J, Rudge P, et al. Acute myelopathy associated with primary infection with human immunodeficiency virus. British Med J 1987:143–144.

78. Dal Pan GJ, Glass JD, McArthur JC, et al. Clinicopathological correlations of HIV-1 associated vacuolar myelopathy: an autopsy based case–control study. Neurology 1994; 44:2159–2164.

79. Rosenblum M, Scheck A, Cronin K, et al. Dissociation of AIDS related vacuolar myelopathy and productive HIV-1 infection of the spinal cord. Neurology 1989; 39:892–896.

80. Radja F, Kay DG, Albrecht S, Jolicoeur P. Oligodendrocyte-specific expression of human immunodeficiency virus type 1 Nef in transgenic mice leads to vacuolar myelopathy and alters oligodendrocyte phenotype in vitro. J Virol 2003; 77(21):11,745–11,753.

81. Brew BJ (ed.). Common spinal cord diseases. In: HIV Neurology. New York: Oxford University Press, 2001:165–173.

82. Eyer-Silva WA, Couto-Fernandez JC, Caetano MR, et al. Remission of HIV-associated myelopathy after initiation of lopinavir in a patient with extensive previous exposure to highly active antiretroviral therapy. AIDS 2002; 16(17):2367–2369.

83. MacGowan D, Scelsa S, Waldron M. An ALS like syndrome with new HIV infection and complete response to antiretroviral therapy. Neurology 2001; 57:1094–1097.

84. Moulignier A, Moulonguet A, Pialoux G, Rozenbaum W. Reversible ALS-like disorder in HIV infection. Neurology 2001; 57:995–1001.

85. von Giesen HJ, Kaiser R, Koller H, Wetzel K, Arendt G, Giesen HJ. Reversible ALS-like disorder in HIV infection. An ALS-like syndrome with new HIV infection and complete response to antiretroviral therapy. Neurology 2002; 59(3):474–475.

86. Pardo CA, McArthur JC, Griffin JW. HIV neuropathy: insights in the pathology of HIV peripheral nerve disease. J Peripher Nerv Syst 2001; 6:21–27.

87. Keswani SC, Pardos CA, Cherry CL. Hoke A, McArthur JC. HIV associated sensory neuropathies. AIDS 2002; 16:2105–2117.

88. Cornblath DR, McArthur JC, Kennedy PGE, Witte AS, Griffin JW. Inflammatory demyelinating peripheral neuropathies associated with human T-cell lymphotropic virus type III infection. Ann Neurol 1987; 21:32–40.

89. Grimaldi LM, Luzzi L, Martino GV, Furlan R, Nemni R, Antonelli A, Canal N, Pozza G. Bilateral eight cranial nerve neuropathy in human immunodeficiency virus. J Neurol 1993; 240:363–366.

90. Brew BJ. The peripheral nervous system complications of human immunodeficiency virus (HIV) infection. Muscle Nerve 2003; 28(5):542–552.

91. Brinley FJ, Pardo CA, Verma A. Human immunodeficiency virus and the peripheral nervous system workshop. Arch Neurol 2001; 58:1561–1566.

92. Markus R, Brew BJ. HIV-1 peripheral neuropathy and combination antiretroviral therapy. Lancet 1998; 352:1906–1907.

93. Boonyapisit K, Katirji B. Severe exacerbation of hepatitis C-associated vasculitic neuropathy following treatment with interferon alpha: a case report and literature review. Muscle Nerve 2002; 25(6):909–913.

94. Authier F, Romain K, Gheradi R. Peripheral neuropathies in HIV-infected patients in the era of HAART. Brain Pathol 2003; 13(2):223–228.

95. Kolson DL, Gonzalez-Scarano F. HIV associated neuropathies: role of HIV-1, CMV, and other viruses. J Peripher Nerv Syst 2001; 6:2–7.

96. Griffin JW, Crawford TO, McArthur JC. Peripheral neuropathies associated with HIV infection. In: Gendelman HE, Lipton SA, Epstein L, Swindells S, eds. The Neurology of AIDS. New York: Chapman and Hall Press, 280–287.

97. Hermann DN, Griffin JW, Hauer P, Cornblath DR, McArthur JC. Epidermal Nerve fibre density and sural nerve morphometry in peripheral neuropathies. Neurology 1999; 53:1634–1640.

98. McArthur JC, Yiannoutsos C, Simpson D, et al. A phase II trial of recombinant nerve growth factor for sensory neuropathy associated with HIV infection. Neurology 2000; 54:1080–1088.

99. Mortin C, Solders G, Sourerborg A, Hansson P. Antiretroviral therapy may improve sensory function in HIV-infected patients: a pilot study. Neurology 2000; 54:2120–2127.

100. Villa A, Foresti V, Confalonieri F. Autonomic nervous system dysfunction associated with HIV infection in intravenous heroin users. AIDS 1992; 6:85–89.

101. Lanska MJ, Lanska DJ, Schmidley JW. Syphilitic polyradiculopathy in an HIV positive man. Neurology 1988; 38:1297–1301.

102. Nemmi R, Sanvito L, Quattrini A, Santuccio G, Camerlingo M, Canal N. Peripheral neuropathy in hepatitis C infection with and without cryoglobulinaemia. J Neurol Neurosurg Psychiatry 2003; 74:1267–1271.

103. deGans J, Portegies P, Tiessens G, Troost D, Danner SA, Lange JM. Therapy for cytomegalovirus polyradiculopathy in patients with AIDS. 1990; 4:421–425.

104. Kim YS, Hollander H. Polyradiculopathy due to cytomegalovirus: report of two cases in which improvement occurred after prolonged therapy and review of the literature. Clin Infect Dis 1992; 17:32–37.

105. Cinque P, Scarpellini P, Vago L, Linde A, Lazzarin A. Diagnosis of central nervous system complication in HIV infected patients: CSF analysis by the polymerase chain reaction. AIDS 1997; 11:1–17.

106. Vinters HV, Kwok MK, Ho HW, Anders KH, Tomiyasu U, Wolfson WL, Robert F. Cytomegalovirus in the nervous system of patients with the acquired immune deficiency syndrome. Brain 1989; 112:245–268.

107. Whitcup SM, Fortin E, Linblad AS, Griffiths P, Metcalf JA, Robinson MR, Manischwetiz, Baird B, Perry C, Kidd IM, et al. Discontinuation of anticytomegalovirus therapy in patients with HIV infection and cytomegalovirus retinitis. JAMA 1999; 282:1633–1637.

108. Roullet E, Assuerus V, Gozlan J, Ropert A, Said G, Baudrimont M, el Amrani M, Jacomet C, Duvivier C, Gonzales-Canali G. Cytomegalovirus multifocal neuropathy in AIDS; analysis of 15 consecutive patients. Neurology 1994; 44:2174–2182.

109. Said G, Lacroix C, Chemouilli P, Goulon-Goeu C, Roullet E, Penaud D, de Broucker T, Meduri G, Vincent D, Torchet M. Cytomegalovirus neuropathy in acquired immunodeficiency syndrome: a clinical and pathological study. Ann Neurol 1991; 29:139–146.

110. Brew BJ (ed.). Infective causes of peripheral neuropathy. In: HIV Neurology. New York: Oxford University Press, 2001:206–207.

111. Carr A, Cooper, DA. Adverse effects of antiretroviral therapy. Lancet 2000; 356:1423–1430.

112. Brew BJ (ed.). Medication-related and nutrition-related peripheral neuropathy. In: HIV Neurology. New York: Oxford University Press, 2001:209–217.

113. Luciano CA, Pardo CA, Carlos A, McArthur JC. Recent developments in the HIV neuropathies. Curr Opin Neurol 2003; 16(3):403–409.

114. Brew BJ, Tisch S, Law M. Nucleoside neuropathy in HIV distal symmetrical neuropathy: relationships to serum lactate and plasma HIV viral loads. AIDS 2003; 17:1094–1096.

18

Gauging the Threats: A Conceptual Framework for Prioritizing Research Directed Toward Intervention

Paul W. Ewald

Department of Biology, University of Louisville, Louisville, Kentucky, U.S.A.

1. INTRODUCTION

Infectious diseases vary greatly in the damage they have inflicted on human populations—smallpox, tuberculosis, and malaria have been much more destructive than acne or the common cold. This simple truth provides a basis for efforts to control emerging infectious diseases by emphasizing the need to distinguish emerging infectious diseases according to the threat that they pose to humans. Critical to this assessment is the breadth of diseases considered. If the breadth is too narrow the greatest infectious threats might fall outside the scope of inquiry and thus fail to be recognized and controlled. This concern draws attention to the value of defining emerging infectious diseases broadly to include diseases that (i) have long been established in human populations but have recently spread from one human population into another, (ii) are newly introduced into humans from other species (zoonoses), and (iii) have long been present in human populations but are newly recognized as infectious.

The vast majority of diseases that have recently emerged according to a narrow definition of emergence—the second of the preceding categories—have caused only a small amount of damage to human populations relative to classic killers, such as smallpox, tuberculosis, and malaria. Such emerging pathogens may cause severe illness in individuals but their spread is generally restricted, because they are poorly adapted to humans and therefore have not evolved the tradeoff between host exploitation and transmission that characterizes well-adapted pathogens. HIV-1 subtype M is the main exception to this generalization. Any general framework for evaluating the relative threats of emerging diseases must therefore be able to explain why HIV emerged to cause a severe pandemic while other pathogens have not. To develop this framework these three categories of emerging diseases are evaluated below with regard to the threat that they pose.

2. CATEGORIES OF EMERGING DISEASES

2.1. Long Established Human Diseases Emerging in a New Human Population

Diseases in this category are transmitted from person to person either directly or indirectly through a biological vector, such as a mosquito, or a nonbiological vehicle such as water. They have been some of the most damaging emerging diseases in human history. Measles and smallpox, for example, decimated native populations in the Americas when they were introduced during the early colonial period (1,2). Syphilis probably caused large amounts of death in previously unexposed populations in Europe as a result of a reciprocal introduction into Europe from the New World (2,3). These diseases were devastating because they were introduced into populations that had no acquired immunity to them and little if any evolved resistance. But such diseases are unlikely to be a great threat in the future for a simple reason: the high degree of transportation that exists today is far greater than the amount needed for global transport of pathogens that have long used humans as primary hosts. So far as is known, the only pathogens of humans that have not already been mixed by human travel are zoonotic, that is, newly introduced into humans from other species.

2.2. Exotic Zoonotic Pathogens

Many examples of recent zoonotic transmission into humans have been documented; the ebola, hantaan, Nipah, H5N1 influenza, West Nile and SARS viruses are widely publicized examples. But none has created problems in humans that amount to anything more than background noise when compared with HIV. The number of deaths over the past year from SARS, for example, was far less than 1% of the number from AIDS.

Most of these zoonotic pathogens have emerged in new human populations only recently because they have little if any potential for transmission from human to human. When zoonotic pathogens infect humans as dead-end hosts, emergence into new human populations depends little on the global transportation of humans. Rather, such emergence depends on the transportation of the hosts from which they can be transmitted, and such hosts may be only accidentally transported by human activities.

The emergence of West Nile virus offers an example. Although the route of transport across the Atlantic is unknown, an infected bird or mosquito was apparently brought into New York and established a transmission cycle between North American mosquitoes and birds, which allowed the virus to spread throughout North America, continuously spilling over into humans through mosquito bites (4–6). So far as is known, little if any transmission can occur from humans to mosquitoes or to other hosts (6). The incidence of West Nile disease in humans is thus tied directly to the spread of infection in the mosquito and avian hosts that maintain the cycle. Although the human infection can be destructive to the individual patients, the virus poses a relatively low threat to the human population as a whole, because dead-end human infections cannot generate a geometrically increasing rate of spread through the human population.

More generally, the threat posed by pathogens that cause dead-end human infections depends on the degree to which humans are in contact with the infected hosts that maintain the cycle. In the case of West Nile virus this contact is low in North America, because modern lifestyle involves living in mosquito-proof dwellings. The best evidence for this conclusion comes from the failure of pathogens that are well-adapted to human–mosquito–human contact to maintain these cycles in human populations in regions with mosquito-proof dwellings; dengue virus, and Plasmodium species, for example, repeatedly enter the United States, but fail to maintain themselves even though evidence indicates that some transmission from human to human via mosquitoes occurs (7–9).

Although West Nile virus has attracted a great deal of attention from researchers and the general public, the numbers of people afflicted bears out the contention that it is a relatively minor threat. In 2002, there were 4161 reported cases of West Nile disease in the United States with 277 deaths. The numbers have been increasing from year to year, because West Nile virus has been gradually spreading westward across North America since 1999 in concert with the movements of the arthropod and vertebrate hosts from which it can be transmitted. But now that the virus has spread throughout virtually all of the contiguous United States, we can expect that the annual morbidity and mortality will tend to stabilize somewhere near the current levels.

Zoonotic pathogens pose the greatest threat when they can be transmitted from one person to another. Even in this case, however, the threat posed is generally low because pathogens that have recently been transmitted to humans are generally not well adapted for transmission between humans. Such pathogens may be able to spread at the onset of the outbreak when control measures are lax and when close contact is possible, for example, in hospitals. Once the outbreak is recognized, however, control measures typically cause probabilities of transmission to drop below that necessary for maintenance of the pathogen in the human population. Outbreaks of ebola, lassa fever, and SARS are examples of this category of pathogen.

Occasionally, however, zoonotic pathogens are transmitted well above this break-even point for spread of infection. Strains of influenza, for example, are sometimes readily transmissible from humans soon after their zoonotic transmission into humans. The impact of such strains is thus vastly greater than the impact for diseases that are incompetent or marginally competent at transmission from human to human. The annual toll for influenza in the United States, for example, usually amounts to approximately 15–100 million cases and 3600 deaths (10).

HIV-1 subtype M is apparently another example of a zoonotic pathogen that could be transmitted well above the break-even point. It was probably transmitted to humans from chimpanzees sometime during the last century or so and has been transmitted from person to person since then (11,12). But even HIV illustrates how zoonotic transfer to humans is generally associated with a low potential for spread from humans at a level sufficient for pandemic spread. None of the other subtypes of HIV-1 and none of the lineages of HIV-2 have shown much if any potential for pandemic spread. For decades they have caused human infections at low frequencies in restricted regions in Africa, infecting relatively few people outside of Africa (13).

Historically the ability to spread from person to person substantially above the break-even point has been the greatest contributor to the overall threat posed by an emerging zoonotic pathogen. The majority of the most deadly human pathogens—smallpox, tuberculosis, yellow fever, typhus, and typhoid, for example—entered humans zoonotically at some time in the past and created problems because they were able to spread geometrically within human populations.

2.3. Longstanding Human Diseases, Newly Recognized as Caused by Infection

Familiar diseases with newly recognized infectious causes are sometimes not considered to be emerging infectious diseases, because they are not emerging in the epidemiological sense. They are emerging, however, in the sense of our understanding of disease causation, and they are some of the most damaging of human diseases. If the overall goal of the health sciences is to improve health, then inclusion of these diseases in considerations of emerging diseases is especially important.

Evolutionary principles, current evidence, and the recent track record of recognizing infectious causation suggest that most of the severe, common diseases of unknown cause are caused by infection (14). Some of the candidate pathogens use humans as primary hosts. Others infect humans zoonotically at high frequency. In contrast to the oft-mentioned examples of newly emerging acute infectious diseases, most of these damaging chronic diseases are already globally distributed and prevalent. These diseases tend to be chronic rather than acute because infectious causation of chronic diseases is more difficult to detect and demonstrate; recognition of infectious causation of longstanding chronic diseases is therefore more likely to be still emerging (14). Some of them—atherosclerosis, for example—are now causing damage in human populations that is comparable to the damage that is merely feared as worst case scenarios for emerging acute infectious diseases.

The emerging recognition that these diseases are caused by infection has great practical significance, because infectious diseases can often be effectively controlled. When a disease of unknown cause becomes recognized as caused by infection, new opportunities for investigation, control, and prevention become apparent, particularly through vaccination, anti-infective compounds, and imposition of barriers to transmission. This generalization has been as true for neurological diseases as it has for diseases in general. Vaccination against polio, the virtual eradication of neurosyphilis through the use of antibiotics, and the prevention of AIDS dementia through protection of the blood supply are three cases in point.

This track record would be largely a matter of historical interest were it not for the fact that the causes of some of the most damaging diseases remain inadequately understood. Infection is known to play a primary causal role in several chronic neurological diseases (Table 1), and evidence already implicates infectious causation for many others, including some of the most damaging neurological diseases (Table 2).

2.4. Relative Threats Posed by the Three Categories of Emergence

The considerations discussed above are summarized in Table 3, which compares the relative threat posed by these three categories of emerging disease. This comparison emphasizes that the greatest potential for improving health arises from controlling diseases that can be maintained in human populations as a result of human-to-human transmission. The large number of such diseases that can be expected in the third category (Table 2) makes this category an important target of research effort during the next few decades. Diseases that are not transmissible from human to human, however, can still pose a great threat if the details of zoonotic transmission and pathol-

Table 1   Chronic Neurological Diseases with Infectious Causes Recognized Over the Past Century

Disease	Infectious cause
Tropical spastic paraparesis	Human T-lymphotropic virus type 1
Neurosyphilis	*Treponema pallidum*
AIDS dementia	HIV, *Toxoplasma gondii, Pneumocystis carinii,*
Sydenham's chorea	Streptococcus pyogenes
Shingles	Varicella zoster virus
Ramsay Hunt Syndrome	Varcella zoster virus
Progressive multifocal leukoencephalopathy	JC virus
Subacute sclerosing panencephalitis (SSPE)	Measles virus
Creutzfeld-Jakob Disease, Kuru, prions	

Table 2   Chronic Neurological Diseases with Suspected Infectious Causes

Disease	Suspected pathogens	References
Amyotrophic lateral sclerosis	Echovirus, *Mycoplasma*	15–17
Alzheimer's disease (sporadic)	*Chlamydia pneumoniae*, Human herpes simplex type 1	18, 19
Multiple sclerosis	*C. pneumoniae*, Epstein Barr virus, endogenous retrovirus	20–22
Schizophrenia	*Toxoplasma gondii*, human herpes simplex bornavirus, endogenous retrovirus	23–29
Bipolar disorder	Bornavirus	30
Bell's palsy	Human herpes simplex type 1, *Mycoplasma, B. burgdorferi*, varicella zoster	31–35
Juvenile onset obsessive compulsive disorder	*Streptococcus pyogenes*	36
Ventricular brain tumors	Simian virus 40	
Systemic lupus Erythematosus	Epstein Barr virus, *T. gondi*	38, 39
Stroke	*C. pneumoniae*, cytomegalovirus	40–42
Fibromyalgia	entrovirus, *Mycoplasma,*	43–44
Chronic fatigue syndrome	Human herpes virus 6, *C. pneumoniae, Mycoplasma, Parvovirus* B19	44–46

Table 3   Categories of Emerging Infectious Diseases.

Category of emergence	Transmissible from humans?	Future threat
Invasion of one human population from another in which it has been long established	Yes	low because such pathogens have already been globally distributed
Exotic zoonotic entrance into a human population	No	Low to moderate depending on contact with the zoonotic host
	Yes	Low to high depending on potential for transmission from human to human and the evolution of virulence
Recently recognized as infectious	Yes or no	Low to high depending on the damage that is already recognized for the disease

ogy result in a high incidence of human disease. Assessments therefore need to be done on a disease-by-disease basis, because the specific details may determine where in this spectrum of threat a particular disease lies.

3. ILLUSTRATIVE EMERGING NEUROLOGICAL DISEASES

3.1. Lyme Disease

Lyme disease illustrates the kind of information that is needed to assess the threat of a newly recognized zoonotic disease. Lyme disease is caused by *Borrelia burgdorferi*, which is transmitted to humans by tick-bite. About 17,000–18,000 new cases of Lyme disease are reported to the CDC each year; its total incidence is estimated at about 100,000 (47). Although these numbers are substantial, they are still low compared with pathogens that are readily transmitted from one person to another (cf. influenza above). The lethality associated with these cases is also low compared with the most damaging long-recognized neurological diseases for which infectious causes are suspected, diseases such as stroke, Alzheimer's, and schizophrenia (Table 4). If one therefore considers only Lyme disease in the strict sense, its threat would be relatively low, largely because of the relatively low probability of acquiring infection and the apparent lack of transmission from person to person.

Several uncertainties need to be resolved, however, to assess with accuracy the threat posed by *B. burgdorferi*. The most important of these uncertainties is the extent to which long-term sequellae of infection are more abundant and damaging than is Lyme disease narrowly defined. This uncertainty emphasizes the need for long-term studies of *B. burgdorferi*-infected patients to determine the spectrum of sequelae of *B. burgdorferi* infections and the probabilities of developing such sequellae.

Another uncertainty is the extent to which *B. burgdorferi* infections can be transmitted from person to person. Transmission from mother to fetus has

Table 4 Deaths per Year in the United States from Neurological Diseases with Known or Suspected Infectious Causes

Disease	Deaths	Year	Reference
Cerebrovascular Diseases	163,601	2001	48
Alzheimer's disease	53,679	2001	48
Schizophrenia	5,000	Recent years	Estimated from 49–51
Amyotrophic lateral Sclerosis	~5,000	Recent years	52
West Nile	277	2002	53
Lyme disease	Rare	Recent years	54

been documented, and the potential for sexual transmission has not been adequately tested (55,56). If person-to-person transmission is common, then Lyme disease, broadly defined, could be much more damaging than is generally presumed, particularly if severe chronic manifestations commonly arise from infections that are inapparent during their early phases. Although the restricted geographic distributions that arise from reported cases can be mustered as evidence against person-to-person transmission, this argument suffers from a circularity: positive tests from patients who live outside areas of recognized zoonotic transmission may be dismissed as false positives, thus making the distribution accord more with dead-end zoonotic transmission than is actually the case (56).

False negatives may also contribute to an underestimate of the threat posed by B. burgdorferi, because *B. burgdorferi* can be identified by polymerase chain reaction, cell culture, and histological methods from patients who are serologically negative (56). The arbitrariness of species classification may compound this underestimate because clinically important infections arise from *Borrelia* that have been classified as closely related species (56).

In sum, if the narrow conception of Lyme disease is largely correct, then Lyme disease poses a relatively small threat because of its restricted potential for person-to-person transmission and restricted transmission to humans from the tick-rodent transmission cycle. If, however, the current conception greatly underestimates the extent of zoonotic infection, morbidity of infection, and person-to-person transmission, then the threat posed by Lyme disease could be great. In this example, the framework for evaluating the threat posed by emerging diseases emphasizes the need for a better understanding of the prevalence of infection with this agent, the spectrum of disease associated with infection, and the transmission of the agents from person to person.

3.2. Schizophrenia and Other Mental Illnesses

Mental illnesses are often separated from neurological diseases under the presumption that the biological basis is different. This separation cannot be justified by evidence and may therefore be counterproductive by artificially limiting the scope of efforts to control neurological illnesses. This limitation is highlighted by the tendency for mental illnesses to be increasingly linked to infectious agents. Schizophrenia provides an illustration.

A neuropathological basis for schizophrenia is evidenced by specific structural changes in the brains of schizophrenics (57,58), and specific functional neurological deficits, such as deficits in prepulse inhibition in the acoustic startle response (59). The underlying causes of these abnormalities and their behavioral correlates are generally presumed to be genetic. Insofar as this generalization is true, schizophrenia could hardly be considered an emerging disease; however, the associations that can be mustered in favor of genetic causation can also be explained by prenatal infectious causation. The reciprocal argument is not true; some of the evidence that suggests infectious causation—such as associations of schizophrenia with season of birth and with particular infectious agents—can be explained only tortuously by genetic causation (24).

Several studies have found an increased prevalence of *Toxoplasma gondii* among schizophrenics (23,24,26,27). Elevated *T. gondii* positivity among first episode schizophrenics and neonates who eventually develop schizophrenia (23,26) is particularly important, because these associations accord with the idea that *T. gondii* causes schizophrenia as opposed to schizophrenia increasing exposure to *T. gondii*. If these associations reflect a causal relationship, then about one-third of schizophrenia would be caused by *T. gondii*.

The natural cycle of *T. gondii* involves transmission from rodents to cats. Humans become infected when they ingest *T. gondii* shed in cat feces or when they ingest undercooked meat from animals that have done so. Human exposure to *T. gondii* thus parallels human exposure to B. burgdorferi in that it represents spillover from a natural cycle that involves a definitive host (a cat or a tick) that acquires infection by feeding on an intermediate rodent as well as by transmission from pregnant women to their fetuses. The potential for spillover into humans is, however, much greater in the case of *T. gondii* because humans are exposed to *T. gondii* from cats or meat much more than to Borrelia from infected ticks. Accordingly, the prevalence of *T. gondii* infections in humans ranges from 0% to nearly 100% (60–62), depending largely on exposure to cats and insufficiently cooked meat.

As is the case with *Borrelia*, several uncertainties apply to estimates of the threat associated with *T. gondii*. As with *Borrelia* the scope of illness caused by *T. gondii* is uncertain. It is generally accepted that prenatal infections with *T. gondii* cause birth defects, miscarriages, mental retardation, and retinal lesions, and that infections identified later in life cause AIDS dementia and schizophrenia-like illness (24,63). The extent to which *T. gondii* causes illness that is currently being diagnosed as schizophrenia is still open to debate. As with *B. burgdorferi*, the occurrence of transmission from person to person outside of pregnancy seems limited but is unclear. *T. gondii* has been found in saliva and urogenital mucus and may therefore be transmitted by intimate contact during kissing or sexual intercourse (64). The threat posed by *T. gondii* as a cause of emerging disease therefore appears to similar to that posed by B. burgdorferi but more extreme, because the potential for transmission of *T. gondii* to humans is greater and the scope of human disease for which *T. gondii* is implicated appears to be more pervasive and damaging. Because the harmfulness of schizophrenia at the population level is far greater than the harmfulness of diseases that are emerging in an epidemiological sense such as Lyme disease or West Nile disease (e.g., for lethality, see Table 4), the possibility of *T. gondii* as an emerging cause of schizophrenia deserves a high priority in the spectrum of emerging diseases. Similar arguments could be made for infectious causation of autism and bipolar disorder, though the evidence for these diseases is more fragmentary.

4. INVESTIGATION AND INTERVENTION: THE OVERALL PICTURE

4.1. Great Imitators?

One of the greatest achievements in modern medicine's efforts to alleviate suffering from neurological diseases was the discovery of penicillin. By preventing syphilitic insanity, treatment of *Treponema pallidum* infections with penicillin reduced by about one-fifth the serious mental illness that existed at the time (65). But rather than considering the possibility that the cause and control of syphilis might offer insight into the cause and control of other severe neurological illnesses, experts put syphilis into its own category. It was labeled The Great Imitator, because it generated chronic illnesses that resembled the real thing— real dementia, real insanity, and real cardiovascular disease.

It is now recognized that *B. burgdorferi*, like *T. pallidum*, is responsible for a much broader array of disease, which encompasses arthritis, dementia, paralysis, meningitis, cranial neuropathies, illnesses that had been diagnosed as multiple sclerosis and motor neuron disease, attention deficit hyperactivity disorder, depression, and multiple sclerosis (66–68). As a consequence, Lyme borreliosis has become known over the past 15 years as "The New Great Imitator" (68–71). Although the use of "Great Imitator" in either case may be appealing, singling out these two pathogens may inhibit rather than advance an understanding of the true spectrum of emerging infectious disease. Group A streptococcal disease could be called a great imitator too, because it can be manifested as arthritis, carditis, chorea, and glomerulonephritis, and probably several other illnesses such as juvenile onset obsessive compulsive disorders (36,72,73). Although Borna disease virus has been studied much less extensively, it been found at elevated frequency in chronic fatigue syndrome, schizophrenia, and bipolar disorder and may be causally linked to these disorders. *Chlamydia pneumoniae* has been similarly linked, perhaps causally, to atherosclerosis, stroke, Alzheimer's disease, multiple sclerosis, asthma, chronic fatigue syndrome, and rheumatoid arthritis (18,45,74,75). Epstein–Barr virus similarly is associated with Hodkins lymphoma, Burkitt's lymphoma and other non-Hodgkins lymphomas, multiple sclerosis, breast cancer, and systemic lupus erythematosus. West Nile virus causes a variety of neurological manifestations, including various forms of paralysis, motor and sensory polyneuropathies, parkinsonian tremors, bradykinesia, and ataxia (76–78). If syphilis deserves the title of Great Imitator then particular disease associated with each of these pathogens could be similarly labeled. Or perhaps the term "imitator" is inappropriate for all of them, including syphilis.

The term imitator makes sense only if we understand the thing being imitated, that is, the model. Then we can clearly identify something else that resembles the model but is distinct from it. Elvis Presley was a real person who was distinct from the Elvis Presley imitators. Acute infectious diseases, such as cholera, malaria or smallpox, and genetic diseases, such as sickle-cell anemia, Huntington's disease or cystic fibrosis, could be appropriately considered models, because each is a real entity defined by its primary cause, either an infectious agent or an allele. In contrast, each chronic disease that syphilis is supposed to be imitating is a category of disease states that are grouped together on the basis of similarities in manifestations rather than a clearly understood etiology. The illnesses that are uncritically accepted as "models" for *T. pallidum* or the other "imitators" mentioned above, may instead be chronic manifestations caused by a variety of persistent infectious agents, of which *T. pallidum* and *B. burgdorferi* are just two. The multiplicity of candidate pathogens being considered as causes for particular categories of chronic illnesses (e.g., for schizophrenia, see Table 2) is just what one would expect to find if the apparent models are actually just umbrella categories for chronic manifestations of a variety of infectious agents.

More generally, the label "Great Imitator" runs counter to the insight that is emerging from the last century of research into the causes of chronic diseases. That is, chronic illnesses have increasingly been recognized as late manifestations of infectious processes (13,14). Perhaps syphilis is not the Great Imitator, but rather the Great Illustrator, because it illustrates a general connection between infection and chronic illnesses for anyone who is willing to think broadly and deeply about the causes of chronic diseases. Recognizing that a particular pathogen can be the common thread connecting a variety of chronic illnesses is the first step toward recognizing that the greatest threat of emerging neurological infections may be those that are already carrying out a degree of damage that is only a worry for infectious agents that have recently been introduced or not yet introduced into new human populations.

4.2. Chronic vs. Acute Emerging Infectious Diseases

Attention to emerging infectious diseases has focused on acute infectious diseases, such as ebola, hantaan, SARS, and West Nile disease. Most acute infectious diseases, however, have very limited potential for spreading in human populations, particularly in wealthy countries, because the global emergence of highly virulent, acute infectious diseases requires special sets of conditions that are rarely met (79). Vectorborne diseases, for example, may be maintained evolutionarily in a highly virulent form, but only a very small proportion of vectorborne pathogens have the characteristics necessary to be transmitted persistently from person to vector to person. No vectorborne pathogen of humans has demonstrated this ability under conditions found in modern wealthy countries, which are characterized by screened houses, air conditioning, and indoor life.

Similarly, severe diarrheal pathogens tend to be waterborne apparently because waterborne transmission allows highly virulent pathogens to be transmitted independently of host mobility (through the activity of attendants and movement of contaminated wash-water into water supplies) (79). For pathogens that are transmitted from person to person by air or direct contact, the newly emergent pathogens would need to have characteristics that enable them to be transmitted readily from sick hosts, particularly durability in the external environment, if they are to maintain transmission cycles. The smallpox virus and tuberculosis bacterium have these characteristics, but the pathogens that have attracted the most public attention in recent years, such as Ebola and SARS, do not

The increasingly recognized importance of infectious causation of chronic diseases emphasizes an irony in the attention devoted to emerging infectious disease over the past two decades. This attention was triggered largely by the AIDS experience, in which a lethal disease arose from an exotic source and spread pandemicly. This experience gave credence to concerns that other exotic diseases might similarly emerge. Concern focused, however, on the most conspicuous examples—acute infectious diseases. But AIDS is a chronic disease syndrome. Its severe chronic effects are in keeping with sexually transmitted diseases in general, which are molded by natural selection to be persistent and thus chronically damaging infections. The irony, therefore, is that the alarm bell was rung in response to an emerging chronic disease syndrome, yet most of the subsequent attention has been devoted to the less threatening acute infectious diseases. The past two decades have not generated a single example of a new globally spreading acute infectious disease that has been highly damaging to human populations, even though such pandemics have been often predicted. In fact there has not been such an example for the entire twentieth century. Pandemics of influenza have occurred, but influenza is not a new acute infectious disease; the danger associated with influenza was recognized long before the recent interest in emerging infectious diseases.

4.3. Interventions

The long-term practical payoff from investigating the causes of disease is generated by improvements in the cure and prevention of disease. Evaluation of research directed toward intervention must therefore take into consideration what can be done if the suspected cause is demonstrated as the true cause. Infectious causes have been the targets of the three greatest medical successes at intervention: vaccination, administration of anti-infectives such as antibiotics, and barriers to transmission. The track record for each category of intervention has been good but variable. Vaccines have been extremely effective for many viral diseases such as measles, smallpox, and polio. Most severe bacterial diseases have been controllable through one or a combination of the three categories of intervention. Control of protozoal diseases has been accomplished by various methods, but has generally been less successful than control of bacterial or viral diseases. Malaria, for example, has been effectively controlled in areas with low to moderate mosquito densities through the suppression of transmission, specifically through the use of insecticides, mosquito-proofing of houses, and the reduction of breeding habitat for mosquitoes. Long-term control of malaria, however, has generally been mediocre in the most malaria-ridden areas.

The considerations presented in this chapter suggest that the greatest potential for improving health through the control of emerging infectious diseases lies in discovering infectious causes of diseases that are already known to be highly damaging in human populations. For the wealthy countries of the world these diseases are as a rule chronic. On the basis of the excellent track record at controlling most infectious diseases through combinations of vaccination, anti-infectives and barriers to transmission, we can expect that most of newly discovered infectious causes of diseases will generally lead to effective control once the infectious causes of these diseases have been identified.

Consider schizophrenia. If one-third of schizophrenia is caused by *T. gondii*, this third could probably be prevented by vaccination of cats and humans. Experimental vaccination of cats in a farm setting illustrates this potential. Vaccination of the cats virtually eliminated *T. gondii* from swine (80). Elimination of *T. gondii* from household settings would be more tractable because the immigration of *T. gondii* into largely indoor household settings (through immigration of cats and rodents) will tend to be less than in farmyard settings.

Similar arguments can be made for the other candidate pathogens listed in Table 2. The control of polio through vaccination serves as a model for the control of amyotrophic lateral sclerosis through vaccination against its candidate enterovirus agent.

Integrating knowledge across the entire spectrum of human disease may lead to recognition of the cost effectiveness of interventions to control any particular disease. This effect occurs because the expected benefit that is necessary to discover and justify an effective intervention against a particular disease needs be less if the target pathogen is known to cause other diseases; for example, the knowledge that *T. gondii* causes birth defects, miscarriages and blindness should reinforce *T. gondii* vaccination for the purpose of preventing schizophrenia. Vaccination against Epstein-Barr virus and *C. pneumoniae* may similarly resolve not only those neurological diseases listed in Table 2 but several other serious diseases as well, such as some breast cancers and lymphomas in the case of Epstein-Barr virus, and atherosclerosis, rheumatoid arthritis, and asthma in the case of *C. pneumoniae*.

4.4. Future Options

The history of infectious causation of neurological disease has proceeded in concert with the recognition of infectious causation in general. Research has identified infectious causes that are most conspicuously infectious first, and those that are less conspicuously caused by infection later as perspectives broaden and skills at detection improve. Medical experts recognized that neurosyphilis, shingles, rabies, and poliomyelitis were infectious neurological diseases early during application of the germ theory of disease, because these diseases are conspicuously associated with an acute phase of disease. Medical experts recognized that tropical spastic paraparesis and progressive multifocal leukoencephalopathy were infectious diseases much later, because the infectious causation of these diseases is much more cryptic. Unlike neurosyphilis, shingles, and poliomyelitis, neither tropical spastic paraparesis or progressive multifocal leukoencephalopathy can be linked to a symptomatic acute phase of illness; the chain of infectious transmission is therefore less apparent.

Although researchers have interpreted familial patterns as evidence of genetic causation for common severe neurological diseases, the familial patterns can often be explained as well or better by infectious causation. Some of the most important of these neurological diseases, such as schizophrenia, are already linked to candidate pathogens (Table 2), but are not considered in discussions of emerging diseases. For others, such as autism and bipolar disorder, epidemiological patterns suggest infectious causation, but there has been almost no effort to identify and evaluate candidate pathogens. Considering that these chronic illnesses are vastly more damaging than the most damaging diseases that meet a more narrow definition of "emerging" (e.g., the acute phases of illness caused by West Nile virus and Lyme disease; see Table 4), it would be wise for any general strategy for controlling emerging neurological diseases to encompass emerging recognition of infectious causes of diseases that have been long established in human populations. Otherwise researchers may be like the fire fighter who conscientiously extinguishes a camp fire while the surrounding forest is ablaze.

ACKNOWLEDGMENTS

I am grateful to Gregory M. Cochran and Levi G. Ledgerwood for their contributions to ideas presented in this chapter.

REFERENCES

1. Bianchine PJ, Russo TA. The role of epidemic infectious diseases in the discovery of America. Allergy Proc 1992; 13:225–232.
2. Guerra F. The European–American exchange. Hist Philos Life Sci 1993; 15:313–327.
3. Rothschild BM, Calderon FL, Coppa A, Rothschild C. First European exposure to syphilis: the Dominican Republic at the time of Columbian contact. Clin Infect Dis 2000; 31:936–941.
4. Johnson RT, Irani DN. West Nile virus encephalitis in the United States. Curr Neurol Neurosci Rep 2002; 2:496–500.
5. Roehrig JT, Layton M, Smith P, Campbell GL, Nasci R, Lanciotti RS. The emergence of West Nile virus in North America: ecology, epidemiology, and surveillance. Curr Top Microbiol Immunol 2002; 267:223–240.

6. Nedry M, Mahon CR. West Nile virus: an emerging virus in North America. Clin Lab Sci 2003; 16:43–49.
7. Centers for Disease Control. Probable locally acquired mosquito-transmitted *Plasmodium vivax* infection—Suffolk County, New York, 1999. Morb Mortal Wkly Rep 2000; 49:495–498.
8. Sunstrum J, Elliott LJ, Barat LM, Walker ED, Zucker JR. Probable autochthonous *Plasmodium vivax* malaria transmission in Michigan: case report and epidemiological investigation. Am J Trop Med Hyg 2001; 65:949–953.
9. Reiter P, Lathrop S, Bunning M, Biggerstaff B, Singer D, Tiwari T, Baber L, Amador M, Thirion J, Hayes J, Seca C, Mendez J, Ramirez B, Robinson J, Rawlings J, Vorndam V, Waterman S, Gubler D, Clark G, Hayes E. Texas lifestyle limits transmission of dengue virus. Emerg Infect Dis 2003; 9:86–89.
10. http://www.cdc.gov/flu/about/disease.htm..
11. Korber B, Muldoon M, Theiler J, Gao F, Gupta R, Lapedes A, Hahn BH, Wolinsky S, Bhattacharya T. Timing the ancestor of the HIV-1 pandemic strains. Science 2000; 288:1789–1796.
12. Santiago ML, Rodenburg CM, Kamenya S, Bibollet-Ruche F, Gao F, Bailes E, Meleth S, Soong SJ, Kilby JM, Moldoveanu Z, Fahey B, Muller MN, Ayouba A, Nerrienet E, McClure HM, Heeney JL, Pusey AE, Collins DA, Boesch C, Wrangham RW, Goodall J, Sharp PM, Shaw GM, Hahn BH. SIVcpz in wild chimpanzees. Science 2002; 295:465.
13. Ewald PW. Plague Time. New York: Free Press, 2000.
14. Cochran GM, Ewald PW, Cochran KD. Infectious causation of disease: an evolutionary perspective. Perspect Biol Med 2000; 43:406–448.
15. Berger MM, Kopp N, Vital C, Redl B, Aymard M, Lina B. Detection and cellular localization of enterovirus RNA sequences in spinal cord of patients with ALS. Neurology 2000; 54:20–25.
16. Nicolson GL, Nasralla MY, Haier J, Pomfret J. High frequency of systemic mycoplasmal infections in Gulf War veterans and civilians with amyotrophic lateral sclerosis (ALS). J Clin Neurosci 2002; 9:525–529.
17. Cermelli C, Vinceti M, Beretti F, Pietrini V, Nacci G, Pietrosemoli P, Bartoletti A, Guidetti D, Sola P, Bergomi M, Vivoli G, Portolani M. Risk of sporadic amyotrophic lateral sclerosis associated with seropositivity for herpesviruses and echovirus-7. Eur J Epidemiol 2003; 18:123–127.
18. Balin BJ, Gérard HC, Arking EJ, et al. Identification and localization of *Chlamydia pneumoniae* in the Alzheimer's brain. Med Microbiol Immunol (Berl) 1998; 187:23–42.
19. Lin WR, Wozniak MA, Cooper RJ, Wilcock GK, Itzhaki RF. Herpesviruses in brain and Alzheimer's disease. J Pathol 2002; 197:395–402.
20. Swanborg RH, Whittum-Hudson JA, Hudson AP. Infectious agents and multiple sclerosis—are *Chlamydia pneumoniae* and human herpes virus 6 involved? J Neuroimmunol 2003; 136:1–8.
21. Haahr S, Munch M. The association between multiple sclerosis and infection with Epstein–Barr virus and retrovirus. J Neurovirol 2000; 6(suppl 2):76–79.
22. Levin LI, Munger KL, Rubertone MV, Peck CA, Lennette ET, Spiegelman D, Ascherio A. Multiple sclerosis and Epstein–Barr virus. JAMA 2003; 289:1533–1536.

23. Buka SL. Potential applications of the National Collaborative Perinatal Project for the study of toxoplasma infections and psychiatric disease. Presented at the Stanley Symposium—Johns Hopkins University meeting "*Toxoplasma* Infection and Schizophrenia," November, 2000, Annapolis, MD, 2000.

24. Ledgerwood LG, Ewald PW, Cochran GM. Genes, germs, and schizophrenia: an evolutionary perspective. Perspect Biol Med 2003; 46:317–348.

25. Yolken RH, Karlsson H, Yee F, Johnston-Wilson NL, Torrey EF. Endogenous retroviruses and schizophrenia. Brain Res Brain Res Rev 2000; 31:193–199.

26. Yolken RH, et al. Antibodies to Toxoplasma gondii in individuals with first-episode schizophrenia. Clin Infect Dis 2001; 32:842–844.

27. Torrey EF, Yolken RH. *Toxoplasma gondii* and schizophrenia. Emerg Infect Dis 2003; 9:1375–1380.

28. Waltrip RW II, Buchanan RW, Carpenter WT Jr, Kirkpatrick B, Summerfelt A, Breier A, Rubin SA, Carbone KM. Borna disease virus antibodies and the deficit syndrome of schizophrenia. Schizophr Res 1997; 23:253–258.

29. Iwahashi K, Watanabe M, Nakamura K, Suwaki H, Nakaya T, Nakamura Y, Takahashi H, Ikuta K. Positive and negative syndromes, and Borna disease virus infection in schizophrenia. Neuropsychobiology 1998; 37:59–64.

30. Dietrich DE, Schedlowski M, Bode L, et al. A viro-psycho-immunological disease—model of a subtype affective disorder. Pharmacopsychiatry 1998; 31:77–82.

31. Morgan M, Nathwani D. Facial palsy and infection: the unfolding story. Clin Infect Dis 1992; 14:263–271.

32. Morgan M, Moffat M, Ritchie L, Collacott I, Brown T. Is Bell's palsy a reactivation of varicella zoster virus? J Infect 1995; 30:29–36.

33. Schirm J, Mulkens PS Bell's palsy and herpes simplex virus. APMIS 1997; 105:815–823.

34. Volter C, Helms J, Weissbrich B, Rieckmann P, Abele-Horn M. Frequent detection of Mycoplasma pneumoniae in Bell's palsy. Eur Arch Otorhinolaryngol 2003. In press.

35. Smith DE. Lyme disease: the cause, diagnosis, and treatment. Clin Lab Sci 1994; 7:286–288.

36. Snider LA, Swedo SE. Post-streptococcal autoimmune disorders of the central nervous system. Curr Opin Neurol 2003; 16:359–365.

37. Vilchez RA, Kozinetz CA, Arrington AS, Madden CR, Butel JS. Simian virus 40 in human cancers. Am J Med 2003; 114:675–684.

38. Lyngberg KK, Vennervald BJ, Bygbjerg IC, Hansen TM, Thomsen OO. Toxoplasma pericarditis mimicking systemic lupus erythematosus. Diagnostic and treatment difficulties in one patient. Ann Med 1992; 24:337–340.

39. James JA, Neas BR, Moser KL, Hall T, Bruner GR, Sestak AL, Harley JB. Systemic lupus erythematosus in adults is associated with previous Epstein–Barr virus exposure. Arthritis Rheum 2001; 44:1122–1126.

40. Kawamoto R, Kajiwara T, Oka Y, Takagi Y. An association between an antibody against Chlamydia pneumoniae and ischemic stroke in elderly Japanese. Intern Med 2003; 42:571–575.

41. Lindsberg PJ, Grau AJ. Inflammation and infections as risk factors for ischemic stroke. 2003; 34:2518–2532.

42. Bucurescu G, Stieritz DD Evidence of an association between *Chlamydia pneumoniae* and cerebrovascular accidents. Eur J Neurol 2003; 10:449–452.

43. Douche-Aourik F, Berlier W, Feasson L, Bourlet T, Harrath R, Omar S, Grattard F, Denis C, Pozzetto B. Detection of enterovirus in human skeletal muscle from patients with chronic inflammatory muscle disease or fibromyalgia and healthy subjects. J Med Virol 2003; 71:540–547.

44. Endresen GK. *Mycoplasma* blood infection in chronic fatigue and fibromyalgia syndromes. Rheumatol Int 2003; 23:211–215.

45. Kerr JR, Bracewell J, Laing I, Mattey DL, Bernstein RM, Bruce IN, Tyrrell DA. Chronic fatigue syndrome and arthralgia following parvovirus B19 infection. J Rheumatol 2002; 29:595–602.

46. Nicolson GL, Gan R, Haier J. Multiple co-infections (*Mycoplasma, Chlamydia,* human herpes virus-6) in blood of chronic fatigue syndrome patients: association with signs and symptoms. APMIS 2003; 111:557–566.

47. Centers for Disease Control. Lyme disease—United States. Morb Mortal Rep 2000; 57(2):29–31.

48. Arias E, Smith BL. Deaths: preliminary data for 2001. Natl Vital Stat Rep 2003; 51(5):1–44.

49. Caldwell CB, Gottesman II. Schizophrenics kill themselves too: a review of risk factors for suicide Schizophr Bull 1990; 16:571–589.

50. Kelly BD, O'Callaghan E, Lane A, Larkin C. Schizophrenia: solving the puzzle. Ir J Med Sci 2003; 172:37–40.

51. Hiroch U, Appleby L, Mortensen PB, Dunn G. Death by homicide, suicide, and other unnatural causes in people with mental illness: a population-based study. Lancet 2001; 358:2110–2112.

52. National Institute of Neurological Disorders and Stroke. http://www.ninds.nih.gov/health_and_medical/pubs/als.htm.

53. http://www.doh.gov.uk/cmo/annualreport2002/westnile.htm.

54. National Institute of Neurological Disorders and Stroke. http://www.ninds.nih.gov/health_and_medical/disorders/lyme_doc.htm.

55. Gardner T. Lyme disease. In: Remington J, Klein J, eds. Infectious Diseases of the Fetus and Newborn Infant. Philadelphia, PA: W.B. Saunders, 2001:519–641.

56. Harvey WT, Salvato P. 'Lyme disease': ancient engine of an unrecognized borreliosis pandemic? Med Hypotheses 2003; 60:742–759.

57. Matsumoto H, et al. Superior temporal gyrus abnormalities in early-onset schizophrenia: Similarities and differences with adult-onset schizophrenia. Am J Psychiatry 2001; 158:1299–1304.

58. Shenton ME, et al. A review of MRI findings in schizophrenia. Schizophr Res 2001; 49:1–52.

59. Curtis CE, et al. Saccadic disinhibition in patients with acute and remitted schizophrenia and their first-degree biological relatives. Am J Psychiatry 2001; 158:100–106.

60. Holliman RE. Toxoplasmosis, behaviour and personality. J Infect 1997; 35:105–110.

61. Jackson MH, Hutchison WM. The prevalence and source of Toxoplasma infection in the environment. Adv Parasitol 1989; 28:55–105.

62. Berdoy M, Webster JP, MacDonald DW. Fatal attraction in rats infected with Toxoplasma gondii. Proc R Soc Lond B Biol Sci 2000; 267:1591–1594.

63. Hill D, Dubey JP. *Toxoplasma gondii*: transmission, diagnosis and prevention. Clin Microbiol Infect 2002; 8:634–640.

64. Terragna A, Morandi N, Canessa A, Pellegrino C. The occurrence of *Toxoplasma gondii* in saliva. Tropenmed Parasitol 1984; 35:9–10.

65. Hotson JR. Modern neurosyphilis: a partially treated chronic meningitis. West J Med 1981; 135:191–200.

66. Shadick NA, Phillips CB, Logigian EL, et al. The long-term clinical outcomes of Lyme disease. Ann Intern Med 1994; 121:560–567.

67. Balcer LJ, Winterkorn JM, Galetta SL. Neuro-ophthalmic manifestations of Lyme disease. J Neuroophthalmol 1997 17:108–121.

68. Fallon BA, Kochevar JM, Gaito A, Nields JA. The underdiagnosis of neuropsychiatric Lyme disease in children and adults. Psychiatr Clin North Am 1998; 21:693–703.

69. Pachner AR. Neurologic manifestations of Lyme disease, the new "great imitator". Rev Infect Dis 1989; 11(suppl 6):1482–1486.

70. Burdash N, Fernandes J. Lyme borreliosis: detecting the great imitator. J Am Osteopath Assoc 1991; 91:573–574, 577–578.

71. Kursawe HK Diagnosis and therapy of neuroborreliosis. On the hunt for the "great imitator". MMW Fortschr Med 2000; 144:33–36.

72. Rullan E, Sigal LH. Rheumatic fever. Curr Rheumatol Rep 2001; 3:445–452.

73. Hilario MO, Terreri MT. Rheumatic fever and post-streptococcal arthritis. Best Pract Res Clin Rheumatol 2002; 16:481–494.

74. Villareal C, Whittum-Hudson JA, Hudson AP. Persistent Chlamydiae and chronic arthritis. Arthritis Res 2002; 4:5–9.

75. Lemanske RF. Is asthma an infectious disease? Thomas A. Neff lecture. Chest 2003; 123(suppl):385–390.

76. Klein C, Kimiagar I, Pollak L, Gandelman-Marton R, Itzhaki A, Milo R, Rabey JM. Neurological features of West Nile virus infection during the 2000 outbreak in a regional hospital in Israel. J Neurol Sci 2002; 200:63–66.

77. Pepperell C, Rau N, Krajden S, Kern R, Humar A, Mederski B, Simor A, Low DE, McGeer A, Mazzulli T, Burton J, Jaigobin C, Fearon M, Artsob H, Drebot MA, Halliday W, Brunton J. West Nile virus infection in 2002: morbidity and mortality among patients admitted to hospital in southcentral Ontario. CMAJ 2003; 168:1399–1405.

78. Leis AA, Stokic DS, Webb RM, Slavinski SA, Fratkin J. Clinical spectrum of muscle weakness in human West Nile virus infection. Muscle Nerve 2003; 28:302–308.

79. Ewald PW. Evolution of Infectious Disease. New York: Oxford University Press, 1994.

80. Mateus-Pinilla NE, et al. 1999. A field trial of the effectiveness of a feline *Toxoplasma gondii* vaccine in reducing T. gondii exposure for swine. J Parasitol 85:855–860.

19

Immediate Responses to New Infections and the Rapid Development of a Vaccine Strategy

**Edwina J. Wright, Catriona A. McLean, and
Steven L. Wesselingh**

*Department of Medicine, Monash University, Melbourne, Australia
and Macfarlane Burnet Institute for Medical Research
and Public Health, Melbourne, Australia*

1. INTRODUCTION

As we have experienced with the recent epidemic of the virulent coronavirus (SARS), new pathogens will continue to challenge us. New pathogens that infect the nervous system provide even greater challenges to clinicians and medical researchers because of the inherent difficulties in the diagnosis and treatment of central nervous system (CNS) infections. In this chapter, we have attempted to provide a guide to the immediate response to a new neurological infectious disease challenge. What would be required to identify and treat affected individuals appropriately and what is required to protect the public. We have also examined the potential for the rapid development of protective vaccines, as ultimately, a vaccination program is the most effective and efficient public health strategy.

2. NEW NEUROLOGICAL INFECTIONS

When confronted by a patient with an undiagnosed CNS infection the clinician may rightly assume that the likeliest cause is a common pathogen that will be identified with further observation and testing of the patient.

In exceptional circumstances, however, the clinician may be dealing with a new infectious disease that is due to: 1) an entirely novel, unknown pathogen, 2) a known pathogen not previously associated with CNS involvement, or 3) a known CNS pathogen not previously encountered in the region, or country. Recent examples of these three scenarios are displayed in Table 1.

2.1. Recognition of a New Neurological Infection

2.1.1. The Role of Individual Clinicians, Disease Registries, Public Health Authorities, and Active Surveillance

Individual clinicians including general practitioners, pediatricians, neurologists, infectious diseases physicians and psychiatrists may be the first to recognize an

Table 1 New Infectious Disease

New infectious disease with CNS involvement	Examples
The infection is due to a newly described pathogen, or due to a pathogen that has not been described previously in humans	Austrlian at lyssavirus infection Australian bat lyssavirus infection causing encephalitis with a rabies-like illness (1) Hendra virus causing encephalitis (2) Nipah virus causing encephalitis (3) Exposure to bovine spongiform encephalopathy agent causing variant Creutzfeldt-Jakob disease (4)
The infection is due to a known pathogen not previously known to involve the nervous system	Epidemic of enterovirus 71 causing neurological disease in children in Bulgaria in 1975 (5) Subsequent outbreaks in Malaysia, Taiwan, and Australia
The infection is due to a known pathogen that has not previously been described in the region/country	Appearance of West Nile virus in the United States (6,7) Appearance of West Nile virus in the United States (6, 7) Appearance of Japanese B encephalitis virus virus in mainland Australia (8)

unfamiliar CNS infectious disease in their patients. Laboratory scientists and infection control practitioners may also note an increase in unusual, or unidentifiable isolates obtained from patients' blood cultures or cerebrospinal fluid within their institution (9).

The importance of reporting unexplained infectious diseases to registries and health departments cannot be overstated. City and State health departments are positioned to observe the common features between individual case reports of unusual infectious diseases and to observe a clustering, or an outbreak of similar cases.

In addition, reporting ostensibly familiar CNS infections may lead to the discovery of a new infectious disease syndrome: in August 1999 an infectious diseases physician from a hospital in Queens, New York reported two patients with encephalitis whose preliminary tests suggested a diagnosis of St Louis Virus encephalitis (6). Subsequently these cases were recognized as the first case reports of West Nile virus (WNV) infection in the United States (7,10).

The failure of notification systems may increase the likelihood that new CNS infectious syndromes will go unrecognized. A recent report from the United Kingdom found that hospitalizations due to viral encephalitis were largely under-reported through both clinical and laboratory notification systems (11). This report also identified six possible clusters of encephalitis of unknown etiology, prompting the authors to ask, "What did we miss?" and to conclude that the extant notification systems in the United Kingdom would fail to recognize the emergence of a new infectious disease.

Active surveillance is important because it can provide evidence to support a causal link between an infectious agent and a specific disease. An example of this was the surveillance of CJD that was established in 1990 by the National CJD Surveillance Unit in the United Kingdom following an epidemic of bovine spongiform encephalopathy (BSE) in cattle. This surveillance led to the first reports, in 1996, of new variant Creutzfeldt–Jakob disease an illness that has been strongly linked to exposure to the agent that causes BSE (4).

More recently the importance of active surveillance for infectious diseases was highlighted following reports of fatal neurodegenerative illnesses in three men who had participated in wild game feasts during the 1990s. Whilst only one man was found to have CJD at postmortem, continued surveillance is ongoing to determine whether there may be a link between CJD and chronic wasting disease (CWD) which, like CJD, is a transmissible spongiform encephalopathy that occurs in deer and elk (12).

2.2. Situations Where New Infectious Diseases Are Likely to be Recognized and Reported

In the setting of threatened, or active bioterrorism, new infections with a predilection for CNS involvement may be recognized by medical practitioners and reported to health authorities. Practitioners may also encounter recognized, albeit rare, CNS infectious diseases including anthrax meningoencephalitis (13) and CNS clostridium botulinum infection following bioterrorist deployment of these pathogens.

A new infectious syndrome may be more readily recognized when a concomitant illness in animals and in the humans who have close contact with them occurs. A recent example of this involved Malaysian pig farmers (3) and Singaporean abattoir workers (14) who developed a systemic illness and encephalitis following exposure to secretions from sick pigs who were infected with a novel paramyxovirus, dubbed the Nipah virus.

Overall a new infectious disease that involves the nervous system stands a greater chance of being detected if the pathogen causes an illness with a high attack rate and a dramatic and rapidly progressive clinical course. As a corollary a new but sporadic and indolent infection involving the CNS could go largely unrecognized for many years. This would be further compounded if the infection predominantly caused psychiatric symptoms.

2.3. Clues to the Possibility of a New Neurological Infectious Disease in an Outbreak Situation

In an outbreak where patients are presenting with an infection of the nervous system there may be some clues indicating that the cause of the outbreak is a new infectious disease.

These clues include: 1) experienced clinicians including infectious diseases physicians, microbiologists, virologists, neurologists and intensive care specialists are unable to recognize the illness; 2) the illness pattern is very uncommon in the age group of the affected patients, for example, young people presenting with a dementing type illness, or elderly people presenting with a chicken-pox, or measles-like illness (15); 3) the illness resembles an illness for which the patients/ the general population have been vaccinated, for example, a polio-, or measles-like illness; 4) the attack-rate or clustering of the disease is entirely uncharacteristic for any known neurotropic pathogen; 5) other clues including the rapidity of the illness progression, the failure to respond to empiric antibiotic or antiviral therapy and absence of diagnostic laboratory features.

3. CLINICAL APPROACH TO THE IDENTIFICATION OF A NEW INFECTIOUS DISEASE IN AN INDIVIDUAL PATIENT

The important aspects that should be ascertained in the history of an individual who has an unusual or undiagnosed neurological infection are outlined in Table 2.

3.1. Clinical Examination

A thorough clinical examination should be undertaken and documented for all patients presenting with an undiagnosed neurological infectious disease. If the patient is alert and cooperative a thorough neurological examination should be made including an assessment of mental status. Subtle evidence of CNS infection may include psychiatric symptoms, which are notably very common in the early stages of variant CJD (20), and symptoms suggestive of a dementing illness. In addition evidence should be sought for involvement of other organ systems including the presence of rash and arthritis.

3.2. Investigations

3.2.1. Blood Tests

Blood should be drawn for full blood examination, urea and electrolytes, liver function tests, serological testing and for viral and bacterial culture. Where possible cerebrospinal fluid should be obtained and sent for microscopy, culture and for PCR analysis for enteroviruses and herpes viruses. CSF should be stored for future analysis. Throat and nasal swabs and fecal and urine samples should be sent for viral culture.

In the setting of an outbreak determining whether respiratory secretions, feces and urine are culture-positive for the pathogen is very important because it will help to guide infection control practices both within the hospital and the home environments. This was borne out with the Nipah virus epidemic where the determination that Nipah virus can be isolated from the upper respiratory tract and the urine shaped the infection control policies throughout the epidemic (21).

The microbiology laboratory should be asked to treat any organism that is cultured from blood or CSF as a potential pathogen to avoid the risk that the isolate would be dismissed as a contaminant.

If a virus or bacteria is isolated, but cannot be identified by a laboratory the isolate should be sent to a state or federal reference laboratory for further testing.

3.2.2. Neuroimaging

Computer tomography (CT) or magnetic resonance imaging (MRI) of the brain or spinal cord is useful to determine the type of pattern of damage, e.g., whether the process is one of demyelination, or vasculitis, or abscess-formation and the site of the infectious process (white or grey matter, basal ganglia, periventricular, meningeal).

3.2.3. Electroencephalogram, Electromyelogram, and Nerve Conduction Studies

In the setting where the patient's illness is not rapidly progressive further testing may be possible to help elucidate the underlying process. For example, electroencephalogram (EEG) testing may be of some use in an encephalitic patient and electromyelogram (EMG) and nerve conduction studies (NCS) may be useful also. A recent example of the usefulness of EMG/NCS was demonstrated when a group of six patients with WNV infection who had developed acute flaccid paralysis were found to have a pathological process involving their anterior horn cells and motor axons (22).

4.   ROLE OF THE NEUROPATHOLOGIST

The role of the neuropathologist in an emerging encephalitis is best perceived as part of a multi-disciplinary approach, involving beside clinicians and molecular pathologists. Adopting a best practice for tissue analysis and storage is essential and an immediate database should be put in place, with all digital images of the macroscopic and microscopic sections made readily available to colleagues. In a situation where diagnostic speed maybe of the essence, this combined approach may provide the fastest diagnosis and allow commencement of appropriate therapy for the individual and prophylactic measures for limiting further spread of disease.

Tissue pathology remains central to understanding the pathogenesis of disease. Preparation of tissue is inexpensive and examination of brain tissue will quickly lead to an overview of the inflammatory nature and micro-anatomical distribution of the process. In the circumstance of a potentially new and infective CNS disease process, brain biopsy and postmortem tissue analysis would be essential.

4.1.   Diagnostic Value of Brain Biopsies and Postmortem Examinations

By their very nature, brain biopsies may be of limited value as they are usually dependent on examination of sections taken from the non-dominant frontal lobe and hence may not represent the topographic extent of disease. An autopsy is much more likely to offer the relevant pathology. Most or all cases with a similar clinical phenotype should be examined for comparison between cases. Patients who have died within a short time of the disease onset are especially important to examine at postmortem as they may show a different cellular response and/or contain visible inclusions or organisms that may no longer be present in patients whose illness was of longer duration.

4.2.   Processing Fresh Tissue and Procedures for Tissue Fixation

Due to the unknown potential infectivity at the time of the initial brain biopsies or postmortems, precautions as per protocols for infectious diseases should be adopted in the laboratory. The decision to utilize fresh tissue should be made in consultation with infectious disease physicians and molecular pathologists. Immediate fixation of residual brain tissue in 10% formaldehyde (for 24 hr) for brain biopsies and 20% formaldehyde (for 10 days) for postmortem tissue with routine processing is advised.

4.3. Tissue Staining and Other Diagnostic Techniques

For both brain biopsy and brain tissue from postmortem the recommended initial stains include hematoxylin and eosin, Luxol fast blue (to detect demyelination), Bielschowsky (to detect axonal damage), gram stain and Periodic Acid Schiff (to detect accumulation of glycoproteins of varying nature, including yeast, fungal hyphae and parasitic cyst wall and evidence of vessel wall destruction). Inclusion bodies should be carefully looked for and routine immunoperoxidase techniques for known viral encephalitides performed if considered appropriate, including those for cytomegalovirus (CMV), herpes simplex, and polyoma virus. Once tissue is embedded in paraffin, sections can also been taken for PCR analysis for detection of specific organisms as available. Following initial examination, the cell types should be qualified with immunoperoxidase studies used for further definition where necessary, including those for T&B lymphocytes, macrophages, microglia and astrocytes. These studies collectively will delineate the cellular and tissue response to the infectious agent. This will help categorize the infective organism.

With the potential for international recognition of the pathology, images could be produced and delivered via the Internet to neuropathologists worldwide for comment and opinion.

5. DEVELOPING A CASE DEFINITION IN THE SETTING OF AN OUTBREAK OF A NEW CENTRAL NERVOUS SYSTEM INFECTION

5.1. Case Definition

In an outbreak setting developing a case definition for a new neurological infectious disease may improve the identification rate of patients who are in the early stages of the disease. In turn, therefore, patients may receive earlier monitoring and treatment. This occurred in the Nipah virus encephalitis outbreak where patients were considered as potentially infected with the (then) unknown pathogen if they were pig farmers and had developed non-specific constitutional symptoms. Such patients were admitted to hospital for observation as it was not uncommon for patients to require ventilatory and intensive care support within hours of presenting with only modest symptoms (A. Kamarulzaman, personal communication).

Table 2 History of Patients

History	Comment
Travel history	Following recent travel a patient may have acquired an entirely novel infection, or an infection that is exotic to the region
Exposure to animals	It is key to establish whether a patient has had significant, or unusual contact with animals.
Occupational exposure • Veterinarian or veterinary nurse • Animal carer/ trainer • Farmer • Abattoir worker • Scientist	If contact with animals has occurred establish whether patient sustained bites or scratches from the animal, whether patient was exposed to the animal's blood, or other secretions and whether the exposure was percutaneous (e.g., a bite), or involved exposure to mucous membranes, or to non-intact skin, or wounds.
Casual exposure • Visit to farm or zoo Owner of exotic animals	Note that new zoonoses may have long incubation periods, e.g., patient developed and died from infection with Australian Bat Lyssa virus 27 months after bite from flying fox (16) For example, monkeys, reptiles
Exposure to sick animals	Recent examples where exposure to secretions and tissues from sick animals has led to new infections involving the nervous system include • Equine morbilliform virus (sick horses) (2) • Nipah virus (sick pigs) (3)
Exposure to sick person	It is important to establish whether the patient has had contact in the recent past with another person who has also experienced a neurological illness, e.g., encephalitis, meningitis, polyneuropathy, etc.
Ingestions of animal products	New variant Creutzfeldt–Jakob disease is an example of a disease that may occur following ingestion of beef from cattle that were infected with agent of BSE. Recent cases of fatal human neurodegenerative disease following ingestion of wild game animals has not established causal link but highlights importance of establishing a history of animal exposure

Unusual dietary intake of insects, molluscs or mammals	Patients who have been incarcerated, or living in conditions of extreme poverty, or travellers who have eaten exotic dishes may have ingested insects, molluscs, rodents and other mammals from which the infectious agent may have been acquired
Exposure to arthropods	A recent important example of an arthropod-acquired infection that involves the CNS and is entirely new to a country (the United States) is the West -Nile Virus virus infection that occurs following a bite from infected mosquitoes
Vaccination history	If a patient has been vaccinated against an infection that causes CNS disease, this helps to refine the differential diagnosis. For example, the first three patients who died from Nipah virus encephalitis had recently received at least two doses of the JE vaccine (3) making the diagnosis of JE less plausible.
	A history of recent immunization with a live-attenuated vaccine is also important. There are recent case reports (17, 18, –19) of patients who developed a yellow-fever like illness following vaccination with the 17D-204 yellow fever vaccine. One of these patients became encephalitic and yellow fever virus was subsequently isolated from both his serum and CSF (18).
Medications including naturopathic and homeopathic medication	These may serve as potential sources of new infectious agents
Receipt of human tissue grafts, organs, blood or plasma products, breast milk and extracts from human tissue.	HIV infection has been well documented to occur following exposure to human organs, blood products and grafts. CJD has occurred following exposure to human pituitary gland and dura mater grafts infected with agent of CJD.
Receipt of animal tissue, organs or grafts	Transplantation of animal organs into humans theoretically may lead to new infectious diseases in humans

In situations where the neurological infectious disease is more slowly progressive a case definition may require that epidemiological, clinical, serological, virological and histopathological criteria be met.

5.2. Establishing Causality

Following the isolation of an organism a causal link between the organism and the disease should be established based upon epidemiological criteria (24). However causality may take many years to prove: a debate still exists regarding the causal link between the BSE prion and variant CJD (23,24).

In the immediate outbreak setting not all criteria may be met to prove causality, but health and government practitioners often need to accept the available evidence and make decisions that may be costly to humans, animals, industry and the country's economy, e.g., the widespread slaughter of cattle, pigs and poultry that have followed the CJD, Nipah and Avian Flu virus epidemics, respectively, in the last decade.

6. TREATMENT

6.1. Supportive Therapy

The management of very sick patients with an undiagnosed infection of the nervous system requires an interdisciplinary approach that includes intensive care physicians, neurologists and infectious disease physicians. Individual patients may require supportive therapy that includes intravenous fluids, blood products (red cell transfusions, fresh frozen plasma and platelets) inotropic and ventilatory support. Plasma exchange may also be required.

6.2. Empiric Antibacterial and Antiviral Therapy

Empiric therapy may be commenced for suspected bacterial, or viral CNS infections. Empiric antibiotic therapy should be comprised of agents with good CSF penetration that have broad activity against aerobes, anaerobes and intracellular pathogens. In an outbreak setting where bioterrorism is being deployed antibiotic therapy should include agents active against clostridium botulinum and Yersinia pestis. As a corollary, empiric antiviral therapy should include agents with good CSF penetration and broad antiviral activity.

An example of a combined empiric antibacterial and antiviral regimen that could be used in *adult* patients who have an undiagnosed, severe CNS illness is the combination of meropenem 500–1000 mg intravenously tds plus ribavirin 30 mg/kg intravenously as a loading dose then 16 mg/kg intravenously every 6 hr for 4 days, then 8 mg/kg every 8 hr for 3 days (25) plus acyclovir 10 mg/kg intravenously every 8 hr. The addition of doxycycline 100 mg every 12 hr to this empiric regimen would cover both anthrax and tularemia in the setting of active, or threatened bioterrorism.

6.3. Directed Antiviral Therapy

Table 3 outlines various antiviral agents that may be used in an outbreak situation including their antiviral spectrum of activity, CSF penetration and published doses that have been used to treat humans with various viral encephalitides.

6.4. Anti-prion Agents

Anti-prion agents that are currently under review include the antimalarial drug quinacrine and the antipsychotic agent chlorpromazine (38).

6.5. Passive Immunization

Recent case reports have documented the successful use of intravenous immunoglobulin therapy for treatment of WNV infection in immunosuppressed patients (39,40). It should be noted that the immunoglobulin described in both case reports came from the same batches that were derived from Israeli donors and had high titers of neutralizing antibodies against WNV.

6.6. Postexposure Prophylaxis

In an outbreak setting persons in close contact with confirmed cases should be considered for postexposure prophylaxis. Table 3 outlines various agents that may be considered for use in an outbreak situation including their antiviral spectrum of activity.

6.7. Vaccination of Close Contacts

Recent case reports have documented the successful use of passive immunization, this therefore should be offered to close contacts in circumstances where the nature of etiologic organism is understood.

It has also been suggested that consideration should be given to the use of vaccines that are already licensed and available for closely related organisms. This needs very careful consideration as there is very limited evidence of this being successful and there is a risk of a partially protective vaccine leading to an atypical infection or even increased immunopathology (41).

7.   INFECTION CONTROL

7.1.   Caring for the Patient in Hospital

For individual patients who present to a hospital with an unidentified infectious disease involving the nervous system universal precautions should be employed when obtaining and handling blood and other fluids or secretions from the patient. Ideally such patients should be managed in a single room. The room should be negatively ventilated and staff should wear protective facemasks and goggles if there is evidence of intercurrent pulmonary disease (42).

In the setting of an outbreak of a suspected new infectious disease that involves the nervous system, if the disease has a high-attack and fatality rate and appears to be spread by person-to-person transmission then infection control measures should meet the strict criteria established for the management of patients with other highly contagious, fatal diseases like viral hemorrhagic fever (42).

These measures include the employment of universal precautions, placing the patient in a single negatively ventilated room, wearing protective face and eye wear, wearing gowns and gloves when entering the patient's room and the use of personal protective respirators if there is the possibility of exposure to aerosolized infectious particles. Decontamination of clothing, objects and surfaces should be undertaken with a registered disinfected or diluted bleach. Soiled linens may be incinerated or autoclaved (42).

7.2.   Caring for the Patient at Home in a Quarantine Situation

In certain circumstances, well exemplified during the recent SARS epidemic (43), the use of quarantine measures may be employed that dictate that the infected patients are cared for at home. In these circumstances, the infection control procedures described above for hospital care should be employed in the home setting, where possible. In turn all up-to-date scientific information regarding the infectiveness of secretions and bodily fluids should continue to inform and modify infection control policies in the setting of an outbreak.

7.3.   Laboratory Precautions

Staff who are collecting and handling patient specimens in the laboratory should use Biological Safety Level II or III facilities and employ appropriate practices (8). These include the use of a BSL II laminar flow hoods, the use of protective eyewear, minimizing the creation of aerosols or droplets and decontaminating infected surfaces (42). Virus isolation must be undertaken at biosafety level 4 (42,44).

8. COORDINATION OF PUBLIC HEALTH, STATE, AND FEDERAL AUTHORITIES

Following September 11, 2001 a number of authors have addressed and devised strategies and paradigms to prepare communities for future bioterrorist attacks (15,45,46). The principals that underlie these strategies should be embraced to prepare for and manage infectious disease outbreaks, including those that result from bioterrorist activities.

In an article written on the preparation for a bioterrorist attack Hoffman observed that a key factor in the successful management of an outbreak, or disaster situation is the ability "for public health and medical experts to assist elected officials in analyzing and interpreting information about an outbreak and in coordinating the public health response to the outbreak" (45).

Key issues that should be considered include (45):

1. Establishing pathways for clear communication between hospitals, health authorities and the public in the setting of a disease outbreak. This includes providing information to health practitioners in the community with written information, information sent via emails or information that may be accessed through websites.
2. Ensuring that mechanisms are in place for accurate disease surveillance, including the capacity for contact-tracing.
3. A knowledge of local state health facilities and laboratories that have the capacity to handle and isolate highly contagious infectious pathogens.
4. Documentation of the availability and sources of antibiotic and antiviral agents.
5. Algorithms for the management of deceased patients including the location of hospitals and medical personnel who would be available to perform postmortems.
6. Knowledge of state legislation that pertains to the ability of state health authorities to adequately perform disease surveillance and investigate and manage an outbreak. This includes an understanding of the capacity to impose quarantine conditions on a community.

9. EDUCATION OF THE PUBLIC

In the initial stages of an outbreak of a new infectious, neurotropic agent, educating the public about the nature and likely cause of the outbreak and providing a management plan for the treatment of those affected and the prevention of further infection is paramount.

Table 3   Antiviral Agents

Agent and in vitro antiviral spectrum	CSF/plasma drug	Does used in treatment of different viral encephalitides
Acyclovir DNA viruses including Herpes simplex virusand varicella-zoster virus	0.3--0.5 (26)	*Herpes virus encephalitis* Adult intravenous regimen: 30 mg/kg/day in 3 three divided doses for 21 days (27) *Neonatal intravenous regimen*: 60 mg/kg/day in 3 three divided doses for 21 days (28) *Small-vessel varicella zoster virus encephalitis* Adult intravenous regimen: 15--30 mg/kg/day in divided doses for 10 days (or longer in immunocompromised patients) (29)
Ganciclovir DNA viruses including cytomegalovirus	25%--70% (30)	*Cytomegalovirus encephalitis* For immunosuppressed patients dual therapy with ganciclovir and foscarnet is recom-
Foscarnet DNA viruses including cytomegalovirus	Approx. 65% (32)	mended at the following doses (31): *Ganciclovir* Adult intravenous induction dose regimen: 5 mg/kg twice daily for 3--6 6 weeks *plus* *Foscarnet* Adult intravenous induction dose regimen: 90 mg/kg twice daily for 3--6 weeks
Ribavirin DNA and RNA viruses -myxo-, paramyxo-, arena-, bunya-, HSV, adeno-, pox- and retro- viruses (35). In vitro activity demon- strated against the fla- viviridae westWest- nile Nile virus (36), Nipah virus (26) and Hendra virus (26)	0.7 (33)	*Nipah virus encephalitis* Adults intravenous regimen: loading dose 30 mg/kg, 16 mg/kg every 6 hours for 4 days, then 8 mg/kg every 8 hours for 3 days (26) *Adult oral regimen*: 2 grams day 1, 1.2 grams tds days 2 to --4, 1.2 grams bd days 5 and 6, then 0.6 grams bd for a further 1 to --4 days (26)
Pleconaril Enteroviruses Rhinoviruses	In rat model high CNS concentra- tions of pleconaril were observed (34)	*Enteroviral encephalitis and chronic enterovi- ral meningoencephalitis* Adult oral regimen: 600 mg, or 1200 mg/day in three divided doses for 7--10 days (36) *Infant and child oral regimen*: 15 mg/kg/day in 3 three divided doses for 7--10 days (36, 37)

The media carry significant responsibility in this situation and need unfettered assistance from health authorities so that the media can provide ongoing accurate information and constructive analysis of the outbreak.

Interestingly the public may be largely counted upon to react with a calm, organized and civil response to a crisis situation such as an infectious diseases outbreak or a bioterrorist attack (48).

10. MANAGEMENT OF OUTBREAKS IN RESOURCE-POOR COUNTRIES

With fewer resources available to them, clinicians and health officials in resource-poor countries may take longer to detect and isolate a new, neurotropic infectious agent and have fewer therapeutic options available. Ideally resource-poor countries should have pre-existing links and extant strategies in place with resource-wealthy countries to enable the joint management of outbreaks in the resource-poor country.

International bodies exist to help identify and manage infectious disease outbreaks including the Global Outbreak Alert and Response Network *http://www.who.int/csr/outbreaknetwork/en/*. This network is auspiced by the World Health Organization and regularly works to contain outbreaks in resource-poor countries

11. RAPID DEVELOPMENT OF PROTECTIVE VACCINE STRATEGIES

Clearly the best way to protect the public from infectious disease is through vaccine strategies. However, most vaccines take 10–15 years of development and testing. We must therefore utilize new developments in molecular biology and genomics to start designing processes that can respond more rapidly to an emerging infectious disease threat to the public (47).

The prevention of infectious disease through the use of vaccines has been one of the most important public health achievements of the twentieth century. In the early part of the 1900s disease such as measles, diphtheria, polio, influenza and pertussis were responsible for millions of deaths among children and adults. As we enter the twenty-first century a substantial amount of infectious disease burden has been reduced in the developed world because of successes in vaccine development and immunization coverage (15).

The two most viable approaches to vaccine development will continue to be live attenuated vaccines, and purified recombinant or native subunit vaccines. These approaches are likely to be complemented by DNA vaccination (48,49). New innovative vaccine vectors will include modified bacterial vectors for the delivery of recombinant protein and DNA, viral vectors, edible oral vaccines based on transgenic plants, and even the possible use of insect vectors (47).

12. MODELS OF RAPID VACCINE DEVELOPMENT

The development of vaccines generally follows a relatively consistent path. Outlined below are the steps that may allow a more rapid development towards a vaccine strategy. There are clear choices along the way, however some pathogens provide limitations if they do not grow in vitro or if there is not an animal model.
Steps involved in the development of a vaccine are:

1. Identification of protective correlates.
2. Rapid identification of key immunogenic and protective antigens.
3. Animal models and use of surrogate markers of protection and safety.
4. Vaccine designs suitable for rapid development are:
   (a) Live attenuated
   (b) Subunit vaccine
   (c) DNA vaccine
   (d) Live vector.

12.1. Identification of Protective Correlates

In order to enable the rapid screening and development of vaccine candidates the protective correlates of wild type disease need to be ascertained. Neutralization, and killing assays can be easily and rapidly developed and utilized to identify both the kinetics and protective nature of the immune response to infection. For example antibodies raised to the H protein after infection with the wild-type measles virus (MV) have MV-neutralizing activity and correlate very well with immunological protection (50).

12.2. Rapid Identification of Key Immunogenic and Protective Antigens

The general availability of genomic sequences of viral and bacterial pathogens and the development of high throughput genomic and proteonomic screening can significantly reduce the time required to identify candidate vaccine antigen (51). Open reading frames of proteins expressed on the surface of pathogens or virulence factors can be quickly identified and screened (52). Rapid advances in bioinformatics have improved our capacity for in silico screening reducing the time needed for in vitro testing. Lead candidates can then be tested in animal models to examine the ability of antigens to elicit a protective immune response.

12.3 Animal Models and Use of Surrogate Markers of Protection and Safety

In vitro models of models of vaccine efficacy cannot at this point replace animal models. The development of animal models is also of critical importance as it is possible that vaccines designed to prevent new life-threatening infections (bioterrorism) may be approved for marketing on the basis of evidence of effectiveness derived from appropriate studies in animals, without well controlled efficacy studies in humans (53,54).

12.4. Vaccine Designs Suitable for Rapid Development

The most successful vaccines have been those that are cheap and easy to deliver, by scarification (vaccinia) or by oral administration (Sabin polio), or less optimally, as combination vaccines delivered by syringe (e.g. triple antigen, MMR). Paradoxically, the highly successful smallpox and polio vaccines are live attenuated viruses, which are sensitive to heat, and hence require some form of cold chain. Live attenuated vaccines tend to be inexpensive to manufacture and, formulate.

Cytotoxic T-cell induction has traditionally required the use of either live viruses or bacteria, vaccine vectors, or the formulation of the antigen in adjuvants which elicited significant site reactions. DNA vaccine technology has changed this. DNA vaccines can elicit cytotoxic T-cell in humans without the toxicity observed with highly active adjuvants. The relatively small number of high affinity T cells "primed" by DNA vaccination are frequently expanded in the vaccine recipient by providing an antigen "boost," most optimally in a form which is also effective at driving CD8+ T-cell proliferation, e.g., from an attenuated poxvirus. The "prime-boost" strategy has been widely adopted by groups seeking to develop new HIV vaccines, but is amenable for use in other cytotoxic T-cell-requiring vaccines (49,55).

The recent observation that attenuated Salmonellae can deliver DNA vaccines, in addition to recombinant proteins, has added momentum to the development of DNA vaccines with oral delivery possible (48).

Immunization strategies that combine different routes of administration or vaccine types frequently result in enhanced protective immune responses. Edible vaccines have considerable potential for use in such "prime-boost" strategies, particularly where multiple antigens or doses are required to induce immunity (56). For example, we found that a single-dose MV-H DNA inoculation followed by multiple MV-H boosters, delivered orally as a plant-derived vaccine, could induce significantly greater quantities of MV-neutralizing antibodies than vaccination with a DNA- or plant-derived vaccine alone. Neutralization titers up to 20 times greater than those considered protective in humans can be achieved (50).

Peptide polymerization, appears to both increase the potency and provide multivalency and can be used to address major technical issues such as immunogen polymorphism.

The significant advantage of the new vaccine strategies is the ease of inserting new antigens into the chosen vectors. With rapid identification of protective antigens these can be simply inserted into the appropriate vector for testing in an animal models.

13. REDUCING BLOCKS TO RAPID VACCINE DEVELOPMENT

13.1. Resources

New vaccine technology is often generated by academic or research institutes and licensed to small biotechnology firms. Such institutions need to both develop access to resources and skills and more quickly forge partnership with larger pharmaceutical companies to rapidly progress new vaccines.

Partnership development in developing country settings is crucial to success for the evaluation and implementation of new vaccines for diseases that predominate in less developed countries. Very significant delays in obtaining political, ethical and regulatory approvals in developing countries can occur. Developing partnerships with less developed countries that can benefit from new vaccines, is crucial to providing global access to new vaccines.

13.2. Measurement of Safety and Efficacy and Regulatory Approval

Unfortunately the development often slows down and often stalls at the point of human safety efficacy. Regulators are aware of this block and are examining options for vaccines designed to prevent new life-threatening infections. It may be possible to obtain provisional approval for distribution on the basis of evidence of effectiveness derived from appropriate studies in animals, without well-controlled efficacy studies in humans.

14. CONCLUSION

In this chapter we have provided a guide to the immediate response to a new neurological infectious disease challenge. For a new CNS disease to be recognized we have described the important roles played by active surveillance, disease registries, and a heightened clinical awareness underpinned by a thorough history and clinical examination and a multidisciplinary clinical, microbiological and pathological approach. Empiric antibacterial and antiviral therapy may be used in certain patients and we have provided examples of potential drugs for empiric and directed therapy. Infection control issues must be addressed early in an outbreak of any new CNS infection and may have broad societal ramification as we have seen recently with the SARS outbreak where quarantine conditions have been frequently invoked in several countries. In outbreak setting coordination of public health, state and federal authorities is paramount and should inform a well-conducted and ongoing education campaign for the public about the outbreak.

Rapid vaccine development is an important part of this strategy. We now have the capacity to rapidly identify protective correlates, identify candidate antigens and rapidly insert them in live vectors, DNA vaccines, or transgenic plants. Developments in immunology, genomics, proteomics and vaccine vectors has been such that there are now no significant obstacles along this path to the point of a viable vaccine strategy. The development often slows down at this point and often stalls at the point of human safety efficacy. However policies are being developed to address these issues. The current concentration of resources on bioterrorism will also help to ensure all the issues identified get adequate attention.

REFERENCES

1. Allworth A, Murray K, Morgan J. A human case of encephalitis due to a lyssavirus recently identified in fruit bats. CDI 1996; 20:504–507.
2. Selvey LA, Wells RM, McCormack JG, et al. Infection of humans and horses by a newly described morbillivirus. Med J Aust 1995; 162:642–645.
3. Chua KB, Goh KJ, Wong KT, et al. Fatal encephalitis due to Nipah virus among pig-farmers in Malaysia. Lancet 1999; 354:1257–1259.
4. Will RG, Ironside JW, Zeidler M, et al. A new variant of Creutzfeldt–Jakob disease in the UK. Lancet 1996; 347:921–925.
5. Shindarov LM, Chumakov MP, Voroshilova MK, et al. Epidemiological, clinical and pathomorphological characteristics of epidemic poliomyelitis-like disease caused by enterovirus 71. J Hyg Emidemiol Microbiol Immunol 1979; 23:284–295.
6. Frankel DH. St Louis encephalitis arrives in New York City. Lancet 1999; 354:925.
7. Briese T, Jia X-Y, Huang C, Grady LJ, Lipkin WI. Identification of a Kunjin/West Nile-like flavivirus in brains of patients with New York encephalitis. Lancet 1999; 354:1261–1262.
8. Hanna JN, Ritchie SA, Phillips DA, et al. Japanese encephalitis in North Queensland, 1998. Med J Aust 1999; 170:533–536.
9. CDC. Recognition of illness associated with the intentional release of a biologic agent. MMWR Morb Mortal Wkly Rep 2001; 50:893–897.
10. CDC. Outbreak of West Nile-like viral encephalitis—New York, 1999. MMWR Morb Mortal Wkly Rep 1999; 48:845–849.
11. Davison KL, Crowcroft NS, Ramsay ME, Brown DWG, Andrews NJ. Viral encephalitis in England, 1989–1998: what did we miss? Emerg Infect Dis [serial online] 2003 February, Vol. 9. Available from: URL: http://www.cdc.gov/ncidod/EID/vol9no2/02-0218.htm.
12. CDC. Fatal degenerative neurologic illnesses in men who participated in wild game feasts—Wisconsin, 2002. MMWR Morb Mortal Wkly Rep 2003; 52:125–127.

13. Lanska DJ. Anthrax meningoencephalitis. Neurology 2002; 59:327–334.

14. Paton NI, Leo YSL, Zaki SR, et al. Outbreak of Nipah-virus infection among abattoir workers in Singapore. Lancet 1999; 354:1253–1256.

15. CDC. Achievements in public health, 1900–1999: impact of vaccines universally recommended for children. Morb Mortal Wkly Rep MMWR 2001; 48:243–248.

16. Hanna JN, Carney IK, Smith GA et al. Australian bat lyssavirus infection: a second human case with a long incubation period. Med J Aust 2000; 172:597–599.

17. Chan RC, Penney DJ, Little D, Carter IW, Roberts JA, Rawlinson WD. Hepatitis and death following vaccination with 17D-204 yellow fever vaccine. Lancet 2001; 358:121–122.

18. Martin M, Tsai TF, Cropp B, et al. Fever and multisystem organ failure associated with 17D-204 yellow fever vaccination: a report of four cases. Lancet 2001; 358:98–104.

19. CDC. Adverse events associated with 17D-204 yellow fever vaccination—United States, 2001–2002. MMWR Morb Mortal Wkly Rep 2002; 51:989–993.

20. Spencer MD, Knight RSG, Will RG. First hundred cases of variant Creutzfeldt–Jakob disease: retrospective case note review of early psychiatric and neurological features. BMJ 2002; 324:1479–1482.

21. Chua KB, Lam SK, Goh KJ, et al. The presence of Nipah virus in respiratory secretions and urine of patients during an outbreak of Nipah virus encephalitis in Malaysia. J Infect 2001; 42:40–43.

22. CDC. Acute flaccid paralysis syndrome associated with West Nile Virus infection-Mississippi and Louisiana, July–August 2002. MMWR Morb Mortal Wkly Rep 2002; 51:825–828.

23. Venters GA. New variant Creutzfeldt–Jakob: the epidemic that never was. BMJ 2001; 323:858–861.

24. Will RG, Knight RSG, Ward HJT, Ironside JW. New variant Creutzfeldt–Jakob disease: the critique that never was. BMJ 2002; 325:102.

25. Chong H-T, Kamarulzaman A, Tan C-T, et al. Treatment of acute Nipah encephalitis with ribavirin. Ann Neurol 2001; 49; 810–813.

26. Laskin OL. Clinical pharmacokinetics of acyclovir. Clin Pharmacokinet 1983; 8:187–201.

27. Levitz RE. Herpes simplex encephalitis: a review. Heart Lung 1998; 27:209–212.

28. Kimberlin DW, Lin CY, Jacobs RF, et al. Safety and efficacy of high-dose intravenous acyclovir in the management of neonatal herpes simplex virus infection. Pediatrics 2001; 108:230–238.

29. Gilden DH, Kleinschmidt-DeMasters, LaGuardia JJ, Mahalingam R, Cohrs RJ. Neurologic complications of the reactivation of varicella-zoster virus. N Engl J Med 2000; 342:635–645.

30. Fletcher C, Sawchuk R, Chinnock R, de Miranda P, Balfour HH Jr. Human pharmacokinetics of the antiviral drug DHPG. Clin Pharmacol Ther 1986; 40:281–286.

31. Anduze-Faris BM, Fillet A-M, Gozlan J, et al. Induction and maintenance therapy of cytomegalovirus central nervous system infection in HIV-infected patients. AIDS 2000; 14:517–524.

32. Hengge UR, Brockmeyer NH, Malessa R, Ravens U, Goos M. Foscarnet penetrates the blood–brain barrier: rationale for therapy of cytomegalovirus encephalitis. Antimicrob Agents Chemother 1993; 37:1010–1014.

33. Connor E, Morrison S, Lane J, et al. Safety, tolerance and pharmacokinetics of systemic ribavirin in children with human immunodeficiency virus infection. Antimicrob Agents Chemother 1993; 37:532–539.

34. Mandell, Douglas and Bennett's Principles and Practice of Infectious Disease. 5th edn. Philadelphia, PA: Churchill Livingstone.

35. Jordan I, Briese T, Fischer N, Lau JY-N, Lipkin WI. Ribavirin inhibits West Nile virus replication and cytopathic effect in neural cells. J Infect Dis 2000; 182:1214–1217.

36. Rotbart HA, Webster AD for the Pleconaril Treatment Registry Group. Treatment of potentially life-threatening enterovirus infections with pleconaril. Clin Infect Dis 2001; 32:228–235.

37. Abzug MJ, Cloud G, Bradley J et al. Double-blind placebo-controlled trial of pleconaril in infants with enterovirus meningitis. Pediatr Infect Dis J 2003; 22:335–341.

38. Korth C, May BCH, Cohen FE, Prusiner SB. Acridine and phenothiazine derivatives as pharmacotherapeutics for prion disease. Proc Natl Acad Sci U S A 2001; 98:9836–9841.

39. Shimoni Z, Niven MJ, Pitlick S, Bulvik S. Treatment of West Nile virus encephalitis with intravenous immunoglobulin. Emerg Infect Dis 2001; 7:759.

40. Hamdan A, Green P, Mendelson E, Kramer MR, Pitlik S, Weinberger M. Possible benefit of intravenous immunoglobulin therapy in a lung transplant recipient with West Nile virus encephalitis. Transpl Infect Dis 2002; 4:160–162.

41. Kanesa-Thasan N, Putnak JR, Mangiafico JA, Saluzzo JE, Ludwig GV. Short report: absence of protective neutralizing antibodies to West Nile virus in subjects following vaccination with Japanese encephalitis or dengue vaccines. Am J Trop Med Hyg, 2002; 66:113–114.

42. CDC. Update: management of patients with suspected viral hemorrhagic fever—United States. MMWR Morb Mortal Wkly Rep 1995; 44:475–479.

43. Ksiazek TG, Erdman D, Goldsmith PHC, et al. A novel coronavirus associated with severe acute respiratory syndrome. N Engl J Med 2003; 348:1953–1966.

44. CDC/National Institutes of Health. Biosafety in Microbiological and Biomedical Laboratories. 3rd edn. Atlanta, GA: U.S. Department of Health and Human Services, Public Health Service, 1993; DHS publication no. (CDC)93-8395.

45. Hoffman RE. Preparing for a bioterrorist attack: legal and administrative strategies. Emerg Infect Dis [serial online] 2003; February:9. Available from: URL: http://www.cdc.gov/ncidod/EID/vol9no2/02-0538.htm.

46. Glass TA, Schoch-Spana M. Bioterrorism and the people: how to vaccinate a city against panic. Clin Infect Dis 2002; 34:217–223.

47. Green BA, Baker SM. Recent advances and novel strategies in vaccine development. Curr Opin Microbiol 2002; 5:483–488.

48. Xiang R, Lode HN, Chao TH, et al. An autologous oral DNA vaccine protects against murine melanoma. Proc Natl Acad Sci U S A 2000 9; 97:5492–5497.

49. Kent SJ, Zhao A, Chandler J, et al. Enhanced T-cell immunogenicity and protective efficacy of a HIV-1 vaccine regimen consisting of consecutive priming with DNA and boosting with recombinant fowlpox virus. J Virol 1998; 72:10180–10188.

50. Webster DE, Thomas MC, Strugnell RA, Dry IB, Wesselingh SL. Appetising solutions: an edible vaccine for measles. From bench to bedside. 2002; 176:434–437.

51. Pizza M, Scarlato V, Masignani V, Giuliani MM, Arico B, Comanducci M, Jennings GT, Baldi, L, Bartolini E, Capecchi B, et al. Identification of vaccine candidates

against serogroup B meningococcus by whole-genome sequencing. Science, 2000; 287:1816–1820.

52. Rappuoli R. Reverse vaccinology, a genome-based approach to vaccine development. Vaccine, 2001; 19:2688–2691.

53. Armand J. Regulatory barrier to new vaccine development…thinking outside the box. In: Brown F, Gust I, eds. Orphan Vaccines—Bridging the Gap. Dev Biol (Basel Karger) 2002; 110:145–148.

54. Rosenthal SR, Clifford JCM. Development of vaccines for bio-warfare agents. In: Brown F, Gust I, eds. Orphan Vaccines—Bridging the Gap. Dev Biol (Basel Karger) 2002; 110:99–105.

55. Ramsay AJ, Kent SJ, Strugnell RA, Suhrbier A, Thomson SA, Ramshaw IA. Genetic vaccination strategies for enhanced cellular, humoral and mucosal immunity. Immunol Rev 1999; 171: 27–44.

56. Tacket CO, Mason HS. A review of oral vaccination with transgenic vegetables. Microbes Infect 1999; 1:777–783.

20

Future Perspectives

Man is embedded in nature. The biologic science of recent years has been making this a more urgent fact of life. The new, hard problem will be coping with the dawning, intensifying realization of just how interlocked we are. The old clung—to notions most of us hold about our special lordship are being deeply undermined.
—*Lewis Thomas 1975*

Humans are unique among all species in their ability to adapt to a remarkable range of environments but this leads to the inevitable consequence of being exposed to many potential pathogens for which they have not developed immune protection. The increasing spectrum of human inhabitation has resulted in newly recognized infections including neurotropic pathogens (1). Each neurological infection included in the current monograph has arisen because of one of the factors associated with emerging infections in general including genetic, biological, social, political, and economic factors (Table 1) (1). For neurological infections, the impact of these variables is incalculable as recently seen with the spread of West Nile virus infection across the North American continent (2) and the recent reports of Nipah virus infections in India and Bangladesh (3). Of interest, among these neuronotropic viral infections, the effects are appreciated immediately, providing an impetus for public health intervention, if available, as evidenced by the rapid development of vaccines for West Nile Virus that appear efficacious in horses and other species (4). Conversely, viruses that are principally gliotropic including HIV usually exhibit an insidious progression and their consequences are not appreciated as promptly (5).

While the emphasis of the present monograph is on emerging neurotropic infectious agents, not all high impact infectious neurological diseases were addressed herein, largely because they represent established epidemics. For example, one neurological infection that continues to cause increasing morbidity and mortality is CNS tuberculosis. Indeed, while *Mycobacterium tuberculosis* (TB) is comparatively well controlled in developed countries, it remains one of

Table 1   Causes of Emerging Infections[a]

Microbial mutation and adaptation
Human susceptibility to infection
Climate and ecosystem change
Human demographics and behavior
Economic development and land use
International travel and commerce
Technology and industry
Public health infrastructure decline
Poverty and social inequality
War, famine, political motivation, and intent to harm

[a]Adapted from Ref. (1).

the principal pathogens globally as nearly one-third of the world's population is infected with TB with 8.4 million people developing active TB disease annually from which 2 million die (6). The resurgence of TB is in part due to the HIV/AIDS epidemic with diminished immune status and greater risk latent infection progressing to active disease although increasing numbers of people living in poverty is another contributing factor (7). Approximately 15% of active tuberculosis is extra-pulmonary, 6% of which is central nervous system tuberculosis (CNS-TB), yielding an annual estimated incidence of 70,000 patients worldwide (8). Of the various forms of TB disease, CNS-TB including tuberculosis meningitis and tuberculoma is the most serious complication, resulting in high levels of morbidity and mortality regardless of locale, and despite the availability of effective treatment. Additionally, there appears to a preponderance of CNS-TB among certain groups including young women and Aboriginals (9). Although CNS-TB accounts for a small percentage of all cases of TB, it remains a serious challenge for health care workers because of the difficulty of diagnosis and the dire consequences of delayed treatment. Given the impact of TB globally, the extraordinary rise in multi-drug resistant (MDR) TB prevalence throughout the world represents an immense health problem (10). Insufficient courses of anti-tuberculous therapies appear to perpetuate the MDR problem with ensuing spread of drug-resistant TB strains, which compounds the already expensive strategy of directly observed therapy for TB. Although the direct impact on MDR TB strains on neurological disease is yet to be fully appreciated, in children it is a recognized problem (11,12). This concern is on the background of grinding poverty together with limited public or governmental resources that has been highlighted in several countries including Russia and Peru (13). In fact, the development of MDR TB heralds a new phase in global infections because of the difficulty in providing the required treatment regimens that will require intensive vigilance and substantial resources to control its spread. Similarly, with greater attempts to treat other potentially drug-resistant pathogens such as HIV-1 or HIV-2, the appearance of more virulent and untreatable viral strains presents a daunting challenge from both public health and clinical perspectives (14). Indeed, HIV drug resistance has already become widespread in developed countries, approaching 75% in some groups (15) with evidence of transmission rates of 10% (16). On the contrary, our diagnostic capabilities remain limited, especially in developing countries where many neurological infectious disease epidemics go unrecognized because of few means to pursue the diagnosis of a new disease. Likewise the developed world has been slow to realize new clinical phenotypes of previously identified pathogens, such as the growing awareness of the diverse clinical presentations of varicella zoster virus (17).

On a more positive front, the growing understanding of genetic susceptibility to infectious diseases will enhance preventative, diagnostic, and treatment opportunities. This is best illustrated by the increasing availability of large-scale genomic studies including the human genome coupled with the study of specific genetic polymorphisms (18). In fact, the full breadth of human genetic diversity is not fully appreciated given that many of the transcriptionally active retro-elements including retrotransposons and endogenous retroviruses were not included in the human genome analyses despite representing approximately 5–8% of the human genome (19). There is no doubt that the increasing genetic information will be complemented by the growing emphasis of the biotechnology sector on the development of new therapies, albeit often too expensive for the developing world and largely focused on a few infectious diseases. However, the potential to develop vaccines promptly, as evidenced by the responses to West Nile virus and SARS bodes well for future epidemics (4). Although treating the underlying cause of a neurological infection is a rational and required approach, neurological therapy can be enhanced in some instances by additional therapeutic intervention in terms of neuroprotective strategies including the use of anti-inflammatory, anti-oxidant, and related interventions. Clinicians dealing with both chronic and acute neurological infections may benefit their patients by considering newer therapeutic strategies established by other neurological fields including stroke, head injury, acute demyelinating polyneuropathy (Guillain–Barre syndrome) as well as chronic diseases such as amyotrophic lateral sclerosis and multiple sclerosis (20–22). For example, the recent implementation of a clinical trial of hyperimmune gammaglobulin in the treatment of West Nile virus-related neurological syndromes may restrict virus production directly together with intrinsic anti-inflammatory effects. In the same way, the use of neuroprotective/anti-inflammatory compounds such as minocycline or a derivative thereof may provide additional neuroprotective benefit in select diseases (23).

Despite the rapid recognition of several neurotropic infectious agents over the past decade, several pathogens and circumstances are looming on the horizon that may become of increasing concern in the next few years. These include the rising numbers of wild cervids with chronic wasting disease and their potential to spread this obscure pathogen to domesticated livestock in North America and possibly to consumers (human or otherwise) of venison. The recent recognition of bovine spongiform encephalopathy in western North America underscores this point, requiring increasing watchfulness for the surfacing of more cases with various presenting phenotypes and the contamination of the food chain. The ongoing appearance of new strains of influenza viruses also represents a disquieting trend, given their rapid spread, especially within the food chain and influenza's possible pathogenic roles in the development of CNS congenital abnormalities, encephalitis and post-infectious encephalomyelitis exhibited by some strains. The Asian influenza A H5N1 strain epitomizes these concerns through its initial appearance in geese in 1996 and subsequent spread to other avian species, largely driven by a series of genetic reassortment events that culminated in spread to humans with ensuing disease (24). In the present context of neurological infections, the emergence of H5N1 is of particular concern because it is neurovirulent in an animal model (25). The recent spread of other influenza strains (H7N3 and H6N2) in North America has the capacity to become major economic and health care predicaments, especially given the immense sizes of the agricultural operations containing hosts for these viruses including poultry and swine that are often in close proximity. Here again, closer attention to incipient trends is needed through international public health institutions. It is also worth bearing in mind that much of the human food supply is derived from oceans, which is replete with microbial organisms. In fact, 95–98% of the oceanic biomass is made up of microbial agents, of which 27 tonnes (the approximate weight of a Blue whale) represent viruses (26). The oceans are also increasingly subject to pollution, amplifying their roles as reservoirs for infection. The development of a neurological syndrome caused by the kainate receptor agonist, domoic acid, resulting from consumption of cultured mussels exposed to domoic acid-producing phytoplankton, reinforces these concerns (27,28).

As we move into an era of greater utilization of allogeneic cells or engineered viruses for therapeutic purposes, it is worth recalling the adage that history ignored can easily repeat itself, as evidenced by the first recognition of the neurovirulence of West Nile virus among cancer patients who received West Nile virus as a chemotherapeutic agent with ensuing neurological morbidity and mortality (29). Finally, as with many infectious diseases, good public measures and optimized socioeconomic conditions, remain the bulwarks of preventing the development and spread of infectious diseases. It has been disconcerting to see the apparent decline in public health scrutiny through the world. This is best illustrated by the demise of the surveillance system established by the Rockefeller Foundation in the Caribbean, South America, Africa, and India beginning in 1971 together with the closing of a research unit in Malaysia maintained by the U.S. army in 1989 (30) and recently increased enthusiasm for outsourcing of government public health activities (31). Indeed, the importance of public health vigilance is underscored by the repeated emergence of Ebola virus, which has been consistently traced to infections acquired by exposure in African forests by single individuals resulting in explosive and fatal epidemics, especially affecting health care workers

(32). There is no question that enhanced surveillance of disease appearance and spread can be monitored with cutting-edge molecular tools followed by vaccine introduction, assuming efficient public health agencies are in place. Similarly, the full beneficial effects of highly effective therapies will be realized only if efforts to prevent or eradicate poverty are concurrently implemented. Thus, we face interesting yet menacing times in the next decade that will require coordinated efforts of clinicians, public health authorities, governments together with expertise in environmental and economic issues to curb and ultimately halt emerging neurological infections as they arise.

REFERENCES

1. Morens DM, Folkers GK, Fauci AS. The challenge of emerging and re-emerging infectious diseases. Nature 2004; 430:242–249.
2. Beasley DW, Davis CT, Guzman H, et al. Limited evolution of West Nile virus has occurred during its southwesterly spread in the United States. Virology 2003; 309:190–195.
3. Enserink M. Emerging infectious diseases. Nipah virus (or a cousin) strikes again. Science 2004; 303:1121.
4. Chang GJ, Kuno G, Purdy DE, Davis BS. Recent advancement in flavivirus vaccine development. Expert Rev Vaccines 2004; 3:199–220.
5. Power C, Johnson RT. Neurovirological and neuroimmunological aspects of HIV infection. Adv Virus Res 2001; 56:579–624.
6. Global Tuberculosis Control. Surveillance, planning, financing. WHO Rep 2003; 316.
7. Bates I, Fenton C, Gruber J, et al. Vulnerability to malaria, tuberculosis, and HIV/AIDS infection and disease. Part 1: Determinants operating at individual and household level. Lancet Infect Dis 2004; 4:267–277.
8. Davis LE. Tuberculous meningitis. In: Davis LE, Kennedy PGE, eds. Infectious Diseases of the Nervous System. Oxford: Butterworth-Heineman 2000:499–520.
9. Arvanitakis Z, Long RL, Hershfield ES, et al. *Mycobacterium tuberculosis* molecular variation in CNS infection: evidence for strain-dependent neurovirulence. Neurology 1998; 50:1827–1832.
10. Wade MM, Zhang Y. Mechanisms of drug resistance in *Mycobacterium tuberculosis*. Front Biosci 2004; 9:975–994.
11. Schaaf HS, Shean K, Donald PR. Culture confirmed multidrug resistant tuberculosis: diagnostic delay, clinical features, and outcome. Arch Dis Child 2003; 88:1106–1111.
12. Shin SS, Hyson AM, Castaneda C, et al. Peripheral neuropathy associated with treatment for multidrug-resistant tuberculosis. Int J Tuberc Lung Dis 2003; 7:347–353.
13. Farmer P. Infections and Inequalities: The Modern Plagues. Berkley, CA: University California Press, 1999:184–210.
14. Weng Y, Siciliano SJ, Waldburger KE, et al. Binding and functional properties of recombinant and endogenous CXCR3 chemokine receptors. J Biol Chem 1998; 273:18288–18291.

15. Richman DD, Morton SC, Wrin T, et al. The prevalence of antiretroviral drug resistance in the United States. AIDS 2004; 18:1393–1401.
16. Simon V, Vanderhoeven J, Hurley A, et al. Evolving patterns of HIV-1 resistance to antiretroviral agents in newly infected individuals. AIDS 2002; 16:1511–1519.
17. Cohrs RJ, Gilden DH, Mahalingam R. Varicella zoster virus latency, neurological disease and experimental models: an update. Front Biosci 2004; 9:751–762.
18. Mira MT, Alcais A, Nguyen VT, et al. Susceptibility to leprosy is associated with PARK2 and PACRG. Nature 2004; 427:636–640.
19. Gifford R, Tristem M. The evolution, distribution and diversity of endogenous retroviruses. Virus Genes 2003; 26:291–315.
20. Alves OL, Doyle AJ, Clausen T, Gilman C, Bullock R. Evaluation of topiramate neuroprotective effect in severe TBI using microdialysis. Ann N Y Acad Sci 2003; 993:25–34.
21. Schwab S, Schwarz S, Spranger M, Keller E, Bertram M, Hacke W. Moderate hypothermia in the treatment of patients with severe middle cerebral artery infarction. Stroke 1998; 29:2461–2466.
22. Mitchell JD, Wokke JH, Borasio GD. Recombinant human insulin-like growth factor I (rhIGF-I) for amyotrophic lateral sclerosis/motor neuron disease. Cochrane Database Syst Rev 2002; 3:CD002064.
23. Friedlander RM. Apoptosis and caspases in neurodegenerative diseases. N Engl J Med 2003; 348:1365–1375.
24. Li KS, Guan Y, Wang J, et al. Genesis of a highly pathogenic and potentially pandemic H5N1 influenza virus in eastern Asia. Nature 2004; 430:209–213.
25. Rowe T, Cho DS, Bright RA, Zitzow LA, Katz JM. Neurological manifestations of avian influenza viruses in mammals. Avian Dis 2003; 47:1122–1126.
26. Suttle CA. The oceans: a frontier of unexplored viral diversity. Am Soc Virol Symp 2004.
27. Teitelbaum JS, Zatorre RJ, Carpenter S, et al. Neurologic sequelae of domoic acid intoxication due to the ingestion of contaminated mussels. N Engl J Med 1990; 322:1781–1787.
28. Stommel EW, Watters MR. Marine neurotoxins: ingestible toxins. Curr Treat Options Neurol 2004; 6:105–114.
29. Johnson RT. Emerging viral infections of the nervous system. J Neurovirol 2003; 9:140–147.
30. Johnson RT. Emerging viral infections. Arch Neurol 1996; 53:18–22.
31. Garrett L. Betrayal of Trust: The Collapse of Global Public Health. New York: Hyperion, 2000:299–480.
32. Feldmann H, Jones S, Klenk HD, Schnittler HJ. Ebola virus: from discovery to vaccine. Nat Rev Immunol 2003; 3:677–685.

Index

RIT - WALLACE LIBRARY
CIRCULATING LIBRARY BOOKS

OVERDUE FINES AND FEES FOR <u>ALL</u> BORROWERS

*Recalled = $1/ day overdue (no grace period)
*Billed = $10.00/ item when returned 4 or more weeks overdue
*Lost Items = replacement cost+$10 fee
*All materials must be returned or renewed by the duedate.